AIDS

Principles, Practices, & Politics

Reference Edition

AIDS

Principles, Practices, & Politics

Reference Edition

Edited by

Inge B. Corless, RN, PhD, FAAN
Chair, Department of Secondary Care
University of North Carolina
Chapel Hill, North Carolina

and

Mary Pittman-Lindeman, DrPH
Director of Planning, Department of Public Health
City and County of San Francisco
San Francisco, California

⬤HEMISPHERE PUBLISHING CORPORATION
A member of the Taylor & Francis Group

New York   Washington   Philadelphia   London

AIDS: Principles, Practices, & Politics

1 2 3 4 5 6 7 8 9 0   E B E B   8 9 8 7 6 5 4 3 2 1 0 9 8

This book was set in Times Roman by EPS Group. The editors were Carolyn Ormes and Allison Brown. Cover design by Renée E. Winfield.

Library of Congress Cataloging-in-Publication Data
AIDS: principles, practices & politics.
   (Series in death education, aging, and health care)
   Includes bibliographies and index.
    1. AIDS (Disease)   2. AIDS (Disease)—Social aspects.
I. Corless, Inge B.   II. Pittman-Lindeman, Mary.
III. Series. [DNLM: 1. Acquired Immunodefiency Syndrome.
2. Politics—United States.   3. Public policy—United
States.   4. Social Environment—United States.
WD 308 A28839]
RC607.A26A3488 1989   616.97'92   88-34780
ISBN 0-89116-716-1

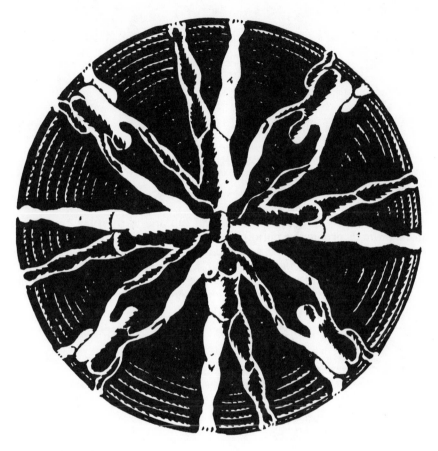

AIDS: An Overview

This single-headed organism with different bodies represents the varied community afflicted with AIDS, men, women, and children and every race, color, and age. They are all caught in the whirling vortex of the epidemic.

This book is dedicated to

ORI SHERMAN

August 30, 1934—August 28, 1988

who chose to see the glass of life as half full and in so doing engaged in an exceedingly productive period of artistic achievement. *AIDS: Principles, Practices, and Politics* is one beneficiary of the flourishing of Ori's artistic creativity. He will be remembered with much love, admiration, and great respect. His work in this book gives voice in another medium to the pain of loss, the fear, the challenge, and the eventual triumph of talent, dedication, inspiration, and the human spirit.

Contents

PART II
PHYSIOLOGICAL ASPECTS

PART III
TREATMENT

PART VI
SOCIOCULTURAL AND ETHICAL ASPECTS

Proposed Public Health Measures   414
Conclusion   421
References   421

35   **Public Schools Confront AIDS**   423
     Elizabeth P. Lamers

     Introduction   423
     Historical Overview   424
     Disease and the Classroom   425
     Scope of the Problem in Schools   426
     Education in the Classroom   429
     AIDS and the News Media   430
     Conclusion   431
     References   431

36   **Hospice and Home Care for Persons with AIDS/ARC: Meeting the
     Challenges and Ensuring Quality**   433
     Jeannee Parker Martin

     Introduction   433
     A Challenge to the Multidisciplinary Approach   434
     Bereavement Support   440
     Ensuring Reimbursement   440
     When Home Care is No Longer Appropriate   442
     Conclusion   444
     References   444

37   **Housing for People with AIDS**   445
     Helen Schietinger

     Introduction   445
     History of the Problem in San Francisco   446
     The Shanti AIDS Residence Program   446
     Problems in Providing Housing   449
     Models of Housing Needed   451
     Summary   453
     Case Study   453

                          PART VIII
                 AIDS AND THE PROFESSIONAL

38   **AIDS: A Special Challenge for Health Care Workers**   461
     Linda Hawes Clever

     Introduction   461
     Infection Control   461

PART IX
POLITICAL ASPECTS

PART X
THE MEDIA AND AIDS

PART XI
THE FUTURE

Contributors

Donald Abrams, MD   Assistant Director, AIDS Clinic, San Francisco General Hospital, San Francisco, California

Terry R. Bard, AB, BAHL, MAHL, OrD Rabbi   Beth Israel Hospital, Boston, Massachusetts

Harvey S. Bartnof, MD   Chief Physician, AVERI, San Francisco, California

Graham Bass, RN, MS   Staff Nurse, St. Vincent's Supportive Care Program, New York, New York

A. E. Benjamin, PhD   Associate Director, Institute for Health and Aging, University of California, S.F., San Francisco, California

Dani P. Bolognese, PhD   James B. Duke Professor, Duke University Medical Center, Durham, North Carolina

Laurel Brodsley, RN, MPH, Phd   Lecturer, English Department, University of California, Los Angeles, California

Rev. Bernard Brown, SJ, PhD   Lecturer, Medical Spirituality, Georgetown University, Washington, D.C.

Cathy Casriel, MSW   Project Director, Narcotic and Drug Research, Inc., New York, New York

Terence Chorba, MD   Medical Epidemiologist, Epidemiology Program Office, Centers for Disease Control, Atlanta, Georgia

Linda Hawes Clever, MD, FACP   Chair, Department of Occupational Health, Pacific Presbyterian Medical Center, San Francisco, California

Marcus A. Conant, MD   Clinical Professor of Dermatology, University of San Francisco Medical Center, San Francisco, California

Ellen C. Cooper, MD, MPH   Director, Antiviral Drug Products, Center for Drug Evaluation and Research, U.S. Food and Drug Administration, Rockville, Maryland

Inge B. Corless, RN, PhD, FAAN   Chair, Department of Secondary Care, School of Nursing, University of North Carolina, Chapel Hill, North Carolina

Donald C. Des Jarlais, PhD   Assistant Deputy Director, New York State Division of Substance Abuse Services, New York, New York

Carole Donovan, RN, MA   Senior Staff Nurse, St. Vincent's Supportive Care Program, New York, New York

Dean F. Echenberg, MD, PhD   Director, Bureau of Communicable Disease Control, Department of Public Health, San Francisco, California

Michael Eller, BA   Research Associate, Howard Brown Memorial Clinic, Chicago, Illinois

Bruce Evatt, MD   Director, Division of Host Factors, Center for Infectious Diseases, Centers for Disease Control, Atlanta, Georgia

Jim Foster   San Francisco Health Commissioner, San Francisco, California

Zelda Foster, MSW   Chief Social Worker, Brooklyn V.A. Medical Center, Brooklyn, New York

Donald P. Francis, MD, DSc   AIDS Advisor to the State of California, Department of Health Services, Centers for Disease Control, Berkeley, California
Samuel Friedman, PhD   Principal Investigator, Narcotic and Drug Research, Inc., New York, New York
Chuck Frutchey   Assistant Director of Education, San Francisco AIDS Foundation, San Francisco, California
Robert Fulton, PhD   Professor of Sociology, Director, Center for Death Education and Research, University of Minnesota, Minneapolis, Minnesota
J. Louise Gerberding, MD   The Medical Service, San Francisco General Hospital, San Francisco, California
Judith Bograd Gordon, PhD   Associate Professor of Sociology, University of New Haven, Lecturer in Psychiatry and Mid-Career Fellow, Bush Center on Child Development and Social Policy, Yale University, New Haven, Connecticut
Margaret Grade   Department of Psychiatry, Langley Porter Psychiatric Hospital, San Francisco, California
Moses Grossman, MD   Professor, Department of Pediatrics, University of California, S.F., San Francisco General Hospital, San Francisco, California
Emmanuel Heller, PhD   Visiting Scientist, Laboratory of Tumor Cell Biology, National Cancer Institute, Bethesda, Maryland
Robert S. Janssen, MD   Medical Epidemiologist, Retrovirus Diseases Branch, Division of Viral Diseases, Center for Infectious Diseases, Centers for Infectious Diseases, Centers for Disease Control, Atlanta, Georgia
Jill G. Joseph, PhD   Assistant Professor, Department of Epidemiology, University of Michigan, Ann Arbor, Michigan
Dobri Kiprov, MD   Director, Plasmapheresis Unit and Clinical Research Immunology, Children's Hospital, San Francisco, California
C. Everett Koop, MD   Surgeon General, U.S. Public Health Service, Department of Health and Human Services, Rockville, Maryland
Elizabeth P. Lamers, MA   Educational Consultant, Malibu, California
A. J. Langlois, PhD   Duke University Medical Center, Durham, North Carolina
Philip R. Lee, MD   Director, Institute for Health Policy Studies, University of California, S.F., San Francisco, California
Calu Lester, PhD (deceased)   Founder, Kapuna West Intercity Child/Family AIDS Network, San Francisco, California
Angie Lewis, RN, MSN   Assistant Director, Nursing Administration, Langley Porter Psychiatric Hospital, San Francisco, California
Dorothy C. H. Ley, MD, FRCP(C), FACP   Chairman, Canadian Medical Association, Committee on the Health Care of the Elderly, Canadian Representative to Board of Directors, International Hospice Institute, Toronto, Ontario, Canada
Randolph Lippert, MD   Children's Hospital, San Francisco, California
Erich H. Lowey, MD   Assistant Professor of Medicine, Department of Medicine, University of Illinois, Peoria, Illinois
H. Kim Lyerly, MD   Resident, Department of Surgery, Duke University Medical Center, Durham, North Carolina
Jonathan M. Mann   Director, Global Programme on AIDS, World Health Organization, Geneva, Switzerland
Jeannee Parker Martin, RN, MPH   Director, Hospice Programs, Visiting Nurses and Hospice of San Francisco, San Francisco, California

Thomas J. Matthews, PhD   Assistant Medical Research Professor, Department of Surgery, Duke University Medical Center, Durham, North Carolina
Robert Miller, MD   Chief, Clinical Service of Neurology, Children's Hospital, San Francisco, California
John C. Moskop, PhD   Associate Professor of Medical Humanities, School of Medicine, East Carolina University, Greenville, North Carolina
Julien S. Murphy, PhD   Assistant Professor, Department of Philosophy, University of Southern Maine, Portland, Maine
Sister Patrice Murphy, SC, RN, MS   Coordinator, St. Vincent's Supportive Care Program, New York, New York
David G. Ostrow, PhD   Associate Professor, Department of Psychiatry, University of Michigan, Ann Arbor, Michigan
Greg Owen, PhD   Senior Research Scientist, Wilder Research Center, St. Paul, Minnesota
Sheila Dollard Pavlis, RN, MSN, CS   Psychiatric Nurse Clinician, In-Patient Division and Infection Control Officer, The Connecticut Mental Health Center, Yale-New Haven Medical Center, New Haven, Connecticut
Richard B. Pearce, PhD   Department of Biological Sciences, University of California, Santa Barbara, California
Leonard I. Pearlin, PhD   Professor, Human Development and Aging Program, Center for Social and Behavioral Sciences, University of California, S.F., San Francisco, California
Kathleen Perry, MSW   Social Worker and Bereavement Counselor, St. Vincent's Supportive Care Program, New York, New York
Wolfgang Pfaeffl, MD, PhD   Department of Nephrology, Klinikum Grosshadern, Munchen, Germany
Mary Pittman-Lindeman, DrPH   Director of Planning and Evaluation, Department of Public Health, City and County of San Francisco, San Francisco, California
Dorothy P. Rice, BA, DrSc (honorary)   Professor in Residence, Department of Social and Behavioral Sciences, University of California, S.F., San Francisco, California
Judith Wilson Ross, MA   Associate, Center for Bioethics, St. Joseph Health System. Orange, California
Michael Samuels, DrPH   Department of Health Administration, School of Public Health, University of South Carolina, Columbia, South Carolina
M. A. Sande, MD   Chief, Medical Service, San Francisco General Hospital, San Francisco, California
Larry Saxxon   Saxxon Quinn Associates, San Francisco, California
Helen Schietinger, RN, MA, MFCC   Global Programme on AIDS, World Health Organization, Geneva, Switzerland
Jerome Schofferman, MD   Medical Director, Hospice of San Francisco, San Francisco, California
Anne A. Scitovsky, MA   Chief, Health Economics Department, Research Institute, Palo Alto Medical Foundation, Palo Alto, California
Betsy Selman, MS   Volunteer Coordinator and Pastoral Counselor, St. Vincent's Supportive Care Program, New York, New York
Shirley J. Semple, MSc   Human Development and Aging Program, Center for Social and Behavioral Sciences, University of California, S.F., San Franciscio, California

Ori Sherman, MA (deceased)   Artist, San Francisco, California
Michael A. Simpson, MD   Director of Program Planning for Clinic Holdings, Pretoria, South Africa
M. Lynn Smiley, MD   Medical Advisor, Department of Antimicrobial Therapy, Burroughs Wellcome Co., Research Triangle Park, North Carolina
Howard Z. Streicher, MD   Senior Staff Fellow, National Cancer Institute, Bethesda, Maryland
Lydia Temoshok, PhD   Assistant Professor of Medical Psychology, Department of Psychiatry, Langley Porter Psychiatric Hospital, San Francisco, California
Heather Turner   Human Development and Aging Program, Center for Social and Behavioral Sciences, University of California, S.F., San Francisco, California
Paul A. Volberding, MD   Chief, AIDS Activities Division, AIDS Outpatient Clinic, San Francisco General Hospital, San Francisco, California
Kazumi Wakabayashi   Shinjuku-ku, Tokyo, Japan
David Watts, MD   Associate Clinical Professor of Medicine, University of California, San Francisco, California
Kent J. Weinhold, PhD   Duke University Medical Center, Durham, North Carolina
Jane Zich, PhD   Assistant Research Psychologist, Department of Psychiatry, University of California, San Francisco, California

Foreword

Throughout the world, there is a need for more dialogue and discussion about AIDS. Despite the extensive media coverage of AIDS during the past several years, despite the thousands of seminars and conferences for all professional groups, despite the thousands of publications for technical and general audiences, there is a need for more information and discussion about AIDS.

This need exists because the educational process is enormously complex and human attitudes and behavior clearly take time to evolve. At one level there is the wisdom of the Latin proverb *Repititio est mater studiorum* [Repetition is the mother of learning]. Facts about AIDS must be repeated, discussed, and questioned. Only then can we expect that the answers may be incorporated fully into a person's understanding of AIDS. At another level AIDS is not a single issue that can be rapidly or even succinctly described. It has vital social, cultural, economic, and political dimensions. People think about AIDS and learn about AIDS in many different ways, and they enter the dialogue from widely varying entry points and perspectives.

In this regard two relevant generalizations have emerged from the worldwide experience with AIDS, particularly during the period 1986–1988. First, to the extent that populations and groups are informed and educated about AIDS, groundless fears recede and simplistic and illusory schemes for AIDS prevention and control are rejected. Second, policies on AIDS prevention and control that have been openly and widely discussed in public and in professional settings are generally more realistic and often more humane than some of the proposals that may have been advanced initially.

For these two reasons and because AIDS is now a part of our world, it is essential that energy and creativity continue to be directed into dialogue and discussion about AIDS. The wide range of authors in this book, *AIDS: Principles, Practices, and Politics* (reference edition), is to be applauded, for the perspectives are accordingly diverse. This book will stimulate thought and it may provoke controversies—both of which are to be hoped. For the danger is not controversy but silence, not open argument but complacency or isolation. This book is an exciting contribution to an ongoing dialogue of local, national, and international importance.

Jonathan M. Mann
Director, Global Programme on AIDS
World Health Organization

Preface

Few diseases in modern times have received the media attention given to Acquired Immune Deficiency Sydrome (AIDS). Whether examined in print or via visual media, a particular slant or "take" on the subject is employed as reporters attempt to present a story. The approach taken in this book is that AIDS is complex and multifaceted. Consequently this volume brings together a broad range of perspectives and incorporates the expertise needed to address the multiple problems inherent in the AIDS epidemic. Although experts in any given field have lengthy and fruitful dialogues with their peers, both in person and in publication, less attention has been given to an exchange of views and expertise that extends beyond disciplinary and geographic boundaries.

This book is also distinctive for its inclusion of visual images that symbolize issues discussed in the text. The editors felt it was important to include the drawings because all of the complexities and nuances associated with HIV infection have not yet been articulated. Art enhances our awareness and gives expression where words may be inadequate. Together, the artist, clinicians, scientists, and public officials present a more complete picture of the different aspects of the AIDS pandemic than would otherwise be possible.

The fundamental questions addressed in these papers apply to a range of issues critical to every society. These include protection of the health of the members of a society, provision of health care, education of health care workers and citizens, and attendant costs. Although the focus of this book is on AIDS, the approaches and solutions suggested are of broader interest and application. Indeed the AIDS pandemic necessitates our confrontation and resolution of many unresolved problems, such as the accessibility and financing of health care.

Our intent is to enhance the knowledge of the reader in a number of fields relevant to AIDS in order to facilitate a more profound appreciation of the problems associated with pandemic. Both microscopic and macroscopic views are necessary to comprehend what is at stake as countries respond to the challenges posed by AIDS.

AIDS: Principles, Practices, and Politics may be helpful to both the educated citizen and the scientist in exploring the scope of the problems associated with AIDS. Moreover, as schools and universities develop courses on AIDS, the present volume may be of use as either a reference or a course text. Indeed, the Table of Contents may serve as a guide for structuring a course. This book will also be useful to any individual who would like a resource on the multiple dimensions of the AIDS pandemic. Although the question of how quickly this material becomes dated is of concern, the papers included in this book address fundamental issues. While statistics change, the problems discussed in this book are rooted in the social structure and will take longer to resolve. *AIDS: Principles, Practices, and Politics* explores these problems and lays a foundation for solutions.

Our lives have been enriched by our work on this project and the friendship and support we have found in each other and those around us. We thank Inge's daughters, Theresa and Patricia, and Mary's husband David, for their loving support throughout the development of this project. Additional organizational support was provided by Maureen Ryan and Rebecca Hughes. We thank both of these special colleagues.

Sandra Tamburrino and Carolyn Ormes, our production editors, truly made it all happen and we thank them. Last, but not least, Kate Roach, our unflappable editor on this project, has earned our respect and friendship. Her belief in this book transformed it from dream to reality. Our work was also enhanced by Ron Wilder, who assumed the editorial task when the book was in production, and we acknowledge his support with much appreciation.

Our thanks as well to all of our colleagues who provided helpful suggestions during the formation of this volume. Finally, we acknowledge our contributors whose insights and wisdom are reflected in these pages. We thank you for sharing our vision and the ardors and delights involved in its development.

Inge B. Corless
Mary Pittman-Lindeman

Introduction

AIDS, the acquired immune deficiency syndrome, is a complex and far reaching phenomenon that encompasses multidisciplinary principles, practices, and politics. The papers included in *AIDS: Principles, Practices, and Politics* address some of the most common, difficult, and distressing issues confronting professionals and the general public. These problems are analyzed by experts and specialists in each area.

To understand AIDS, the book first explores the AIDS retrovirus, originally termed LAV, lymphadenopathy virus, by Luc Montagnier and his co-workers at the Pasteur Institute in France; HTLV-III by Robert Gallo and his colleagues at the National Institutes of Health in Washington, D.C.; and ARV, AIDS-related virus, by Jay Levy and his associates at the University of California, San Francisco. Standardizing the virus name to human immunodeficiency virus (HIV) has been complicated further by discoveries of new viruses or sets of viruses, such as LAV-II/HIV-II. Given the concern for the immense devastation in terms of human lives that has occurred as a result of the rapid spread of HIV infection, the international research community has set aside the debate over terminology and scientific primacy in favor of international cooperation and a global effort to combat AIDS.

Efforts at the development of a cure have resulted in the identification of drugs that delay progression of some of the manifestations of the disease but do not eliminate the virus or resolve the underlying immune deficiency. Thus efforts to contain HIV infection have emphasized preventive measures. These efforts at prevention have taken two major approaches that are addressed in this text: developing a vaccine and educating the public about the disease.

While these efforts are moving forward, there are a number of questions that confront professionals, researchers, the public, and persons with HIV disease that are discussed in this test. First, to what extent is HIV infection spreading? Discussions of the epidemiology are presented for various risk categories. The danger from AIDS is not limited to gays and intravenous drug users, as is apparent from the development of seropositivity in transfusion recipients and in the partners of virus-exposed individuals. In addition, in Africa, AIDS appears to be largely heterosexually transmitted. It is difficult to estimate the true extent of the problem in Africa due to malnutrition, the effects of which are similar to AIDS, and to the lack of appropriate laboratory facilities to test for infection. The repeated use of needles without intermittent disinfection in some public health clinics in Africa may also serve as a source of disease transmission. Transfusions, frequently given for malaria and during child birth, may have abetted disease transmission. The Surgeon General of the United States has taken the position, based on the findings of AIDS investigators, that children and adolescents must be alerted to the danger of infection with HIV as a result of sexual intercourse or intravenous drug use. The potential for the virtual elimination of a generation of young people is a real and present danger in the United States, Africa, and other high prevalence locations.

Second, why do some people who test positive for exposure to the virus develop AIDS rapidly while others do not? The extent to which cofactors are necessary for the development of the disease in an individual is not clear at this time. The obverse of this question is why is it that some who test positive do not develop AIDS? The other possibility, of course, and one almost too dreadful to contemplate, is that everyone who tests positive will eventually develop AIDS. Many feel that it is only a matter of time.

Third, what social and health care resources are necessary to deal with the epidemic? The resources required to care for those with AIDS, particularly as the number of patients increases, will have profound economic, social, and personal impact. The illness and death of so many persons in the prime of their working lives will have vast demographic implications not only for the current economy but also for the support of the aging population.

The observation that the AIDS epidemic highlights all the weaknesses and gaps in the health care system of the United States is well taken. If there is one silver lining to the gray cloud of AIDS is may be a rationalization of the health care system with guarantees of access to all individuals. If, however, the demands for care are greater than available resources, some painful choices will be necessary. How and for whom should limited resources be utilized? And who will make such determinations? In a related issue, will national health insurance be enacted if private companies refuse to enroll clients?

The needs of the person with AIDS and his or her care givers are not uniform. The medical and social needs will vary, depending not only on whether the person with AIDS is a pregnant woman, a child, an intravenous drug user, a hemophiliac, a gay man, a transfusion recipient, or the partner of a seropositive individual, but also on the contextual and situational factors pertaining to that individual. The availability of health care and other support services as well as the political milieu and the presence of informed care givers all affect care giving. The presence of professional care givers cannot be assumed. Decreases in the number of students electing to enter the nursing profession combined with a fear of disease transmission, pressures by family, friends, and colleagues, and a concern with career may decrease the availability of professional care givers at the very time when the need is greatest.

Hospice programs face a more difficult challenge in providing care for persons with AIDS than for people with other terminal illnesses. The capacity of hospice programs to respond to the AIDS epidemic will depend in large measure on the availability of other needed resources such as housing. Unfortunately, the current Medicare reimbursement mechanism for hospice care (which emphasizes home care) may prove inadequate to the needs of persons with AIDS who lose their homes when their landlords learn of their illness; who become impoverished by their health care needs before Medicaid covers their costs; or who may or may not have family members, friends, or lovers willing to act as care givers. This situation is not dissimilar to the Medicare recipient living alone or with a partner in frail health who has housing but no one who can assume the role of continuous care giver.

One resource that has been developed as a result of the AIDS epidemic is a volunteer "buddy" and support program, which provides emotional and practical support for persons with AIDS. This type of resource will also need financial support to maintain the organization, even though the major portion of care giving is provided by volunteers.

Fourth, do we have an adequate approach to dealing with the ethical dilemmas posed by AIDS? Concerns exist regarding the ethics and decision-making process that will be used to establish public policy in the area of HIV testing and reporting. Many serious concerns are raised by the specter of a society that searches out and isolates those who are infected with the HIV virus and restricts their civil liberties. On the other hand, the call for the safety of the public's health poses a challenge that requires careful balancing between the needs of the community and the civil liberties of the individual. Thus, far, the balance has been leaning toward the protection of civil liberties, but federal proposals for mandatory testing may be indicative of a change in emphasis.

With the exponential growth in research information, new programs, and public policies related to this epidemic, it would be impossible to adequately cover all topics of interest. Topics not addressed include the legal implications of the pandemic, certain aspects of public policy, information on HIV-II, and other issues. The ramifications of infection including HIV dementia, the Belle Glade phenomenon, the role of corporate leaders in educating their employees, as well as other subjects, will be included in the next volume. The topics included in this book represent the breadth of the issues that must be considered when contemplating the meaning of the AIDS pandemic.

Where it has been difficult to achieve an international accord on the use of nuclear arms, the emergence of a retrovirus may foster setting aside political differences to develop the concerted efforts necessary to control the pandemic and preserve life. It is our hope that by examining some of the principles, practices, and politics associated with AIDS this book makes a contribution to those efforts.

1

AIDS Overview

Paul A. Volberding

INTRODUCTION

Since first observed in 1981, the acquired immune deficiency syndrome (AIDS) has become an enormous medical, social, and political problem that requires major commitments of human and financial resources to resolve. As a new disease that primarily affects young adults and that has very high mortality, AIDS has generated intense public and medical interest. Under pressure to act as quickly as possible to find a cure or vaccine for AIDS, medical researchers have sometimes been overly optimistic about the implications of their findings. As a consequence the public and people with AIDS have sometimes been misdirected toward false hopes or confused by revised interpretations based on new data. Although a cure or a vaccine has not yet been found, much has been learned about the epidemiology, routes of transmission, natural history, and clinical manifestations of AIDS. We now know that the life-threatening diseases associated with AIDS are end-stage manifestations of infection with the human immunodeficiency virus (HIV). As we learn more about the life cycle of HIV, it is becoming possible to develop and test antiviral drugs and immune system modulators to halt progression of the retroviral infection and correct the immune deficiency.

DEFINITION OF AIDS

The Centers for Disease Control (CDC) defined AIDS for surveillance purposes as a syndrome characterized by unusual opportunistic infections and rare malignancies in otherwise healthy individuals with no other reason for immune system compromise.[1] Although somewhat restrictive, this definition enabled public health officials to monitor the rapidly expanding AIDS epidemic even before its cause was known.

In 1983–84 the retrovirus that causes the underlying immune deficiency was independently identified by researchers in France and the United States. Variously called LAV by Luc Montagnier of the Pasteur Institute,[2] HTLV-III by Robert Gallo of the National Institutes of Health,[3] and ARV by Jay Levy of the University of California, San Francisco,[4] the retrovirus was renamed in 1986 by an international committee on nomenclature[5] and is now known as HIV. Once the virus was cultured and sensitive viral antibody tests were developed, it became possible to understand much more fully the nature, transmission, and epidemiology of AIDS and related clinical syndromes.

HIV infection produces a spectrum of clinical manifestations ranging from no symptoms in some infected individuals to rapid disease progression in others,

1

with death from opportunistic infections or rare malignancies. Within this clinical spectrum, several syndromes have been defined, including the persistent generalized lymphadenopathy syndrome (PGL),[6-8] the AIDS-related complex (ARC),[9,10] and the acquired immune deficiency syndrome (AIDS).[11-13] At first thought to represent discrete manifestations of response to the virus, these syndromes are now understood to be clinical stages of progressive retroviral damage to the immune system.

The CDC recently proposed a new classification system for HIV infection, in which the clinical manifestations of AIDS are categorized as Stage IVC (secondary infectious diseases) and Stage IVD (secondary malignancies).[14] The CDC surveillance definition of AIDS may soon be extended to include severe wasting (Stage IVA, constitutional disease) and dementia (Stage IVB, neurological disease).

MAGNITUDE OF THE EPIDEMIC IN THE UNITED STATES

In the United States more than 35,000 AIDS cases and more than 20,000 AIDS deaths have been recorded.[15] By the end of 1991, these numbers are expected to increase to 270,000 cases and 179,000 deaths.[16] Because the AIDS-related complex (ARC) is not currently a reportable condition in this country, the actual number of people with symptoms of acquired immune deficiency not included in the surveillance definition for AIDS is unknown. However, it is estimated that 10 times the number of people with AIDS may have ARC.

When AIDS was first described in 1981, 95% of cases were among homosexual or bisexual males; today that percentage has fallen to about 73% of all AIDS cases. Intravenous drug users (IVDUs) account for approximately 17% of cases. Recently, the CDC has begun to differentiate in its reporting between homosexual and bisexual men who are not intravenous drug users (66%) and those who are (8%). Combining homosexual and heterosexual AIDS patients who have a history of intravenous drug use, 25% of AIDS patients may be classified in this group. With evidence of rapid spread of HIV among IVDUs in certain cities,[17-21] the proportion of AIDS cases in this risk group may be expected to increase in future years.

Although white males are disproportionately represented among AIDS cases overall, more than two-thirds of heterosexual IVDUs with AIDS and three-quarters of the children with AIDS are black or Hispanic.[22] The majority of pediatric AIDS cases result from perinatal transmission from infected mothers who are themselves IVDUs or the sexual partners of IVDUs. In the United States, 8% of AIDS cases are women and 92% are men, but in Central Africa, where AIDS has been transmitted primarily among heterosexuals, the ratio of male to female cases is 1.1 male to 1.0 female. To date, only 4% of AIDS cases in the United States have resulted from heterosexual contact, but this percentage is expected to increase by 1991.

The case fatality rate for AIDS is 50%, which means that at any given time approximately half the people diagnosed with AIDS have died. Among patients with the opportunistic infections and rare cancers included in the CDC surveillance definition of AIDS, the two-year mortality approaches 90% and the ultimate mortality is close to 100%.[23] In patients with ARC the two-year mortality is still low, but because many of these patients progress to AIDS, the ultimate mortality may be quite high.

The magnitude of the epidemic is most apparent when measured on a local scale. In San Francisco, a city of 700,000 people, 3,300 AIDS cases have already been reported and 18,000 cumulative cases are expected by the early 1990s. In the cities and hospitals where the majority of AIDS cases are diagnosed and treated, health care resources and systems are already overburdened by the complex medical, psychological, and social needs of AIDs patients. Estimates of the average lifetime costs of care per AIDS patient range from $50,000 to $150,000.[24-26] Costs are lower at San Francisco General Hospital, where a comprehensive system of AIDS patient care was developed. The San Francisco General Hospital model emphasizes coordination among multidisciplinary medical, psychosocial, and nursing staff in an outpatient care setting, integration of inpatient and outpatient care, and close cooperation with voluntary community agencies in providing psychosocial support, home care, and educational services.[27,28] Lifetime hospital charges at this hospital are about $30,000,[29] but when out-of-hospital costs are included, the cost of care is probably $50,000 to $70,000.

Evidence is accumulating that a majority of people with HIV infection will eventually manifest some symptoms of disease[30,31] and more than half may progress to ARC or AIDS (G. Rutherford, personal communication, 1987). Since 1 to 2 million people in the United States may currently be infected with HIV, and millions more in Africa and other nations, the full impact of AIDs in terms of morbidity, mortality, and socioeconomic costs has only begun to be felt.

TRANSMISSION OF HIV

HIV is transmitted by blood and by direct contact of genital or rectal mucosa with infected semen or vaginal secretions. Although HIV may be found in virtually any body fluid, only blood, semen, and vaginal and cervical secretions are thought to be important in viral transmission. HIV has been detected in saliva and tears, but there is no evidence that the virus is transmitted through these fluids.

Sexual transmission of the virus can occur through vaginal, anal, and possibly oral intercourse. Infected males can transmit the virus to male or female sexual partners, and infected females can transmit the virus sexually to males and perinatally to their unborn infants. Although it is theoretically possible for females to transmit the virus to female sexual partners, lesbians who are not bisexual and do not use intravenous drugs are considered to be at low risk for HIV infection.

In the United States, viral transmission through blood transfusion is less problematic now that blood is being tested for HIV antibodies. However, among intravenous drug users, blood-borne transmission takes place through sharing hypodermic syringes contaminated with infected blood. Because infected intravenous drug users also can transmit the virus sexually, this group may constitute a bridge for viral transmission into the wider heterosexual population.

Health care workers have been concerned about the risks of occupational infection with HIV. Recently, three cases of occupational transmission of HIV following mucocutaneous exposure to infected blood were reported to the CDC. In general, however, studies show that the risks of transmission of the virus to health care workers are very low.[32-34] At San Francisco General Hospital, for example, 300 health care workers agreed to be tested for HIV antibodies. Of the 253 health care workers without other risk factors (i.e., heterosexual, non-IV drug users), not one was found to be infected with HIV despite 5 years of working with hundreds of AIDS patients. Of 84 health care workers who stuck themselves with needles contaminated by HIV-infected blood, none showed evidence of viral infection. Clearly, if health care workers do not become infected with HIV following years of intense close contact with AIDs patients, the risk to the general public from casual contact with infected individuals is virtually nonexistent. Studies of household contacts of AIDS patients also demonstrate that casual transmission of the virus does not occur.[35-37]

The risk of HIV transmission varies considerably among different populations. Homosexual men and intravenous drug users who share needles are at very high risk for HIV infection. Heterosexuals who have had long-term monogamous sexual relationships and who do not use intravenous drugs or share needles still have a very low risk of HIV infection in most parts of the world. The determinants of an individual's infectiousness or susceptibility to HIV infection are unknown at this time. The role of possible cofactors, such as concurrent viral infections or venereal diseases, nutrition, and recreational drug use, in facilitating viral transmission or infection also is unclear.

When introduced into a susceptible population, HIV can be spread very rapidly. In San Francisco, serum samples collected in 1978 from a large group of homosexual men with histories of venereal disease were tested retrospectively for HIV antibodies. This cohort has now been followed for several years by the San Francisco Health Department. Although in 1978 only 4% of serum samples had been infected with HIV, by 1984, 50% of this cohort tested seropositive to the virus, and by 1986, 75% were infected.[38] The epidemiology of AIDs in Central African countries and possibly in other parts of the world suggests that heterosexual populations may be as susceptible to rapid infection with HIV as the homosexual population in San Francisco.[39-43] Retrospective studies document rapid spread of HIV among intravenous drug users as well. In New Jersey seroprevalence rates among IVDUs rose from 11% in 1977, to 27% in 1979, to 58% in 1984.[44] Similar rates of increase among IVDUs have been reported in European cities[45,46] and in San Francisco.[47]

PATHOGENESIS AND NATURAL HISTORY OF AIDS

Retroviral infection occurs when HIV attaches to the T4 antigen on the surface of a cell. Many cells appear to carry the antigen, including T-helper lymphocytes, macrophages, and possibly glial cells in the central nervous system. It is not yet known whether infection requires exposure to the naked virus or to cells infected with the virus. After penetrating the nucleus of the cell, the retrovirus integrates its genetic material into that of the cell through the action of a unique enzyme, reverse transcriptase, and can begin to replicate itself.

At various lengths of time following infection, HIV begins to destroy the T-helper cell population, possibly by lysing (disintegrating) these cells following viral replication, or by disrupting hormones responsible for normal cell functioning, or by infecting and destroying the stem cells needed to replenish the T-cell population. Although we do not have good measures of immune competence, the absolute number of T-helper cells is often used as a shorthand for measuring the degree of immune damage caused by this virus. As the immune system is destroyed, patients gradually begin to manifest the variety of symptoms collectively referred to as AIDS-related complex, or ARC. With further immune deficiency, opportunistic infections or Kaposi's sarcoma appear as the overt clinical manifestations of AIDS.

HIV may penetrate the central nervous system very early in the disease process. Evidence for this comes from clinical observations of aseptic meningitis in patients who experience the acute retroviral syndrome within a few weeks following infection.[48] The presence of HIV in the central nervous system has been confirmed by viral culture of cerebral spinal fluid.[49] It is not known whether the dementias and neurologic syndromes associated with AIDS are caused directly by viral infection of brain cells or indirectly through the action of lymphokines or other secreted factors in the brain.

Within eight weeks following infection with HIV, 50% of infected people show a positive result on the ELISA antibody test.[50] Almost all individuals seroconvert within six months following infection. First developed to screen donated blood, the HIV antibody test has also been used to detect the presence of the virus in populations and to monitor the rate of viral transmission in large cohorts of people at risk for infection. The ELISA test, with Western Blot confirmation, is most commonly used, although sensitive and accurate immunofluorescence assays also are available.[51] Regardless of the technique, when properly used in populations with high prevalence of the virus, the antibody test is highly accurate. In populations with low prevalence of the virus, however, the ELISA test produces some false positives.[52] Recombinant antigens are currently being developed to decrease some of the problems associated with HIV antibody testing.

Antibodies to HIV do not appear to function in the same way as antibodies to many other viruses. The hepatitis virus antibody, for example, appears as the antigen disappears, and the presence of the antibody implies immunity to the virus. By contrast, the HIV antibody and antigen appear almost simultaneously, and the presence of antibody implies ongoing viral infection rather than immunity. Thus, a positive HIV antibody test implies that an individual is actively infected, presumably for life, and represents a continuous contagious risk to others through sexual, parenteral, or perinatal routes of transmission.[53-55]

In the past, it was estimated that perhaps 5–10% of people infected with HIV would develop AIDS,[56] but recent evidence suggests that those estimates were much too low. In one study of patients with diffuse lymphadenopathy (mild ARC), 50% of patients developed AIDS within 5 years following HIV infection.[57] It now seems very likely that the majority of infected people will go on to experience some degree of immune deficiency and perhaps overt AIDS. Based on the estimated numbers of people presently infected with the virus, it is anticipated that we will be dealing with an AIDS epidemic for the next 5 to 10 years, regardless of any preventive measures now taken to stop viral spread.

CLINICAL MANIFESTATIONS OF AIDS

Following infection with HIV, many people remain asymptomatic and healthy, often unaware that they are infected, yet capable of transmitting the virus to others. Why some people rapidly develop AIDS following infection and others live in apparent homeostasis with the virus for many years is still unknown. In certain people various chronic symptoms may be present for some time before an opportunistic infection or cancer appears, but many patients initially manifest Kaposi's sarcoma or an opportunistic infection.

Some infected people experience an acute flulike illness within a few weeks following infection. This acute retroviral syndrome lasts for a mean of eight days and is characterized by fevers, sweats, malaise, lethargy, swollen glands, and other nonspecific symptoms.[58] A transitory erythematous macular rash (reddish patches) is seen in about 50% of these patients. As the immune system becomes progressively impaired, other clinical manifestations may appear, including persistent generalized lymphadenopathy (PGL), oral candidiasis, and oral hairy leukoplakia. In people with PGL, the onset of oral candidiasis or hairy leukoplakia signals an increased risk of rapid progression to AIDS.[59]

The clinical forms of AIDS vary among risk groups; AIDS does not give rise to the same diseases in homosexual men as in heterosexuals. For example, Kaposi's sarcoma is seen at diagnosis in gay men in 30–50% of cases.[60] By contrast, only 2% of hemophiliacs with AIDS have Kaposi's sarcoma. Similarly, *Pneumocystis carinii* pneumonia (PCP), which accounts for more than 50% of all initial AIDS diagnoses in this country, is relatively more common in heterosexuals infected through blood transfusions than among gay men. Lymphocytic interstitial pneumonitis is very rarely seen in adults with AIDS, but it is a common diagnosis in children with AIDS. These differences have not yet been explained. Regional differences also occur in the clinical manifestations of AIDS.[61] In the United States, PCP is the most common opportunistic infection, seen more frequently than esophageal candidiasis and cryptococcal meningitis. In Africa and Haiti, however, PCP is less common than other infections. *Candida* infection and cryptococcal meningitis are the most common AIDS-related infections in Africa and *Candida* and tuberculosis are seen more frequently in Haiti. To some degree, the types of infections manifested in different parts of the world reflect the microorganisms most frequently found in those regions. It is not yet known whether there are genetic influences on the manifestations of AIDS or regional differences in the AIDS virus itself that might cause different reactions to different tissues and, thus, different clinical manifestations of disease.

As the epidemic evolves, changes are taking place in its clinical manifestations. In the United States, the incidence of Kaposi's sarcoma, which accounted for 48% of AIDS cases in 1981, accounted for only 18% of cases in 1986. To understand these changes, we will need ongoing epidemiologic surveillance.

Opportunistic Infections

Opportunistic infections are the most common presenting clinical manifestations that establish a diagnosis of AIDS. These infections are characterized by an aggressive clinical course, resistance to therapy, and a high rate of relapse. Among the infections associated with AIDS are parasitic infections (e.g., PCP, cryptosporidiosis, toxoplasmosis), bacterial infections (e.g., *Mycobacterium avium intracellulare*), viral infections (e.g., invasive cytomegalovirus, invasive herpes simplex virus), and fungal infections (e.g., cryptococcal disease, histoplasmosis).

PCP is the most common opportunistic infection, seen in 55–60% of AIDS patients, and is by far the most common initial presenting diagnosis in AIDS. PCP usually presents with a diffuse pneumonitis. Symptoms include shortness of breath, nonproductive cough, dyspnea (labored breathing) on exertion, chest tightness, and often high fever. At the time of diagnosis, chest x-rays usually are abnormal, showing some increase in bronchovascular/interstitial markings in more than 95% of cases. Although a diagnosis of PCP once required doing a bronchoscopy, it is now diagnosed at many hospitals on the basis of careful microscopic observation of induced sputum. This technique decreases the need for expensive and invasive testing of patients and allows more rapid outpatient diagnosis of this infection.

The standard drugs used to treat PCP are trimethoprim/sulfamethoxazole and pentamidine administered intravenously, orally, or by inhalation. Unfortunately, most patients become allergic to or intolerant of these medications and they must be discontinued. Dapsone, a drug now being tested for use in treating PCP, appears to have substantial activity especially when combined with trimethoprim/sulfamethoxazole.

Malignancies

Several cancers are associated with HIV infection, including Kaposi's sarcoma and various lymphomas. Kaposi's sarcoma, central nervous system lymphomas, and high grade peripheral B-cell lymphomas are believed to result directly from the immune deficiency caused by HIV infection. Other cancers, such as Hodgkin's lymphoma, may not be directly attributable to HIV infection, but their clinical course is definitely altered by it. Hodgkin's lymphoma is seen with increased incidence in homosexual men and follows an aggressive clinical course.

Kaposi's sarcoma (KS), the second most common clinical manifestation of AIDS, is a multicentric disease process that produces reddish or violaceous lesions in various regions of the body simultaneously. Often the lesions are distributed in a striking linear pattern, following the paths of lymphatic drainage. Although the cell of origin is uncertain, tumors appear to arise from the lymphatic endothelium. The earliest KS lesions resemble many other types of lesions commonly seen on the body. At more advanced stages of disease, however, the appearance of the lesions is so striking and typical that biopsy often is not necessary to make the diagnosis. Visceral KS is common, but often clinically silent. In contrast, pulmonary KS is less common, but more aggressive. Generally, patients with pulmonary KS have an extremely poor prognosis.

Unlike many other manifestations of AIDS, KS can be quite disfiguring. In addition to visible lesions, lymphedema of the face or the lower extremities, caused by lymphatic obstruction by the tumor, frequently occurs. AIDS patients with KS are usually the most stigmatized and isolated, often rejected by employers, friends, and family members. Although patients with KS usually die of opportunistic infections rather than the cancer itself, much of the morbidity associated with AIDS is caused by this visible tumor.

Chemotherapeutic agents have some activity against KS, but because they may further impair cellular immunity and increase the risk of infection, their use is controversial. Radiation therapy is used primarily for palliation, to reduce painful lesions of the feet, erosive oral lesions, and areas of extensive lymphedema.

Despite the development of efficacious treatments to control the opportunistic infections and cancers that result from AIDS, their impact on AIDS-related mortality will be minimal until the underlying immune deficiency can be corrected.

ANTIVIRAL THERAPY AND IMMUNE SYSTEM STIMULATION

General Considerations

Several experimental therapies are being developed to correct the underlying immune dysfunction and to interrupt and neutralize the retroviral infection process. The goals of antiviral drug development are both preventive and therapeutic. These drugs might be used to prevent viral transmission by reducing the infectiousness of people already carrying the virus or by reducing the susceptibility of people not yet exposed to it. An important goal is to prevent further progression of disease in infected people. In people with AIDS or ARC, it may be possible to reverse established disease and restore immune function. Much more needs to be learned, however, about the mechanisms of HIV transmission, its natural history, and the pathogenesis of immune deficiency before truly effective antiviral drugs can be developed. Moreover, many practical and economic issues must be resolved before an antiviral drug can be distributed to the millions of people at risk or already infected. For these reasons, efficacious antiviral agents are not expected to be available for many years.

To reduce infectiousness, an antiviral drug would have to markedly decrease viral replication and concentration in semen, blood, and vaginal secretions. To reduce susceptibility to infection, the drug would have to block attachment of the virus to the T4 antigen on cells or neutralize the effects of possible cofactors. To prevent disease progression or to reverse established disease, an antiviral drug must block viral replication without compromising the restoration of normal immune function. The drug also must be capable of crossing the blood-brain barrier to treat infected cells in the central nervous system.

Ideally, to prevent retroviral damage to the immune system, treatment should start almost immediately following infection. However, widespread use of an HIV antigen or antibody test to identify individuals as soon as possible following infection raises several concerns, including potential risks to civil rights and the needless trauma that many people who test false positive will undergo. This last concern is especially relevant if the tests are used in populations with low viral prevalence.

Those issues aside, antiviral drug treatment of infected people poses many other difficulties. Treatment may need to continue for 10 or more years and possibly for life. Experience with other chronic illnesses, such as hypertension, suggests that long-term compliance with drug treatment is extremely difficult to maintain. An antiviral drug for HIV, therefore, must be convenient to take, orally administered, have minimal toxicity and no subjective side effects, and must be inexpensive so that large numbers of people can afford to take it continuously for many years. Thus far, no experimental agent to treat HIV that has been clinically tested meets all of these requirements.

For ethical reasons, the first anti-HIV experimental drugs were tested in patients with advanced disease. Even if a drug is active against HIV, this may be difficult to demonstrate in patients whose immune systems are already severely compromised. Although there is still concern about testing experimental drugs in infected people who are relatively healthy, researchers today are designing clinical trials of drugs in healthier patients to see if a drug such as zidovudine (formerly AZT) might prevent progression of disease.

Immune System Modulators

Attempts to restore immune function through immune system modulators have thus far been unsuccessful. Interferon, an antiviral drug with anticancer properties, also stimulates the immune system. In our tests, however, interferon showed no evidence of activity against cytomegalovirus or other viruses, modest activity against Kaposi's sarcoma, and no evidence of boosting the immune system.[62] The most potent immune stimulator that we have tested is recombinant interleuken-2, the lymphokine of the immune system. Even at very high doses, however, this drug showed no benefit.

Several factors may explain why immune stimulators have been unsuccessful in correcting the immune deficiency in AIDS. First, by the time a person has AIDS, the immune deficiency may be so severe that correction is impossible. Second, newly produced T-lymphocytes may themselves become infected with HIV. Third, the worst possibility, immune stimulation may actually exacerbate the immune deficiency by causing cells infected with HIV to proliferate and produce more virus.

Antiviral Agents

Most experimental drug treatments for AIDS focus on decreasing replication of the virus once infection has occurred. Because HIV requires reverse transcriptase to replicate itself within cells, several antiviral drugs are being designed to target this and other enzymes. Drugs like interferon may act to prevent, delay, or slow down the assembly of intact viruses following transcription within the cell.

Suramin was the first antiviral agent against HIV tested in the United States.[63-67] Unfortunately, suramin proved to have no efficacy and considerable toxicity; it led to the death of a number of patients who had not yet developed AIDS. Two of our patients became adrenal insufficient during the trial and still have no detectable adrenal function. Although HIV was no longer detectable in viral cultures of five patients treated with suramin, the disease continued to progress in four of these patients. Tests of HPA 23, the French drug that drew Rock Hudson and many other Americans to Paris when it was first used there, had similar disappointing results in clinical trials. HPA 23 had no effect on clinical outcome even when the virus appeared to be inhibited.

Zidovudine (formerly called azidothymidine or AZT) is the first drug that has showed clear benefits in slowing down, but not preventing, the progression of AIDS. Under the brand name Retrovir (Burroughs Wellcome), zidovudine recently received FDA approval for prescription to AIDS patients who meet certain eligibility requirements. A simple analogue of thymidine, zidovudine is difficult to synthesize and expensive to produce.

Initially developed as a potential antineoplastic (tumor) agent, zidovudine was later found to be very active against HIV in vitro. In a double-blind placebo clinical trial in patients with AIDS and ARC, patients receiving the drug had significantly reduced mortality during the trial compared with those who received the placebo.[68] The trial was terminated at the end of six months, after 16 deaths had occurred among patients receiving the placebo and only 1 death among patients receiving zidovudine. In comparing patients receiving placebo or zidovudine in terms of serious events experienced during the course of the trial (e.g., development of opportunistic infections or Kaposi's sarcoma, or death), researchers found that after the first six weeks of the study, drug recipients appeared to experience fewer serious events than placebo recipients. These indirect indications of zidovudine's effectiveness against HIV are supported by the observation of slightly increased levels of T-helper cells during the study in patients receiving the drug compared with those on placebo.

Zidovudine has considerable toxicity. Hemoglobin levels often drop dramatically in patients receiving this drug. By the end of the clinical trial, 25% of AIDS patients taking zidovudine required regular blood transfusions to maintain hemoglobin. With the problem of an already limited blood supply in this country, the prospect of thousands of people taking zidovudine on a continuous basis and becoming transfusion-dependent is worrisome but may be reduced when the drug is used in less advanced HIV infections.

The cost for one year's supply of zidovudine has been estimated to be about $10,000. The high cost alone makes this a less than ideal drug for lifelong use by thousands of infected people in the United States and may preclude its use altogether in Third World countries with few health care resources. Our experience with zidovudine has helped us to appreciate that even if a drug is active against HIV in vivo, we may have other problems when we try to use it on a large scale.

Research for effective treatments is very important and must go forward, but education remains our most potent weapon to halt the spread of AIDS. Both homosexuals and heterosexuals must be encouraged to follow safer sex guidelines, which include decreasing the number of sexual partners, getting to know partners well before having sexual contact, and using condoms. Among our most pressing tasks is the development of adequate means of communicating information about AIDS to intravenous drug users, members of minority groups, adolescents, and others at risk for HIV infection. In addition to preventing further viral spread, widespread education about AIDS can help to reduce the stigma, discrimination, and psychosocial distress that have so often accompanied an AIDS diagnosis.

REFERENCES

1. *The Case Definition of AIDS Used by the CDC for National Reporting (CDC-Reportable AIDS)*. 1985. (Document No. 0312S). Atlanta, GA: Centers for Disease Control.

2. Barre-Sinoussi, F.; Chermann, J. C.; Rey, F.; Nugeyre, M. T.; Chamaret, S.; Gruest, J.; Daugier, C.; Axler-Blin, C.; Vezinet-Brun, F.; Rouzioux, C.; Rosenbaum, W.; Montagnier, L. 1983. Isolation of a T-lymphotropic retrovirus from a patient at risk for acquired immune deficiency syndrome (AIDS). *Science* 220: 868–871.

3. Gallo, R. C.; Salahuddin, S. Z.; Popovic, M.; Shearer, G. M.; Kaplan, M.; Haynes, B. F.; Palker, T. J.; Redfield, R.; Oleske, J.; Safai, B.; White, G.; Foster, P.; Markham, P. 1984. Frequent detection and isolation of cytopathic retroviruses (HTLV-III) from patients with AIDS and at risk for AIDS. *Science* 224: 500–503.

4. Levy, J. A.; Hoffman, A. D.; Kramer, S. M.; Landis, J. A.; Shimabukuro, J. M.; Oshiro, L. S. 1984. Isolation of lymphocytopathic retroviruses from San Francisco patients with AIDS. *Science* 225: 840–842.

5. Coffin, J.; Haase, A.; Levy, J. A.; Montagnier, L.; Oroszian, S.; Teich, N.; Temin, H.; Toyoshima, K.; Varmus, H.; Vogt, P.; Weiss, R. 1986. Human immunodeficiency viruses. *Science* 232: 697.

6. Pinn-Wiggins, V. W. 1985. Follow-up at 4½ years on homosexual men with generalized lymphadenopathy. *New England Journal of Medicine* 313: 1542.

7. Sirianni, M. C.; Rossi, P.; Scarpati, B.; Ragona, G.; Seminara, R.; Bonomo, G.; Aiuti, F. 1985. Immunological and virological investigation in patients with lymphadenopathy syndrome in a population at risk for acquired immunodeficiency syndrome (AIDS); with particular focus on the detection of antibodies to human T-lymphotropic retroviruses (HTLV-III). *Journal of Clinical Immunology* 5: 261–268.

8. Abrams, D. I.; Mess, T.; Volberding, P. A. 1985. Lymphadenopathy: Endpoint or prodrome? Update of a 36-month prospective study. *Advances in Experimental Medicine and Biology* 187: 73–84.

9. Morris, L.; Distenfeld, A.; Amorosi, E.; Karpatkin, S. 1982. Autoimmune thrombocytopenic purpura in homosexual men. *Annals of Internal Medicine* 96: 714–717.

10. Abrams, D. I.; Kiprov, D. D.; Goedert, J. J.; Sarngadharan, M. G.; Gallo, R. C.; Volberding, P. A. 1986. Antibodies to human T-lymphotropic virus type III and development of the acquired immunodeficiency syndrome in homosexual men presenting with immune thrombocytopenia. *Annals of Internal Medicine* 104: 47–50.

11. Gottlieb, G. J.; Ragaz, V.; Vogel, J. V.; Friedman-Kien, A.; Rywkin, A. M.; Weiner, E. A.; Ackerman, A. B. 1981. A preliminary communication on extensively disseminated Kaposi's sarcoma in young homosexual men. *American Journal of Dermatopathology* 3: 111–114.

12. Rivin, B. E.; Monroe, J. M.; Hubschman, B. P.; Thomas, P. A. 1984. AIDS outcome: A first follow-up. *New England Journal of Medicine* 311: 857.

13. Jaffe, H. W.; Bregman, D. J.; Selik, R. M. 1984. Acquired immunodeficiency syndrome in the United States: First 1,000 cases. *Journal of Infectious Diseases* 148: 339–345.

14. Centers for Disease Control. 1986. Classification system for human T-lymphotropic virus type III/lymphadenopathy-associated virus infections. *Morbidity and Mortality Weekly Report* 20: 334–340.

15. Centers for Disease Control. 11 May 1987. *AIDS Weekly Surveillance Report—United States.*

16. National Academy of Sciences. 1986. *Confronting AIDS*. Washington, DC: National Academy Press, p. 8.

17. Weiss, S. H.; Ginzberg, H. M.; Goedert, J. J., et al. 1985. Risk of HTLV-III exposure and AIDS among parenteral drug abusers in New Jersey [Abstract]. *The International Conference on the Acquired Immunodeficiency Syndrome*. Philadelphia, PA: American College of Physicians.

18. Robertson, J. R.; Bucknall, A. B. V.; Welsby, P. D.; Roberts, J. J. K.; Inglis, J. M.; Peutherer, J. F.; Brettle, R. P. 1986. Epidemic of AIDS-related virus (HTLV-III/LAV) infection among intravenous drug users. *British Medical Journal* 292: 527–529.

19. Angarano, G.; Pastore, G.; Monno, L.; Santantono, J.; Luchese, N.; Schiraldi, O. 1985. Rapid spread of HTLV-III infection among drug addicts in Italy. *Lancet* 2: 1302.

20. Rodrigo, J. M.; Serra, M. A.; Aguilar, E.; Del Olmo, J. A.; Gimeno, V.; Aparisi, L. 1985. HTLV-III antibodies in drug addicts in Spain. *Lancet* 2: 156–157.

21. Chaisson, R. E.; Moss, A. R.; Onishi, R.; Osmond, D.; Carlson, J. R. 1987. Human immunodeficiency virus infection in heterosexual intravenous drug users in San Francisco. *American Journal of Public Health* 77: 169–172.

22. Centers for Disease Control. 11 May 1987. *AIDS Weekly Surveillance Report—United States.*

23. Moss, A. R.; McCallum, G.; Volberding, P. A.; Bacchetti, P.; Dritz, S. 1984. Mortality associated with mode of presentation in the acquired immune deficiency syndrome. *Journal of the National Cancer Institute* 73: 1281–1284.

24. Hardy, A.; Rauch, K.; Echenberg, D. F.; Morgan, W. M.; Curran, J. W. 1986. The economic impact of the first 10,000 cases of AIDS in the United States. *Journal of the American Medical Association* 225: 209–211.

25. Kizer, K. W.; Rodriguez, J.; McHolland, G. F.; Weller, W. 1986. *A Qualitative Analysis of AIDS in California.* Sacramento, CA: California Department of Health Services.

26. Scitovsky, A. A.; Rice, D. P.; Showstack, J.; Lee, P. R. 1986. *Estimating the Direct and Indirect Economic Costs of the Acquired Immune Deficiency Syndrome, 1985, 1986, and 1990.* (Task order 282-85-0061.) Atlanta, GA: Centers for Disease Control.

27. Volberding, P. A. 1985. The clinical spectrum of the acquired immunodeficiency syndrome: Implications for comprehensive patient care. *Annals of Internal Medicine* 103: 729–733.

28. Abrams, D. I.; Dilley, J. W.; Maxey, L. M.; Volberding, P. A. 1986. Routine care and psychosocial support of the patient with acquired immunodeficiency syndrome. *Medical Clinics of North America* 70: 707–720.

29. Scitovsky, A. A.; Cline, M.; Lee, P. R. 1986. Medical care costs of patients with AIDS in San Francisco. *Journal of the American Medical Association* 256: 3103–3106.

30. Abrams, D. I., et al. Lymphadenopathy: Endpoint or prodrome? See ref. 8.

31. Abrams, D. I., et al. Antibodies to human T-lymphotropic virus type III. See ref. 10.

32. McCray, E. 1986. Occupational risk of the acquired immunodeficiency syndrome among health care workers. *New England Journal of Medicine* 314: 1127–1132.

33. Henderson, D. K.; Saah, A. J.; Zak, B. J.; Kaslow, R. A.; Lane, H. C.; Folks, T.; Blackwelder, W. C.; Schmitt, J.; LeCamera, D. J.; Masur, H.; Fauci, A. S. 1986. Risk of nosocomial infection with human T-cell lymphotropic virus type III/lymphadenopathy-associated virus in a large cohort of intensively exposed health care workers. *Annals of Internal Medicine* 104: 644–647.

34. Moss, A.; Osmond, D.; Bacchetti, P.; Gerberding, J.; Sande, M.; Volberding, P.; Levy, J. A.; Carlson, J.; Casavant, C.; Conant, M. 1986. Risk of seroconversion for the acquired immune deficiency syndrome (AIDS) in San Francisco health workers. *Journal of Occupational Medicine* 28: 821–824.

35. Friedland, G. H.; Saltzman, B. R.; Rogers, M. F.; Kahl, P. A.; Lesser, M. L.; Mayers, M. M.; Klein, R. S. 1986. Lack of transmission of HTLV-III/LAV infection to household contacts of patients with AIDS or AIDS-related complex with oral candidiasis. *New England Journal of Medicine* 314: 344–349.

36. Mann, J. M.; Quinn, T. C.; Francis, H.; Nzilambi, N.; Bosenge, N.; Bila, K.; McCormick, J. B.; Ruti, K.; Asila, P. K.; Curran, J. W. 1986. Prevalence of HTLV-III/LAV in household contacts of patients with confirmed AIDS and controls in Kinshasa, Zaire. *Journal of the American Medical Association* 256: 721–724.

37. Fischl, M. A.; Dickinson, G. M.; Scott, G. B.; Klimas, N.; Fletcher, M. A.; Parks, W. 1987. Evaluation of heterosexual partners, children, and household contacts of adults with AIDS. *Journal of the American Medical Association* 256: 640–644.

38. Rutherford, G. W.; Echenberg, D. F.; O'Malley, P. M.; Darrow, W. W.; Wilson, T. E.; Jaffe, H. W. 1986. The natural history of LAV/HTLV-III infection and viraemia in homosexual and bisexual men: A 6-year follow up study [Abstract P99]. *Abstracts of the Second International Conference on AIDS.* Paris.

39. Mann, J. M.; Francis, H.; Quinn, T. C. 1986. Surveillance for AIDS in a central African city: Kinshasa, Zaire. *Journal of the American Medical Association* 255: 3255–3259.

40. Piot, P. T.; Quinn, T. C.; Taelman, H.; Feinsod, F. M.; Minlangu, K. B.; Wobin, O.; Mbendi, N.; Mazebo, P.; Ndangi, K.; Stevens, W.; Kalambayi, K.; Mitchell, S.; Bridts, C.; McCormick, J. B. 1984. Acquired immunodeficiency syndrome in a heterosexual population in Zaire. *Lancet* 2: 65–69.

41. Clumeck, N.; Van de Perre, P.; Carael, M.; Rouvroy, D.; Nzaramba, D. 1985. Heterosexual promiscuity among African patients with AIDS. *Lancet* 2: 182.

42. Van de Perre, P.; Rouvroy, D.; Lepage, P.; Bogaerts, J.; Kestelyn, P.; Kayihigi, J.; Hekker,

A. C.; Butzler, J. P.; Clumeck, N. 1984. Acquired immunodeficiency syndrome in Rwanda. *Lancet* 2: 62–65.

43. Kreiss, J. K.; Koech, D.; Plummer, F. A.; Holmes, K. K.; Lightfoote, M.; Piot, P.; Ronald, A. R.; Ndinya-Achola, J. O.; D'Costa, L. J.; Roberts, P.; Ngugi, E. N.; Quinn, T. C. 1986. AIDS virus infection in Nairobi prostitutes: Spread of the epidemic to east Africa. *New England Journal of Medicine* 314: 414–418.

44. Weiss, S. H., et al. Risk of HTLV-III exposure and AIDS among parenteral drug abusers in New Jersey. See ref. 17.

45. Angarano, G., et al. Rapid spread of HTLV-III infection among drug addicts in Italy. See ref. 19.

46. Rodrigo, J. M. HTLV-III antibodies in drug addicts in Spain. See ref. 20.

47. Chaisson, R. E. Human immunodeficiency virus infection in heterosexual intravenous drug users in San Francisco. See ref. 21.

48. Cooper, D. A.; Gold, J.; Maclean, P.; Donovan, B.; Finlayson, R.; Barnes, T. G.; Michelmore, H. M.; Brooke, P.; Penny, R. 1985. Acute AIDS retrovirus infection: Definition of a clinical illness associated with seroconversion. *Lancet* 1: 537–540.

49. Ho, D. D.; Rota, T. R.; Schooley, R. T.; Kaplan, J. C.; Allan, J. D.; Groopman, J. E.; Resnick, L.; Felsenstein, D.; Andrews, C. A.; Hirsch, M. C. 1985. Isolation of HTLV-III from cerebrospinal fluid and neural tissues of patients with neurological syndromes related to the acquired immunodeficiency syndrome. *New England Journal of Medicine* 313:1493–1497.

50. Melbye, M. 1986. The natural history of human T-lymphotropic virus III infection: The cause of AIDS. *British Medical Journal* 292: 5–12.

51. American Medical Association Council on Scientific Affairs. 1985. Status report on the acquired immunodeficiency syndrome: Human T-cell lymphotropic virus type III testing. *Journal of the American Medical Association* 254: 1342–1345.

52. National Institutes of Health. 7–9 July 1986. *The Impact of Routine HTLV-III Antibody Testing of Blood and Plasma on Public Health*. Draft report on a consensus conference, Bethesda, MD.

53. Markham, P. D.; Salahuddin, S. Z.; Popovic, M.; Patel, A.; Veren, K.; Fladager, A.; Orndorff, S.; Gallo, R. C. 1985. Advances in the isolation of HTLV-III from patients with AIDS and AIDS-related complex and from donors at risk. *Cancer Research* 45 (Suppl): 4588s.

54. Groopman, J. E. 1985. Clinical spectrum of HTLV-III in humans. *Cancer Research* 45 (Suppl): 4649–4651s.

55. Centers for Disease Control. 1986. Recommendations for assisting in the prevention of perinatal transmission of human T-lymphotropic virus type III/lymphadenopathy-associated virus and the acquired immunodeficiency syndrome. *Morbidity and Mortality Weekly Report* 34: 721–726; 731–732.

56. Sivak, S. L., and Wormser, G. P. 1985. How common is HTLV-III infection in the United States? *New England Journal of Medicine* 313: 1352.

57. Abrams, D. I., et al. Lymphadenopathy: Endpoint or prodrome? See ref. 8.

58. Cooper, D. A., et al. Acute AIDS retrovirus infection. See ref. 48.

59. Metroka, C. E.; Cunningham-Rundles, S.; Krim, M., et al. 1984. Generalized lymphadenopathy in homosexual men: An update of the New York experience. *Annals of the New York Academy of Science* 407: 400–411.

60. Des Jarlais, D. C.; Marmor, M.; Thomas, P.; Chamberland, M.; Zolla-Pazner, S.; Sencer, D. J. 1984. Kaposi's sarcoma among four different AIDS groups. *New England Journal of Medicine* 310: 1119.

61. Volberding, P. 1986. AIDS—Variations on a theme of cellular immune deficiency. In J. C. Gluckman and E. Vilmer (eds.). *Acquired Immunodeficiency Syndrome*. Paris: Elsevier, pp. 191–198. (International Conference on AIDS, Paris, June 23–25).

62. Groopman, J. E.; Gottlieb, M. S.; Goodman, J.; Mitsuya, R. T.; Conant, M. A.; Prince, H.; Fahey, J. L.; Derezin, M.; Weinstein, W.; Casavant, C.; Rothman, J.; Rudnick, S. A.; Volberding, P. A. 1984. Recombinant alpha 2 interferon therapy of Kaposi's sarcoma associated with acquired immunodeficiency syndrome. *Annals of Internal Medicine* 100: 671–676.

63. Broder, S.; Yarchoan, R.; Collins, J. M.; Lance, H. C.; Markham, P. P.; Klecker, R. W.; Redfield, R. R.; Mitsuya, H.; Hoth, D. F.; Gellman, E.; Groopman, J. E.; Resnick, L.; Gallo, R. C.; Myers, C. E.; Fauci, A. S. 1985. Effects of suramin on HTLV-III/LAV infection presenting Kaposi's sarcoma or AIDS-related complex: Clinical pharmacology and suppression of virus in vivo. *Lancet* 2: 627–630.

64. Levine, A. M.; Gill, P. S.; Cohen, J.; Hawkins, J. G.; Formenti, S. C.; Aguilar, S.; Meyer,

P. R.; Krailo, M.; Parker, J.; Rasheed, S. 1985. Suramin antiviral therapy in the acquired immunodeficiency syndrome. Clinical, immunologic, and virologic results. *Annals of Internal Medicine*
105: 32–37.
    65. Rouvroy, D.; Bogaerts, J.; Habyarimana, J. B.; Nzaramba, O.; Van de Perre, P. 1985.
Short-term results with suramin for AIDS-related conditions. *Lancet* 1: 878–879.
    66. Stein, C. A.; Saville, W.; Yarchoan, R.; Broder, S.; Gellman, E. P. 1986. Suramin and
function of the adrenal cortex. *Annals of Internal Medicine* 104: 286–287.
    67. Kaplan, L. D.; Wolfe, P. R.; Volberding, P. A.; Feorino, P.; Levy, J. A.; Abrams, D. I.;
Kiprov, D.; Wong, R.; Kaufman, L.; Gottlieb, M. S. 1987. Lack of response to suramin in patients
with AIDS and AIDS-related complex. *American Journal of Medicine* 82: 615–619.
    68. Fischl, M. A.; Richmond, D. D.; Grieco, M. H.; Gottlieb, M. S.; Volberding, P. A.; Laskin,
O. L.; Leedom, J. M.; Groopman, J. E.; Mildvan, D.; Schooley, R. T.; Jackson, G. G.; Durack,
D. T.; King, D., the AZT Collaborative Working Group. In press. The efficacy of 3′-azido-3′-
deoxythymidine (azidothymidine) in the treatment of patients with AIDS and AIDS-related complex:
A double-blind placebo-control trial. *New England Journal of Medicine*.

I

THE AIDS VIRUS

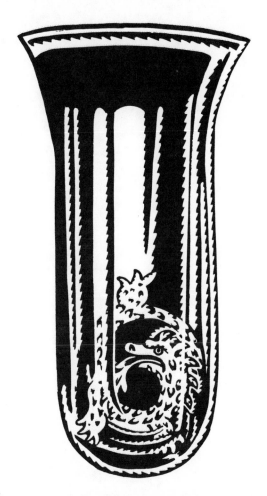

The AIDS Virus
The AIDS virus can be likened to the dragon of the fairy tale which ravages the countryside, killing all in his path before he is subdued. Here he is, isolated in a test tube.

2

Human Retroviruses and Human Disease

Howard Z. Streicher and Emmanuel Heller

INTRODUCTION

The story of retroviruses provides fascinating insights into both disease processes and basic biology. Animal retroviruses were first discovered as agents that could produce sarcomas in chickens by Peyton Rous at the Rockefeller Institute in 1911. Interest in virally induced tumors was heightened in the early 1950s by the work of Ludwig Gross, who demonstrated the vertical and horizontal transmission of tumor-causing viruses in mice.[1] Naturally occurring feline leukemia caused by a retrovirus was described by William Jarrett and Max Essex in the 1960s. A brilliant insight into the nature of these viruses came with the prediction of a DNA intermediary form of the RNA tumor virus by Howard Temin and proved independently by the discovery of the enzyme reverse transcriptase by Temin and Baltimore in 1970.[2] The study of the molecular biology of *onc* genes carried by some of the animal retroviruses provided insights into the regulation of cellular growth and malignant transformation. The search for human retroviruses, however, proved to be more difficult. As often happens, the solution of difficult problems provides exciting and unexpected results.[3]

GENERAL BIOLOGY

In this paper we consider first some of the general features of retroviruses that characterize their remarkable biology and then discuss the human retroviruses in more detail. Human retroviruses were first discovered in the late 1970s.[4] Within 6 years, four distinct virus groups have been described, in vitro systems for their study developed, modes of transmission and geographic prevalence determined, their genomes analyzed and sequenced, and the molecular mechanisms of their effects on cells partially unraveled and, most importantly, linked to the cause of two fatal human diseases—HTLV-I with adult T-cell leukemia (ATL) and HTLV-III with acquired immune deficiency syndrome (see Table 1 for a description of nomenclature).

Retroviruses are enveloped viruses that carry their genetic information in the form of single-stranded RNA and reproduce by budding from the membrane of an infected cell (see Fig. 1). The unique feature of these viruses is the replication of the viral genome by the formation of a double-stranded DNA copy of the viral genome. This process is catalyzed by the special viral polymerase, reverse transcriptase (RT), from which the group derived its name. The inner core of the virus is composed of virally encoded structural proteins (core or gag proteins)

17

Table 1   Human retroviruses

Group A	Group B
HTLV-I (STLV-I)	HIV-1: [HTLV-III or LAV]
HTLV-II	numerous strains, e.g., HLTV-III$_B$, LAV-1, HTLV-III$_{RF}$
	HIV-2: [HTLV-IV]
	(STLV-III)
	several strains, e.g., LAV-2, SBL-6669

The human retroviruses are T-lymphotropic. Related simian T-lymphotropic viruses (STLV-I and STLV-III) are indicated in parentheses. Alternate generic names are indicated in square brackets. HIV-1 and HIV-2 (human immunodeficiency viruses) are generic names for *each* subgroup.

that enclose the genes of the virus and the RT. The outer envelope proteins (env) are incorporated into a lipid membrane acquired from the cell membrane during the budding process. The simplest form of a retrovirus contains the three genes that encode these three proteins necessary for viral replication: *gag* (core proteins); *pol* (polymerase or RT); and *env* (envelope proteins). These genes are flanked at each end by viral elements, called long terminal repeats (LTRs), that form the site of integration into the host cell genome and contain control sequences for viral replication (Fig. 2).

The life cycle of a retrovirus helps us understand some of the unique features of this group of viruses. The cycle includes the following:

1. Entry of a virus into a cell mediated by the viral *env* proteins attaching to a specific cell receptor. These proteins are important determinants of viral targets and are themselves usually the target sites for neutralizing antibody.

2. Formation of double-stranded DNA provirus and integration of the provirus into the host cell genome where it becomes part of the cell's DNA. Thus, infection is maintained for the life of the cell and through daughter cells may endure for the life of the organism.

3. Control of expression of viral genes by the LTRs. These sequences (300–900 base pairs) flank both ends of the provirus and form the sites of covalent attachment or boundary with cellular DNA.

4. The life cycle is completed by budding of the virus from the cell membranes.

The life cycle of a retrovirus is shown in Fig. 2.

Viral Genomes

It is useful to consider one classification or grouping of retroviruses according to the organization of their genome. It is this organization that determines the mechanisms that allow the virus to affect cellular function. The vast majority of animal retroviruses contain only the three genes necessary for replication (*gag*, *pol*, and *env*) (Fig. 3). This type of virus is often known as chronic leukemia virus, because the viruses produce disease after a relatively long period of infection and viral replication. Copious replication results in many new random integration events into the DNA of the target cells with occasional chance in-

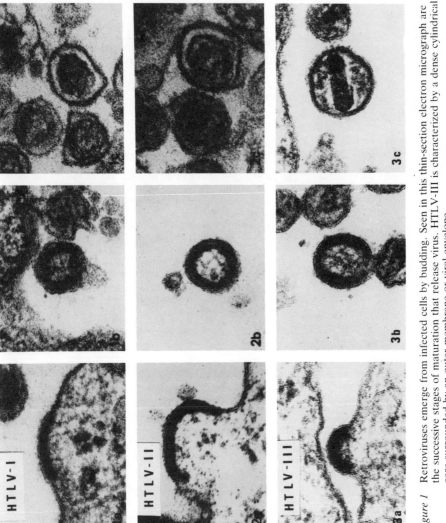

Figure 1 Retroviruses emerge from infected cells by budding. Seen in this thin-section electron micrograph are the successive stages of maturation that release virus. HTLV-III is characterized by a dense cylindrical core surrounded by an outer membrane or viral envelope.

HTLV-I

HTLV-II

HTLV-III

19

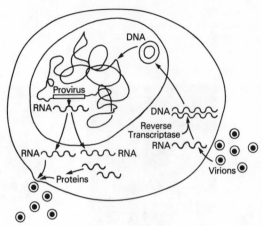

Figure 2 Life cycle of a retrovirus. Virions enter the
cell by binding to a specific cellular receptor.
The outer membrane and core proteins are
removed once the viruses are inside the cell.
The viral enzyme, reverse transcriptase,
transcribes viral RNA (the viral genome
depicted in Fig. 3) to double-stranded DNA.
This form of the virus (called the provirus)
can then become part of the host cell's genes
in the nucleus of the cell. Proviral DNA is
transcribed to make the viral genome and
messenger RNA that directs the production
of new viral proteins. This viral RNA and
new viral proteins assemble at the cell membrane and are released by budding, thus
completing the viral life cycle.

tegration of the viral LTR into a region that may promote expression of nearby
cellular genes critical to cell growth. The malignancies they produce are monoclonal expansions of this single event. Although they are known to cause disease
in many species of animal and are readily identified in chickens and mice, this
type of virus has not been found in humans.

During the 1970s a group of viruses that rapidly produced tumors at a high
frequency in all infected animals were analyzed. It was found that these viruses
had replaced part of the animals' genomes with a cellular gene. Identification

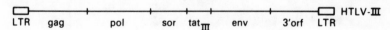

Figure 3 A scheme of the genes of HTLV-III: LTR—long terminal repeat; *gag*—core
proteins; *pol*—reverse transcriptase or polymerase; *env*—envelope; *sor*—
short opened reaching frame; 3' orf—3' opened reading frame; *tat* ₁₁₁—trans-
acting gene of HTLV-III. Not shown are additional regulator genes recently
described, such as trs and the R gene. Each gene may code for several proteins, which are often denoted by their molecular weight: gp 120 and gp 41 for
the outer and transmembrane envelope proteins, p24 and p17 of the *gag*
protein.

of these genes, known as *onc* genes, has provided insights into the study of mechanisms controlling cellular growth and differentiation. For example, the sequencing of a gene called *v-sis*, found in the simian sarcoma virus, led to its identification as part of the human PDGF receptor gene, which is involved in cell growth. The loss of control of expression of these genes or the expression of an altered gene product presumably leads to cellular transformation. Although of great interest for the study of basic mechanisms, retroviruses containing *onc* genes are not usually replication-competent, rarely produce naturally occurring disease, and have also not been found in humans.

Human Retroviruses

As it turns out, the human tumor viruses HTLV-I and HTLV-II do not replicate extensively and are difficult to detect by electron microscopy. Fundamental innovations such as the development of sensitive assays to detect RT and the discovery of TCGF (T-cell growth factor), or IL2, to allow the growth and expansion of normal and malignant T cells in culture provided the essential tools that led to the discovery of the first human retrovirus, human T-cell lymphotropic virus, or HTLV-I, in 1978.[5] This human retrovirus was isolated from a patient with an aggressive form of mycosis fungoides, a malignancy of the T4 cell. Serendipitously, halfway around the world, Takasuki and colleagues in Japan described a form of aggressive T4 cell leukemia, adult T-cell leukemia (ATL), that was found in high prevalence clustered in regions of southern Japan.[6] In a strong international collaboration, the groups of Dr. Gallo and Dr. Takatsuki were able to identify the newly isolated retrovirus as the cause of this disease. In 1982 Dr. Gallo's NIH Laboratory of Tumor Cell Biology again identified a second human retrovirus isolated from a patient with a T-cell variant of hairy cell leukemia.[7] This virus proved to be similar to HTLV-I and also infects T4 cells. Both of these viruses were able to transform normal T cells in tissue culture and thus provided in vitro models of malignant transformation by human retroviruses.[8]

By 1982 several features of these viruses strongly suggested that a human retrovirus might be the cause of a newly emerging epidemic of immune deficiency disease. In the period 1982–84 a third human retrovirus was isolated and proved to be causally associated with this increasingly visible epidemic, now named acquired immune deficiency syndrome (AIDS).[9,10] In 1985 a fourth human virus, HTLV-IV or LAV-2, very closely related to the simian T-cell lymphotropic virus, STLV-III, was described.[11,12]

Although these four groups of human retroviruses are distinct, they share many common biologic features. The major target is the T4 lymphocyte; they directly cause pathology of this cellular subset as well as the central nervous system; and they are transmitted by intimate sexual contact, by blood products, by intravenous drug abuse, by transfusions, and perinatally from mother to child. In addition, they appear to have an African origin, with each group having a closely related simian virus, STLV-I or STLV-III. They all contain extra genes, one or more of which codes for a protein that regulates virus expression in *trans* (*tat* genes), and expression of virus by infected T cells appears to depend on immune stimulation.

Human Immune Deficiency Virus

The idea that AIDS was caused by a new human retrovirus was proposed by Gallo based on (1) the epidemiology strongly suggesting a new, rapidly increasing infectious agent because the disease was transmitted by transfusion, factor VIII preparations, as well as sexual contact; (2) the disease specifically involving the T4 cells—the same cell targeted by HTLV-I; (3) the possibility of an African origin similar to that proposed for HTLV-I; (4) the observation of Essex and co-workers that immune deficiency is the most common outcome of infection by the feline leukemia retrovirus (FeLV); and (5) reports that HTLV-I can cause some alterations in T-cell function. However, the extensive and unexpected cytopathogenic effects of this new virus presented an obstacle to further progress.[13]

The next major advance was the ability of Popovic and co-workers in Gallo's lab to grow the virus in cloned leukemic human T4 cell lines. This allowed the comparison of individual isolates and demonstrated that these isolates represented a single new virus that was the cause of AIDS. Sufficient virus and viral proteins were made to initiate specific new epidemiology studies, establish more specific tests for antiviral antibodies in blood and blood products, characterize proteins of the virus, and advance biologic and molecular characterization and cloning of the virus (14–17).

Viral Genome and Protein

Since 1984 the genome has been completely sequenced from many isolates, and the protein products of the virus have been identified. In addition to the usual retrovirus genes, HIV codes for five additional genes, making it the most complex retrovirus known. These genes for the most part appear to be important for the regulation of virus replication (see Fig. 3).[18] At least 14 protein products are made from these genes. Some of these viral proteins—the *gag*, *env*, *pol*, and possibly *sor* products—are part of the virus structure. The others appear to be regulatory proteins. They are made by the virus inside an infected cell but are not found in the virus particle. The viral genome holds the key to understanding the behavior of the virus. The envelop protein on the outside of the virus allows the virus to bind to the T4 molecule and penetrate the cell. It is the site to which antibodies must bind to prevent infection of a cell and so is a major focus of efforts to develop a vaccine. The viral RT produced by the *pol* gene is a unique viral enzyme. Blocking its action by inhibitors such as the drug azidothymidine (AZT) has, so far, been the most successful approach to chemotherapy. A thorough understanding of other viral proteins, such as the *tat* gene protein, that are essential to viral replication presents many possibilities for new and effective therapies.[19]

When the sequences of virus isolates from many individuals are compared, a striking degree of variation is found. There are not, however, just a few identifiable and distinct strains, as is the case with influenza, but a continuous variation ranging from 1–2% to 15–20% of the genetic sequences and proteins. These differences are most evident in the viral envelope.[20,21] Because the viral RT tends to be "error prone," it is assumed that these changes occur during the transcription of viral RNA to the DNA form. This variation may present difficulties in developing vaccines that work for a broad range of viruses (group-specific response). So far, most experimental vaccines have produced type-specific antibodies that neutralize the virus used to immunize a given animal. Sera from infected individuals contain antibodies that neutralize most virus variants tested. In addition, the viruses obtained from a single infected individual appear to be variants that are closely related, even if they have been exposed to many different sources of virus. This suggests that there is some protection from further infection.

Cytopathic Effect

Infection of T4 lymphocytes by HIV leads to a cytopathic effect in tissue culture. This in vitro effect closely corresponds to the depletion of these T4 cells in vivo. In infected patients progressive and continuous loss of T4 cells is associated with the characteristic opportunistic infections and eventual death described as AIDS. The loss of T4 cells and resulting immune impairment are most probably a direct result of the death of virus-infected cells. However, the precise mechanism by which this occurs and the factors or cofactors that lead to profound impairment are not known. We know that infected cells per se do not produce virus but require stimulation or immune activation results for virus production and cell death. The T4 molecule not only is required for infection but also appears to participate in bringing about the death of the cell. When virus is produced in cells lacking lacking T4, the cells are generally not killed by the virus. The interaction of viral envelope protein and T4 between cells may result in the formation of multinucleated giant cells characteristic of viral infection. In addition, virus-infected cells may produce factors that lead to further immune suppression.[22–24]

HIV-Associated Disease

The spectrum of clinical disease associated with HIV infection has expanded to include many conditions not considered in the original epidemiologic definition of AIDS. We recognize many modes of virus infection, such as immune deficiency with opportunistic infection, impaired immune regulation with autoimmunity and hypergammaglobulinemia, neurologic disease with dementia, lung disease with lymphocytic interstitial pneumonia, lymphomas, Kaposi's sarcoma, congenital defects, and a wasting syndrome sometimes called slim disease. Serologic testing has resulted in appreciation of the extensive clinical features and the ability to stage the disease based on evidence of HIV infection, T-cell numbers, and clinical presentation. Two observations should be kept in mind: first, the disease is progressive; second, in any group infected by virus, the majority will develop some disease, and, owing to the varied latency period, the number of persons developing the syndrome will increase with time. These considerations make prevention and treatment all the more urgent.[25]

PREVENTION AND TREATMENT

Three avenues are available to control the epidemic of immune deficiency disease. They are not mutually exclusive. The first is public health measures that minimize the risk of exposure to the virus and subsequent infection. Transmission of virus has been attributed in virtually every instance to intimate sexual contact, blood products by transfusion or by use of clotting factors, intravenous drug abuse, or maternal-fetal transmission. A handful of cases have been attributed to accidental exposure to infected blood by needle stick or skin contact, predominantly in health care workers. Education, identification of infected blood products, behavioral changes such as the use of latex prophylactics and avoidance of shared needles, and identification of infected individuals who may transmit the virus have become highly debated social concerns. Understanding the biology of the causal agent and its epidemiology should provide the basis for implementing effective and intelligent public health measures.[26]

Second, vaccines that produce protective immune responses have been the most effective historical means of controlling virus infection. The elimination of smallpox as a human disease; prevention of measles, rubella, and polio; and our annual "flu shots" attest to the power of this approach. Several candidate HIV vaccines are or will be approved for human testing after being evaluated in primates. Several difficulties must be overcome in the development of a vaccine: the lack of apparent naturally occurring immunity, virus heterogenity, and the limitation of animal models for testing.[27,28]

Third, drug therapy based on a rational understanding of the virus must be developed. The end of this decade may well be marked by advances in antiviral therapy. A number of drugs have undergone clinical trials in AIDS patients. The most successful, AZT, was licensed in 1987. A pioneering effort by Drs. Sam Broder, Robert Yarchoan, and Hiroaki Matsuya at the National Cancer Institute brought the drug from an obscure experimental compound into clinical trials. This drug, as well as others, 2,3-dideoxycytidine, for example, that are currently undergoing clinical trials block the critical activity of the unique viral enzyme RT. AZT has proved useful in prolonging life, improving immunologic function, reversing some of the disease processes, and preventing virus replication. It is not a cure but a very promising beginning.

CONCLUDING REMARKS

Six years into the AIDS pandemic, what visions come to mind? The alarmist feels panic and fear. Globally, there are now more than 50,000 AIDS cases and an estimated 5–10 million HIV-infected individuals and potential for significant increases every year. Unbounded extrapolations predict that the human race is threatened with extinction because no natural protective factors are operative and no treatments or preventive measures are available. Of course, this will not happen. Human history has been marked by episodic plagues and has survived. AIDS is only a recent virulent expression of one of these natural phenomena, and it has turned up at a time when science has already accumulated a vast store of information on the nature of its causative agent, a retrovirus. There is optimism that the AIDS pandemic is only a problem of nature's tinkering and that it will be stopped and overcome through education, public health measures, and research.

The study of the molecular biology of the virus, that is, its life cycle, its genes, and their products, has revealed that HIV is a complicated retrovirus. The viral genome has eight genes—genes concerned with producing structural proteins that make up the physical components of the viral particle, and genes that regulate the production of structural protein. The presence of regulatory genes implies that the viral life cycle is prone to extraviral stimuli and that the environmental factors determine the fate of the virus. Retroviruses can establish one of two relationships with their host cell, latent or replicating. The control of this latter cell-virus relationship, in the case of HIV, may prevent destruction of the host cell and prevent disease.

These aspects of HIV have relevance for our further understanding of gene regulation in all biological systems and, in particular, in cell differentiation and malignancy, both of which involve the influence of environmental factors on preprogrammed gene activity. The study of HIV molecular biology will also be relevant to the science of "vaccinology" in general, and of course, the search for a vaccine against AIDS. Several problems are associated with an HIV vaccine. Basically, there is so far no evidence that a protective immune response is possible. To find out whether a protective immune response is feasible, several problems must be addressed: the heterogeneity of the virus, the long latency between infection and disease, the destruction or dysfunction of critical cells of the immune system, and the lack of animal models for AIDS. Despite these many problems, a number of candidate vaccines have been produced and are being studied in both animals and man. Knowledge of the molecular biology of HIV will also signpost the search for new antiviral drugs.

We still know relatively little of the pathogenesis of HIV infection. Is the virus transmitted as free virus or cell-associated virus, and which cell types in the recipient initiate infection? Are some individuals relatively resistant to infection? Are there strain differences that correlate with pathogenesis? What causes the activation of virus production? What are the nature of the immune dysfunction and the mechanism of immune cell destruction leading to immunodeficiency?

These questions and future research will shed light on the specific pathogenesis in AIDS and will also reveal new information and give better understanding of the interrelationships of the various components of the immune system. They will open up new vistas on other immune deficiency diseases and will reaffirm the role of the immune system in homeostasis. They will also lead to new treatments for the restoration of a damaged immune system, perhaps by utilizing hematopoietic growth factors; will encourage the study of related environmental factors, such as stress, to well-being; and will encourage a search for new treatments of viral diseases and opportunistic infection.

The neuropathies that are associated with AIDS will focus attention on all viral-induced neuropathies and to other diseases in which dementia manifests itself, such as Alzheimer's disease. These studies may shed further light on the relationship between neural cells that carry out brain functions and glial cells that help to support the brain's neural network.[30,31] Pharmacologists will be given a further opportunity to develop drugs that cross the brain barrier.

Malignancies that are associated with AIDS include Kaposi's sarcoma (KS) and lymphomas. Classically, KS is known to develop in older men of East European and Mediterranean origin. In Africa KS has appeared with high prevalence in young persons, and in the United States KS has appeared in AIDS victims. Is the common denominator in these KS cases immune deficiency arising from aging (classical), HIV infection and other infectious agents (Africa), or HIV infection (U.S.)? Comparative study of these several KS entities will be informative with regard to the underlying pathogenesis of this cutaneous vascular malignancy and of the factors involved in producing neoangiogenesis in embryology, in malignancies in general, and in the pathophysiology of tissue injury. AIDS-associated lymphomas will stimulate studies of the role of HIV in B-cell transformation and have already led to the discovery of a new human herpesvirus, human B-lymphotropic virus (HBLV).[32,33]

The last subject we wish to mention is the epidemiology of HIV infection. An overview of this subject seems to have implications for general medical hygiene, sexual mores, and sexually transmitted diseases (STDs). AIDS transmission basically involves access of HIV to the blood system. This can take place via shared needles as in IV drug abusers, via contaminated blood as in hemophiliacs, transplacentally to the fetus, or via contaminated needles frequently used in routine medical practice in Third World countries, as well as through sexual activity, especially when this involves trauma. Control and prevention of HIV infection therefore necessitates measures directed to medical hygiene that must include using sterile needles whenever needles are employed, ensuring HIV-free blood for transfusion, and advocating and adopting safer sex procedures. Only a concerted global effort of education can address these problems, and it is hoped that the World Health Organization can and will coordinate these efforts. The results that will be achieved for the control of AIDS will also benefit those afflicted with other STDs whose spread is definitely bidirectional and independent of sexual preference.

At the beginning of this paper we stated that the search for human retroviruses proved difficult despite the fact that the first retrovirus was discovered 70 years earlier and a large number of similar retroviruses were subsequently found in various animal species. The 1980s have produced two distinct groups of human retroviruses and have shown them to be linked with two distinct human diseases, malignancies and AIDS. It is perhaps not unexpected that these human retroviruses have been discovered. The experience gained from the study of animal retroviruses had paved the way—in particular, the discovery in 1970 of the RT enzyme and development of assays for this enzyme that increased the sensitivity by which the retroviruses could be detected. The discovery of how to grow human lymphocytes in vitro permitted the isolation and growth of those human retroviruses associated with T4 lymphocytes. These successes not only have confirmed our long belief that human retroviruses exist but now open up the field to search for human retroviruses in association with other human diseases.

REFERENCES

1. Gross, L. *Oncogenic Viruses*, 3d Ed. Pergamon Press, Oxford, U.K., 1983.

2. Baltimore, D. RNA-dependent DNA polymerase in virions of RNA tumor viruses. *Nature* 226:1209. Temin, H. M., and Mizutani, S. RNA-dependent DNA polymerase in virions of Rous sarcoma virus. *Nature* 226:1211, 1970.

3. Gallo, R. C. The AIDS virus, January 1987, and The first human retrovirus, December 1986, *Sci. Am.*

4. Poiesz, B. J.; Ruscetti, F. W.; Gazdar, A. F.; Bunn, P. A.; Minna, J. D.; Gallo R. C. Detection and isolation of type-C retrovirus particles from fresh and culture lymphocytes of a patient with cutaneous T-cell lymphoma. *Proc. Natl. Acad. Sci. USA* 77:7415–7419, 1980.

5. Ibid.

6. Uchiyama, Takashi; Yodoi, Junji; Sagawa, Kimitaka; Takatsuki, Kiyoshi; Uchino, Haruto. Adult T-cell leukemia: Clinical and hematologic features of 16 cases. *Blood* 50(3):481–492, 1977.

7. Kalyanaraman, V. S.; Narayanan, R.; Feorino, P.; Ramsey, R. B.; Palmer, E. L.; Chorba, T.; McDougal, S.; Getchell, J. P.; Holloway, B.; Harrison, A. K.; Cabradilla, C. D.; Telfer, M.; Evatt, B. Isolation and characterization of a human T cell leukemia virus type II from a hemophilia-A patient with pancytopenia. *EMBO J.* 4(6):1455–1460, 1985.

8. Wong-Staal, F.; Gallo, R. C. The family of human T-lymphotropic leukemia viruses: HTLV-I as the cause of adult T cell leukemia and HTLV-III as the cause of acquired immunodeficiency syndrome. *Blood* 65:253–263, 1985.

9. Popovic, M.; Sarngadharan, M. G.; Read, E.; Gallo, R. C. Detection, isolation and continuous production of cytopathic retroviruses (HTLV-III) from patients with AIDS and pre-AIDS. *Science* 224:497–500, 1984.

10. Barre-Sinoussi, F.; Chermann, J. C.; Rey, R.; et al. Isolation of a T-lymphotropic retrovirus from a patient at risk for acquired immune deficiency syndrome (AIDS). *Science* 220:868–871, 1983.

11. Kanki, P. J.; Barin, F.; M'Boup, S.; Allan, J. S.; Romet-Lemonne, J. L.; Marlink, R.; Melane, M. F.; Lee, T. H.; Arbeille, B.; Denis, F.; Essex, M. New human T-lymphotropic retroviruses related to simian T-lymphotropic virus type III (STLV-III). *Science* 232:238–243, 1986.

12. Clavel, F.; Guetard, D.; Brun-Vezinet, F.; Chamamet, S.; Rey, M. A.; Santos-Ferreira, M. O.; Laurent, A. G.; Dauguet, C.; Katlama, C.; Rouzious, C.; Klatzmann, D.; Champalimaud, J. L.; Montagnier, L. Isolation of a new human retrovirus from West African with AIDS. *Science* 233:343–346, 1986.

13. Wong-Staal, F.; Gallo, R. C. Human T-lymphotropic retroviruses. *Nature* 317:395–403, 1985.

14. Gallo, R. C.; Salahuddin, S. Z.; Popovic, M.; et al. Frequent detection and isolation of cytopathic retroviruses (HTLV-III) from patients with AIDS and at risk for AIDS. *Science* 224:500–503, 1984.

15. Popovic, *Loc. cit.*

16. Barre-Sinoussi, *Loc. cit.*

17. Shaw, G. M.; Hahn, B. H.; Arya, S. K.; Groopman, J. E.; Gallo, R. C.; Wong-Staal, F. Molecular characterization of human T-cell leukemia (lymphotropic) virus type III in the acquired immune deficiency syndrome. *Science* 226:1165–1171, 1984.

18. Arya, K. S.; Gallo, R. C. Three novel genes of human T-lymphotropic virus type III: Immune reactivity of their products with sera from acquired immune deficiency syndrome patients. *Proc. Natl. Acad. Sci. USA* 83:2209–2213, 1986.

19. Mitsuya, H.; Broder, S. Strategies for antiviral therapy in AIDS. *Nature* 325:773–778, 1987.

20. Hahn, B. H.; Shaw, G. M.; Taylor, M. E.; Redfield, R. R.; Markham, P. D.; Salahuddin, S. Z.; Wong-Staal, F.; Gallo, R. C.; Parks, E. S.; Parks, W. P. Genetic variation in HTLV-III/LAV over time in patients with AIDS or at risk for AIDS. *Science* 232:1548–1553, 1986.

21. Starcich, B. R.; Hahn, B. H.; Shaw, G. M.; McNeely, P. D.; Modrow, S.; Wolf, H.; Parks, E. S.; Parks, W. P.; Josephs, S. F.; Gallo, R. C.; Wong-Staal, F. Identification and characterization of conserved and variable regions in the envelope gene of HTLV-III/LAV, the retrovirus of AIDS. *Cell* 45:637–648, 1986.

22. Zagury, D.; Cheynier, R.; Bernard, J.; Leonard, R.; Feldman, M.; Sarin, P. S.; Gallo, R. C. Cytopathogenic mechanisms which lead to cell death of HTLV-III infected cells. In Chandra, P. (ed.) *New Experimental Modalities in the Control of Neoplasia.* Plenum, New York, 1986, pp. 357–361.

23. Lifson, J. D.; Reyes, G. R.; McGrath, M. S.; Stein, B. S.; Engleman, E. G. AIDS retrovirus induced cytopathology: Giant cell formation and involvement of CD4 antigen. *Science* 232:1123–1127, 1986.

24. Dalgleish, A. G.; Beverley, P. C. L.; Clapham, P. R.; Crawford, D. H.; Greaves, M. F.; Weiss, R. A. The CD4 (T4) antigen is an essential component of the receptor for the AIDS retrovirus. *Nature* 312:763–767, 1984.

25. Gallo, R. C.; Streicher, H. Human T-lymphotropic retroviruses (HTLV-I, II, and III): The biological basis of adult T-cell leukemia/lymphoma and AIDS. In Broder, S. (ed.) *AIDS: Modern Concepts and Therapeutic Challenges.* Marcel Dekker, New York, 1986, pp 1–21.

26. Robert-Guroff, M; Gallo, R. C. A virological perspective on the acquired immunodeficiency syndrome. In Cole, H. M., and Lundberg, G. D. (eds.) *AIDS—From the Beginning.* AMA, Chicago, 1986, pp XXVII–XXXI.

27. Matthews, T. J.; Langlois, A. J.; Robey, W. G.; Chang, N. T.; Gallo, R. C.; Fischinger,

P. J.; Bolognesi, D. P. Restricted neutralization of divergent human T-lymphotropic virus type III isolates by antibodies to the major envelope glycoprotein. *Proc. Natl. Acad. Sci. USA* 83:9709–9713, 1986.

28. Putney, S. D.; Matthews, T. J.; Robey, W. G.; Lynn, D. L.; Robert-Guroff, M.; Mueller, W. T.; Langlois, A. J.; Ghrayeb, J.; Petteway, S. R. Jr.; Weinhold, K. J.; Fischinger, P. J.; Wong-Staal, F.; Gallo, R. C.; Bolognesi, D. P. HTLV-III/LAV neutralizing antibodies to and *E. coli* produced fragment of the human envelope. *Science* 234:1392–1395, 1986.

29. Yarchoan, R.; Broder, S. Development of antiretroviral therapy for the acquired immunodeficiency syndrome and related disorders. *N. Engl. J. Med.* 316:557–564, 1987.

30. Gartner, S.; Markovits, P.; Markovitz, D.; Kaplan M. H.; Gallo, R. C.; Popovic, M. The role of mononuclear phagocytes in HTLV-III/LAV infection. *Science* 233:215–219, 1986.

31. Gartner, S.; Markovits, P; Markovitz, D.; Betts, R. F.; Popovic, M. Virus isolation from the identification of HTLV-III/LAV producing cells in brain tissue from an AIDS patient. *JAMA* 256:2365–2371, 1986.

32. Salahuddin, S. Z.; Ablashi, D. V.; Markham, P.; Josephs, S. F.; Sturzenegger, S.; Kaplan, M.; Halligan, G.; Biberfeld, P.; Wong-Staal, F.; Kramarsky, B.; Gallo, R. C. Isolation of a new virus, HBLV, in patients with lymphoproliferative disorders. *Science* 234:596–601, 1986.

33. Josephs, S. F.; Salahuddin, S. A.; Ablashi, D. V.; Schachter, F.; Wong-Staal, F.; Gallo, R. C. Genomic analysis of the human B-lymophotropic virus (HBLV). *Science* 234:601–603, 1986.

3

Prospects for Development of a Vaccine Against HTLV-III-Related Disorders

**Thomas J. Matthews, H. Kim Lyerly, Kent J. Weinhold,
A. J. Langlois, and Dani P. Bolognesi**

The acquired immune deficiency syndrome (AIDS) is a highly lethal new disease, first reported in 1981.[1] In 1982 this predominantly blood-borne disorder was officially designated an epidemic by the Centers for Disease Control,[2] and by May 1984 a human retrovirus designated HTLV-III* was unequivocally established as the etiological agent.[3-6] By the end of that year, a blood test (ELISA) was licensed to screen individuals who had been exposed to the virus. The etiology and diagnosis of the problem were largely resolved in record time, but the remaining larger issues of prevention and treatment of the disease stand before us.

These are formidable challenges. To date more than 25,000 cases of AIDS have been reported with nearly half resulting in fatalities. Equally important is the overwhelming number of individuals, as many as 2 million in the United States and 10 million worldwide, who have been infected to date with HTLV-III and remain asymptomatic but can nonetheless transmit the virus as effectively as their diseased counterparts. This healthy virus-carrier state, the extent of which is uncertain, raises the alarming possibility that there will be no obvious barriers between infected and uninfected individuals. As would be expected, both the virus and the disease are finding their way to the general population in a steady fashion,[7,8] and in spite of the acute public awareness of this problem we are faced with a rapidly expanding infectious agent, which requires the development of strict countermeasures. These include improved detection of the virus, prevention of its further spread, and ultimately elimination of it from the population.

In attempting to devise preventive strategies against human retroviruses, one is immediately drawn to the issue of previous experience with animal retroviruses. Fortunately, the available information indicates that vaccination against retroviruses is an achievable goal. However, counter to that optimism, the possibility of developing a vaccine against human retroviruses, notably HTLV-III, is dependent on the ability to overcome considerable obstacles. The purpose of

---

*The Executive Committee of the International Committee on Taxonomy of Viruses (ICTV) has endorsed the name human immunodeficiency virus (to be abbreviated HIV) recently proposed by a majority of the members of a study group of ICTV as appropriate for the retrovirus isolates implicated as the causative agents of acquired immune deficiency syndrome [(1968) *Science* 232:1486, and *Nature* 321:644].

this discussion is to review these issues and to outline a general course for developing effective preventive measures against HTLV-III.

RETROVIRUSES—ANTIGENS THAT ELICIT IMMUNITY TO INFECTION

The viral component responsible for the salient immunobiological features of retroviruses is its major exterior glycoprotein (gp) (for review see ref. 9). First, the gp is required for infection and mediates attachment of the virus to the host cell surface. It is also the viral component most directly involved in the phenomenon of interference as it relates to attachment of virus receptors at the cell surface. Finally, the gp specifies the pattern of neutralization by antiviral antibodies. Consistent with these properties is its strategic location on the outer surface of virion,[10] as is illustrated in Fig. 1.

Another antigen in the envelope of the virion is a hydrophobic transmembrane protein (tmp), which noncovalently anchors the gp to the particle.[10] The tmp can either contain or be devoid of carbohydrate, but in every case the degree of glycosylation is considerably less than that of the exterior gp. The tmp can also be a target for neutralizing antibodies, but this is generally weak unless complement is present.[11]

The viral gp and tmp are also present in infected cells, concentrated at the sites of virus budding but also distributed on other areas of the cell surface.[12] As such, the envelope components represent a cellular target for immune attack.[13]

Animals infected with retroviruses usually respond with easily detectable humoral immunity against the virus envelope components. For the most part, these are selective for the infecting agent—i.e., they are *type-specific*.[14] This is one of the three immunogenic domains of the external gp. The others represent determinants that are common to all viruses of a given species (*group*) or extend to those in widely different species (*interspecies*).[9] It is only in rare cases that animals respond to these latter domains under natural conditions, with the exception of antibodies to the tmp, which are directed predominantly to highly conserved regions of the molecule.[15,16] On the other hand one can immunize animals with virus or purified envelope components and obtain antibody responses that are much broader in their reactivity than natural antibodies.[9] This is particularly the case when heterologous species are employed. Thus, potent neutralizing as well as cytotoxic antibodies that display strong group- and interspecies-specific reactivity can be raised artificially against gp.

VACCINATION AGAINST RETROVIRUS INFECTIONS

As noted above, immunization with gp elicits strong neutralizing antibodies as well as antibodies that are cytotoxic for infected cells. Mice immunized with purified gp can indeed resist substantial challenges of infectious leukemogenic virus.[17] The immune response associated with protection exhibits both type- and group-specific reactivity.[17,18]

Although monomeric gp is capable of inducing protective immunity, relatively large quantities of purified antigen were required to accomplish this reproducibly.[17] In other animal systems, notably the cat's, similar attempts were not

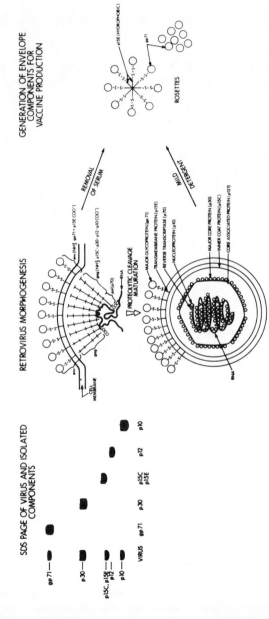

Figure 1 Morphogenesis, structure, and composition of a typical murine leukemia retrovirus. The surface components gp71 (gp) and p15E (tmp) derived from the *env* gene of the virus can be recovered in homogeneous form as either multimers (rosettes) or monomers as a result of shedding from the cell surface or treatment with mild, nonionic detergents.

31

successful. On the other hand the use of gp linked to the tmp so as to form multimeric aggregates (Fig. 1) resulted in a much more effective immunogen in both the mouse[18] and cat.[19] It is likely that a similar principle is involved in the use of viral components from cell culture supernatants following serum starvation.[20] This is the basis for a vaccine against feline leukemia virus that has been licensed for use in cats.

Recently, it appears from work by Morein and colleagues[21] that the capture of virus envelope components (gp and tmp) by glycoside lattices through hydrophobic interaction with tmp generates a multimeric matrix structure (ISCOM; immune-stimulating complex) that is an unusually powerful immunogen. When compared to monomeric gp, an ISCOM preparation containing an equal amount of gp elicits at least a 10-fold increase in the protective endpoint.[22] It may be that these complex structures are more easily recognized, presented, taken up, and processed by macrophages for antigen presentation to the immune system. In a recent report Kleiser and colleagues[23] showed that similar results could be obtained, even in the absence of tmp, provided appropriate aggregates of gp could be formed.

SPECIAL CONSIDERATIONS FOR DEVELOPMENT OF A VACCINE AGAINST HTLV–III

A major challenge for developing a successful immunogen against HTLV-III relates to the issue of genomic diversity in this family of viruses.[24] It is now well recognized that most of the variability occurs in the exterior glycoprotein portion of the envelope gene.[25] The significance of the extensive variability in certain regions of the exterior glycoprotein gp120 is not apparent in the antiviral immune responses occurring in patients. Said otherwise, there is no evidence of a hypervariable immune response that mirrors the genomic changes. However, the presence or absence of humoral antiviral immunity has not correlated with viral infection or the development of AIDS,[26] and the significance of its role remains occluded.

The biological properties of the antibodies in patients also reveal perplexing features. Serum samples from individuals in various stages of infection and disease progression have been tested for their ability to neutralize the infectivity of HTLV-III. Curiously, neutralizing antibodies can be found in late stages of disease (AIDS), and virus-exposed asymptomatic patients generally exhibit lower titers than are present in individuals with immune abnormalities (LAS) or AIDS. Other studies show that it can take several months from virus exposure, as measured by Western blot reactivity to HTLV-III, before neutralizing antibody becomes detectable. These results are indicative of the possible situation that neutralizing antibody may arise too late under natural conditions for it to be effective in preventing the establishment of clinical infection.

A second major concern relates to the mode of transmission of the virus. More specifically, does the infectious material consist of free virus, virus-infected cells, or both? It is likely that each is a possibility and that none are mutually exclusive. A corollary to this situation is how the virus spreads within the host after the initial infection; again, is it as free virus or via cell-to-cell contact? The probability that both mechanisms are involved is reasonably high. With these considerations in mind, a successful vaccine against HTLV-III infection would have to be capable of eliciting not only neutralizing antibodies but also an immune response that could destroy infected cells. Although the presence of virus-specific cellular immunity has been weak or absent,[18] antibodies that are cytolytic in the presence of complement[18] or that mediate antibody-dependent cellular cytotoxicity (ADCC) (for review see ref. 27) have been documented in animal models.

Cytophilic antibodies that mediate ADCC are particularly noteworthy. When used in passive immune therapy studies, they were extremely effective in preventing the outgrowth of large numbers of virus-infected tumor cells.[27] Under optimal conditions, as many as 2×10^7 tumor cells, where the lethal dose is 1,000 cells, were rejected in the presence of relatively small quantities of antiviral antibodies.[28] In this context, recent studies by two independent laboratories failed to detect the presence of cytotoxic antibodies[29,30] in individuals seropositive for HTLV-III, although antibodies that functioned in ADCC were observed.[30]

A third issue to consider is the extensive layer of carbohydrate that covers the HTLV-III exterior gp. There are 32 potential glycosylation sites on the molecule such that as much as 40% of its apparent molecular weight on SDS gels, 120,000 daltons (gp120),[31,32] consists of polysaccharide side chains.[33] This raises the important question of whether the sugar umbrella represents a detriment to vaccine development, because it masks epitopes on the protein backbone that are potential targets for neutralization. A corollary is whether deglycosylated forms of the gp might be better or at least equally effective immunogens. This possibility has indeed been suggested by the studies of Elder and colleagues[34] and is consistent with a number of studies with animal retroviruses, including lentiviruses, that show that the targets for neutralization reside on the protein backbone.[35-37] This is not to say that glycosylation is not essential for certain antigenic features of the molecule. For instance, glycosylation is necessary for the appropriate folding of the protein, especially for epitopes consisting of noncontiguous regions as has been described in studies with the GIX gp of murine retroviruses.[38]

APPROACHES FOR A VACCINE AGAINST HTLV–III DISEASE

Aside from the question of what constitutes an effective human vaccine are the issues of safety, homogeneity, quantity, and economy. Such considerations lead one immediately toward molecular engineering approaches for primary emphasis. This is not unlike the current strategies for developing vaccines against hepatitis B or herpesviruses.[39-41] To be decided initially is whether the method of choice for HTLV-III vaccine material is recombinant products made in bacteria, yeast, or mammalian cells. This would depend on the role carbohydrate plays in the immunogenicity of the gp. Recent studies by Putney et al.[42] clearly demonstrate that carbohydrate-free fragments produced in bacteria generate neutralizing antibodies comparable to those elicited by the native molecule. However, the antibody response induced by various forms of gp120 developed to date is characteristically type-specific.[43] Although the search has been intense, the identity of a common epitope among all strains that would serve as a target for virus neutralization remains elusive. One might thus be faced with the difficult task of a cocktail of immunogens originating from representative strains.

An additional target of opportunity that should be exploited in this regard is the specific site that binds to the CD4 receptor on the surface of T lymphocytes.[44] Recent studies have suggested that this is indeed a conserved region of the molecule,[45] although its precise location remains to be determined. This site is important not only for attachment of gp120 leading to virus infection, but also to the formation of multinucleated giant cells,[46] which represent one of the features of HTLV-III cytopathology. Of note is the demonstration that the presence of carbohydrate is required for binding, suggesting that a conformational rather than a linear determinant may be involved. On the other hand recent evidence that a pentapeptide may block the binding reaction[47] points to the likelihood that a linear sequence does form part of the binding domain.

Thus, if linear epitopes can be demonstrated that are effective targets for neutralization, the use of synthetic peptides becomes immediately feasible. Those that are either shared or unique among the various isolates can be mapped according to their biological properties. Based on current experience with synthetic peptides as immunogens, it is likely that chemical modifications and/or special modes of presentation will be necessary to generate protective immune responses against live virus challenges.[48] As indicated above for the native gp, one may wish to consider the ISCOM approach for both the peptide and recombinant materials.

Another promising strategy would be to use infectious recombinant viruses. Typically a nonessential region of vaccinia virus, a classical vaccine virus with a known safety record, would be used as the locus for the desired gene, which would then be expressed under the control of vaccinia promoters. The resulting construct would consist of autonomously replicating vaccinia virus, which would also express large amounts of properly processed inserted antigen.[49,50] An attractive feature would be that several related gp regions could be introduced in sequence, as has been recently demonstrated.[51] Since there are a number of considerations that might mitigate against using vaccinia as a vector (i.e., prior immunization of the population, possibly pathogenicity in immunosuppressed individuals), nonpathogenic strains of herpes- or adenoviruses may also be considered.

A final possibility is the use of antiidiotypes as immunogens. An antiidiotype represents the internal image of the relevant epitope within the antigen combining regions of the antibody. In several experimental systems a proper combination of native antigen and antiidiotype to the neutralizing antibody induces a powerful and long-lasting protective response within several compartments of the immune system.[52]

ANIMAL MODELS FOR PRECLINICAL VACCINE TESTING

An additional challenge toward developing a successful vaccine is an appropriate animal model where efficacy and safety can be evaluated. To date the chimpanzee is the only species that can be infected with the standard human

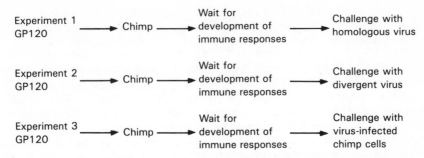

Figure 2   Hypothetical scheme for evaluating candidate vaccine antigens. Parallel studies should focus on: 1) Other viral antigens necessary (or desirable) to achieve protective response, 2) Approaches to maximize the immunogenicity of viral subunits: role of adjuvants, 3) Role of cell mediated immunity in protection, 4) Impact of routes of immunization and challenge, 5) Role of passively administered antibodies in protection, and 6) Assessment of immunotoxicity of viral subunit immunogens

isolates in such a manner as to at least establish persistent viremia.[53,54] Unfortunately, the chimp does not develop the full-blown syndrome of AIDS, but a few immunological abnormalities are noted. Although imperfect, it is adequate for testing the power of a vaccine preparation to resist challenge by free virus and/or virus-infected cells. At the present time some promising immunogens are available that, in other animal species, have raised neutralizing antibodies. These are represented by the native gp120 in purified form,[55,43] a recombinant gp120 expressed in mammalian cells,[56] and are recombinant envelope products produced in bacteria[42] and yeast.[57]

The major drawbacks for vaccine testing of the chimp model are the scarcity of the animals, their expense and difficulties in handling, and the designation of the chimp as an endangered species. Efforts to find a smaller and more plentiful animal that can be infected with the human isolates would thus represent a major breakthrough in this regard. In this context the close resemblance of STLV-III with HTLV-III and particularly with HTLV-IV indicate that the further development of the experimental models in rhesus macaques and African green monkeys will add a great deal to our knowledge in the meantime. Valuable lessons concerning the nature of immunity required to protect against infection can also be gained by exploiting other animal virus models, particularly those of the ruminant lentiviruses, but not excluding either the feline or murine systems which have been so instructive thus far.

Independent of which model is used for testing, the issues of genomic diversity and mode of transmission will have to be seriously considered. Hence, the model must be amenable to challenge with different substrains of HTLV-III including those that exhibit the greatest degree of diversity. In addition, inclusion of infected cells in the challenge will have to be addressed, as will issues such as mode of presentation, routes of inoculation, appropriate adjuvant, and intense immunologic monitoring of the inoculated animals (Fig. 2) with particular attention to both neutralizing antibodies and cell-mediated immunity.

CONCLUSIONS

Although difficult, the problems associated with devising a successful vaccine against HTLV-III are not insurmountable. The heterogeneity among the virus isolates is balanced by conserved regions that are potential targets for immune attack. One of these that can be highlighted is the region responsible for binding to the CD4 receptor on the target cell surface.[45] An important issue to consider is that whereas natural antibodies against retroviruses are extremely narrow in their specificity, antibodies raised artificially are much more broadly reactive. Presumably the same situation is operative with HTLV-III, and it will be incumbent on the vaccine strategies to highlight the conserved regions. In that context the mode of antigen presentation will be critical in order to achieve the desired response. In the same vein, the elicitation of immune responses that are effective in dealing with virus-infected cells is an attainable goal. Both cytotoxic and cytophilic antibodies can be obtained in response to immunization with retroviruses, and, as noted earlier, these are extremely active in clearing infected cells in model systems. The most important in this regard, however, is the role of cell-mediated immunity, particularly virus-specific cytotoxic lymphocytes. Vaccine strategies must take note of this critical element of the immune response and define the segments of the viral gene products that elicit cell-mediated immunity and the optimal mode of presentation to achieve the desired goal. If one considers other virus models, the possibility that internal virus components as well as those associated with the envelope are operative must be seriously considered.[58,59]

An issue that has not been mentioned thus far is the role of secretory immunity. Most viruses that are pathogenic in man enter through mucous membranes. There is substantial evidence that secretory immunity is an effective barrier during the early stages of viral infection.[60] Insofar as HTLV-III is concerned, there is a good possibility that epithelial surfaces are involved in virus transmission, particularly where sexual involvement is the primary mode. Indeed, there is evidence for the presence of a secretory immune response to HTLV-III when one examines saliva of infected individuals.[61] The role of secretory IgA as a line of defense against HTLV-III infection needs to be explored.

This discussion has been limited to the possibility of development of a vaccine against the human retroviruses associated with AIDS. However, exclusion of all the necessary public health and educational measures should not detract from their critical value in stemming the tide of infection with this agent in the human population. Likewise, the use of immunoprophylaxis with antiviral antibodies or chemoprophylaxis mediated by antiviral compounds could be very effective means to reduce virus load and prevent the onset of disease if applied sufficiently early after exposure. Indeed, it is the combined role of all approaches to prevention that will be necessary to make a significant impact on this disease.[62]

In conclusion, though the AIDS epidemic may eventually prove to be one of the most severe devastations by an infectious agent to affect mankind, it remains fortunate that it has occurred during a period when the biomedical community has the opportunity to deal with it. One must find considerable comfort in the vast knowledge that exists about retroviruses in general and their human counterparts in particular and expect that effective countermeasures against these agents will be developed. In like manner our rapidly expanding knowledge of how the immune system functions will no doubt lead to specific approaches to restore the damage the virus has perpetrated. In both areas modern biotechnology is likely to provide the methodology and capability of dealing with this problem on a world scale.

As we progress down the avenues to control this disease, valuable principles will be gained that will apply to other human diseases associated with retroviruses. Because some of these are malignant neoplasms,[63] the opportunity to control a cancer by direct attack on the etiological agent clearly presents itself. The possibility that other widespread diseases such as autoimmune and degenerative syndromes might also involve this group of agents[64] further highlights the valuable by-product of the intense studies in HTLV-III and AIDS.

REFERENCES

1. Gottlieb, M. S.; Schroff, R.; Schanker, H. M.; et al. *Pneumocystis carinii* pneumonia and mucosal candidiasis in previously healthy homosexual men: Evidence of a new acquired cellular immunodeficiency. *N. Engl. J. Med.* 305:1425, 1981.

2. Curran, J. W.; Morgan, W. M.; Hardy, A. M.; et al. The epidemiology of AIDS: Current status and future prospects. *Science* 229:1352–1357, 1985.

3. Popovic, M.; Sarngadharan, M. G.; Read, E.; et al. Detection, isolation and continuous production of cytopathic retroviruses (HTLV-III) from patients with AIDS and pre-AIDS. *Science* 224:497, 1984.

4. Gallo, R. C.; Salahuddin, S. Z.; Popovic, M.; et al. Frequent detection and isolation of cytopathic retroviruses (HTLV-III) from patients with AIDS and at risk for AIDS. *Science* 224:500, 1984.

5. Schupbach, J.; Popovic, M.; Gilden, R. V.; et al. Serological analysis of a sub-group of human T-lymphotropic retroviruses (HTLV-III) associated with AIDS. *Science* 224:503, 1984.

6. Sarngadharan, M. G.; Popovic, M.; Bruch, L.; et al. Antibodies reactive with human T-lymphotrophic retroviruses (HTLV-III) in the serum of patients with AIDS. *Science* 224:506, 1984.

7. Wong-Staal, F.; Gallo, R. C. Human T-lymphotropic retroviruses. *Nature* 317:395–403, 1985.

8. Barnes, D. M. Military statistics on AIDS in the U.S. *Science* 233:283, 1986.

9. Schafer, W.; Bolognesi, D. P. Mammalian C-type oncornaviruses: Relationship between viral structural and cell surface antigens and their possible signficance in immunological defense mechanisms. *Contemp. Top. Immunobiol.* 6:127–167, 1977.

10. Bolognesi, D. P.; Montelaro, R. C.; Frank, H.; et al. Assembly of type-C oncornaviruses: A model. *Science* 199:183–186, 1978.

11. Fischinger, P. J.; Schafer, W.; Bolognesi, D. P. Neutralization of homologous and heterologous oncornaviruses by antisera against the p15(E) and gp71 polypeptides of Friend murine leukemia virus. *Virology* 71:169–178, 1976.

12. Schwarz, H.; Hunsmann, G.; Moennig, V.; et al. Properties of mouse leukemia viruses. XII. Immunoelectron microscopic studies on viral structural antigens on the cell surface. *Virology* 69:169–178, 1976.

13. Hunsmann, G.; Claviez, M.; Moennig, V.; et al. Properties of mouse leukemia viruses. X. Occurrence of viral structural antigens on the cell surface as revealed by a cytotoxicity test. *Virology* 69:157–168, 1976.

14. Ihle, J.N.; Lee, J. C.; and Janna, M. G. Jr. Characterization of natural antibodies in mice to endogenous leukemia virus. In *The Biology of Radiation Carcinogenesis* (J. M. Yuhan, R. W. Tennant, and J. D. Regan, eds.). Raven Press, New York, 1976, pp. 261–273.

15. Thiel, H.-J.; Broughton, E. M.; Matthews, T. J.; et al. Interspecies reactivity of type-C and D retroviruses p15E proteins. *Virology* 111:270–274, 1981.

16. Thiel, J.; Schwarz, H.; Bolognesi, D.; et al. The role of antibodies against the transmembrane protein p15E in immunotherapy against AKR leukemia: A model for studies in human AIDS. *Proc. Natl. Acad. Sci. USA* 84:5893–5897, 1987.

17. Hunsmann, G.; Moenning, V.; Schafer, W. Properties of mouse leukemia viruses. IX. Active and passive immunization of mice against Friend leukemia with isolated viral gp71 glycoprotein and its corresponding antisera. *Virology* 66:327–329, 1975.

18. Hunsmann, G.; Schneider, J.; Schulz, A. Immunoprevention of Friend virus-induced erythroleukemia by vaccination with viral envelope glycoprotein complexes. *Virology* 113:602–612, 1981.

19. Hunsmann, G.; Pedersen, N. C.; Theilen, G. H.; et al. Active immunization with feline leukemia virus envelope glycoprotein suppresses growth of virus induced feline sarcoma. *Med. Microbiol. Immunol.* 171:233–241, 1983.

20. Lewis, M. G.; Mathes, L. E.; Olson, R. G. Protection against feline leukemia by vaccination with a subunit vaccine. *Infect. Immun.* 34:888–894, 1981.

21. Morein, B.; Sundquist, B.; Hoglund, S.; et al. Iscom, a novel structure for antigenic presentation of membrane proteins from enveloped viruses. *Nature* 308:457–462, 1984.

22. Osterhaus, A.; Weijer, K.; Uytdehaag, F.; et al. Induction of protective immune response in cats by vaccination with feline leukemia virus ISCOM. *J. Immunol.* 135:591–596, 1985.

23. Kleiser, C.; Schneider, J.; Bayer, H.; et al. Immunoprevention of Friend leukemia virus-induced erythroleukaemia by vaccination with aggregated gp70. *J. Gen. Virol.* 67:1901–1907, 1986.

24. Hahn, B. H.; Gonda, M. A.; Shaw, G. M.; et al. Genomic diversity of the acquired immune deficiency syndrome virus HTLV-III: Different viruses exhibit greatest divergence in their envelope genes. *Proc. Natl. Acad. Sci. USA* 82:4813–4817, 1985.

25. Starcich, B. R.; Hahn, B. H.; Shaw, G. M.; et al. Identification and characterization of conserved and divergent regions in the envelope genes of HTLV-III/LAV, the retrovirus of AIDS. *Cell* 45:637–648, 1986.

26. Robert-Guroff, M.; Brown, M.; Gallo, R. C. Neutralizing antibodies in patients with AIDS and ARC. *Nature* 316:72, 1985.

27. Iglehart, J. D.; Weinhold, K. J.; Ward, E. C.; et al. Prospects for the immunological management of lethal tumors. *Cancer Invest.* 1(5):409–421, 1983.

28. Matthews, T. J.; Weinhold, K. J.; Langlois, A. J.; et al. Immunologic control of a retrovirus associated murine adenocarcinoma. VI. Augmentation of antibody dependent killer following quantitative and qualitative changes in peritoneal cells. *JNCI* 75:703–708, 1985.

29. Nara, P. L.; Robey, W. G.; Gonda, M. A.; et al. Absence of cytotoxic antibody to HTLV-III-infected cells in man and its induction in animals after infection or immunization with purified gp120. *Proc. Natl. Acad. Sci. USA* 84:3797–3801, 1987.

30. Lyerly, H. K.; Weinhold, K. J.; Matthews, T. J.; et al. HTLV-III$_B$ glycoprotein (gp120) bound to CD-4 determinants on normal lymphocytes serves as target for immune attack. *Proc. Natl. Acad. Sci. USA* 84:4601–4605, 1987.

31. Allan, J. S.; Coligan, J. E.; Barin, F.; et al. Major glycoprotein antigens that induce antibodies in AIDS patients are encoded by HTLV-III. *Science* 228:1091–1094, 1985.

32. Robey, W. G.; Safai, B.; Oroszlan, S.; et al. Characterization of envelope and core structural gene products of HTLV-III with sera from AIDS patients. *Science* 228:593–595, 1985.

33. Ratner, L.; Haseltine, W.; Patarca, R.; et al. Complete nucleotide sequence of the AIDS virus, HTLV-III. *Nature* 313:277–284, 1985.

34. Elder, J. H.; McGee, J. S.; Alexander, S. Carbohydrate side chains of Rauscher leukemia virus envelope glycoproteins are not required to elicit a neutralizing antibody response. *J. Virol.* 57 (1):340–342, 1986.

35. Bolognesi, D. P.; Collins, J. J.; Leis, J. P.; et al. Role of carbohydrate in determining the immunochemical properties of the major glycoprotein (gp71) of Friend murine leukemia virus. *J. Virol.* 16:1453–1463, 1975.

36. Schafer, W.; Fischinger, P. J.; Collins, J. J.; et al. Role of carbohydrate in biological functions of Friend murine leukemia virus gp71. *J. Virol.* 21:35–40, 1977.

37. Montelaro, R. C.; West, M.; Issel, C. J. Antigenic reactivity of the major glycoprotein of equine infectious anemia virus, a retrovirus. *Virology* 136:368–374, 1984.

38. Pierotti, M.; DeLeo, A. B.; Pinter, A.; et al. The G_{IX} antigen of murine leukemia virus: An analysis with monoclonal antibodies. *Virology* 112:450, 1981.

39. Valenzuela, P.; Coit, D.; Kuo, C. H. Synthesis and assembly in yeast of hepatitis B surface antigen particles containing the polyalbumin receptor. *Bio/Technology* 3:317–320, 1985.

40. Valenzuela, P.; Coit, D.; Medina-Selby, M. A.; et al. Antigen engineering in yeast: Synthesis and assembly of hybrid hepatitis B surface antigen–herpes simplex 1 gD particles. *Bio/Technology* 3:323–326, 1985.

41. Berman, P. W.; Gregory, T.; Crase, D.; et al. Protection from genital herpes simplex virus type 2 infection by vaccination with cloned type 1 glycoprotein D. *Science* 227:1490–1492, 1985.

42. Putney, S. D.; Matthews, T. J.; Robey, W. G.; et al. HTLV-III/LAV neutralizing antibodies to an *E. coli* produced fragment of the virus envelope. *Science* (in press).

43. Matthews, T. J.; Langlois, A. J.; Robey, W. G.; et al. Restricted neutralization of divergent

HTLV-III/LAV isolates by antibodies to the major envelope glycoprotein. *Proc. Natl. Acad. Sci. USA* 83:9709–9713, 1986.

44. Lifson, J. D.; Reyes, G. R.; McGrath, M. S.; et al. AIDS retrovirus-induced cytopathology: Giant cell formation and involvement of CD4 antigen. *Science* 232:1123–1127, 1986.

45. Matthews, T. J.; Weinhold, K. J.; Lyerly, H. K.; et al. Interaction between HTLV-III$_B$ envelope gp120 and CD4: Role of carbohydrate in binding and cell fusion. *Nature* 84:5424–5428, 1987.

46. Lifson, J. D.; Feinberg, M. B.; Reyes, G. R.; et al. Induction of CD4-dependent cell fusion by the HTLV-III/LAV envelope glycoprotein. *Nature* 323:725–728, 1986.

47. Pert, C. Personal communication.

48. Tainer, J. A.; Getzoff, E. D.; Alexander, H.; et al. The reactivity of anti-peptide antibodies is a function of the atomic mobility of sites in a protein. *Nature* 312:127–134, 1984.

49. Paoletti, E.; Lipinskas, B. R.; Samsonoff, C.; et al. Construction of live vaccines using genetically engineered poxviruses: Biological activity of vaccinia virus recombinants expressing the hepatitis B virus surface antigen and the herpes simplex virus glycoprotein D. *Proc. Natl. Acad. Sci. USA* 81:193–197, 1984.

50. Macket, M.; Smith, G. L.; Moss, B. Vaccinia virus: A selectable eukaryotic cloning and expression vector. *Proc. Natl. Acad. Sci. USA* 79:7415, 1982.

51. Perkus, M. E.; Piccini, A.; Lipinskas, B. R.; Paoletti, E. Recombinant vaccinia virus: Immunization against multiple pathogens. *Science* 229:981–984, 1985.

52. McNamara, M.; Kohler, H. T-cell helper circuits. *Immunol. Rev.* 79:87, 1984.

53. Gajdusek, D. C.; Amyx, H. L.; Gibbs, C. J. Jr.; et al. Infection of chimpanzees by human T-lymphotrophic retroviruses in brain and other tissues from AIDS patients. *Lancet* i:55–56, 1985.

54. Fultz, P. N.; McClure, H. M.; Swenson, R. B.; et al. Persistent infection of chimpanzees with human T-lymphotropic virus type III/lymphadenopathy-associated virus: A potential model for acquired immunodeficiency syndrome. *J. Virol.* 58:116, 1986.

55. Robey, W. G.; Arthur, L. O.; Matthews, T. J.; et al. Prospect for prevention of human T-cell lymphotropic virus infection: Purified 120,000 dalton envelope glycoprotein induces neutralizing antibody. *Proc. Natl. Acad. Sci. USA* (in press).

56. Lasky, L. A.; Groopman, J. E.; Fennie, C. W.; et al. Neutralization of the AIDS retrovirus by antibodies to a recombinant envelope glycoprotein. *Science* 233:209–212, 1986.

57. Levy, J. Personal communication.

58. Holt, C. A.; Osorio, K.; Lilly, F. Friend virus-specific cytotoxic T lymphocytes recognize both *gag* and *env* gene-encoded specificities. *J. Exp. Med.* 164:211–226, 1986.

59. Townsend, A. R. M.; Gotch, F. M.; Davey, J. Cytotoxic T cells recognize fragments of influenza nucleoprotein. *Cell* 42:457–467, 1985.

60. Chanock, R. M. Local antibody and resistance to acute viral respiratory tract disease. In *The Secretory Immunologic System* (D. H. Dayton, P. A. Small, R. M. Chanock, H. E. Kaufman, and T. B. Tomasi, eds.). U.S. Government Printing Office, Washington, D.C., 1971.

61. Essex, M. Personal communication.

62. Coolfont Report: A PHS plan for prevention and control of AIDS and the AIDS virus. *Public Health Rep.* 101:341, 1986.

63. Gallo, R. C.; Wong-Staal, F. Current thoughts on the viral etiology of certain human cancers: The Richard and Hinda Rosenthal Foundation Award Lecture. *Cancer Res.* 44:2743–2749, 1984.

64. Hauser, S. L.; Aubert, C.; Burks, J. S.; et al. Analysis of human T lymphotropic virus sequences in multiple sclerosis tissue. *Nature* 322:176–177, 1986.

II

PHYSIOLOGICAL ASPECTS

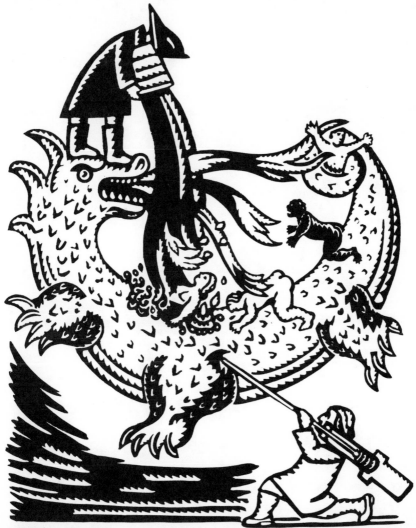

Physiological Aspects
The fire-breathing dragon scorches the victims who ride his back, while valiant attempts are made to extinguish his death-dealing fire and subdue his vigorous assaults.

4

HIV Infection and AIDS—Definition and Classification of Disease

M. Lynn Smiley

HIV INFECTION

Infection with the retrovirus that causes AIDS, the human immunodeficiency virus (HIV), may be diagnosed serologically and/or virologically. Infection may be asymptomatic as well as symptomatic. Serologic evidence for HIV infection includes a positive enzyme-linked immunosorbent assay (ELISA) which is confirmed by Western blot or immunofluorescence.[1,2] Another means of diagnosing HIV infection is by isolating the virus from blood, body fluids, or host tissues.[3–5] Virus isolation techniques are not readily available and are expensive, relatively insensitive, and time-consuming, thus limiting their practical applicability. Virus isolations are a research tool for defining HIV infection. It is hoped that sufficiently sensitive antigen assays applicable directly to patients' specimens might eventually replace the time-consuming virus isolation techniques.[6,7]

There are two situations in which serology may be negative in patients who have HIV infection. Early in the course of infection, there might occur a seronegative, but virus-positive, healthy carrier state.[8,9] Late in severe disease, HIV antibody may be lost because of severe immune deficiency, but virus can often be recovered at this stage.

HIV–INDUCED DISEASE

In general, infection with HIV can result in a spectrum of subclinical and clinical manifestations. The majority of persons infected with HIV are asymptomatic "healthy carriers." When symptoms or signs develop as a result of HIV infection, the person has HIV-induced disease. The clinical manifestations of HIV infection may be a direct result of the viral infection or the result of a secondary condition occurring as a consequence of immune dysfunction. HIV-induced disease—i.e., symptomatic infections such as progressive generalized lymphadenopathy (PGL), AIDS-related complex (ARC), AIDS, or AIDS-dementia complex—occurs in a subset of infected individuals. There are more precise classifications of HIV-induced disease than such terms as PGL or ARC, which are discussed below. The development of standardized and accurate classification systems for HIV-induced disease may eventually allow for the elimination of such vague terms as ARC.

It is not understood what determines which particular patient will go on to develop serious disease after infection. During seroconversion, an acutely infected person might develop a mononucleosislike illness and/or an aseptic meningitis that resolves.[9-11] Acute encephalopathy has been reported coincident with seroconversion.[12] During the asymptomatic healthy-carrier state, some patients might have measurable immunologic abnormalities, such as reduced CD4+ T-helper lymphocytes or cutaneous anergy. Other HIV-infected individuals might develop symptomatic neurologic disease before any signs of opportunistic infections or neoplasms.[13] In addition to infectious, neoplastic, and neurologic complications, autoimmune phenomena such as thrombocytopenia have been associated with HIV infection. The pathogenesis of this remains obscure.

CDC CASE DEFINITION FOR AIDS

Prior to the discovery of HIV as the etiologic agent of AIDS,[1,3-5] a working definition for the diagnosis of full-blown AIDS was derived by the Centers for Disease Control (CDC). This case definition is intended primarily for epidemiologic surveillance purposes (Table 1). In the United States only the patients with the more severe manifestations of HIV infection are reported to the CDC. Since its first description the definition was subsequently modified several times.[14] The most recent modifications are described below (Table 2). This case definition is highly specific and applicable to patients in countries where HIV serologic testing and the required usually invasive diagnostic procedures are readily available in the health care delivery system.

A weakness in this CDC AIDS case definition is the absence of neurological disease. Under the present definition patients with positive HIV tests who die of subacute encephalitis felt to be caused by HIV (where other etiologies have been excluded) and who have only subclinical immune abnormalities will not be reportable as patients with AIDS. The spectrum of neurologic disease is reviewed in Chapter 5.

CLASSIFICATION SYSTEMS FOR HIV INFECTION AND DISEASE

As described above, persons with HIV infection may have a variety of manifestations ranging from asymptomatic infection to severe immune deficiency

Table 1 Centers for Disease Control surveillance definition of the acquired immune deficiency syndrome

---

Presence of reliably diagnosed disease at least moderately indicative of underlying cellular immunodeficiency (Kaposi's sarcoma in a patient <60 years of age, *Pneumocystis* pneumonia, other opportunistic infections).

Absence of known causes of underlying immunodeficiency and of any other reduced resistance reported to be associated with the disease (immunosuppressive therapy, lymphoreticular malignancy)[a]

---

[a]Specific conditions that must be excluded in a child are: (1) primary immunodeficiency diseases—severe combined immunodeficiency, DiGeorge syndrome, Wiskott-Aldrich syndrome, ataxia-telengiectasia, graft versus host disease, neutropenia, neutrophil function abnormality, agammaglobulinemia, or hypogammaglobulinemia with raised IgM; (2) secondary immunodeficiency associated with immunosuppressive therapy, lymphoreticular malignancy, or starvation.

Source: Reprinted from *MMWR 34*, 373–375, 1985.

Table 2   Modification of the CDC case definition for AIDS[14,15]

I. Infections considered at least moderately predictive of underlying cellular immune deficiency are as follows:

  A. Protozoal and helminthic infections

   1. Cryptosporidiosis, intestinal, causing diarrhea for > 1 month
   2. *Pneumocystis carinii* pneumonia
   3. Strongyloides, causing pneumonia, CNS infection, or disseminated infection
   4. Toxoplasmosis, causing CNS infection or pneumonia
   5. Isosporiasis, intestinal, causing diarrhea for >1 month

  B. Fungal infections

   1. Candidiasis, causing esophagitis or bronchial or pulmonary infections
   2. Aspergillosis, causing CNS or disseminated infection
   3. Cryptococcus, causing pulmonary, CNS, or disseminated infection
   4. Histoplasmosis, disseminated

  C. Bacterial infections

   1. Atypical mycobacteriosis (species other than *Mycobacterium tuberculosis* or *Mycobacterium leprae*), causing disseminated infection

  D. Viral infection

   1. Cytomegalovirus, causing pulmonary, gastrointestinal tract, or CNS infection
   2. Herpes simplex virus, causing chronic mucocutaneous infection with ulcers persisting >1 month or pulmonary, gastrointestinal tract, or disseminated infection
   3. Progressive multifocal leukoencephalopathy presumed to be caused by a papovavirus
   4. In children, congenital infections, e.g., toxoplasmosis or herpes simplex virus infection in the first month after birth or cytomegalovirus infection in the first 6 months after birth must be excluded

II. Malignancies

  A. Kaposi's sarcoma in patients <60 years of age
  B. Non-Hodgkin's lymphoma of high-grade pathogenic type (diffuse, undifferentiated) or of B-cell or unknown immunologic phenotype
  C. Patients who have a lymphoreticular malignancy diagnosed >3 months after the diagnosis of an opportunistic disease used as a marker for AIDS will no longer be excluded as AIDS cases

III. In the absence of the opportunistic diseases required by the case definition, a histologically confirmed diagnosis of chronic lymphoid interstitial pneumonitis in a child (<13 years of age) will be considered indicative of AIDS unless HIV serology is negative

IV. To increase the specificity of the case definition, patients will be excluded as AIDS cases if they have a negative result on testing for serum antibody to HIV, have no other type of HIV test with a positive result, and do not have a low number of T-helper lymphocytes or a low T-helper to T-suppressor ratio. In the absence of laboratory test results, patients satisfying all other criteria in the definition will continue to be included.

Source: MMWR 34, 373–375, 1985.

and/or neurologic disease. As knowledge about HIV infection increases there is an increasing need for a classification system for HIV infection. Because the natural history of HIV infection has yet to be defined, no classification schema has been reported to give prognostic implications. The results of many ongoing natural history studies, such as the one reported by Polk and colleagues,[16] will be useful in further refining currently available classification systems. Since the epidemic has been under way less than a decade, the possible long-term sequelae such as malignancies and chronic degenerative and autoimmune diseases may eventually occur in HIV-infected persons.[17]

To date four classification systems have been described.[18,19,26,32] Equivalences among these published classification systems for HIV infection can be found. The utility of these systems, in particular the predictive value of progression over the hierarchy of stages preceding the development of frank AIDS, needs to be validated in different cohorts of patients. The first published classification system[18] is hierarchical and stratifies patients into seven groups (categories 1 through 7). This schema is based on clinical manifestations (Table 3).

The next classification system to be published is the Walter Reed staging system.[19] This schema is also hierarchical and represents an effort to provide an objective scale of disease progression. It has special merit because it is based on current concepts of the immunopathogenesis of AIDS.[20-23] The Walter Reed stages are defined according to virologic/serologic evidence of HIV infection, CD4 + T-helper lymphocyte subset depletion, loss of cutaneous delayed hypersensitivity, and appearance of opportunistic infections (Table 4). There are several drawbacks to this system. It was not designed to be used in the pediatric population, and the cost for doing the required laboratory studies is high, thus limiting its usefulness to research studies. Many such studies using this staging system are ongoing.[24,25]

One of the strengths of this system is that it provides a useful tool for studying the natural history of "early" HIV infection. If various clinical trials are to be undertaken in patients during the early stages of infection, it would be useful to evaluate which subclinical markers are indicative of disease progression. For more broad applicability, such as in developing countries, it would be important to develop a similar staging system that describes early events in HIV infection without requiring expensive and sophisticated laboratory support.

Table 3 Proposed stratification of HIV-related illness for clinical trials

Category		Clinical features
1		Asymptomatic
2		Immune thrombocytopenic purpura (ITP)
3		Unexplained palpable lymphadenopathy at two or more noncontiguous, noninguinal sites of >4 months' duration
	A	Systemic symptoms absent
	B	Fevers low grade (<38.5°C), intermittent, or continuous for >1 month or night sweats (4 or more nights in the last month)
4		Minor opportunistic infection (OI), unexplained thrush or herpes zoster in individuals <60 years of age
	A	No adenopathy
	B	Adenopathy as above
5		Systemic prodrome defined as intermittent or continuous fevers >38.5°C for 1 or more months or watery diarrhea 2 or more weeks or sustained weight loss more than or 10% of body weight; no etiology established.
6		AIDS with Kaposi's sarcoma, no OI

Table 4 Walter Reed staging classification for HIV infection

Stage	HIV Ab &/or HIV VI	LN	No. T4	DHS	Thrush	OI
WR-0	−	−	>400	NL	−	−
WR-1	+	−	>400	NL	−	−
WR-2	+	+	>400	NL	−	−
WR-3	+	+/−	<400	NL	−	−
WR-4	+	+/−	<400	P	−	−
WR-5	+	+/−	<400	C and/or	+	−
WR-6	+	+/−	<400	P or C	+/−	+

HIV Ab, antibody to HIV; HIV VI, virus isolation from blood; LN, lymphadenopathy; T4, T-helper lymphocytes; DHS, delayed hypersensitivity skin testing; NL, normal; P, partial anergy (intact response to at least one of the four test antigens (mumps, *Candida*, tetanus, *Trichophyton*); C, complete anergy; OI, opportunistic infection.
Source: Redfield.[19] Reprinted by permission of the *New England Journal of Medicine* (314:131, 1986).

In addition to a classification schema designed for epidemiologic surveillance purposes, an urgent need exists for the development, evaluation, and validation of an objective system for classifying clinical stages of HIV disease progression. Such a staging system will be necessary for the proper conduct of controlled clinical trials of antiviral agents, biological response modifiers, and vaccines that are recognized to have potential activity against HIV disease.

HIV infections with symptoms (T° > 38°C for 3 weeks, unexplained weight loss >10% of body weight, night sweats for 3 weeks, or chronic diarrhea for more than 1 month) are further designated by the addition of the letter B (e.g., WR-5B). When Kaposi's sarcoma occurs, it is designated by adding the letter K after the appropriate stage (e.g., WR-5K). The occurrence of other neoplasms is designated by adding the letter N after the appropriate stage (e.g., WR-4N). If neurologic disease is present, it is designated by adding the letters CNS (e.g., WR-3CNS).

The most recent classification system proposed by the CDC along with a panel of expert consultants[26] is described in Table 5. Included in the group of consultants were authors of the other classification systems described above.[18,19] This system is primarily for public health purposes and does not imply that there is any change in the case definition for AIDS previously established by the CDC (see above). The classification system does not alter the case reporting of patients with AIDS, which continues to be based on the case definition (Table 1).

Patients are grouped, according to the clinical expression of disease, into one of four principal groups designated by Roman numerals I through IV. Like the schema reported by Haverkos et al.[18] and the Walter Reed staging system,[19] the CDC's system is hierarchical and is based on clinical manifestations. Unlike the Walter Reed staging classification, subclinical markers of HIV infection (i.e., cutaneous anergy, T-helper lymphocyte depletion) are not included. The CDC system could describe pediatric as well as adult cases. It should be emphasized that this system is not explicitly intended to have prognostic significance or to designate severity of illness.

Table 5 Summary of classification system for human immunodeficiency virus

Group I	Acute infection
Group II	Asymptomatic infection[a]
Group III	Persistent generalized lymphadenopathy[a]
Group IV	Other disease
Subgroup A	Constitutional disease
Subgroup B	Neurologic disease
Subgroup C	Secondary infectious diseases
Category C-1	Specified secondary infectious diseases listed in CDC surveillance definition for AIDS[b]
Category C-2	Other specified secondary infectious diseases
Subgroup D	Secondary cancers[b]
Subgroup E	Other conditions

[a]Patients in groups II and III may be subclassified on the basis of a laboratory evaluation.
[b]Includes patients whose clinical presentation fulfills the definition of AIDS used by CDC for national reporting.

PEDIATRIC AIDS

The clinical features of pediatric AIDS might include chronic weight loss (failure to thrive), chronic diarrhea, hepatosplenomegaly, lymphadenopathy, interstitial pneumonia, CNS involvement such as microcephaly and psychomotor retardation, and opportunistic infections. These are discussed in greater detail in Chapter 18. There are several noteworthy differences between pediatric and adult AIDS. Chronic parotid swelling and lymphocytic interstitial pneumonitis[27–30] are found in pediatric AIDS but only rarely in adult AIDS, whereas Kaposi's sarcoma is frequently found in adult cases but is only rarely reported in the pediatric population. Pediatric patients with HIV infection are also predisposed to serious bacterial infections (meningitis, pneumonia) by common organisms, not qualifying strictly as "opportunistic" infections.

The definition of AIDS in infants and children varies from that originally described for adults.[31] The original CDC classification underestimated the number of pediatric patients with AIDS. Both adults and children with AIDS have some common features, but important differences exist that are noteworthy. Recognizing the features specific to the pediatric population, the pediatric definition used by the CDC for epidemiologic surveillance was recently revised.[31] These revisions have been incorporated into the definition as outlined in Tables 1 and 2.

A second, more precise system for defining pediatric AIDS has been proposed by Ammann.[32] This particular definition is based on immunologic and virologic criteria as well as on epidemiologic and clinical data (Table 6). This system was designed to be consistent with the methodology used by the World Health Organization (WHO) in defining primary immunodeficiency disorders. Again, it must be emphasized that the applicability of this staging system in the developing world is limited because of the lack of widespread availability of virus isolation and HIV antibody assays. Ammann suggests that the CDC definition for pediatric AIDS was too restrictive because of the necessity for the presence of opportunistic infection, hence the most severe form of HIV-induced disease. He therefore recommends that the diagnostic "label" AIDS be made relatively

Table 6 Proposed classification of pediatric cases of the acquired immune deficiency syndrome (AIDS)

Epidemiology—history of risk factor
Immunology—polyclonal hypergammaglobulinemia and T-cell immunodeficiency
Virology—antibody to AIDS retrovirus or viral isolation
Exclusions—primary immunodeficiency, adenosine deaminase deficiency, and nucleoside phosphorylase deficiency

---

Source: Reproduced, with permission, from Ammann, A. J. The Acquired Immunodeficiency Syndrome in infants and children. *Ann. Intern. Med.* 103:734, 1985.

early in the course of HIV-induced disease. Clinical features associated with the full-blown syndrome as seen in adult patients are not required. In this classification schema, the presence of four features would establish a diagnosis of pediatric AIDS (Table 6). A more detailed classification schema proposed for pediatric AIDS is shown in Table 7.

CLASSIFICATION OF AIDS IN THE DEVELOPING WORLD

It is estimated that there are several million HIV-infected persons in Africa.[33] The epidemiology of HIV infection and the clinical features of HIV-induced disease may vary in different countries depending on cultural differences and endemic diseases. The clinical manifestations seen in African patients with AIDS resemble Haitian cases with prominent gastrointestinal and dermatologic symptoms and opportunistic infections such as cryptococcosis, toxoplasmosis, and mycobacterial infections. In contrast, in the United States, generalized lymphadenopathy and *Pneumocystis carinii* pneumonia (PCP) are more commonly reported than in African patients. In the United States and Europe, 63% of all

Table 7 Classification of pediatric cases of the acquired immune deficiency syndrome (AIDS)

Epidemiology	Immunology		Enzymes[a]	AIDS-related retrovirus	Clinical symptoms and signs	Diagnosis
	B Cell	T Cell				
+	nl[b]	nl	nl	neg	nl	nl
+	nl	nl	nl	pos	nl	at risk
+	abn	nl	nl	pos	nl	at risk
+	abn	abn	nl	pos	nl	AIDS
+	abn	abn	nl	pos	abn	AIDS
−	abn	abn	def/nl	neg	nl/abn	1° immunodef
−	abn	abn	def/nl	pos	nl/abn	1° immunodef with 2° inf

[a]Adenosine deaminase and purine nucleoside phosphorylase.
[b]nl, normal; abn, abnormal; def, deficient; neg, negative; pos, positive; 1°, primary; 2°, secondary; inf, infection.
Source: Reproduced, with permission, from Ammann, A. J. The Acquired Immunodeficiency Syndrome in infants and children. *Ann. Intern. Med.* 103:734, 1985.

AIDS patients eventually develop PCP, but only 14% of African patients diagnosed in Europe were found to have this particular opportunistic infection.[34–36] As more studies are done in tropical countries, it is likely that HIV-infected patients will manifest other endemic infections, such as leishmaniasis, leprosy, malaria, filariasis, and other parasitic and bacterial infections.[33] In developing countries diagnostic procedures are limited. The definition of AIDS previously established by the CDC and WHO requires sophisticated laboratory diagnoses of opportunistic infections and malignancies.[14,37] Especially important in children is the exclusion of other known causes of immune deficiency.

The WHO recently developed a definition for AIDS in Africa, where sophisticated diagnostic equipment and virologic methods may not be available (Table 8). This clinical case definition was found to be 93% specific with a positive predictive value of 82% for HIV-seropositive hospitalized patients in Zaire.[38] In a recent study reported from Uganda and Tanzania, HIV antibody was found in all patients who presented with chronic diarrhea and weight loss of more that 10 kg.[39–41] Likewise in Zaire, the positive predictive value for HIV infection in hospitalized patients with weight loss and oral thrush was 97%.[42,43] It is expected that this definition will be updated as more research is done in these populations. At present a tool such as this classification schema can be used for valuable epidemiologic surveillance. Although pediatric HIV disease in Africa resembles that in the United States,[44–51] it is difficult to distinguish HIV-associated disease in Africa on clinical grounds, where failure to thrive, malnutrition, and pulmonary disease are common pediatric problems. Therefore, this classification schema is somewhat more inclusive for children than it is for adults.

CONCLUSIONS

Infection with HIV can result in a spectrum of subclinical and clinical manifestations ranging from asymptomatic infection to severe immune deficiency and/or neurologic disease. When symptoms or signs develop either as a direct result of HIV infection or as a consequence of immune abnormalities, the person has HIV-induced disease. The various classification systems described above reflect what is known to date about the spectrum of HIV-induced disease. As more is learned about this infection, descriptions such as the "AIDS-related complex" are vague and, for the most part, not meaningful. It is hoped that more widespread use of classification systems for HIV infection and disease will lead to replacement of such imprecise terms. It is extremely important for ongoing and future clinical research endeavors to use a staging system to define their study population. What would result would be further development of accurate classification schema.[52] The optimal staging system would be applicable to different cohorts of patients, including children, and hopefully be useful in developing countries as well. Once a classification system is fully developed and well standardized, much more can be learned about disease progression, prognostication, and therapeutic interventions. This would allow for comparisons of data from various research centers in order to exchange information expeditiously and develop answers to the pressing problems posed by this tragic epidemic.

Table 8 Provisional WHO clinical case definition for AIDS where diagnostic resources are limited[37]

Adults

AIDS in an adult is defined by the existence of at least two of the major signs associated with at least one minor sign, in the absence of known causes of immunosuppression such as cancer or severe malnutrition or other recognized etiologies.

Major signs
  (a) Weight loss >10% of body weight
  (b) Chronic diarrhea >1 month
  (c) Prolonged fever >1 month (intermittent or constant)

Minor signs
  (a) Persistent cough for >1 month
  (b) Generalized pruritic dermatitis
  (c) Recurrent herpes zoster
  (d) Oropharyngeal candidiasis
  (e) Chronic progressive and disseminated herpes simplex infection
  (f) Generalized lymphadenopathy

The presence of generalized Kaposi's sarcoma or cryptococcal meningitis is sufficient by itself for the diagnosis of AIDS.

Children

Pediatric AIDS is suspected in an infant or child presenting with at least two major signs associated with at least two minor signs in the absence of known causes of immunosuppression.

Major signs
  (a) Weight loss or abnormally slow growth
  (b) Chronic diarrhea >1 month
  (c) Prolonged fever >1 month

Minor signs
  (a) Generalized lymphadenopathy
  (b) Oropharyngeal candidiasis
  (c) Repeated common infections (otitis, pharyngitis, and so forth)
  (d) Persistent cough >1 month
  (e) Generalized dermatitis
  (f) Confirmed maternal LAV/HTLV-III infection

Reprinted from *Weekly Epidemiological Record*, 7 March 1986 (Global Programme on AIDS, World Health Organization), with permission.

REFERENCES

1. Sarngadharan, M. G.; Popovic, M.; Bruch, L.; et al. Antibodies reactive with human T-lymphotropic retroviruses (HTLV-III) in the serum of patients with AIDS. *Science* 224:506–508, 1984.
2. Sandstrom, E. G.; Schooley, R. T.; Ho, D. D.; et al. Detection of human anti-HTLV-III antibodies by indirect immunofluorescence using fixed cells. *Transfusion* 25:308–312, 1985.
3. Barre-Sinoussi, F.; Chermann, J. C.; Rey, F.; et al. Isolation of a T-lymphotropic retrovirus from a patient at risk for acquired immune deficiency syndrome. *Science* 220:868–871, 1983.
4. Levy, J. A.; Hoffman, A. D.; Kramer, S. M.; et al. Isolation of lymphocytopathic retroviruses from San Francisco patients with AIDS. *Science* 225:840–842, 1984.

5. Gallo, R. C.; Salahuddin, S. Z.; Popovic, M.; et al. Frequent detection and isolation of cytopathic retroviruses (HTLV-III) from patients with AIDS and at risk for AIDS. *Science* 224:500–503, 1984.

6. Allain, J. P.; Paul, D. A.; Laurian, Y.; Senn, D. Serological markers in early stages of human immuno-deficiency virus infection in hemophiliacs. *Lancet* ii:1233–1236, 1986.

7. Goudsmit, J.; deWolf, F.; Paul, D. A.; et al. Expression of human immunodeficiency virus antigen (HLV-Ag) in serum and cerebrospinal fluid during acute and chronic infection. *Lancet* ii:177–180, 1986.

8. Salahuddin, S. Z.; Groopman, J.; Markham, P. D.; et al. HTLV-III in symptom-free sero-negative persons. *Lancet* ii:1418–1420, 1984.

9. Ho, D. D.; Sarngadharan, M. G.; Resnick, L.; et al. Primary Human T-Lymphotropic Virus Type III infection. *Ann. Intern. Med.* 103:880–883, 1985.

10. Cooper, D. A.; Gold, J.; MacLean, P.; et al. Acute AIDS retrovirus infection. Definition of a clinical illness associated with seroconversion. *Lancet* i:537–540, 1985.

11. Tucker, J.; Ludlam, C. A.; Craig, A.; et al. HTLV-III infection associated with glandular-fever-like illness in a haemophiliac (letter). *Lancet* i:585, 1985.

12. Carne, C. A.; Smith, A.; Elkington, S. G.; et al. Acute encephalopathy coincident with seroconversion for anti-HTLV III. *Lancet* ii:1206–1208, 1985.

13. Ho, D. D.; Rota, T. R.; Schooley, R. T.; et al. Isolation of HTLV-III from cerebrospinal fluid and neural tissues of patients with neurologic syndromes related to the acquired immunodeficiency syndrome. *N. Engl. J. Med.* 313:1493–1497, 1985.

14. Centers for Disease Control. Revision of the case definition of Acquired Immunodeficiency Syndrome for national reporting—United States. *MMWR* 34:373–375, 1985.

15. Centers for Disease Control. Revision of the case definition of Acquired Immunodeficiency Syndrome for national reporting—United States. *Ann Intern. Med.* 103:402–403, 1985.

16. Polk, B. F.; Fox, R.; Brookmeyer, R.; et al. Predictors of the acquired immunodeficiency developing in a cohort of seropositive homosexual men. *N. Engl. J. Med.* 316:61–66.

17. Francis, D. P.; Jaffe, H. W.; Fultz, P. N.; et al. The natural history of infection with the lymphadenopathy-associated virus Human T-Lymphotropic Virus Type III. *Ann. Intern. Med.* 103:719–722, 1985.

18. Haverkos, H. W.; Gottlieb, M. S.; Killen, J. Y.; Edelman, R. Classification of HTLV-III/LAV related diseases. *J. Infect. Dis.* 152:1095, 1985.

19. Redfield, R. R.; Wright, D. C.; Tramont, E. C. The Walter Reed staging classification for HTLV-III/LAV infection. *N. Engl. J. Med.* 314:131–132, 1986.

20. Dalgleish, A.G.; Beverley, P. C. L.; Clapham, P. R.; et al. The CD4 (T4) antigen is an essential component of the receptor for the AIDS retrovirus. *Nature* 312:763–767, 1984.

21. Klatzman, D.; Barre-Sinoussi, F.; Nugeryre, M. T.; et al. Selective tropism of lymphadenopathy associated virus (LAV) for helper T lymphocytes. *Science* 255:59–63, 1984.

22. Gottlieb, M. S.; Groopman, J. F.; Weinstein, W. M.; et al. The Acquired Immunodeficiency Syndrome. *Ann Intern. Med.* 99:208–220, 1983.

23. Gottlieb, M. S.; Schroff, R.; Schanker, H. M.; et al. *Pneumocystis carinii* pneumonia and mucosal candidiasis in previously healthy homosexual men. *N. Engl. J. Med.* 305:1425–1431, 1981.

24. Redfield, R. R.; Wright, D. C.; Rhoades, J.; Burke, D. S. The natural history of HTLV-III/LAV infection. Presented at the International Conference on AIDS, Paris, June, 1986.

25. Smiley, L.; White, G. C.; Matthews, T. J.; Weinhold, K. J.; Bolognesi, D. P. Natural history of HTLV-III/LAV infection in hemophiliacs. Presented at the 26th Interscience Conference on Antimicrobial Agents and Chemotherapy, New Orleans, La., October, 1986.

26. Centers for Disease Control. Classification system for Human T-Lymphotropic Virus Type III/Lymphadenopathy Associated Virus Infection. *MMWR* 35:334–339, 1986.

27. Rubenstein, A.; Sicklick, M.; Gupta, A.; et al. Acquired immunodeficiency with reversed T4/T8 ratios in infants born to promiscuous and drug-addicted mothers. *JAMA* 249:2350–2356, 1983.

28. Ammann, A. J. Is there an acquired immunodeficiency syndrome in infants and children? *Pediatrics* 72:430–432, 1983.

29. Hellmann, D.; Cowan, M. J.; Ammann, A. J.; et al. Chronic active Epstein-Barr virus infection in two immunodeficient patients. *J. Pediatr.* 103:585–588, 1983.

30. Joshi, V. V.; Oleske, J. M.; Minnefor, A. B.; et al. Pathology of suspected acquired immune deficiency syndrome in children: A study of eight cases. *Pediatr. Pathol.* 2:71–87, 1984.

31. Centers for Disease Control. Education and foster care of children infected with Human T-Lymphotropic Virus Type III/Lymphadenopathy-Associated Virus. *MMWR* 34:517–521, 1985.

32. Ammann, A. J. The acquired immunodeficiency syndrome in infants and children. *Ann Intern. Med.* 103:734–737, 1985.

33. Quinn, T. C.; Mann, J. M.; Curran, J. W.; Piot, P. AIDS in Africa: An epidemiologic paradigm. *Science* 234:955–963, 1986.

34. Centers for Disease Control. Update:Acquired Immunodeficiency Syndrome—Europe. *MMWR* 35:35, 1986.

35. Centers for Disease Control. Update:Acquired Immunodeficiency Syndrome—United States. *MMWR* 35:17, 1986.

36. Brunet, J. B.; Ancelle, R. A. The international occurrence of the Acquired Immunodeficiency Syndrome. *Ann. Intern. Med.* 103:670, 1985.

37. World Health Organization. Occupational health leading work related diseases and injuries. *Weekly Epidemiol. Res.* 61:69, 1985.

38. Colebunders, R., et al., Paper presented at the International Conference on AIDS, Paris, 1986.

39. Kamradt, T.; Niese, D.; Vogel, F. Slim disease (AIDS). *Lancet* ii:1425, 1985.

40. Marquart, K. H.; Muller, H. A. G.; Sailer, J.; Moser, R.; et al., Slim Disease (AIDS). *Lancet* ii:1186, 1985.

41. Lloyd, G.; et al. Paper presented at the International Conference on AIDS, Paris, 1986.

42. Dewit, S.; et al. Paper presented at the International Conference on AIDS in Africa, Brussels, Belgium, 1985.

43. Cran, S.; Dewit, S.; Clumeck, N. Paper presented at the International Conference on AIDS in Africa, Brussels, Belgium, 1985.

44. Lapoint, N.; Michaud, J.; Pekovic, D.; et al. Transplacental transmission of HTLV-III Virus (letter). *N. Engl. J. Med.* 312:1325, 1985.

45. Ziegler, J. B.; Johnson, R. O.; Cooper, D. A.; et al. Postnatal transmission of AIDS-associated retrovirus from mother to infant. *Lancet* i:896, 1985.

46. Scott, G. B.; Fischl, M. A.; Klimes, N.; et al. Mothers of infants with the acquired immunodeficiency syndrome. Evidence for both symptomatic and asymptomatic carriers. *JAMA* 253:363, 1985.

47. Rogers, M. F. AIDS in children: A review of the clinical, epidemiologic, and public health aspects. *Pediatr. Infect. Dis.* 4:230, 1985.

48. Cowan, M. J.; Hellman, D.; Chudwin, D.; Wara, D. W.; et al., Maternal transmission of acquired immune deficiency syndrome. *Pediatrics* 73:382, 1984.

49. Pahwa, S.; Kaplan, M.; Fikrig, S.; et al., Spectrum of human T-cell lymphotropic virus type III infection in children. Recognition of symptomatic, asymptomatic seronegative patients. *JAMA* 255:2299, 1986.

50. Oleske, J.; Minnefor, A.; Cooper, R.; et al., Immune deficiency syndrome in children. *JAMA* 249:2345, 1983.

51. Scott, G. B.; Buck, B. E.; Leterman, J. G.; et al. Acquired immunodeficiency syndrome in infants. *N. Engl. J. Med.* 310:76, 1984.

52. Solomon, S. L.; Curran, J. W. Public health applications of a classification system for Human Immunodeficiency Virus infection. *Ann. Intern. Med.* 106:319, 1987.

5

HIV and the Nervous System

Robert S. Janssen

Systemic opportunistic infections and cancers in unusual hosts heralded the onset of the epidemic of acquired immune deficiency syndrome (AIDS) in 1981, and within a year, neurologic infections and cancers were described.[1] Although secondary nervous system illness became evident, primary human immunodeficiency virus (HIV) effects on the nervous system were initially obscured because of the difficulty of neurologically evaluating patients with overwhelming systemic illness.[2] Snider et al.[3] first analyzed the neurologic complications of AIDS and described a dementia syndrome called subacute encephalitis. Initial clinical and pathologic data suggested that subacute encephalitis was caused by cytomegalovirus[3,4]; however, in 1985, Shaw and co-workers[5] demonstrated HIV DNA and RNA in brains of patients with subacute encephalitis or AIDS encephalopathy. These data suggested that HIV might be the causative agent of encephalopathy in many AIDS patients. Since that time, studies have described other neurologic problems probably due to HIV infection, and some recent studies have addressed issues of pathogenesis. This chapter reviews the clinical manifestations of HIV infection and some of the recent work on mechanisms of neurologic disease caused by HIV.

HIV ENCEPHALOPATHY

HIV encephalopathy has been referred to as subacute encephalitis, AIDS encephalopathy, and AIDS dementia complex. It occurs in 5–10% of AIDS patients,[3,6,7] and as many as 42% of AIDS patients have neuropathologic evidence of HIV encephalopathy at autopsy.[8] The clinical syndrome of HIV encephalopathy is one of dementia and motor and behavioral abnormalities in a variety of combinations and has been described in detail by Navia et al.[9] Symptoms and signs of HIV encephalopathy occur most frequently after the diagnosis of AIDS; 67% of patients in one study had AIDS prior to neurologic symptoms.[9] Memory loss or forgetfulness manifested by difficulty remembering names or historical details and loss of concentration are the most frequent early symptoms. Impaired concentration can account for some of the memory loss, and it becomes most apparent when the patient is asked to complete a multistep task. Behavioral changes such as lethargy, loss of sexual drive, withdrawal from social and business contacts, and diminished emotional responsiveness can occur early in the illness. Early motor symptoms include unsteady gait, leg weakness, and tremor. Neurologic examination demonstrates primarily motor slowing, subtle cognitive impairment, slowed verbal responses, and blunted affect in the less affected patients. In some patients, particularly those with AIDS-related complex (ARC), subtle cognitive changes are detectable only by formal neuropsychologic testing.[10,11] In mildly impaired patients, neurologic examination frequently demonstrates inattention and mild recent memory loss. HIV encephalopathy is a progressive disease in AIDS patients[9] and perhaps progresses more slowly in ARC patients.[11] Navia et al.[9] reported that over half of the AIDS patients they studied developed severe global mental impairment within 2 months of the onset of neurologic symptoms; however, none of the ARC patients in one study developed severe dementia by the time of evaluation.[11] Late manifestations of HIV encephalopathy include severe dementia, psychomotor slowing, and severe ataxia. Some patients also develop other problems, such as leg weakness, urinary and fecal incontinence, or seizures. Evaluation by computed tomography (CT) or magnetic resonance imaging (MRI) reveals cortical atrophy in the majority of patients, which can precede the onset of cognitive symptoms.[9] However, in patients with subtle cognitive abnormalities, MRI can be normal.[11] Cerebrospinal fluid (CSF) can be normal or demonstrate elevated protein, mononuclear pleocytosis, oligoclonal bands,[9] or antibodies to HIV.[12-14] In some patients with HIV encephalopathy, HIV can be cultured from CSF; in later stages of infection, HIV can be more difficult to culture.[15]

Pathologically, patients with AIDS encephalopathy show brain atrophy and histologic changes in white matter and subcortical structures with relative sparing of the cortex. White matter pallor, inflammatory infiltrates with lymphocytes and macrophages, multinucleated giant cells, and astrocytosis are frequently present. Severity of neuropathologic abnormalities does not always correlate with severity of clinical symptoms, since some of these pathologic findings occur in patients without any cognitive abnormalities. Navia et al.[16] reported that only 5 of 24 nondemented AIDS patients had histologically normal brains at autopsy. The high percentage of neuropathologic abnormalities compared with clinical symptoms may reflect the fact that HIV encephalopathy is frequently subclinical, but it may also reflect selection bias in the autopsy series, since it is unlikely that every patient who died of AIDS had an autopsy.

PROGRESSIVE ENCEPHALOPATHY IN CHILDREN

Progressive encephalopathy in children with AIDS has been reported.[17,18] It is characterized by loss of motor milestones in younger children and loss of higher cortical function in older children as well as weakness, pyramidal tract signs, and acquired microcephaly. CT scan in most of these children shows cortical atrophy, and in some, calcification of the basal ganglia. Lumbar puncture demonstrates normal protein, glucose, and cell count. Pathologically, children with progressive encephalopathy have brain atrophy, glial nodules, and white matter degeneration similar to that described in adults.

ACUTE ENCEPHALOPATHY OR MENINGITIS

Acute encephalopathy or meningitis has been associated with seroconversion[19-21] or as occurring later in the course of HIV infection.[3,6] Ho et al.[21] reported on two patients who presented with symptoms of headache, myalgias, fever, and stiff neck consistent with viral meningitis. CSF was normal on initial lumbar puncture, but a second lumbar puncture a few days later showed a lymphocytic pleocytosis and elevated protein. No etiology could be established, but the illnesses corresponded to seroconversion to HIV. Carne et al.[19] and Piette et al.[20] have reported patients who presented with fever, malaise, mood changes, confusion, and memory loss coincident with seroconversion to HIV. Lumbar punctures in most instances were abnormal, with pleocytosis and elevated protein. All these patients had self-limited illnesses.

In addition to reports of illness coincident with seroconversion, atypical aseptic meningitis or acute encephalopathy have been reported at later stages of HIV infection. Levy et al.[6] had seen 17 patients with recurrent meningitis with cranial nerve palsies and pyramidal tract signs. We have seen 1 patient in a cohort of 43 patients with persistent lymphadenopathy who had an acute onset of fever, memory loss, and headache, who, 6 months later, had not fully recovered cognitive function.[11] At this time none of the patients reported to have had acute meningitis or encephalopathy have had AIDS.

MYELOPATHY

Spinal cord disease has been described in AIDS patients with and without AIDS dementia complex.[2,22,23] These patients complain primarily of lower-extremity weakness, paraparesis and/or gait ataxia, and urinary incontinence. Most have concurrent dementia, but spinal cord disease may not be evident on examination. Petito et al.[2] have described pathologic changes in the spinal cord that show vacuolation of the posterior and lateral columns, hence the name vacuolar myelopathy. The severity of the pathologic abnormalities in the spinal cord has correlated with that in the forebrain. Selective degeneration of the gracile tract of unknown etiology has also been reported.[23] Other spinal syndromes have been described but are not well delineated pathologically.

PERIPHERAL NEUROPATHY

Peripheral neuropathies associated with HIV infection have occurred in at least three types: distal symmetric polyneuropathy (DSPN), mononeuropathy multiplex (MM), and inflammatory demyelinating neuropathy (IDP).

DSPN is a sensorimotor illness with symptoms of distal painful dysesthesias and, to a lesser degree, leg weakness. Navia et al.[9] reported that 48% of their AIDS patients had peripheral neuropathies characterized by burning, painful dysesthesias, or numbness. DSPN occurs more frequently in patients with AIDS than in patients with HIV infection who do not have AIDS.

Lipkin et al.[24] described a group of LAS patients who had a sensorimotor neuropathy with an MM pattern; a variety of single nerves or roots were involved. Some of these patients had spontaneous resolution of symptoms, and others responded to plasmapheresis. MM in AIDS patients has not been reported.

Cornblath et al.[25] reported IDP in a series of patients with progressive weakness and LAS or asymptomatic HIV infection. Patients present with progressive muscle weakness, sometimes acute, with mild sensory complaints and areflexia. These patients are distinguished from patients with Guillain-Barré syndrome (GBS) by a CSF pleocytosis, which is unusual in GBS. Like GBS, nerve biopsy shows inflammatory demyelination. In the HIV-infected patients, symptoms can be transitory, but they also have responded to plasmapheresis. IDP can mimic

GBS, and Cornblath et al.[25] recommended that GBS patients with risk factors for HIV exposure should be screened for HIV infection.

ETIOPATHOGENESIS

When it became clear that AIDS patients were developing encephalopathy of unknown etiology, investigators explored the hypothesis that HIV caused the illness. Initially, HIV DNA was demonstrated in brains of patients with encephalopathy.[5] Later, HIV was cultured from CSF and brain from AIDS and ARC patients with neurologic complaints,[12,14] and patients with neurologic symptoms had increased HIV antibody production in the CSF.[13] All of these studies support the idea that HIV in some way causes encephalopathy.

To better understand the pathogenesis of HIV encephalopathy, investigators have worked to identify the cell types in the brain that are infected by HIV. Studies have detected HIV nucleic acids or antigens in brains of patients with encephalopathy, primarily in multinucleated giant cells of the macrophage cell line.[16,26-29] If HIV primarily infects macrophages in the brain and not neural or glial cells, then how does it cause brain dysfunction? Perhaps infected macrophages secrete factors that cause local neural or glial cell function. On the other hand HIV may infect neural cells but be too rare to easily detect or may exist in a difficult-to-detect form. Perhaps replication of HIV in neural or glial cells in the CNS is defective but able to disrupt cellular function. The white matter pallor may represent myelin dysfunction and thus neural dysfunction, but of what etiology? Navia et al.[16] separated demented patients neuropathologically into two groups: those with and those without multinucleated cells. They have detected HIV antigen or nucleic acid only in brains with multinucleated cells, which raises the possibility that another as yet undetected agent or mechanism might be causing dementia in some AIDS patients.

Clinical reports of meningitis and encephalopathy concident with seroconversion to HIV suggest that HIV travels to the CNS, at least in some patients, very early in the course of infection. Patients with asymptomatic HIV infection have also been shown to have antibody to HIV in their CSF.[15,30,31] How HIV travels to the CNS early in infection is unknown.

Although many patients at autopsy have neuropathologic evidence of HIV encephalopathy, varying tissue tropism of HIV might explain why some AIDS patients have no clinical neurologic abnormalities and, on neuropathology, have normal brains. Recent data suggest that HIV isolates from patients with HIV encephalopathy grow better in macrophage/monocyte cell lines in vitro than in lymphocytes, suggesting there might be a relatively neurotropic strain of HIV and a relatively lymphotropic strain of HIV. The more neurotropic strain might cause HIV encephalopathy, and the more lymphotropic strain might not cause neurologic abnormalities. Although in vitro studies suggest the existence of strains with different tissue tropisms, data are preliminary.

The etiology of vacuolar myelopathy is unknown, but HIV has been cultured from the spinal cord of one patient with vacuolar myelopathy.[12] Vacuolar myelopathy may be caused by direct HIV invasion of the spinal cord, by a metabolic abnormality, or by some yet to be determined factor.

The etiology of peripheral neuropathies in HIV infection is also unclear. DSPN in AIDS patients could be due to drug therapy, metabolic factors, or

HIV infection. Ho et al.[11] isolated HIV from a sural nerve biopsy from a patient with IDP, but in situ hybridization in biopsies from other patients were negative for HIV.[25] Whether the virus itself causes demyelination or stimulates an immune attack on Schwann cells or there is some other factor remains to be determined.

CONCLUSION

Although neurologic diseases in AIDS patients were initially thought to be due to secondary infections or cancers, evidence is accumulating that multiple neurologic abnormalities are due to direct HIV infection of neural tissues. HIV infection seems to be related to an acute meningitis or encephalopathy associated with seroconversion to HIV, to subtle cognitive abnormalities in patients with ARC, and to severe encephalopathy, mainly in patients with AIDS. Thus, HIV probably causes a spectrum of illnesses of the CNS. However, the pathogenesis of these disorders remains entirely unknown. In addition, whether HIV has a direct effect in the pathogenesis of myelopathy and peripheral neuropathy remains to be demonstrated. Ongoing research will answer some of the initial questions, but much more research into the neurologic manifestations of HIV infection is needed.

REFERENCES

1. Horowitz, S. L.; Benson, D. F.; Gottlieb, M. S.; et al. Neurological complications of gay-related immunodeficiency disorder. *Ann. Neurol.* 1982; 12:80 (abstract).

2. Petito, C. K.; Navia, B. A.; Cho, E. S.; Jordan, B. D.; George, D. C.; Price, R. W. Vacuolar myelopathy pathologically resembling subacute combined degeneration in patients with the acquired immunodeficiency syndrome. *N. Engl. J. Med.* 1985; 312:874–879.

3. Snider, W. D.; Simpson, D. M.; Nielsen, S.; Gold, J. W. M.; Metroka, C. E.; Posner, J. B. Neurological complications of acquired immune deficiency syndrome: Analysis of 50 patients. *Ann. Neurol.* 1983; 14:403–418.

4. Nielsen, S. L.; Petito, C. K.; Urmacher, C. D.; Posner, J. B. Subacute encephalitis in acquired immune deficiency syndrome: A postmortem study. *Am. J. Clin. Pathol.* 1984; 82:678–682.

5. Shaw, G. M.; Harper, M. E.; Hahn, B. H.; et al. HTLV-III infection in brains of children and adults with AIDS encephalopathy. *Science* 1985; 227:177–182.

6. Levy, R. M.; Bredesen, D. E.; Rosenblum, M. L. Neurological manifestations of the acquired immunodeficiency syndrome (AIDS): Experience at UCSF and review of the literature. *J. Neurosurg.* 1985; 62:475–495.

7. Koppel, B. S.; Wormser, G. P.; Tuchman, A. J.; Maayan, S.; Hewlett, D. Jr.; Daras, M. Central nervous system involvement in patients with acquired immune deficiency syndrome (AIDS). *Acta Neurol. Scand.* 1985; 71:337–353.

8. Levy, R. M.; Bredesen, D.E.; Rosenblum, M. L.; Davis, R. L. Postmortem neuropathology in the acquired immunodeficiency syndrome (AIDS) (abstract). Congress of Neurological Surgeons, New Orleans, September 1986.

9. Navia, B. A.; Jordan, B. D.; Price, R. W. The AIDS dementia complex. I. Clinical features. *Ann. Neurol.* 1986; 19:517–524.

10. Grant, I.; Atkinson, J. H.; Hesselink, J. R.; et al. Evidence for early central nervous system involvement in the acquired immunodeficiency syndrome (AIDS) and other human immunodeficiency virus (HIV) infections. *Ann. Intern. Med.* 1987; 107:828–836.

11. Janssen, R. S.; Saykin, A. J.; Kaplan, J.; et al. Neurologic complications of lymphadenopathy syndrome associated with HIV infection. *Ann. Neurol.* 1988; 23:49–55.

12. Ho, D. D.; Rota, T. R.; Schooley, R. T.; et al. Isolation of HTLV-III from cerebrospinal fluid and neural tissues of patients with neurologic syndromes related to the acquired immunodeficiency syndrome. *N. Engl. J. Med.* 1985; 313:1493–1497.

13. Resnick, L.; diMarzo-Veronese, F.; Schupbach, J.; et al. Intra-blood-brain-barrier synthesis of HTLV-III-specific IgG in patients with neurologic symptoms associated with AIDS or AIDS-related complex. *N. Engl. J. Med.* 1985; 313:1498–1504.

14. Levy, J.; Shimabukuro, J.; Hollander, H.; Mills, J.; Kaminsky, L. Isolation of AIDS-associated retroviruses from cerebrospinal fluid and brain of patients with neurological symptoms. *Lancet* 1985; ii:586–588.

15. Resnick, L.; Berger, J. R.; Shapshak, P.; Tourtellotte, W. W. Early penetration of the blood-brain-barrier by HIV. *Neurology* 1988; 38:9–14.

16. Navia, B. A.; Cho, E. S.; Petito, C. K.; Price, R. W. The AIDS dementia complex. II. Neuropathology. *Ann. Neurol.* 1986; 19:525–535.

17. Epstein, L. G.; Sharer, L. R.; Joshi, V. V.; Fojas, M. M.; Koenigsberger, M. R.; Oleske, J. M. Progressive encephalopathy in children with acquired immune deficiency syndrome. *Ann. Neurol.* 1985; 17:488–496.

18. Belman, A. L.; Ultmann, M. H.; Horoupian, D.; et al. Neurological complications in infants and children with acquired immune deficiency syndrome. *Ann. Neurol.* 1985; 18:560–566.

19. Carne, C. A.; Smith, A.; Elkington, A. G.; et al. Acute encephalopathy coincident with seroconversion for anti-HTLV-III. *Lancet* 1985; ii:1206–1208.

20. Piette, A. M.; Tusseau, F.; Vignon, D.; et al. Acute neuropathy coincident with seroconversion for anti-LAV/HTLV-III. *Lancet* 1985; i:852 (letter).

21. Ho, D. D.; Sarngadharan, M. G.; Resnick, L.; diMarzo-Veronese, F.; Rota, T. R.; Hirsch, M. S. Primary human T-lymphotropic virus type III infection. *Ann. Intern. Med.* 1985; 103:880–883.

22. Goldstick, L.; Mandybur, T. I.; Bode, R. Spinal cord degeneration in AIDS. *Neurology* 1985; 35:103–106.

23. Rance, N.E.; McArthur, J. C.; Cornblath, D. R.; Landstrom, D. L.; Griffin, J. W.; Price, D. L. Gracile tract degeneration in patients with sensory neuropathy and AIDS. *Neurology* 1988; 38:265–271.

24. Lipkin, W. I.; Parry, G.; Kiprov, D.; Abrams, D. Inflammatory neuropathy in homosexual men with lymphadenopathy. *Neurology* 1985; 35:1479–1483.

25. Cornblath, D.R.; McArthur, J.C.; Kennedy, P. G. E.; Witte, A. S.; Griffin, J. W. Inflammatory demyelinating peripheral neuropathies associated with human T-cell lymphotropic virus type III infection. *Ann. Neurol.* 1987; 21:32–40.

26. Koenig, S.; Gendelman, H. E.; Orenstein, J. M.; et al. Detection of AIDS virus in macrophages in brain tissue from AIDS patients with encephalopathy. *Science* 1986; 233:1089–1093.

27. Wiley, C. A.; Schrier, R. D.; Nelson, J. A.; Lampert, P. W.; Oldstone, M. B. A. Cellular localization of human immunodeficiency virus infection within the brains of acquired immune deficiency syndrome patients. *Proc. Natl. Acad. Sci. USA* 1986; 83:7089–7093.

28. Gartner, S.; Markovits, P.; Markovitz, D. M.; Betts, R. F.; Popovic, M. Virus isolation from and identification of HTLV-III/LAV-producing cells in brain tissue from a patient with AIDS. *JAMA* 1986; 256:2365–2371.

29. Gabuzda, D. H.; Ho, D. D.; de la Monte, S. M.; Hirsch, M. S.; Rota, T. R.; Sobel, R. A. Immunohistochemical identification of HTLV-III antigen in brains of patients with AIDS. *Ann. Neurol.* 1986; 20:289–295.

30. Goudsmit, J.; Wolters, E. C.; Bakker, M.; et al. Intrathecal synthesis of antibodies to HTLV-III in patients without AIDS or AIDS related complex. *Br. Med. J.* 1986; 292:1231–1234.

31. Hollander, H.; Levy, J. A. Neurologic abnormalities and recovery of human immunodeficiency virus from cerebrospinal fluid. *Ann. Intern. Med.* 1987; 107:692–695.

6

Parasites and Other Cofactors for AIDS

Richard B. Pearce

On the basis of epidemiological, clinical, and in vitro studies, it has been suggested that acquired immune deficiency syndrome (AIDS) is opportunistic, requiring prior or concomitant stimulation of the immune system in addition to a cytopathic retrovirus.[1-5] Several cofactors have been proposed as agents that chronically provoke the immune system and that account for the selective appearance of AIDS among individuals within the known risk groups.[6-12]

The idea that a lymphotropic virus might benefit from various environmental or endogenous stimuli that activate the cells in which the virus resides is not new,[13-17] but the notion has been given scientific support by many recent and diverse studies. A clearer understanding of the biology and global distribution of animal and human lymphotropic viruses and the effects of parasitism and other mitogenic influences on the immune system have made it possible to formulate a specific and readily testable hypothesis about the role of the environment in the development of lymphotropic viral-induced diseases including AIDS.

NULL HYPOTHESIS

There is no etiological association between parasites or other causes of immunosuppression and T-cell activation (such as pregnancy, exposure to foreign blood proteins, and opiates) and diseases linked to lymphotropic viruses. The apparent origin of AIDS in parasite endemic regions, its seroepidemiological link with parasites, and its rapid spread through the homosexual community in which parasites are endemic are fortuitous.

BURKITT'S LYMPHOMA, EBV, AND MALARIA

It is now widely accepted that the B-cell tropic Epstein-Barr virus (EBV) is a principal but insufficient "cause" of Burkitt's tumor, a B-cell lymphoma largely confined to tropical Africa, India, and New Guinea.[15,18-20] EBV can be repeatedly isolated from patients with Burkitt's lymphoma and is a strong inducer of B-cell proliferation. However, the virus is also common in developed nations as a cause of mononucleosis and perhaps other syndromes[21] but where Burkitt's lymphoma is virtually absent. EBV has also been linked to nasopharyngeal carcinoma.[22] These observations have led several researchers to propose that environmental factors play a key role in determining disease outcome for EBV-infected individuals.

In 1969 Denis Burkitt proposed that Burkitt's tumor resulted from an interaction between "some virus or viruses" and a "reticuloendothelial system altered by chronic and heavy infection by malaria or other parasites."[23] In support of his argument, Burkitt evoked two lines of evidence: *geographical restriction* of the tumor to areas where malaria was holoendemic, and *chronic immune stimulation* provided by the parasites, which, Burkitt argued, rendered the host susceptible to virus-induced B-cell neoplasia.

Modern clinical and immunological studies have since established that malaria is immunosuppressive in animals and humans.[24-27] Malaria has been shown to increase the rate of lymphatic tumors in mice infected with the Moloney virus.[16] In humans, malaria has been found to reduce several parameters of cellular immunity.[28,29] It was recently demonstrated that humans acutely infected with malaria exhibit a reversible depression of the OKT4/OKT8 ("helper"/"suppressor") T-cell ratio.[25] This study also showed that the ability of the patients' T cells to restrict EBV-stimulated growth of B cells was greatly diminished but that after successful treatment for malaria, normal immune function returned. The authors of the report suggested that malaria might predispose to Burkitt's lymphoma by permitting unrestrained B-cell replication which, in time, could lead to a somatic (chromosomal crossover) mutation and growth of a monoclonal B-cell tumor.

Additional, albeit less direct, evidence in support of a role for malaria in Burkitt's lymphoma can be seen in an earlier analysis of the frequencies of sickle cell trait in Nigerians. Because sickled erythrocytes are less susceptible to invasion by the malaria parasite, a lower frequency of Burkitt's lymphoma in sickle cell populations would be expected if the parasite were a major cofactor for Burkitt's lymphoma. In a study of Nigerians, the frequency of the sickle trait in healthy subjects was found to be significantly greater than that in a group of Burkitt's lymphoma patients from the same tribe and region.[30] The absence of malaria in groups with sickle cell anemia may have protected them from chronic antigenic stimulation and B-cell lymphoma. In Uganda a study using neighborhood controls matched for age, sex, and tribe also showed an inverse relationship between the presence of the sickle trait and Burkitt's lymphoma, but it was not significant at $p = 0.16$.[31]

It is certainly possible that parasites other than malaria may predispose to tumors in the small percentage of sickle cell patients who did develop Burkitt's lymphoma in these two studies. Parasitic diseases such as schistosomiasis and onchocerciasis have been associated with various viral and neoplastic diseases in Africa, including lymphoreticular tumors, Kaposi's sarcoma, and hepatitis B.[32-36]

ADULT T–CELL LEUKEMIA, HTLV–I, AND PARASITES

The first human T-cell tropic retrovirus, HTLV-I, was isolated in 1978 from a 28-year-old black male U.S. resident with cutaneous T-cell lymphoma.[37,38] Since that time serosurveys have disclosed that HTLV-I is geographically restricted and that it is present in clinically well individuals as well as patients with adult T-cell lymphoma/leukemia (ATLL), a distinct leukemic disorder found in the HTLV-I endemic regions.[39-42]

HTLV-I is confined chiefly to three tropical regions of the world: the southern coastal regions of Japan; the Caribbean, including the coastal regions of South America; and equatorial Africa.[39,41,43-45] Small foci have also been found in the coastal regions of Niigata Prefecture, Japan[44]; Italy[47]; Alaska; and Lapland.[48]

Frequencies for antibody to HTLV-I in populations living in the endemic regions of Japan range from 0.9% in Sado Island in the north to 37% in Nagasaki Prefecture in the south.[46,49-51] HTLV-I is virtually absent in all other northern regions and mountainous areas in the south[51,53] as well as Taiwan[54] and China.[55] HTLV-I antibodies are uniformly detected in patients with ATLL,[56,57] and the virus can be grown from T cells of both ATLL patients[58,59] and symptomless antibody carriers.[60]

A nationwide survey conducted in Japan has confirmed that ATLL is restricted to HTLV-I endemic areas, namely, the southern ports of Kagoshima and Nagasaki, the Goto Islands, Okinawa, and the coastal regions of Kochi and the Kii peninsula.[61,62]

The striking geographical overlap between the natural range of Bancroftian filariasis and HTLV-I in each of the ATLL endemic regions prompted Tajima and co-workers to speculate that the two are etiologically associated.[63] The idea is supported by a 1981 serosurvey of residents of the Goto Islands showing that individuals with high titers of antifilarial antibody have a significantly greater risk of being seropositive for HTLV-I than those without antifilarial antibody.[64] In the study, 50% of males and 71% of females with high levels of filarial antibody were seropositive for HTLV-I. The rates are more than three times the background level.

Other Japanese researchers subsequently reported finding an association between HTLV-I antibody and *Strongyloides stercoralis* among residents of Okinawa.[65] In this serosurvey 60% of 166 *Strongyloides* carriers were HTLV-I antibody-positive compared to only 20% of 2962 controls not harboring the parasite when examined. Both groups of researchers concluded provisionally that parasites may predispose to HTLV-I infection or growth within the body by chronically activating T cells.

A low-frequency HTLV-I endemic region has been recently found in Sado Island on the western coast of Honshu in northern Japan.[46] Though no studies have yet investigated a possible link with parasitism there, the area is unique among temperate northern prefectures in that it has a semitropical climate and a history of filariasis.[66]

Thus HTLV-I is confined to the regions of Japan that are also endemic for parasites and is several times more prevalent in groups exposed to or harboring parasites than in random blood donors. It is unlikely that HTLV-I is predisposing to parasite infection, as both species of parasite thus far linked to the virus in Japan are nonopportunistic; that is, they readily infect and cause disease in healthy individuals who, solely by chance, acquire them through a mosquito bite (filaria) or via contaminated water (*Strongyloides*). Although it is possible that insects carry HTLV-I, the association between parasites and HTLV-I seropositivity is not likely to be simply a vectorial one, as *Strongyloides* is not insect vectored. Moreover, filaria has been found to have immunosuppressive potential in vitro,[67] and *Strongyloides* is reported to cause a chronic immunosuppressive syndrome in humans.[68]

HTLV-I is also endemic in Africa, particularly equatorial regions.[69,70] Based on stringent confirmatory criteria, the highest rate of HTLV-I seropositivity in

Table 1 Association between HTLV-I and HIV antibody with various parasitic diseases in Venezuela[44,88]

Region	HTLV-I Ab Rate		HIV Ab Rate		Endemic Parasitic Disease
Aragus	4/43	9%	—		Leishmaniasis
Guarico	6/40	15%	—		Chagas disease
Zulia	7/51	14%	—		Malaria, Chagas disease
T. F. Amazonas	7/51	14%	9/224	4%	Malaria
Caracas	1/102	1%	0/211[a]	0%	None

[a]Control sera from Caracas and other cities in Venezuela.

one serosurvey was 21% for Ugandan blacks both with and without Burkitt's lymphoma.[45] Ten percent of Burkitt's patients from Ghana and 8% of normal controls were also found to be seropositive for HTLV-I. In Kenya an overall rate of 31% has been reported for HTLV-I, with the highest rates consistently appearing in rural tribes.[71] The notable exception is the Falashas from Ethiopia, in whom a seropositivity of 37% has been reported.[72] HTLV-I is far less prevalent (<1–2%) in nonequatorial regions of Africa.[45]

The islands of the Caribbean and the northern areas of South America represent the third major focus for HTLV-I. HTLV-I rates ranging from 4% to 33% have been reported for the French West Indies,[73,74] and a survey in Venezuela found rates ranging from 1% in urban Caracas to 14% percent for both the Yanomami Indians living in the Federal Territory of Amazonas (southern Venezuela) and non-Indians living in the coastal state of Zulia.[44]

As in southern Japan, parasitic disease has been found to be a strong risk factor for HTLV-I antibody positivity in Africa and the Caribbean/South American regions.

In Ghana individuals with antibody to P. faciparum malaria were found to be nearly four times more likely to have HTLV-I than nonparasitized individuals.[75] HTLV-I seropositivity also strongly correlated with malaria antibody in a study of rural Kenyans,[71] and a study of native Venezuelan Indians found that HTLV-I seropositivity rates are highest in those with parasitic disease or who live in areas endemic for parasites (Table 1).

A small HTLV-I cluster has recently been found in Apulia, southern Italy.[47] Viral antibodies were present in 8% of sera from the area but were not found elsewhere in Italy. Two cases of HTLV-I-positive ATLL have been identified in the region. As recently as a few decades ago, malaria was highly prevalent in low-lying coastal regions of Italy, including Apulia. Also, a single case of "smoldering" T-cell lymphoma associated with HTLV-I has been reported from Sicily,[76] another malarial region.

AIDS, HIV, AND PARASITES

Since 1983 several closely related lymphotropic retroviruses have been repeatedly isolated from patients with AIDS and related conditions—e.g., persistent generalized lymphadenopathy and thrombocytopenia. The viruses, termed lymphadenopathy-associated virus (LAV), immune deficiency-associated virus

(IDAV), human T-cell lymphotropic virus (HTLV-III), and AIDS-related virus (ARV) appear to be variants of a family of viruses that are cytopathic for lymphocytes bearing the OKT4 phenotypic marker.[77-83] In agreement with recently proposed nomenclature the term human immunodeficiency virus (HIV) will be adopted here.

Two geographical foci for AIDS exist—one in central Africa, the other in Haiti. AIDS also appears throughout the Free World in several specific risk groups not confined by geography: emigrants from the endemic areas of Haiti and Africa and their spouses and offspring, male homosexuals and bisexuals, intravenous drug users and their spouses or offspring, hemophiliacs and their spouses and offspring, and recipients of blood. AIDS appears infrequently in others not known to be associated with any risk group.

Reported seropositivity rates for HIV vary considerably from region to region within Africa, but, overall, as many as 25% of asymptomatic Africans living in Zaire, Uganda, Kenya, and Rwanda have been infected.[71,84] The frequency of HIV antibody in normal Caribbean populations has not been well characterized. However, in one report,[85] 7% of Haitian immigrants living in French Guyana and, in another report,[86] 9% of Haitians working in the Dominican Republic were seropositive. In Venezuela the rate of HIV seropositivity has been found to range from less than 1%[87] to 13.3%, the highest being in native Indians living in malarial regions.[88] In contrast blood donors from several urban areas of Venezuela revealed no HIV-positive cases.

Not unexpectedly, the frequency of HIV seropositivity in risk groups outside of tropical areas varies considerably. The year in which blood is tested is an important determinant of seroprevalence, as the incidence of the viruses within risk groups is increasing. However, from numerous reports published over the past 4 years it is clear that between 25% and 60% of sexually active homosexuals living in developed nations are seropositive for HIV,[89-93] and as many as 80% of hemophiliacs and IV drug users in the United States and Europe have been exposed to the virus.[94-98]

Several recent studies have identified parasites as a risk factor for being HIV-seropositive. In rural Zaire and Kenya HIV seroprevalence has been found to be strongly and significantly linked to malaria seropositivity.[71,84,99] In Kenya the estimated HIV prevalence for the region is 21%; however, an HIV antibody rate of 80% was reported for subjects with shistosomiasis.[71] A study of a Zairian control (non-AIDS) population showed that the seropositivity rate for HIV ranged from 19% to 23%.[84] This estimate is biased, however, as 12 of the 26 subjects, including all but one of the viral-positive cases, had been hospitalized for various infectious diseases, including three with tuberculosis and two with acute malaria. Similarly, a recent survey in Zaire found a greater rate of HIV seropositivity in Africans with tuberculosis (but without AIDS) than in noninfected controls.[100]

Venezuelans with malaria are also at high risk for HIV seropositivity. Volsky and co-workers[87] recently reported an HIV prevalence rate of 41% for Venezuelans living in rural Tachira, where parasites are most prevalent (Table 1). This report is also significant for its mention of a case in which HIV was isolated from a patient with acute malaria. The finding that the AIDS virus itself could be isolated from a Venezuelan without other risk factors argues against the notion that positive antibody tests for HIV in tropical regions are only artifacts caused by some kind of nonspecific action by parasites on B cells or antibodies.[101,102]

Numerous case reports of Africans with AIDS cite prior or concurrent infection with nonopportunistic parasites.[100,103-105] For example, in one study of 17 Africans with AIDS, 9 had reported previous parasitic infections, including ankylostomiasis, schistosomiasis, amebiasis, ascaridiasis, and filariasis.[103]

Haitians with AIDS have been reported to harbor one or more of the intestinal parasites *Giardia lamblia*, *Entamoeba histolytica*, *Loa loa*, and *Strongyloides steroralis*.[106] Also, parasites are endemic in Haiti and among Haitian immigrants. A clinical study of recent Haitian immigrants found that 72% were positive for one or more of 12 species of intestinal parasite.[107] Parasitic disease is also a major health problem for the Haitian immigrant community of Belle Glade, Florida, where the rate of AIDS may be the highest of any comparable-sized community in the world.[108]

Overshadowed by AIDS is the epidemic of amebiasis and giardiasis which appeared suddenly among homosexual men living in major cities in the United States and Europe during the years immediately preceding the outbreak of AIDS.[109-113] Although precise incidence studies are lacking, several surveys of venereal disease and clinic volunteer populations place the current frequency of intestinal protozoal infections at 60% or higher among homosexuals, most of whom report no symptoms.[114,115]

In San Francisco the number of officially recorded cases of amebiasis (infection with *Entamoeba histolytica*) among men rose 10-fold between 1977 and 1984, far out of proportion to the increases (and in some cases decreases) in other sexually transmitted diseases. The rate of giardiasis has also increased rapidly (San Francisco Department of Health). Among intestinal parasites commonly isolated from homosexual men but not reported are *Endolimax nana*, *Iodamoeba butschlii*, *Dientamoeba fragilis*, and *Entamoeba coli*.

It has been suggested that the epidemic of gastrointestinal parasites in urban homosexual populations may have paved the way for AIDS.[1,6,12] To explore this further, Dr. Donald Abrams, codirector of the AIDS Clinic at San Francisco General Hospital, and I collaborated on a study of the parasite prevalence in homosexual men with either of two AIDS-related conditions (ARC)—persistent lymphadenopathy syndrome (LAS) or immune thrombocytopenic purpura (ITP). We found 80% and 82% of the patients in each group, respectively, harbored at least one species of parasite (Table 2). *Endolimax nana* was the most frequently found amoeba. The frequency of parasites in the two groups combined was significantly greater than that previously reported for either a predominantly homosexual[115] or heterosexual[116] population.

Over half of the subjects in each group presented with more than one parasite (Table 3). In two patients initially found to have only *E. nana*, an additional 12 stool samples were obtained. During this period of further testing the patients were requested not to engage in sexual practices that might expose them to feces. In one patient *E. hartmanni* was detected with and without *E. nana*. In the second patient *E. hartmanni* was found in stools 4–9 and *E. histolytica* in stools 10–15.

Thus, homosexuals with ARC have a very high incidence of parasitism. Given the low diagnostic accuracy of stool tests for amebiasis (approximately 80% for

Table 2 Frequency of intestinal parasites in homosexual men with Lymphadenopathy Syndrome (LAS) and Immune Thrombocytopenic Purpura (ITP) compared to predominantly homosexual (health fair) and heterosexual (multiphasic) historical control groups

	Percent infected			
Parasite	LAS ($n = 75$)	ITP ($n = 17$)	Health fair ($n = 105$)	Multiphasic ($n = 415$)
Any parasite	80	82	59	14
Potential pathogen	49	47	31	6
Endolimax nana	61	59	38	7
Entamoeba histolytica	37	41	27	1
Entamoeba hartmanni	37	41	25	2
Entamoeba coli	21	24	17	4
Iodamoeba butschlii	7	6	18	1
Giardia lamblia	1	0	5	2
Dientamoeba fragilis	1	6	1	3

three samples) and *Giardia* (<30%), it is likely that all patients were, or had been, carriers of parasites.

In addition to our findings, cases of AIDS among homosexuals frequently report a history of, or concomitant infection with, nonopportunistic parasites.[117-128]

SAIDS, STLV–III, AND PARASITES

An AIDS-like condition has also been identified in nonhuman primates. Its clinical manifestations include malignant lymphoma, lymphocytic nodules (lymphadenopathy), diarrhea, depression of in vitro lymphocyte responses to mitogens, and a susceptibility to opportunistic bacterial and protozoal infections. The similarity of the diseases in monkeys to AIDS in humans has led to the use of the acronym "SAIDS" for "simian AIDS." Transmissibility of the disease experimentally and naturally suggests a viral component, and several candidates have been proposed. Among macaques raised at the New England Regional Primate Center in Southborough, Massachusetts, 85% with lymphoma or lymphoproliferative disease were judged seropositive for HTLV-I.[129] More recently a virus similar to but antigenically distinct from HIV and HTLV-I has been isolated from macaques and African green monkeys[129-131] and is termed simian T-lymphotropic virus type 3 (STLV-III).

Table 3 Frequency of multiple parasitic infections in patients with Lymphadenopathy Syndrome (LAS) and Immune Thrombocytopenic Purpura (ITP)

	Number and percent (%) infected	
Number of different protozoa detected	LAS ($n = 75$)	ITP ($n = 17$)
None	15 (20)	3 (18)
1	19 (25)	4 (24)
2	19 (25)	2 (12)
3	13 (17)	6 (35)
4	8 (11)	1 (6)
5	1 (1)	1 (6)

Whether in the wild or maintained in experimental colonies, primates, even when judged "healthy," are known to harbor numerous parasites including nematodes, protozoa, helminths, cestodes, and trematodes.[132-134] Simian malaria is infrequently mentioned as a cause of illness in primates maintained for experimental studies, yet when sera of monkeys imported from malarial areas are examined, up to two-thirds are positive for antimalarial antibodies.[135] The earliest recorded outbreak of SAIDS occurred between 1969 and 1971, when 23 rhesus monkeys housed at the National Center for Primate Biology (now the California Primate Research Center in Davis) developed a Burkitt's-like tumor.[136] Forty-three percent of these animals had been previously infected with simian malaria (*Plasmodium cynomolgi*). Subsequent reports from this facility have documented additional cases of lymphoma as well as opportunistic infections. In one instance a retroorbital tumor developed in a 1-year-old female monkey whose father and maternal grandmother had been inoculated with malaria. Six months later her mother acquired widespread lymphomatous tumors and gastrointestinal *Mycobacterium avium*.[137] Another early report from the Davis facility related the unusual occurrence of disseminated toxoplasmosis among macaques housed there.[138] All four animals were infected with numerous parasites including *Strongyloides*, *Balantidium*, and amoebae. In addition, two of these four animals had been experimentally inoculated with malaria.

More recently macaques with SAIDS from this and other primate centers have been reported to be concurrently infected with *Entamoeba histolytica*, *Giardia lamblia*, or *Trichomonas*.[131,139,140] Thus, not only are monkeys in general at risk for parasites, but animals with SAIDS have a documented history of having been infected with malaria or intestinal parasites.

BOVINE LEUKEMIA, BLV, AND PARASITES

Bovine leukemia is thought to be caused by bovine leukemia virus (BLV), a lymphotropic retrovirus that shares genetic organization and considerable nucleotide homology with HTLV-1 and, to a lesser extent, HIV.[141,142] In one report it was observed that leukemic cattle were frequently infected with *Trypanosome theileri*.[143] A later study[144] found that the incidence of trypanosomes in leukosis herds was significantly higher than in leukosis-free cattle (70.8% of the animals with leukosis were positive for *T. theileri* compared to 28.7% of the nonleukosis animals $p < 0.001$). The authors of the report suspected that single rather than serial sampling underestimated the true incidence of parasites by as much as 30% and that a rate of 100% parasite positivity was possible for the leukosis herd. Others have reported an association between bovine leukemia and babesiosis in Africa.[14] Interestingly, BLV is also prevalent in southern Japan and Venezuela, where up to 50% of herds in a particular region may be infected.[145]

ARE LYMPHOTROPIC VIRUSES OPPORTUNISTIC?

There is now strong evidence that T-lymphotropic viruses demand T-cell activation and perhaps concomitant immunosuppression to reproduce within the organism. The propagation of lymphotropic viruses in vitro requires the continued presence of mitogenic factors such as phytohemagglutinin and human T-cell growth factor (interleukin-2).[38,146] Antigenic stimulation of lymphocytes in culture is obligatory for HIV reproduction, which ultimately leads to cell death.[147] The authors of this last report remarked that antigens such as malaria, semen, or blood proteins could serve as cofactors for AIDS conceivably by facilitating the entry of HIV into the cell or by activating provirus in already infected cells.

Also in support of the notion that immunostimulation might be necessary for the growth of HIV are several studies in monkeys. In order to infect monkeys with HIV it has been found necessary to coinject allogeneic cells, inject large volume of AIDS serum, or infect autogeneic cells in vitro (with mitogenic factors), then reintroduce the virally infected cells into the animal.[148,149]

If AIDS is opportunistic one would expect to find immune abnormalities in individuals from groups at risk for AIDS but who do not have AIDS and who are seronegative for the HIV. The fact is, marked and unusual immune abnormalities do occur in asymptomatic, seronegative homosexual men, hemophiliacs, heroin users, pregnant women, neonates, and recipients of blood.[3,7,150-155]

Studies from Hungary,[156] Sweden,[157] Finland,[3] and the United States[158-160] have shown that a large percentage of homosexual men have reversed OKT4/OKT8 ratios even though they are seronegative for HIV. As early as 1982 a study from New York found that 80% of a volunteer group of homosexual men had reversed T-cell ratios.[122] However, serosurveys of blood obtained from New York homosexuals at that time indicate that HIV incidence was 20–30%.[158] Homosexuals lacking evidence for exposure to HIV have also been found to have autoimmune neutropenia,[162] autoantibodies against lymphocytes,[163] and elevated cytotoxic T-lymphocyte activity against foreign lymphocytes.[164] Clearly some factor other than HIV must be responsible for immune abnormalities, as it is unlikely that all such cases represent viral infection without the production of detectable antibody.

Some evidence suggests that immunologically normal individuals exposed to the AIDS virus may be able to avoid infection. For instance, it has been reported that for Scottish hemophiliacs who were inadvertently exposed to factor VIII contaminated with HIV, seroconversion was related to preexisting immunosuppression.[165] A role for iatrogenic immunosuppression in the subsequent development of AIDS has also been proposed.[166]

A study of 96 individuals at risk for AIDS from whom HIV could be cultured revealed that 4 had no detectable antibody. Each was also found to be immunologically normal.[167] Two were homosexual partners of AIDS cases, and two were female partners of AIDS cases from other known risk groups. Since no immune abnormalities or antibodies to HIV were seen in these four, it may be that they had successfully suppressed viral replication even though the virus could be grown from T cells under the special conditions of cell culture.

Recently Krohn and co-workers reported that the rate of HIV seroconversion is less among Finnish homosexual men who were immunologically normal at initial testing than among those who were immunosuppressed.[168] Since immunosuppression was seen in the absence of HIV, the researchers looked for clinical and demographic differences between immunocompromised and nonimmunocompromised men. The rates of sexually transmitted diseases and viruses were comparable between the two groups. However, immunosuppressed men seronegative for HIV were more likely than nonimmunosuppressed, seronegative men to have reported diarrhea and to have had the intestinal parasite *Giardia lamblia*. In mice, *Giardia* has been shown to suppress humoral and cellular immune responses.[169]

DO PARASITES PROMOTE LYMPHOTROPIC VIRAL INFECTION OR REPLICATION?

Parasites, including schistosomes, malaria, filaria, amoebae, and trypanosomes, are mitogenic for T lymphocytes.[26,67,170-175] In addition to being immunostimulatory, parasites are able to subvert the cell-mediated and humoral immune responses of their hosts.[176,177] Some of the consequences of parasitic infection include hyperglobulinemia,[178] the production of autoantibodies,[179] elaboration by activated lymphocytes of suppressor factors,[24,180] interference with macrophage migration inhibition,[181] increase in interferon production,[26] induction of anergy to skin antigens,[29] allograft tolerance,[27] and predisposition to viral infections[16] and tumors.[32-34,182,183] In specific reference to parasites most likely to infect tropical and homosexual risk groups for AIDS, malaria and amoebae have been shown to reduce delayed hypersensitivity in humans,[29,184] and amebiasis is associated with anti-DR (anti-antigen-presenting cell) autoantibodies[185] and suppressor factors.[170,180]

COFACTORS IN OTHER RISK GROUPS

Obviously parasites do not explain why AIDS appears in all groups exposed to HIV. However, individuals in every known risk group for AIDS are also at risk of immunostimulation, immunosuppression, or both (Table 4).

Hemophiliacs have reversed T-cell ratios, most likely caused by their regular exposure to the foreign clotting factors.[150,186] In an early study, 66% of asymptomatic hemophiliacs receiving factor VIII were immunodeficient, but only half were seropositive for HIV.[150] As mentioned above, this immunocompromised state may predispose hemophiliacs to HIV seroconversion and perhaps fulminant AIDS. Today the majority of hemophiliacs in the United States and England have been exposed to HIV ($\approx$80%), and yet the rate of AIDS is still low, a fact that has led some to argue that "susceptibility factors may be involved" in the transition from seropositivity to disease.[187] With the introduction of heat treat-

Table 4 Members of risk groups for AIDS with preexisting immunosuppression/stimulation caused by various nonviral factors

Risk group (with AIDS)	Parasites?	Prior immuno-suppression?
Homosexual	Yes	Yes
Haitian	Yes	Yes
African	Yes	Yes
SAIDS	Yes	Yes
Opiate users	NA[a]	Yes
Blood	NA	Yes
Hemophiliacs	NA	Yes
Pregnant	NA	Yes

[a]NA = not applicable

ment and blood screening for HIV, hemophiliacs are not apt to come into contact with HIV.

Opiates bind to T lymphocytes, and it has been suggested that this may contribute directly to the chronic state of subclinical immunosuppression seen in those addicted to IV drugs.[152] Cases of transfusion-associated AIDS are of particular interest. Although cited as evidence against the need to postulate cofactors for the development of AIDS, transfusion studies actually support the theory. Blood from a single donor is routinely fractionated and given to many different recipients, and yet AIDS develops in only a small number of recipients. For instance, in one report, blood from 22 donors who later developed AIDS had been transfused into 122 recipients.[188] Of the 41 who could be followed up (i.e., who did not die from the condition for which they were hospitalized or who could not be located), only 2 had developed AIDS (follow-up averaged 3 years for the group). Also to be considered is the rarity with which two or more cases of AIDS can be traced to a single donor.[187-190] If HIV is not opportunistic, what would account for its being unable to cause AIDS in at least the majority of those exposed to the virus via transfusion? The answer may be found by recognizing that blood transfusions are themselves immunosuppressive. Transfusions are often given to patients before transplant surgery in order to raise a patient's tolerance to the allograft by lowering T-cell-mediated immune responses. Interestingly, one of the largest studies of transfusion AIDS found that the average number of units transfused was 15.9 units, several times the usual transfused quantity.[191]

Lastly, pregnant women in third trimester and their fetuses are immunosuppressed by virtue of factors that depress T-cell function.[153] This natural response presumably increases the mother's tolerance to paternal-derived fetal proteins. In this light it should be mentioned that women with AIDS who do not report themselves as belonging to a known risk group but who do report having had sexual intercourse with a member of a risk group or an individual with AIDS have very often become pregnant at the time of, or immediately prior to, their diagnoses. Newborns of pregnant women are also immunosuppressed and are at special risk for AIDS.[154,192]

DISCUSSION

The appearance of Burkitt's lymphoma, ATLL, and AIDS in areas where parasites abound; the direct relationship between parasite antibody titers and HTLV-I and HIV; and the regular isolation of nonopportunistic parasites from individuals with AIDS, monkeys with SAIDS, and cattle with bovine leukemia support a direct role for parasites in the development of diseases associated with lymphotropic viruses. The entry of the AIDS virus into nonparasitized groups may have been facilitated by other immunostimulatory factors (e.g., exposure to opiates or foreign proteins, pregnancy, neonatalism).

It should not come as a surprise to the naturalist that viruses that infect the cells of the immune system should also benefit from chronic stimulation of those cells. Indeed, a case can be made for vertebrate retroviruses *arising* from transposable genetic elements of lymphocytes,[193] perhaps under the evolutionary pressure of parasites.

Though largely a forgotten medical problem in industrialized nations, parasites take a large toll in human suffering and life throughout most of the world. Perhaps as many as 1 billion people are infected with one or another of the more debilitating parasites. In India, Africa, and South America parasitic diseases such as onchocerciasis, malaria, filariasis, shistosomiasis, trypanosomiasis (Chagas disease), amebaisis, giardiasis, strongylodiasis, and enterobius are major health concerns. Even in developed countries such as Portugal, Spain, Italy, and the western and southern United States, malaria was a formidable problem as recently as 40 years ago.

Though studies never intended to show it, HTLV-I has been linked in every instance to regions where malaria was, or continues to be, prevalent, whereas in neighboring regions without the parasite HTLV-I is absent. This includes the southern United States, California, Alaska, Africa, southern Japan, the Caribbean, and southern Italy. In each area, low-lying coastal regions are affected, whereas communities in higher, dryer areas, sometimes no more than a few kilometers away, remain free of the virus. It is likely that the frequency of HTLV-I in endemic regions is diminishing as the result of parasite eradication efforts. The smallest clusters, such as those in coastal Italy, Alaska, and Sado Island, Japan, are in regions that have been relatively free of parasites for several decades. In contrast viral prevalence is still quite high in regions where parasites thrive.

In Venezuela HTLV-I has infected both native Indian and Hispanic populations, although the two do not, as a rule, intermarry. Here parasitism is ubiquitous in areas where HTLV-I and HIV have been detected. However, in urban Caracas, where medical care for parasitic diseases such as malaria, Chagas disease, and leishmaniasis is readily available (and where parasite vectors are largely absent), HTLV-I and HIV are not found.

HTLV-I is restricted to regions of southern Japan that, in recent years, were highly endemic for filaria and other parasites. It has been suggested that Portuguese mariners may have brought HTLV-I to the southern ports of Japan in the 16th century.[194] Given the ability of the virus to pass from person to person though sexual contact,[195] one would have expected that HTLV-I would have moved out of southern Japan to the northern island of Honchu, to the Chinese mainland, and even to continental Europe as a consequence of human migration, warfare, and trade during the centuries following its presumed introduction there. That this hasn't happened suggests that regional forces are conspiring to restrict the spread of the virus. In short, what may have limited further spread of HTLV-I and ATLL throughout northern Japan may have been the absence of parasitism outside the HTLV-I regions. If this is true, the rate of HTLV-I and ATLL in southern Japan should decrease in the next 10–20 years as parasites become less prevalent.

AIDS is prevalent in Haiti but not in the Dominican Republic, even though the two countries share the same island and, to a great extent, the same Haitian farm labor force. A recent survey found that approximately 9% of Haitian migrant workers in the Dominican Republic are seropositive for HIV.[86] The same study also found that the rate of HIV in male prostitutes in the Dominican Republic is 10%, but less than 1% in venereal disease and drug clinic patients. Again, the question looms: Why are HTLV-I and HIV prevalent in Haiti and Haitians but the viruses and associated diseases virtually absent in the Dominican Republic despite the seemingly open opportunity for spread? Perhaps it is because Dominicans enjoy a high standard of living with good medical care and a low prevalence of parasitic disease, whereas Haiti is one of the poorest of the Caribbean nations and has a high rate of parasitic disease. The first suggestion that parasites may predispose to full-blown AIDS in homosexual men[1] was made before serosurveys in Africa and Venezuela indicated that the two are strongly linked and was not, therefore, based on knowledge that such an epidemiological association was likely. In other words it was not a case of the theory trying to fit the known facts, but of one that was subsequently supported by them. Biggar[99,101] and others[102] contend that parasites may be nonspecifically increasing the reactivity of antibody to T-lymphotropic viruses and for this reason present an apparent etiological association between the two. However, sera from patients with malaria have been found not to cause false-positive reactions with commercial ELISA HIV antibody kits.[196] Also, in one study of hospitalized Africans (some with parasites), HTLV-I and HIV antibodies were detected and confirmed in different individuals.[84] If parasites are causing false-positive antibody reactions, they do so discriminantly. Lastly, HIV itself has been isolated from a rural Venezuelan with chronic malaria but no other risk factor for AIDS.[88]

Studies of the possible etiological relationship between parasites and lymphotropic viruses are warranted, as it may be possible to limit the spread of HTLV-I and HIV along with their associated diseases by eliminating parasites in individuals and by taking reasonable measures to prevent entry of the viruses into regions of the world where parasites are increasing (e.g., malaria in India and Southeast Asia) but where these viruses are apparently not yet endemic. The first public health measures to be taken in Western societies should be in the diagnosis and treatment of intestinal parasites in homosexual men whose infectious plight persists in consequence of minimal gastrointestinal symptoms,[114] risky sexual practicies, and ignorance or neglect of the problem by public health officials[112] and private physicians.[113]

REFERENCES

1. Pearce, R. B. Intestinal protozoal infections in AIDS. *Lancet*, 1983; ii:51.

2. Levy, J. A.; and Zeigler, J. L. Acquired immunodeficiency syndrome is an opportunistic infection and Kaposi's sarcoma results from secondary immune stimulation. *Lancet*, 1983; ii:78–80.

3. Krohn, K.; Ranki, A.; Antonen, J; et al. Immune functions in HTLV-III antibody positive homosexual men without clinical AIDS. *Lancet*, 1984; ii:746–747.

4. Greenwood, B. M. AIDS in Africa. *Immunol. Today*, 1984; 5:293–294.

5. Gallo, R. C. The family of human lymphotropic retroviruses called HTLV: HTLV-I in adult T-cell leukemia (ATL), HTLV-II in hairy cell leukemias, and HTLV-III in AIDS. Kaplan Memorial Lecture, in: *Retroviruses in Human Lymphoma/Leukemia*, M. Miwa et al. (eds.), Japan Sci. Soc. Press, Tokyo, 1985.

6. Pearce, R. B.; Abrams, D. I. AIDS and parasitism. *Lancet*, 1984; i:1411.

7. Daul, C. B.; Mann, M. Y.; Andes, W. A.; deShazo, R. D. In vitro effects of commercial factor VIII concentrates on normal immunocompetent cell function. International Conference on AIDS, Atlanta, April 14–17, 1985; Session 15, p. 47.

8. Sonnabend, J. A.; Saadoun, S. The acquired immunodeficiency syndrome: A discussion of etiological hypotheses. *AIDS Res.*, 1983/84; 1:107–120.

9. Shearer, G. M. Immunosuppression and recognition of class II (Ia) antigens: Possible factor in the etiology of acquired immune deficiency syndrome. *Proceedings of the New York University Symposium on Epidemic Kaposi's Sarcoma and Opportunistic Infections in Homosexual Men*, Mar. 17–19, 1983.

10. Quinn, T. C., Piot, P., McCormick, J. B., et al. Serologic and immunologic studies in patients with AIDS in North America and Africa: The potential role of infectious agents as cofactors in Human Immunodeficiency Virus infection. *JAMA*, 1987; 257: 2617–2621.

11. Goedert, J. J.; Sarngadharan, M. G.; Biggar, R. J.; et al. Determinants of retrovirus (HTLV-III) antibody and immunodeficiency conditions in homosexual men. *Lancet*, 1984; ii:711–715.

12. Archer, D. L.; Glinsman, W. H. Enteric infections and other cofactors in AIDS. *Immunol. Today*, 1985; 6:292–295.

13. Dalldorf, G. Lymphomas of African children: With different forms or environmental influences. *JAMA*, 1962; 181:1026.

14. Weipers, W. L.; Jarrett, W. F. H.; Martin, W. B.; et al. Lymphosarcoma in domestic animals. *Br. Emp. Cancer Campaign Res.*, 1964; 42:682–686.

15. Krüger, G.; O'Conner, G. T. Epidemiological and immunological considerations on the pathogenesis of Burkitt's tumor. In: Grundmann, E., Tulinius, H. *Current Problems in the Epidemiology of Cancer and Lymphomas*. Springer-Verlag, Berlin, 1972, p. 212.

16. Wederburn, N. 1970. Effect of concurrent malarial infections on development of a virus-induced lymphoma in BALB/C mice. *Lancet*, 1970; ii:1114–1116.

17. Ulbright, T.; and Cruz, D. J. Kaposi's sarcoma: Relationship with hematologic, lymphoid and thymic neoplasia. *Cancer*, 1981; 47:963–973.

18. Burkitt, D. The discovery of Burkitt's lymphoma. *Cancer*, 1983; 51:1777–1786.

19. Grundmann, E.; Tulinius, H. *Current Problems in the Epidemiology of Cancer and Lymphomas*. Springer-Verlag, Berlin, 1972.

20. Venkitaraman, A. R.; John, T. J.; Rangad, F.; Singh, A. D.; Date, A.; Lenoir, G. Epstein-Barr virus associated with Burkitt's lymphoma in India. *Trop. Geogr. Med.*, 1983; 35:273–277.

21. Shearer, W. T.; Ritz, J.; Finegold, M.; et al. Epstein-Barr virus associated proliferations of diverse clonal origins after bone marrow transplantation in a 12-year-old patient with severe combined immunodeficiency. *N. Engl. J. Med.*, 1985; 312:1151–1159.

22. Zhu, X. X.; Zeng, Y.; Wolf, H. Detection of IgG and IgA antibodies to EBV membrane antigen in sera from patients with nasopharyngeal carcinoma and from normal individuals. *Int. J. Cancer*, 1986; 37:689–692.

23. Burkitt, D. Etiology of Burkitt's lymphoma—an alternative hypothesis to a vectorial virus. *JNCI*, 1969; 42:19–28.

24. Khansari, N; Segre, M.; Segre, D. Immunosuppression in murine malaria: A soluble immunosuppressive factor derived from *Plasmodium berghei*-infected blood. *J. Immunol.*, 1981; 127:1889–1893.

25. Whittle, H. C.; Brown, J.; Marsh, K.; Greenwood, B. M.; Seidelin, P.; et al. T-cell control of Epstein-Barr virus-infected B cells is lost during *P. falciparum* malaria. *Nature*, 1984; 312:449–450.

26. Ojo-Amaize, E. A.; Vilcek, J.; Cochrane, A. H.; Nussenzweig, P. S. *Plasmodium berghei* sporozoites are mitogenic for murine T cells, induce interferon, and activate natural killer cells. *J. Immunol.*, 1984; 133:1005–1009.

27. Wedderburn, N.; Campa, M.; Tosta, C. E.; Henderson, D. C. The effect of malaria on the growth of two syngenic transplantable murine tumors. *Ann. Trop. Med. Parasitol.*, 1981; 75:597–605.

28. Greenwood, B. M.; Bradley-Moore, A. M.; Palit, A. Immunosuppression in children with malaria. *Lancet*, 1972; i:169–172.

29. Tanphaichitra, D. Cellular immunity in amebiasis, malaria and other intracellular infections in the tropics. *Clin. Res.*, 1979; 27:481A.

30. Pike, M. C.; Morrow, R. H.; Kissuule, A.; Mafigiri, J. Burkitt's lymphoma and sickle cell trait. *Br. J. Prev. Soc. Med.*, 1970; 24:39–41.

31. Williams, A. O. Hemoglobin genotypes, ABO blood groups, and Burkitt's tumor. *J. Med. Genet.*, 1966; 3:177.

32. Cheever, A. W.; Kamel, I. A.; Elwi, A. M.; Mosimann, J. E.; Danner, R.; Sippel, J. E. *Schistosoma mansoni* and *S. haematobium* infections in Egypt. III. Extrahepatic pathology. *Am. J. Trop. Med. Hyg.*, 1978; 27:55–60.

33. Daneshmend, T. K.; Homeida, M.; Satir, A. A.; Vandervelde, E. M. Increased hepatitis B infection in hepatosplenic schistosomiasis in the Sudan. *East Afr. Med. J.*, 1984; 61:133–135.

34. Edington, G. M.; Von Lichtenberg, F.; Nwabuebo, J.; Taylor, J. R.; Smith, J. H. Pathological effects of schistosomiasis in Ibadan, western state of Nigeria. *Am. J. Trop. Med. Hyg.*, 1970; 19:982–994.

35. Williams, E. H.; Williams, P. H. A note on an apparent similarity of distribution of

onchocerciasis, femoral hernia, and Kaposi's sarcoma in the West Nile District of Uganda. *East Afr. Med. J.*, 1966; 43:208–209.

36. Smith, J. H.; Kamel, I. A.; Elwi, A.; Von Lichtenberg, F. A quantitative post mortem analysis of urinary schistosomiasis in Egypt. *Am. J. Trop. Med. Hyg.*, 1974; 23:1054–1069.

37. Poiesz, B. J.; Ruscetti, F. W.; Gazdar, A. F.; Bunn, P. A.; Minna, J. D.; Gallo, R. C. Detection and isolation of type C retrovirus particles from fresh and cultured lymphocytes of a patient with cutaneous T-cell lymphoma. *Proc. Natl. Acad. Sci. USA*, 1980; 77:7415–7419.

38. Gallo, R. C.; Wong-Staal, F. Retroviruses as etiologic agents of some animals and human leukemias and lymphomas and as tools for elucidating the molecular mechanism of leukemogenesis. *Blood*, 1982; 60:545–557.

39. Gallo, R. C.; Sarin, P. S.; Blattner, W. A.; Wong-Staal, F.; Popovic, M. T-cell malignancies and human T-cell leukemia virus. *Semin. Oncol.*, 1984; 11:12–17.

40. Wong-Staal, F.; Gallo, R. C. The family of human T-cell lymphotropic leukemia viruses: HTLV-I as the cause of adult T-cell leukemia and HTLV-III as the cause of acquired immuno-deficiency syndrome. *Blood*, 1985; 65:253–263.

41. Blattner, W. A.; Blayney, D. W.; Robert-Guroff, M.; Sarngadharan, M. G.; et al. Epidemiology of human T-cell leukemia/lymphoma virus. *J. Infect. Dis.*, 1983; 147:406–414.

42. Gallo, R. C.; Blattner, W. A.; Reitz, M. S.; Ito, Y. HTLV: The virus of adult T-cell leukemia in Japan and elsewhere. *Lancet*, 1982; i:683.

43. Blattner, W. A.; Gibbs, W. N.; Saxinger, C.; Robert-Guroff, M.; Clark, J.; et al. Human T-cell leukemia/lymphoma virus associated lymphoreticular neoplasia in Jamaica. *Lancet*, 1983; ii:61–64.

44. Merino, F.; Robert-Guroff, M.; Clark, J.; et al. Natural antibodies to human T-cell leukemia/lymphoma virus in healthy Venezuela populations. *Int. J. Cancer*, 1984; 34:501–506.

45. Saxinger, W.; Blattner, W. A.; Levine, P. H.; et al. Human T-cell leukemia virus (HTLV-I) antibodies in Africa. *Science*, 1984; 225:1473–1476.

46. Aoki, T.; Miyakoshi, H.; Kolde, H.; Yoshida, T.; Ishikawa, H.; et al. Seroepidemiology of human T-lymphotropic retrovirus type-I (HTLV-I) in residents of Niigata prefecture, Japan. Comparative studies by indirect immunofluorescence microscopy and enzyme-linked immunosorbent assay. *Int. J. Cancer*, 1985; 35:301–306.

47. Manzari, V.; Gradilone, A.; Barillari, G.; et al. HTLV-I is endemic in southern Italy: Detection of the first infectious cluster in a white population. *Int. J. Cancer*, 1985; 36:557–559.

48. Robert-Guroff, M.; Clark, J.; Lanier, A. P.; et al. Prevalence of HTLV-I in arctic regions. *Int. J. Cancer*, 1985; 36:651–655.

49. Tajima, H.; Tominaga, S.; Suchi, T.; et al. Epidemiological analysis of the distribution of antibody to adult T-cell leukemia virus associated antigen: Possible horizontal transmission of adult T-cell leukemia virus. *Gann*, 1982; 73:893–901.

50. Clark, J. W.; Robert-Guroff, M.; Ikehara, O.; et al. Human T-cell leukemia-lymphoma virus type I and adult T-cell leukemia-lymphoma virus in Okinawa. *Cancer Res.*, 1985; 45:2849–2852.

51. Karitani, Y.; Kobayashi, T.; Koh, T.; et al. Adult T-cell leukemia on the east coast of Kii peninsula—presentation of an anti-ATLA-negative case. *Jpn. J. Clin. Oncol.*, 1983; 13:269–280.

52. Taguchi, H.; Fujishita, M.; Miyoshi, I.; Mizobuchi, I.; Nagasaki, A. HTLV antibody positivity and incidence of adult T-cell leukemia in Kochi prefecture, Japan. *Lancet*, 1983; ii:1029.

53. Hinuma, Y.; Chosa, T.; Komoda, H.; Mori, I.; Suzuki, M.; et al. Sporadic retrovirus (ATLV)-seropositive individuals outside Japan. *Lancet*, 1983; i:824–825.

54. Pan, I.-H.; Chung, C.; Komoda, H.; et al. Seroepidemiology of adult T-cell leukemia virus in Taiwan. *Jpn. J. Cancer Res. (Gann)*, 1985; 76:9–11.

55. Zeng, Y.; Lan, X. Y.; Fang, J.; et al. HTLV antibody in China. *Lancet*, 1984; i:799.

56. Blayney, D. W.; Jaffe, E. S.; Blattner, W. A.; et al. The human T-cell leukemia lymphoma virus associated wih American adult T-cell leukemia lymphoma. *Blood*, 1983; 62:401–405.

57. Bunn, P. A.; Schechter, G. P.; Jaffe, E.; et al. Clinical course of retrovirus-associated adult T-cell lymphoma in the United States. *N. Engl. J. Med.*, 1983; 309:257–264.

58. Reitz, M. S.; Kalyanaraman, V. S.; Robert-Guroff, M.; Popovic, M.; et al. Human T-cell leukemia/lymphoma virus: The retrovirus of adult T-cells leukemia/lymphoma. *J. Infect. Dis.*, 1983; 147:399–404.

59. Kinoshita, K.; Amagakaki, T.; Yamada, Y.; et al. Adult T-cell leukemia associated antigen (ATLA) and anti-ATLA antibodies in patients with Hodgkin's disease in the Nagasaki district. *Jpn. J. Clin. Oncol.*, 1983; 13:309–312.

60. Tochikura, T.; Iwahashi, M.; Matsumoto, T.; et al. Effect of human serum anti-HTLV

antibodies on viral antigen induction in in vitro cultured peripheral lymphocytes from adult T-cell leukemia patients and healthy virus carriers. *Int. J. Cancer*, 1985; 36:1–7.

61. The T- and B-cell Malignancy Study Group. Statistical analysis of immunologic, clinical, and histopathologic data on lymphoid malignancies in Japan. *Jpn. J. Clin. Oncol.*, 1981; 11:15–38.

62. Suchi, T.; Tajima, K. Spectrum of malignant lymphomas in Japan, with special reference to adult T-cell leukemia-lymphoma and its epidemiology. In: *Pathogenesis of Leukemias and Lymphomas: Environmental Influences*, edited by I.T. Magrath, G.T. O'Conner, and B. Ramot. Raven Press, New York, 1984, pp. 75–83.

63. Tajima, K.; Tominaga, S.; Shimizu, H.; Suchi, T. A hypothesis on the etiology of adult T-cell leukemia/lymphoma. *Gann*, 1981; 72:684.

64. Tajima, K.; Fujita, K.; Tsukidate, S.; Oda, T.; Tominaga, S.; et al. Seroepidemiological studies on the effects of filarial parasites on infestation of adult T-cell leukemia virus in the Goto Islands, Japan. *Gann*, 1983; 74:188–191.

65. Nakada, K.; Kohakura, M.; Komoda, H.; Hinuma, Y. High incidence of HTLV antibody in carriers of *Strongyloides stercoralis*. *Lancet*, 1984; i:633.

66. Sasa, M.; Kanda, T.; Mitsui, G.; Shirasaka, A.; Chinzei, H. The filariasis control programs in Japan and their evaluation by means of epidemiological analysis of the microfilaria survey data. In: *Recent Advances in Research on Filariasis and Schistosomiasis in Japan*. University of Tokyo Press, Tokyo, and University Park Press, Baltimore, 1970, pp. 3–72.

67. Piessens, W. F.; Partono, F.; Hoffman, S. L.; Ratiwayanto, S.; Piessens, P. W.; et al. Antigen-specific suppressor T lymphocytes in human lymphatic filariasis. *N. Engl. J. Med.*, 1982; 307:144–148.

68. Gill, G. V.; Bell, D. R. Strongyloidiasis and impaired immunity. *Lancet*, 1984; i:858.

69. Hahn, B. H.; Shaw, G. M.; Popovic, M.; et al. Molecular cloning and analysis of a new variant of human T-cell leukemia virus (HTLV-Ib) from an African patient with adult T-cell leukemia/lymphoma. *Int. J. Cancer*, 1984; 34:613–618.

70. Williams, C. K. O.; Alabi, G. O.; Junaid, T. A.; et al. Human T-cell leukemia virus associated lymphoproliferative disease. Report of two cases in Nigeria. *Br. Med. J.*, 1984; 288:1495–1496.

71. Biggar, R. J.; Johnson, B.; Oster, C.; et al. Regional variation in prevalence of antibody against human T-lymphotropic virus types I and III in Kenya, East Africa. *Int. J. Cancer*, 1985; 35:763–767.

72. Ben-Ishai, Z.; Haas, M.; Triglia, D.; et al. Human T-cell lympotropic virus type-I antibodies in Falashas and other ethnic groups in Israel. *Nature*, 1985; 315:665–666.

73. Schaffar-Deshayes, L.; Chavance, M.; Monplaisir, N.; Courouce, A.; Gessain, A.; et al. Antibodies to HTLV-I p24 in sera of blood donors, elderly people and patients with hemophilic diseases in France and in French West Indies. *Int. J. Cancer*, 1984; 34:667–670.

74. De-Thé, G.; Gessain, A.; Gazzolo, L.; et al. Comparative seroepidemiology of HTLV-I and HTLV-III in the French West Indies and some African countries. *Cancer Res.* (Suppl.), 1985; 45:4633s–4636s.

75. Biggar, R. J.; Saxinger, C.; Gardnier, C.; et al. Type-I HTLV antibody in urban and rural Ghana, West Africa. *Int. J. Cancer*, 1984; 34:215–219.

76. Vilmer, E.; Le Deist, F.; Fischer, A.; et al. Smouldering T-lymphoma related to HTLV-I in a Sicilian child. *Lancet*, 1985; ii:1301–1302.

77. Brun-Vézinet, F.; Rouzioux, C.; Barre-Sinoussi, F.; et al. Detection of IgG antibodies to lymphadenopathy-associated virus in patients with AIDS or lymphadenopathy syndrome. *Lancet*, 1984; i:1253–1256.

78. Levy, J. A.; Hoffman, A. D.; Kramer, S. M.; et al. Isolation of lymphotropic retroviruses from San Francisco patients with AIDS. *Science*, 1984; 225:840–842.

79. Popovic, M.; Sarngadharan, M. G.; Read, E.; Gallo, R. C. Detection, isolation, and continuous production of cytopathic retroviruses (HTLV-III) from patients with AIDS and pre-AIDS. *Science*, 1984; 224:497–500.

80. Sanchez-Pescador, R.; Power, M. D.; Barr, P. J.; et al. Nucleotide sequence and expression of and AIDS-associated retrovirus. *Science*, 1985; 227:484–492.

81. Gallo, R. C.; Salahuddin, S. Z.; Popovic, M.; Shearer, G. M.; Kaplan, M.; et al. Frequent detection and isolation of cytopathic retroviruses (HTLV-III) from patients with AIDS and at risk for AIDS. *Science*, 1984; 224:500–503.

82. Vilmer, E.; Barre-Sinoussi, F.; Rouziouz, C.; Gazengel, C.; Brun-Vézinet, F.; et al. Isolation of new lymphotropic retrovirus from two siblings with hemophilia B, one with AIDS. *Lancet*, 1984; i:753–757.

83. Kalyanarman, V. S.; Cabradilla, C. D.; Getchell, J. P.; et al. Antibodies to the core protein of lymphadenopathy-associated virus (LAV) in patients with AIDS. *Science*, 1984; 225:321–324.

84. Gazzolo, L.; Robert-Guroff, M.; Jennings, A.; et al. Type-I and type-III HTLV antibodies in hospitalized and out-patient Zairians. *Int. J. Cancer*, 1985; 36:373–378.

85. Gazzolo, L.; Gessain, A.; Robin, Y.; et al. Antibodies to HTLV-III in Haitian immigrants in French Guiana. *N. Eng. J. Med.*, 1984; 311:1253.

86. Koenig, R. E.; Pittaluga, J.; Bogart, M.; et al. Detection of antibodies to AIDS-associated retroviruses (ARV) in the Dominican Republic. International Conference on AIDS, Atlanta, April 14–17, 1985, p. 67.

87. Volsky, D. J.; Yin, T. W.; Stevenson, M.; Dewhurst, S.; et al. Antibodies to HTLV-III/LAV in Venezuelan patients with acute malarial infections. *N. Engl. J. Med.*, 1986; 314:647.

88. Rodriguez, L.; Dewhurst, S.; Sinangil, F.; et al. Antibody to HTLV-III/LAV among aboriginal Amazonian Indians in Venezuela. *Lancet*, 1985; ii:1098–1100.

89. Hehlmann, R.; Kreeb, G.; Erfle, V.; et al. Antibodies to HTLV-III in patients with the acquired immunodeficiency syndrome or lymphadenopathy syndrome in West Germany. *Lancet*, 1984; ii:1094.

90. Cooper, D. A.; Gold, J.; May, W.; et al. The spectrum of clinical and immunological response to ARV infection. International Conference on AIDS, Atlanta, April 14–17, 1985, p. 44.

91. Moss, A. R.; Osmond, D.; Bachetti, P.; et al. One year follow-up of men exposed to AIDS in San Francisco. International Conference on AIDS, Atlanta, April 14–17, 1985, p. 83.

92. Vogt, M. W.; Schüpbach, J.; Bhushan, R.; et al. Antibodies to HTLV-III in Swiss patients with AIDS, AIDS related complex (ARC), AIDS risk groups and in refugees from central Africa. International Conference on AIDS, Atlanta, April 14–17, 1985, p. 52.

93. Cheingsong-Popov, R.; Weiss, R. A.; Dalgleish, A.; et al. Prevalence of antibody to human T-lymphotropic virus type III in AIDS and AIDS-risk patients in Britain. *Lancet*, 1984; ii:477–480.

94. Gürtler, L. G.; Wernicke, D.; Eberle, J.; et al. Increase in prevalence of anti-HTLV-III in hemophiliacs. *Lancet*, 1984; i:240–241.

95. Kitchen, L. W.; Barin, F.; Sullivan, L.; et al. Aetiology of AIDS—antibodies to human T-cell leukemia virus (type III) in haemophiliacs. *Nature*, 1984; 312:367–369.

96. Spira, T. J.; Des Jarlais, D. C.; Marmor, M.; et al. Prevalence of antibody to lymphadenopathy-associated virus among drug-detoxification patients in New York. *N. Engl. J. Med.*, 1984; 311:467–468.

97. Mortimer, P. P.; Pereira, M. S.; Jesson, W. J.; Vanderveld, E. M. Antibody to HTLV-III in British homosexuals, hemophiliacs and drug addicts. International Conference on AIDS, Atlanta, April 14–17, 1985, p. 85.

98. Weiss, S. H.; Ginzberg, H. M.; Goedert, R. J.; et al. Risk for HTLV-III exposure and AIDS among parenteral drug abusers in New Jersey. International Conference on AIDS, Atlanta, April 14–17, 1985, p. 66.

99. Biggar, R. J.; Gigase, P. L.; Melbye, M.; et al. ELISA HTLV retrovirus antibody reactivity associated with malaria and immune complexes in healthy Africans. *Lancet*, 1985; ii:520–523.

100. Francis, H.; Mann, J.: Quinn, T.; Curran, J.; et al. Immunological profile of AIDS and other parasitic infections in Africa and their relationship to HTLV-III infection. International Conference on AIDS, Atlanta, April 14–17, 1985, p. 50.

101. Biggar, R. J. The AIDS problem in Africa. *Lancet*, 1986; i:79–82.

102. Hunsmann, G.; Schneider, J.; Wendler, I.; Fleming, A. F. HTLV positivity in Africans. *Lancet*, 1985; ii:952–953.

103. Clumeck, N.; Sonnet, J.; Taelman, M.; et al. Acquired immunodeficiency syndrome in African patients. *N. Engl. J. Med.*, 1984; 310:492–497.

104. Piot, P.; Quinn, T.; Taelman, H.; et al. Acquired immunodeficiency syndrome in a heterosexual population in Zaire. *Lancet*, 1984; ii:65–69.

105. Edwards, D.; Harper, P. G.; Pain, A. K.; et al. Kaposi's sarcoma associated with AIDS in a woman from Uganda. *Lancet*, 1984; i:631.

106. Pitchenick, A. E.; Fischl, M. A.; Dickinson, G. M.; et al. Opportunistic infections and Kaposi's sarcoma among Haitians, evidence of a new acquired immunodeficiency state. *Ann. Intern. Med.*, 1983; 98:227–284.

107. Moore, J. D.; Buster, S. H. Intestinal parasites in Haitian entrants. *J. Infect. Dis.*, 1984; 150:965.

108. Whiteside, M. E.; Witmum, B.; Tavris, B.; Macleod, C. Outbreak of no identifiable risk AIDS in Belle Glade, Florida. International Conference on AIDS, Atlanta, April 14–17, 1985, W-84 poster, p. 84.

109. Chin, A. T. L.; Gerken, A. Carriage of intestinal protozoal cysts in homosexuals. *Br. J. Vener. Dis.*, 1984; 60:193–195.

110. Imperato, P. J. Conclusions about amebiasis. *Bull. N.Y. Acad. Med.*, 1981; 57:240.

111. Fodor, T. Unanswered questions about the treatment of amebiasis. *Bull. N.Y. Acad. Sci.*, 1981; 57(3):224.

112. Kean, B. H. Clinical amebiasis in New York City: symptoms, signs, and treatment. *Bull. N.Y. Acad. Med.*, 1981; 57:207.

113. Dritz, S. K. Medical aspects of homosexuality. *N. Engl. J. Med.*, 1980; 302:463–464.

114. Ortega, H. B.; Borchardt, K. A.; Hamilton, R.; Ortega, P.; Mahood, J. Enteric pathogenic protozoa in homosexual men from San Francisco. *Sex. Transm. Dis.*, 1984; 11:59–63.

115. Markell, E. K.; Havens, R. F.; Kuritsubo, R. A. Intestinal parastic infections in homosexual men at a San Francisco health fair. *West. J. Med.*, 1983; 139:177–178.

116. Markell, E. K.; Kuritsubo, R. A. Intestinal protozoan infections: Prevalence in the San Francisco Bay Area. *West. J. Med.*, 1981; 135:188–190.

117. Ziegler, J. L.; Drew, W. L.; Miner, R. C.; Mintz, L.; et al. Outbreak of Burkitt's-like lymphoma in homosexual men. *Lancet*, 1982; ii:631–632.

118. Golden, J. *Pneumocystis* lung disease in homosexual men—medical staff conference. *West. J. Med.*, 1982; 11:400–407.

119. Gottlieb, M. S.; Schroff, R.; Schanker, H. M.; et al. *Pneumocystic carinii* pneumonia and mucosal candidiasis in previously healthy homosexual men. *N. Engl. J. Med.*, 1981; 305:1425–1431.

120. Hymes, K. B.; Cheung, T.; Greene, J. B.; et al. Kaposi's sarcoma in homosexual men— a report of eight cases. *Lancet*, 1981; ii:598–600.

121. Miller, J.; Barrett, R. E.; Britton, C. B.; et al. Progressive multifocal leukoencephalopathy in a male homosexual with T-cell immune deficiency. *N. Engl. J. Med.*, 1982; 307:1436–1437.

122. Kornfeld, H.; Vande Stouwe, R. A.; Lange, M.; et al. T-lymphocyte subpopulations in homosexual men. *N. Engl. J. Med.*, 1982; 307:729–731.

123. Seigal, F. P.; Lopez, C.; Hammert, G. S.; et al. Severe acquired immunodeficiency in male homosexuals manifested by chronic perianal ulcerative herpes simplex lesions. *N. Engl. J. Med.*, 1981; 305:1439.

124. Follansbee, S. E.; Busch, D. F.; Wofsy, C.; et al. An outbreak of *Pneumocystic carinii* pneumonia in homosexual men. *Ann. Intern. Med.*, 1982; 96:705–713.

125. Gerstoft, J.; Malchon-Møller, A.; Bygbjerg, I.; et al. Severe acquired immunodeficiency in European homosexual men. *Br. Med. J.*, 1982; 285:17–19.

126. Soave, R.; Danner, R. L.; Honig, C. L.; et al. Cryptosporidiosis in homosexual men. *Ann. Intern. Med.*, 1984; 100:504–511.

127. Marmor, M.; Friedman-Kien, A.; Laubenstein, L.; et al. Risk factors for Kaposi's sarcoma in homosexual men. *Lancet*, 1982; i:1083–1086.

128. René, E.; Régnier, B.; Seimot, A. G.; et al. Gastrointestinal infections during AIDS. *Lancet*, 1984; i:915.

129. Homme, T.; Kanki, P. J.; King, N. W.; Hunt, R. D. Lymphoma in macaques: Association with virus of human T lymphotropic family. *Science*, 1984; 225:716–718.

130. Hunt, R. D.; Blake, B. J.; Chalifoux, L. V.; Sehgal, P. K.; King, N. W.; Letvin, N. L. Transmission of naturally occuring lymphoma in macaque monkeys. *Proc. Natl. Acad. Sci. USA*, 1983; 80:5085–5089.

131. Daniel, M. D.; Letvin, N. L.; King, N. W. Isolation of T-cell tropic HTLV-III like retrovirus from macaques. *Science* 1985; 228:1201–1204.

132. Arambulo, P. V.; Abass, J. B.; Walker, J. S. Silver leaf-monkeys (*Presbytis cristatus*). II. Gastrointestinal parasites and their treatment. *Lab. Anim. Sci.*, 1974; 24:299–302.

133. Reardon, L. V.; Rininger, B. F. A survey of parasites in laboratory primates. *Lab. Anim. Care.*, 1968; 18:577–580.

134. Van Riper, D. C.; Day, P. W.; Fineg, J.; Prine, J. R. Intestinal parasites of recently imported chimpanzees. *Lab. Anim. Care*, 1966; 16:360–362.

135. Le Bras, J.; Larouze, B.; Geniteau, M.; Andrieu, B.; Dazza, M. C.; Rodhain, F. Malaria, arbovirus, and hepatitis infections in *Macaca fascicularis* from Malaysia. *Lab. Anim.*, 1984; 18:61–64.

136. Stowell, R. E.; Smith, E. K.; España, C.; Nelson, V. G. Outbreak of malignant lymphoma in rhesus monkeys. *Lab. Invest.*, 1971; 25:476–479.

137. Manning, J. R. S.; Griesemer, R. A. Spontaneous lymphoma of the nonhuman primate. *Lab. Anim. Sci.*, 1974; 24:204–210.

138. Wong, M. M.; Kozek, W. J. Spontaneous toxoplasmosis in macaques: A report of four cases. *Lab. Anim. Care*, 1974; 24:273–277.

139. Fine, D. L. Mason-Pfizer monkey virus and simian AIDS. *Lancet*, 1984; i:335.

140. Hendrickson, R. V.; Maul, D. H.; Osborn, K. G.; et al. Epidemic of acquired immunodeficiency in rhesus monkeys. *Lancet*, 1983; i:388–390.

141. Ferrer, J. F.; Piper, C. E.; Abt, D. A.; et al. Natural mode of transmission of the bovine C type leukemia virus (BLV). *Comp. Leuk. Res.*, 1975; 43:235.

142. Ehleringer, J. R.; Schulze, E. D.; Ziegler, H.; et al. Bovine leukemia virus-related antigens in lymphocyte cultures infected with AIDS-associated viruses. *Science*, 1985; 227:1482–1484.

143. Malmquist, W. A. *Preliminary Report of Progress for 7/1/64–6/30/65.* Animal Disease and Parasite Research Division, USDA, Washington, D.C., 1965.

144. Hare, W. C. D.; Soulsby, E. J. L.; Abt, D. A. Bovine trypanosomiasis and lymphocytosis parallel studies. In: *Comparative Leukemia Research 1969, Bibl. Haematol.* No. 36, ed. R. M. Dutcher. Karger, Basel, pp. 504–517, 1970.

145. Onions, D. Animal models: Lessons from feline and bovine leukemia virus infections. *Leuk. Res.*, 1985; 9:709–711.

146. Gallo, R. C.; Sarin, P. S.; Gelmann, E. P.; Robert-Guroff, M.; Richardson, E.; et al. Isolation of human T-cell leukemia virus in acquired immune deficiency syndrome (AIDS). *Science*, 1983; 220:865–868.

147. Zagury, D.; Bernard, J.; Leonard, R.; et al. Long-term cultures of HTLV-III infected T-cells: A model of cytopathology of T-cell depletion in AIDS. *Science*, 1986; 231:850–853.

148. Francis, D. P.; Ferino, P. M.; et al. Infection of chimpanzees with lymphadenopathy-associated virus. *Lancet*, 1984; ii:1276–1277.

149. Alter, H. J.; Eichberg, J. W.; Masur, H.; et al. Transmission of HTLV-III infection from human plasma to chimpanzees: An animal model for AIDS. *Science*, 1984; 226:549–552. Pearce, R. B. Intestinal protozoal infections and AIDS. *Lancet*, 1983; ii:51.

150. Tsoukas, C.; Gervais, F.; Shuster, J.; et al. Association of HTLV-III antibodies and cellular immune status of hemophiliacs. *N. Engl. J. Med.*, 1984; 311:1514–1515.

151. Rogers, J. S.; Raich, P. C. Altered cellular immunity in hemophilia. *Clin. Res.*, 1983; 31:321a.

152. Layon, J.; Idris, A.; Warzynski, M.; et al. Altered T-lymphocyte subsets in hospitalized intravenous drug abusers. *Arch. Intern. Med.*, 1984; 14:1376–1380.

153. Horne, C. H. W.; Armstrong, S. S.; Thomson, A. W.; Thompson, W. D. Detection of pregnancy associated alpha-2-glycoprotein (PAG), an immunosuppressive agent, in IgA producing plasma cells and in body secretions. *Clin Exp. Immunol.*, 1983; 51:631–638.

154. Baley, J. E.; Schacter, B. Z. Mechanisms of diminished natural killer cell activity in pregnant women and neonates. *J. Immunol.*, 1985; 134:3042–3045.

155. Kessler, C. M.; Schulof, R. S.; Goldstein, A. L. Abnormal T-lymphocyte subpopulations associated with transfusion of blood-derived products. *Lancet*, 1983; i:911–912.

156. Hollan, S. R.; Füst, G.; Nagy, K.; et al. Immunological and virological studies in AIDS risk groups in Hungary. International Conference on AIDS, Atlanta, April 14–17, 1985, p. 70.

157. Bibberfeld, G.; Bottiger, M.; Karlsson, A.; et al. HTLV-III antibodies and T-cell subpopulations in homosexual men in Sweden. International Conference on AIDS, Atlanta, April 14–17, 1985; W-49 Poster, p. 80.

158. Giorgi, J.; Nishanian, P. G.; Afrasiabi, R. T-cell subset alterations in homosexual men: Relationship to HTLV-III/LAV infection. International Conference on AIDS, Atlanta, April, 14–17, 1985, W-61 poster, p. 82.

159. Frazer, I. R.; Mackay, I. R.; Gust, E. D.; et al. Deficient cell-mediated immunity in healthy homosexual men negative for antibody to HTLV-III virus. International Conference on AIDS, Atlanta, April 14–17, 1985, p. 33.

160. Sirianni, M. C.; Rossi, P.; Scarpati, B.; et al. Immunological and virological investigation in patients with lymphadenopathy syndrome and in a population at risk for AIDS, with particular focus on the detection of antibodies to HTLV-III. *J. Clin. Immunol.*, 1985; 5:261.

161. Marmor, M.; Elsadr, W.; Zolla-Panzer, S.; et al. HTLV-III seropositivity and its relationship to disease in a prospective study of homosexual males. International Conference on AIDS, Atlanta, April 14–17, 1985, session 8, p. 27.

162. Minchinton, R. M.; Frazer, I. Idiopathic neutropenia in homosexual men. *Lancet*, 1985; i:936.

163. Kiprov, D. D.; Anderson, R. E.; Morand, P. R.; et al. Antilymphocyte antibodies and

80   R. B. PEARCE

seropositivity for retroviruses for groups at high risk for AIDS. *N. Engl. J. Med.*, 1985; 312:1517–1518.

164. Tung, K. S. K.; Koster, F.; Bernstein, D. C.; et al. Elevated allogeneic cytolytic T-lymphocyte activity in peripheral blood leukocytes of homosexual men. *J. Immunol.*, 1985; 135:3163–3171.

165. Ludlam, C. A.; Tucker, J.; Steel, C. M.; et al. Human T-lymphotropic virus type III (HTLV-III) infections in seronegative haemophiliacs after transfusion of factor VIII. *Lancet*, 1985; ii:233–236.

166. Cohen, J.; Winearls, C.; Olivera, D.; Williams, G. Opportunistic AIDS. *Lancet*, 1984; ii:1209–1210.

167. Salahuddin, S. Z.; Groopman, J. E.; Markham, P. D. HTLV-III in symptom-free seronegative persons. *Lancet*, 1984; ii:1418–1420.

168. Ranki, A.; Valle, S.; Antonen, J.; et al. Immunosuppression in homosexual men seronegative for HTLV-III. *Cancer Res.*, 1985; 45 (Suppl.):4616s.

169. Anders, R. F.; et al. Giardiasis in mice: Analysis of humoral and cellular immune responses to *Giardia muris*. *Parasite Immunol.*, 1982; 4:47–57.

170. Diamanstein, T.; Klos, M.; Gold, D.; Hahn, H. Interaction between *Entamoeba histolytica* and the immune system. I. Mitogenicity of *E. histolytica* extracts for human peripheral T-lymphocytes. *J. Immunol.*, 1981; 126:2084–2086.

171. Feldmeier, H.; Gastl, G. A.; et al. Relationship between intensity of infection and immunomodulation in human schistosomiasis. I. Lymphocyte subpopulations and specific antibody responses. *Clin. Exp. Immunol.*, 1985; 60:225–233.

172. Feldmeier, H.; Gastl, G. A.; et al. Relationship between intensity of infection and immunomodulation in human schistosomiasis. II. NK cell activity and in vitro lymphocyte proliferation. *Clin. Exp. Immunol.*, 1985; 60:234–240.

173. Kamal, K. A.; Higashi, G. I. Suppression of mitogen-induced lymphocyte transformation by plasma from patients with hepatosplenic *Schistosomiasis mansoni*: Role of immune complexes. *Parasite Immunol.*, 1982; 4:283.

174. Troye-Blomberg, M.; Sjoholm, P. E.; Perlmann, H.; Patarroyo, M. E.; Perlman, P. Regulation of the immune response in *Plasmodium falciparum* malaria. I. Non-specific proliferative responses in vitro and characterization of lymphocytes. *Clin. Exp. Immunol.*, 1983; 53:335–344.

175. Wellhausen, S. R.; Manfield, J. M. Lymphocyte function in experimental African trypanosomiasis. II. Splenic suppressor cell activity. *J. Immunol.*, 1979; 122:818–824.

176. Mitchell, G. F. Invited review. Host-parasite responses. *Pathology*, 1981; 13:659–667.

177. Nussenzweig, R. S. Parasitic disease as a cause of immunosuppression. *N. Engl. J. Med.*, 1982; 306:423–424.

178. Carswell, F.; Hughes, A. O.; Palmer, R. I.; et al. Nutritional status, globulin titers, and parasitic infections of two populations of Tanzanian school children. *Am. J. Clin. Nutr.*, 1981; 34:1292–1299.

179. Salem, E.; Zaki, S. A.; et al. Autoantibody in amoebic colitis. *J. Egypt Med. Assoc.*, 1973; 56:113–118.

180. Kobiler, D.; Mirelman, D. A lectin activity in *Entamoeba histolytica* trophozoites. *Arch. Invest. Med.*, 1983; 98:227–284.

181. Ghadirian, E.; Mearovitch, E. Macrophage requirement for host defense against experimental hepatic amoebiasis in the hamster. *Parasite Immunol.*, 1982; 4:219–225.

182. Cheever, A. W. Schistosomiasis and neoplasia. *JNCI*, 1978; 61:13.

183. Davies, D. H.; et al. The biological significance of the immune response with special reference to parasites and cancer. *J. Parasitol.*, 1980; 66:705.

184. Vinayak, V. K.; Jain, P.; Gupta, B.; et al. Cellular and humoral immune responses in amoebic patients. *Trop. Geogr. Med.*, 1980; 32:298–302.

185. De Simone, C.; Cilli, A.; Zanzoglu, S.; et al. Anti-Ia reactivity in sera from subjects with *Entamoeba histolytica* infection. *Trans. R. Soc. Trop. Med. Hyg.*, 1984; 78:64–68.

186. Jason, J.; Hilgartner, M.; Holman, R. C.; et al. Immune status of blood product recipients. *JAMA*, 1985; 253:1140–1145.

187. Curran, J. W.; and Barker, L. F. The acquired immunodeficiency syndrome associated with transfusions: The evolving perspective. *Ann. Intern. Med.*, 1984; 100(2):298–299.

188. Perkins, H. A.; Samson, S.; Rosenschein, S.; et al. Risk of AIDS from blood donors who subsequently develop AIDS. International Conference on AIDS, Atlanta, April 14–17, 1985, session 13, p. 46.

189. Wykoff, R. F.; Perl, E. R.; Saulsbury, F. I. Immunological dysfunction in infants infected through transfusion of HTLV-III. *N. Engl. J. Med.*, 1985; 312:294–296.

190. Feorino, P. M.; Jaffe, H. W.; Palmer, E.; et al. Transfusion-associated acquired immunodeficiency syndrome: Evidence for persistent infection in blood donors. *N. Engl. J. Med.*, 1985; 312:1293–1296.

191. Curran, J. W.; Lawrence, D. N.; Jaffe, H. W.; et al. Acquired immunodeficiency syndrome associated with transfusions. *N. Engl. J. Med.*, 310:69–75.

192. Vilmer, E.; Fischer, A.; Grischelli, C.; et al. Possible transmission of a human lymphotropic retrovirus (LAV) from mother to infant with AIDS. *Lancet*, 1984; ii:229–230.

193. Shimotohno, K.; Temin, H. M. Evolution of retroviruses from cellular movable genetic elements. Cold Spring Harbor Symposium on RNA Retroviruses, 1979.

194. Gallo, R. C.; Sliski, A.; Wong-Staal, F. Origin of HTLV. *Lancet*, 1983; ii:962–963.

195. Hinuma, Y.; Chosa, T.; Komoda, H.; et al. Sporadic retrovirus (ATLV)-seropositive individuals outside Japan. *Lancet*, 1983; i:824–825.

196. Greenberg, A. E.; Schable, C. A.; Sulzer, A. J.; et al. Evaluation of serological cross-reactivity between antibodies to plasmodium and HTLV-III/LAV. *Lancet*, 1986; ii:247–249.

TREATMENT

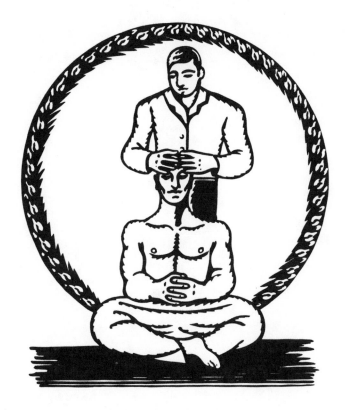

Treatment
A relaxed patient receives a head message and radiates a halo of renewed energy.

7

Treatment Issues in AIDS

Ellen C. Cooper

BACKGROUND

Acquired immune deficiency syndrome (AIDS) presents one of the most complex therapeutic challenges of any disease ever described. While fundamentally a systemic viral infection, its hallmark is a profound immune deficiency that leaves the human host susceptible to many opportunistic infections (OIs) that eventually lead to death in most patients. The most common AIDS-defining OI in the United States is pneumonia due to *Pneumocystis carinii*, a ubiquitous parasite that causes life-threatening pulmonary infection in the immunocompromised host. Other organisms causing OIs in patients with AIDS include cytomegalovirus (CMV), *Mycobacterium avium intracellulare* (MAI), *Toxoplasma gondii*, *Cryptococcus neoformans*, *Candida albicans*, and *Cryptosporidium*. In addition, individuals infected with the human immunodeficiency virus (HIV)* are at increased risk for developing malignancies, the most common by far being Kaposi's sarcoma (KS). It is not understood why some HIV-infected individuals develop KS, often months or even years before developing their first major opportunistic infection, while others are spared this manifestation of the disease. Epidemiologic evidence suggests the role of a cofactor, which may be particularly prevalent in the male homosexual population.[1]

Once an infected individual develops an AIDS-defining opportunistic infection, median life expectancy is reported as a year or less, while individuals with cutaneous KS as their only AIDS-defining condition have a somewhat longer survival.[2] Individuals infected with HIV may also die of their infection before they develop classic AIDS, for instance, from a progressive wasting syndrome resulting in death without the diagnosis of an OI, or from complications of HIV infection of the brain causing a debilitating neurologic syndrome called AIDS-dementia complex (both of these conditions were added to the CDC surveillance definition of AIDS in August 1987).[2a]

Thus it is apparent that treatment of persons with AIDS requires a multifaceted approach. First and foremost, in a destructive disease process thought to be dependent on continued viral replication, the retroviral infection must be

---

*The primary etiologic agent of AIDS. The virus is also referred to as HTLV-III (human T-lymphotropic virus), LAV (lymphadenopathy-associated virus), and ARV (AIDS-related virus).

I thank Dr. Robert Yarchoan of the Clinical Oncology Program, National Cancer Institute, National Institutes of Health, Bethesda, Maryland, and Dr. H. Clifford Lane of the Laboratory of Immunoregulation, National Institute of Allergy and Infectious Diseases, National Institutes of Health, Bethesda, Maryland, for their helpful comments and critical review of the manuscript. I also thank Ms. Betty McRoy for her technical assistance.

controlled in order for any additional treatment to have lasting benefit. An ideal antiviral therapy would be capable of eliminating the virus from the body, but no such agent is available today even in an experimental stage. HIV appears to integrate into the host DNA of some cells it infects[3] where it presumably remains and is inaccessible to existing compounds that act on actively replicating viruses. This so-called provirus may remain latent for long periods of time in some cells, while in others it produces copies of itself and viral proteins in enormous quantities. The result is a lytic (destructive) infection which kills the cell and releases many virions into the extracellular environment that are then able to infect other susceptible host cells. It is also believed that the virus may move from cell to cell directly, without an extracellular phase. An effective antiviral agent could presumably act at one or both phases by inhibiting the process of viral replication itself or by interfering with viral penetration into uninfected cells. Because there is little optimism that an agent that can selectively destroy integrated viral DNA will be developed in the foreseeable future, it is presumed that antiviral treatment will need to be chronic, probably lifelong. Therefore it is important that it be relatively nontoxic and available in a convenient formulation for outpatient administration (e.g., oral). It should also cross the blood-brain barrier in sufficient quantity to inhibit viral replication in the central nervous system.

The second aspect of AIDS that may require treatment is the immune deficiency that develops sometime after initial infection with HIV but is always present to a significant extent once an AIDS-defining opportunistic infection develops. The immune deficiency is primarily cellular, although humoral (contained in serum) immunity is also affected.[4] It may be that in earlier stages of HIV infection, effective treatment of the retroviral infection alone will halt progression of the disease and specific immunotherapy will not be required, but no such agent has yet been demonstrated to accomplish this goal.

For persons with more advanced disease, effective control of the virus may not permit sufficient recovery of immune cells such that specific immunotherapy is not needed. However, some researchers believe that if an effective nontoxic antiretroviral agent is developed, even the most advanced patients may be able to recover without additional immunotherapy, as long as a minimum critical number of uninfected thymic and stem cells remain.

There are at least three approaches that may be taken in attempting to restore immune function in patients with AIDS. One is passive administration of immune elements (such as immune globulins or white blood cells) with the hope that these substances will provide protection from infection with the multitude of organisms to which the AIDS patient is susceptible. The second approach is to attempt active immunostimulation with an agent having the ability to activate mature lymphocytes and/or induce growth and differentiation of uninfected lymphocyte precursors or stem cells. No such agent has yet been shown to be clinically effective in this manner, although several lymphokines, including interleukin 2 and gamma interferon, have been studied in small numbers of patients.[5,6] One concern with this general approach has been that lymphocyte stimulation, in the absence of effective antiviral therapy, may accelerate the disease process by making the newly activated lymphocytes more susceptible to infection with HIV, as has been observed in vitro.[7]

A third approach is to replace the major elements of the destroyed immune system by transplanting uninfected stem cells from a healthy person into the infected person (e.g., bone marrow transplant and/or thymic transplant). While this approach has a number of appealing aspects, transplantation has two important limitations: (1) the need for an HLA-compatible donor (i.e., one with similar histocompatibility locus antigens, also known as "tissue transplant" antigens), and (2) the need to control the retroviral infection in the recipient before and after transplantation without causing unacceptable toxicity to the transplanted cells, resulting in a failure of engraftment (some antiretroviral agents currently under study are quite toxic to blood cells). Bone marrow transplantation (BMT) is also an expensive procedure, with certain risks to the donor (primarily general anesthesia) and to the patient (if the donor is not an identical twin, there is the possibility of graft versus host disease). Progress has been made in the past few years in reducing the potential for this complication in recipients of allogeneic (genetically different) marrow by depleting the donor marrow of mature T cells, but some studies indicate that this approach may increase the likelihood of graft failure and/or an increased incidence of opportunistic infections.[8,9]

Another facet of treating AIDS patients is the need for effective specific therapies to treat the opportunistic infections. The infections that are AIDS-defining are frequently disseminated and life-threatening, and some of them, such as cytomegalovirus (CMV), may exacerbate the immunologic defects in these patients.[10] These infections are most commonly caused by environmental parasites, fungi, mycobacteria, and viruses, which generally require a functional cellular immune response in the host for resistance, rather than by the more usual pathogenic bacteria, although serious bacterial infections can also occur in patients with AIDS.[11] As there are many relatively nontoxic antibiotics available, and AIDS patients respond reasonably well to specific antibiotic therapy for bacterial infections, these are not usually fatal. However, there are fewer antiparasitic, antifungal, antimycobacterial, and antiviral agents available, and they are generally more toxic. In addition, since most of the opportunistic infections tend to be both severe and recurrent, intensive initial therapy is required, and prolonged "suppressive" regimens appear necessary after infection with many organisms.[12]

An additional complication of treating OIs in AIDS patients is the much higher incidence of adverse effects after administration of certain drugs, in particular sulfa-containing agents such as trimethoprim/sulfamethoxazole for *Pneumocystis carinii* pneumonia (PCP).[13] Medications causing hematologic toxicity are also likely to be less well tolerated in AIDS patients because of their already compromised hematologic status secondary to the HIV infection itself.[14]

Comprehensive medical management of AIDS patients requires the use of drugs and other therapies for the treatment of KS and the other malignancies that afflict them. Indolent, cutaneous KS does not usually require treatment unless it poses a cosmetic problem, and in that case localized radiation therapy is often temporarily effective.[15] If symptomatic visceral KS develops, more aggressive systemic chemotherapy can be used, although it is not always efficacious. Alpha-interferon is also under investigation for the treatment of KS in AIDS and has been shown to have preliminary evidence of efficacy, particularly in patients without a prior history of an OI.[16] B-cell lymphomas, especially of the central nervous system, are the second most common AIDS-associated malignancy. This condition is usually fatal within 1 year despite intensive chemotherapy, which is particularly difficult to administer to already immunocompromised individuals.[17]

An additional aspect of the medical treatment of HIV-infected individuals is the frequent need for symptomatic therapy: (1) for debilitating manifestations of the underlying infection(s) (e.g., fever, headache, diarrhea); (2) for global reactions to the disease process, both organic and reactive (e.g., depression, anxiety, insomnia); and (3) for treatment of side effects (e.g., nausea, vomiting, rashes) of the potent medications often required to treat the primary and secondary manifestations of the disease.

Finally, a special aspect of the treatment of patients with HIV infection is the management of babies and young children with AIDS. While many of the treatment issues in AIDS apply to pediatrics as well, there are several potentially important differences in the pathogenesis and manifestations of the two disease processes that may require refocusing the issues somewhat. Briefly, these differences include the following[18]:

1. An immunologically immature host infected with HIV at a very early stage of development;

2. A generally more rapid progression to death of infected children compared with adults;

3. More frequent and more severe bacterial infections; and

4. An unusual lung disease called lymphoid interstitial pneumonitis as a common disease manifestation.

THE ISSUES

One very important issue that will arise in the management of HIV-infected persons as effective antiviral therapies are developed is the decision as to when in the course of the disease to initiate treatment. The answer is not simple for at least two important reasons, and will probably vary with the particular agent under consideration. First of all, the natural history of HIV infection in terms of the risk of developing AIDS is not well established at this time. While some infected persons clearly develop AIDS rather rapidly (within a couple of years), in natural history studies reported to date,[19,20] the majority of asymptomatic patients have not progressed to AIDS after 4–5 years, and varying proportions have developed symptomatic disease. It may be that the immune systems of some individuals can effectively contain the virus early during infection and AIDS will not develop. On the other hand, another 5 years of follow-up may indicate that most, if not all, infected persons will experience progressive deterioration.

At this time, however, the existence of a latent but relatively benign lifelong infection with HIV remains a possibility in some individuals and certainly has precedent in other human viral infections caused by herpes simplex virus, Epstein-Barr virus, hepatitis B virus, and so on. Persons who are naturally able to control the virus, even if only temporarily, may be better off without specific antiviral therapy, which carries the risk that treatment may interfere with the ongoing natural host immune response. Such early intervention may actually do harm by permitting the disease to progress more rapidly should the infected individual become unable to continue antiretroviral therapy for some reason (e.g., toxicity, resistance to the drug, drug interactions).

A second reason why it is unclear at what stage of infection initiation of specific antiretroviral therapy will be beneficial is that many of the antiretroviral drugs tested in people have significant toxicities. Zidovudine (approved generic name for azidothymidine, or AZT), for instance, has been demonstrated to have benefit in prolonging life in certain patients with AIDS or advanced ARC when given for 6 months or less. However, it has significant bone marrow toxicity, which could limit its efficacy when it is taken for longer periods of time. For example, the dose may have to be reduced to subtherapeutic levels or discontinued frequently owing to severe anemia or granulocytopenia (depressed white blood cell count), or the recovery of lymphocyte number and function may eventually be inhibited by the toxicity of the drug itself. On the other hand, less advanced patients may experience less hematologic toxicity from zidovudine and therefore be able to tolerate it for longer periods, deriving a net benefit.

The argument for initiation of antiretroviral therapy in asymptomatic patients rests primarily on the twin assumptions that if the spread of the viral infection is halted early, destruction of the immune system will not occur and AIDS will not develop, and that antiretroviral drugs may have a better chance of working in patients with more intact immune systems. At this time there is no way of clearly identifying those asymptomatic infected individuals who will progress to AIDS and who therefore are more likely to benefit from early antiviral therapy than those infected individuals who are unlikely to progress, at least in the near term, and for whom the toxicities of prolonged antiviral therapy may outweigh the benefits. It has been reported that asymptomatic persons who are viremic (i.e., have virus in the blood) are at higher risk of progression[21,22] but this logical risk factor has not been thoroughly evaluated and, in any event, will be difficult to study rigorously until a reliable, interpretable method for culturing patients or assessing "viral load" is established. Several new antigen capture assays that are being developed hold some hope in this regard.[23,24]

Various laboratory immune parameters, such as elevated plasma levels of acid-labile alpha interferon,[25,26] decreased gamma interferon production by lymphocytes in vitro after stimulation with antigen,[27] declining plasma levels of erythrocyte complement 3B receptors together with triple positive Coombs test,[28] and high serum levels of antilymphocyte antibodies,[29] have been reported by different investigators to be associated with risk of progression, but they have not been studied prospectively in large numbers of individuals. A lower absolute T-helper/inducer (CD4 or T4) cell count in the peripheral blood is generally acknowledged to be correlated with risk of progression, but this association has not yet been studied closely in asymptomatic individuals over the entire spectrum of CD4 counts. In any event it is unlikely that this parameter alone will be a good early discriminator for antiviral intervention in the individual patient because destruction of T-helper/inducer cells is a consequence of HIV infection, and the aim of identifying patients early as candidates for antiretroviral therapy is to prevent this destruction.

A second issue in the treatment of HIV-infected persons involves the concept of immunorestoration: whether it is useful, and if so, at what stage of the disease it may be necessary and what might be the best approach.

Once HIV infection has progressed to the point where clinical immuno-suppression exists (manifested as an OI or neoplasm), it will likely be more difficult for antiviral treatment alone to restore health than at earlier stages of disease. As previously discussed, if HIV exists in an integrated but latent state to any significant extent in infected humans, the current and foreseeable types of antiretroviral agents will not eradicate the virus from the body. In most infections, and particularly in viral infections, the aim of antiinfective therapy is to reduce the replication of organisms and associated tissue destruction while the host immune response is developing. Organisms not destroyed by the anti-infective agent are then eliminated or held in check by the body's own newly developed immunity, cellular immune responses being of primary importance in most viral infections.[30] HIV impairs the ability of the body to develop effective cellular immunity by destroying the T-helper/inducer cells, which are critical for this function.

There is no known immunomodulator capable of restoring lost T-helper/inducer cell function. Bone marrow transplantation has theoretical promise[31] but has practical problems that will probably restrict widespread application even if it proves efficacious in individual patients. While pharmacologic doses of lymphokines such as interferon and interleukin-2 can be administered to humans, it is unlikely that such a monolithic approach will be of long-term benefit in restoring as complex and intricate a biological mechanism as the immune system (although certainly something would be learned in the attempt). It would seem that an effective immunorestorative agent needs to stimulate the differ-entiation, production, and maturation of cellular immune elements that are destroyed by HIV and thereby restore the patient's own ability to resist oppor-tunistic infections.

Because there is no proven or even promising therapy that will completely restore immunocompetence in patients with AIDS, passive immunoprophylaxis has been attempted in the form of immunoglobulin injections. This form of therapy has not been demonstrated to be particularly helpful in adults, probably because they have normal or elevated levels of immunoglobulins, which generally contain antibodies against multiple pathogens acquired earlier in life. In the pediatric population, where there has not been prior exposure to multiple an-tigens, gamma globulin may be of some benefit in preventing serious bacterial infections.[32] Whether a type of hyperimmune globulin made up of neutralizing or other antibodies to HIV will be of greater benefit remains to be seen.

A second form of passive immunotherapy, aimed at restoring cellular im-munity, consists of the repeated transfusion of peripheral blood lymphocytes from a compatible donor.[33] This approach has been further refined to involve the transfer of CD4 cell-enriched populations of lymphocytes cultured in vitro to very high numbers under special conditions before transfusion to the HIV-infected recipient. While this procedure is technically less risky to the donor than bone marrow transplantation and therefore can be performed more fre-quently, it has not been shown to be of proven benefit and has a disadvantage similar to BMT in requiring an HLA-compatible donor. Some investigators feel that intensive lymphocyte therapy may transfer a sufficient quantity of stem cells to essentially substitute for bone marrow transplantation, but this possibility remains unproved in humans at this time. For any cellular therapy to be effective, it is generally felt that inhibition of HIV replication must be achieved, or infection and destruction of the transferred lymphocytes will occur. Here again, the question of optimal dosage of an antiviral agent is critical, particularly for an agent such as zidovudine whose primary toxicity is hematologic.

A third major issue in treating HIV-infected patients involves therapies for opportunistic infections. Once an OI is diagnosed, initial treatment is usually reasonably straightforward for those infections for which there exist effective and relatively safe drug(s). Special problems in AIDS patients include the generally increased severity of such infections, their high likelihood of recurrence even after successful acute treatment, and the increased incidence of adverse reactions to standard medications.

The treatment of opportunistic infections is further complicated by the fact that for a number of OIs, no approved, effective therapy exists, in part because many of these infections were relatively rare prior to the AIDS epidemic. Examples include infection with *Mycobacterium avium intracellulare* and *Cryptosporidium*. When these infections were recognized as pathogenic in the context of AIDS several years ago, many physicians felt justified in administering experimental therapies based on in vitro susceptibility data or the sparsest of anecdotal reports of apparent efficacy. Thus a number of unproven experimental agents have become available for the "treatment" of certain OIs through a mechanism previously referred to as "compassionate INDs" (investigational new drug applications), under which unapproved drugs were made available on a case-by-case basis to patients with a particular disease. One problem with this approach, particularly in the context of the AIDS pandemic, is that after several years it is still not clear whether some of these experimental agents are truly efficacious or in fact harmful, and it becomes increasingly difficult to carry out well-controlled clinical trials, either because it is generally deemed "unethical" to withhold active drug from some patients in a placebo-controlled trial because of presumed but not proven or well-characterized efficacy, or because interest in the drug is lost, even for conducting controlled trials, because of apparent but not established lack of effectiveness. On balance, it is probably a greater disservice to patients now and in the future to permit the use of unproven drugs on a "compassionate" basis in lieu of adequately controlled, appropriately designed clinical trials in which safety and efficacy can be determined over a relatively limited period of time. The likely consequences of widespread use of unproven drugs in a disease as complex as AIDS include delayed development and approval (if ultimately demonstrated to be efficacious), excessive polypharmacy (administering several drugs concurrently), and the real risk of additional toxicity not justified by any benefit to the patient.

For many opportunistic infections, chronic "prophylaxis" or suppressive therapy is another important issue in the treatment of patients with HIV infection. For certain infections, such as cerebral toxoplasmosis, cryptococcosis, and CMV retinitis, chronic low-dose therapy following acute treatment is generally accepted as necessary because of the very high relapse rate when therapy is discontinued. For other infections, notably PCP, the value of either primary or secondary prophylaxis is less clear for several reasons. After an initial episode of PCP, the relapse or recurrence rate is under 50% (although the proportion of patients who develop a second episode may increase in patients on zidovudine if life expectancy is increased signficantly); acute treatment of a second episode (particularly if detected early) is usually successful; there is concern that resistant organisms may develop with prolonged use of subtherapeutic doses usually given for prophylaxis; and the available drugs most appropriate for prophylaxis, such as trimethoprim sulfamethoxazole (TMP-SMX) and pyrimethamine sulfamethionine, contain sulfa components, which are poorly tolerated in many patients with AIDS. New therapies, notably aerosolized pentamidine, have been enthusiastically embraced for PCP prophylaxis in some parts of the country, but no controlled trials have been reported to date. A controlled trial of TMP-SMX for PCP prophylaxis was reported recently by Fischl et al.,[34] in which HIV-infected patients with a history of KS were randomly assigned to receive either TMP-SMX twice a day or no treatment. Sixty patients were enrolled and followed for at least 2 years. The patients taking chronic TMP-SMX experienced significantly fewer episodes of PCP and had prolonged survival compared to the untreated group. Fifty percent (15) of the patients on TMP-SMX experienced adverse events, primarily skin rashes, but only five had reactions severe enough to necessitate drug discontinuation.

As alluded to previously, another concern in the treatment of patients with AIDS is polypharmacy, or the concurrent administration of a number of drugs, particularly on a chronic basis. When chronic antiretroviral therapy becomes commonplace, the problem of drug interactions from concomitant therapy will become more prominent. Many of the drugs used to treat OIs have significant toxicity at the doses required, and administration of two or more drugs at the same time can be expected to result in additive or even synergistic toxicity, and also possibly to result in diminished efficacy for one or the other agent because of competition for similar enzymatic, metabolic, or excretory pathways in the body. A recent report of in vitro antagonism between zidovudine and ribavirin is a good example.

On the other hand, in vitro testing of agents against HIV shows that some combinations of drugs may result in synergistic (more than additive) efficacy.[35,36] Several such combinations of agents are being considered for human trials, and at least two have already begun. In these situations, the administration of the second drug is based on a sound scientific rationale under which it is hoped that either efficacy will be improved or toxicity will be reduced or both. Appropriate combinations of proven antiretroviral agents may also be tested, when available, to see if lower and therefore less toxic doses of each drug are effective when administered concurrently, and also to determine whether potential resistance to the drugs by the virus can be prevented or reduced by combining agents with different mechanisms of action. This latter approach has proven utility in the treatment of certain other infections (e.g., tuberculosis)[37] but remains to be established for viral infection, including HIV. A third rationale for combined therapy is the use of an antiretroviral with an immunomodulator in patients with various degrees of immunodeficiency. Again, the aim is to achieve efficacy that cannot be obtained by either therapy alone.

Certain public health aspects of AIDS, such as prevention of transmission of the virus, are very important but have not generated treatment issues per se until recently. As clinically efficacious antiretroviral agents become available, questions regarding their usefulness in reducing the probability that an infected individual will transmit the virus to others and their potential role as "prophylactics" if taken immediately before or after exposure to a potential source of infection will surely be raised.

SPECIFIC ANTIRETROVIRAL AGENTS

The antiretroviral drug zidovudine (which is marketed under the trade name Retrovir and manufactured by Burroughs Wellcome Company) is a nucleoside analog that has been demonstrated to delay death and increase the time to development of OIs in certain patients with advanced AIDS-related complex (ARC) or "early" AIDS/OI. In early 1985 it was shown to markedly reduce evidence of HIV replication at low concentrations in laboratory assays,[38] and it appeared reasonably nontoxic in early short-term animal studies. Zidovudine was administered to human beings for the first time in July 1985 at the National Cancer Institute (NCI) in a small pilot study designed to obtain pharmacokinetic data and to study tolerance (toxic effects), first at low doses, and then at higher doses as tolerated, in patients with AIDS or advanced ARC.[39] Although this phase I study, performed largely under the direction of Drs. Samuel Broder and Robert Yarchoan at the NCI, was not designed primarily to study the possible efficacy of the drug, some preliminary but encouraging signs of a beneficial effect were noted, such as increases in the number of helper T cells in the peripheral blood, weight gains, improved sense of well-being, improved neurologic function in patients with deficits at entry, and clearing of minor fungal infections in two patients without specific antifungal therapy.

These results encouraged Burroughs Wellcome, in collaboration with university and government scientists, to plan and sponsor a larger multicenter placebo-controlled trial in similar types of patients, that is, certain patients with AIDS or advanced ARC. The goal was to determine if the drug was truly efficacious, or whether the apparent benefits that had been seen in the uncontrolled phase I trial were either part of the natural waxing and waning of the disease or due to a "placebo effect" (merely the fact of receiving a potentially helpful drug may cause a patient to feel better, not due to any specific action of the drug itself). Although significant toxicities from zidovudine, primarily hematologic in nature, were seen in the phase I trial, they were felt to be manageable by blood transfusions and/or temporary reduction or discontinuation of therapy.

Enrollment in the planned 6-month, 12-center, placebo-controlled trial began in February of 1986 and was complete by the end of June. Two hundred eighty-one patients were enrolled and randomized to receive either zidovudine or a matching but inert placebo. To be eligible, patients with AIDS were required to have recovered from a first episode of PCP within the previous 3 months, and patients with "advanced" ARC were required to have documented oral thrush and/or recent significant unexplained weight loss, plus one other ARC symptom, such as persistent unexplained fever or diarrhea. All patients were also required to have an absolute T-helper cell (CD4) count less than 500/mm^3 and cutaneous anergy (lack of responsiveness) to four specific antigens.

An independent Data Safety Monitoring Board composed of approximately eight individuals (physicians, scientists, ethicists, and statisticians) had the responsibility of reviewing significant toxicity and efficacy data from the trial (such as deaths, incidence of opportunistic infections, and hematologic data) on a bimonthly basis to decide whether or not the trial should be terminated early because of unacceptable toxicity or overwhelming efficacy. On September 10, 1986, the Board convened for a special meeting at the company's request to review the mortality data that had accumulated over the previous month showing an apparent marked imbalance in the number of deaths in the two treatment groups, occurring predominantly in AIDS patients. Eight days later, after a more thorough review of additional data supplied by the company, both the board and the FDA were convinced that the results were real and apparently due to the drug. At this time, 17 patients receiving placebo and one on zidovudine had died, and the board recommended to Burroughs Wellcome that the placebo be discontinued. It was deemed unethical to continue administering an inactive substance to patients in the face of such strong evidence of efficacy.

The following week a protocol was written that would allow persons with AIDS who had recovered from a histologically confirmed episode of PCP and who met certain laboratory criteria to receive zidovudine under a company-sponsored "Treatment IND." This protocol was submitted to the FDA on September 26, 1986, and was approved within 2 working days.

The National Institutes of Health provided administrative support for this project, and as of this writing (March 1987), over 4000 patients have received zidovudine free of charge from Burroughs Wellcome under the Treatment IND. During the last quarter of 1986, the company further collected, compiled, and analyzed the data from the placebo-controlled trial in order to submit an NDA (new drug application) to the Food and Drug Administration requesting permission to market the drug based on the efficacy demonstrated in the trial. Zidovudine was approved by the FDA on March 19, 1987, "for the management of certain adult patients with symptomatic HIV infection (AIDS and advanced ARC) who have a history of cytologically confirmed *Pneumocystis carinii* pneumonia or an absolute CD4 (T4-helper/inducer) lymphocyte count of less than 200/mm^3 in the peripheral blood before therapy is begun."

Because important unanswered questions remained regarding zidovudine and and its use in HIV-infected patients, a number of other clinical trials were initiated after the company's placebo-controlled trial in AIDS/post-PCP and advanced ARC patients ended in September 1986. In addition, those patients still receiving zidovudine in an uncontrolled extension of this study continue to be monitored closely. Under the NIH-sponsored AIDS Clinical Trial Group (ACTG) program, a placebo-controlled trial in asymptomatic patients with KS was begun in December 1986 along with a large dose-comparison study in AIDS/post-PCP patients (zidovudine at 250 mg every 4 h compared with a lower dose that is hoped will provide the same benefit with less toxicity). A number of other studies are also under way, sponsored by NIH, Burroughs Wellcome, and others, including trials in HIV-infected patients with primarily neurologic manifestations (AIDS-dementia complex), in asymptomatic HIV-infected individuals, and in earlier ARC patients with minimal symptoms and higher CD4 cell counts.

It is desirable to conduct placebo-controlled trials in many of these groups of patients, particularly those with a good short-term prognosis, as the risk-to-benefit ratio of zidovudine has yet to be determined in less ill patients. As discussed previously in this chapter, the toxicity of the drug when administered over many months may reduce the potential benefit the drug appears to have in halting the replication of the virus. The most efficient study design to determine whether or not a drug will be of more benefit than harm is to compare a group of treated patients with a similar group of untreated (or control) patients in a double-blind, randomized trial. It is ethical to do this when the drug is of unknown value in a particular group of patients. Data safety and monitoring boards will review the data from the trials on a periodic basis much as they did for Burroughs Wellcome's placebo-controlled trial.

Another antiviral drug that inhibits HIV replication in some laboratory assays is ribavirin,[40] also a nucleoside analog, which exhibits in vitro activity against a broad range of viruses, including respiratory syncytial virus (RSV), influenza viruses, and herpes simplex virus. It has been tested in humans in various formulations for a number of years and is approved for use in aerosol form in hospitalized infants and young children with serious RSV pulmonary infection.

Placebo-controlled studies of the oral formulation of ribavirin at two doses (600 and 800 mg per day) for 6 months were begun early in 1986 in asymptomatic HIV-infected patients with the chronic lymphadenopathy syndrome (LAS) and CD4 count less than 500/mm^3 and in more advanced patients with at least one ARC symptom (fever, malaise, diarrhea, night sweats, weight loss). Although the manufacturer, ICN Pharmaceutical, Inc., announced in early 1987 that the drug delayed progression to CDC-defined AIDS in the LAS study, FDA failed to confirm this claim during its review of the data submitted to the agency by the company. No efficacy was demonstrated in the ARC study. As of April 1988, neither of these studies has been published in peer-reviewed scientific journals. Smaller, uncontrolled trials of the drug are currently under way to determine whether higher doses can be tolerated in various groups of HIV-infected patients.

No other antiretroviral agents have been tested in placebo-controlled efficacy trials. Suramin, a complex antitrypanosomal agent in human use for years but not approved in the United States, was identified early by NCI scientists as having activity against HIV in the laboratory.[41] Extensive phase I testing in AIDS and ARC patients over 1½ years identified a maximum tolerated dose, but some patients developed serious side effects, such as adrenal insufficiency, and no clinical efficacy was seen.[42] A placebo-controlled trial was never begun, so it is unclear to what extent adverse events were disease-related rather than caused by the drug. The NIH has recommended that suramin no longer be studied alone for its antiretroviral effects in this disease.[42]

HPA 23, a complex heteropolyanion (compound) developed at the Pasteur Institute in Paris, was discovered to have antiretroviral activity against HIV in vitro and was given to HIV-infected individuals in France beginning in 1983. Early reports of clinical improvement in a few patients generated much interest in the drug,[43] and a phase I trial was conducted in this country in the fall/winter of 1985–86. Very little further information has been reported.[44]

Foscarnet (sodium phosphonoformate) is an antiviral drug manufactured in Sweden that was initially studied in topical formulation against herpes simplex virus. It also has activity in vitro against CMV and HIV[45] and is currently undergoing studies in Europe in a parenteral formulation. Other antiretroviral drugs, including other nucleoside analogs, are in earlier stages of testing. One of these drugs, dideoxycytidine, a potent inhibitor of HIV replication in vitro, produces a painful peripheral neuropathy after several months of daily treatment, which necessitates discontinuation of the drug. It is currently being studied in different dosing regimens, including weekly alternation with zidovudine. No clinical benefits have been reported to date.

The approval of zidovudine for the treatment of certain patients with advanced

HIV infection raises major issues regarding the testing of other experimental antiretroviral therapies. The design of trials for determining the efficacy and safety of new drugs will be guided by both regulatory and ethical concerns in addition to scientific imperatives. It will be important to compare new agents with zidovudine in those patients for whom the approved drug is indicated (been shown to be of benefit). For other groups of HIV-infected patients for whom there is no approved therapy, placebo-controlled trials will continue to be ethical and in fact, highly desirable, but they may be difficult to implement and complete if many patients at earlier stages of infection choose to risk taking zidovudine or other drugs even though benefit has not been established.

The specific agents discussed above are believed to act primarily by inhibiting reverse transcriptase, an enzyme critical for retroviral replication. Other approaches to controlling the spread of infection within the host include the use of agents that interfere with the ability of HIV to attach to and penetrate uninfected target cells. It appears that the virus enters the cell after binding to the CD4 molecule,[46] so considerable research has focused on exploring inhibitors of CD4 receptor binding including monoclonal antibodies. AL721, an investigational agent that has been reported to inhibit HIV in cell culture,[47] is said to act by changing the "fluidity" of the cell (or virus) membrane and thus altering critical receptor configuration. Another approach to antiretroviral therapy that is being actively pursued in the laboratory at this time is the use of synthetic oligonucleotides complementary to viral RNA or proviral DNA, aimed at inhibiting viral replication by interfering with gene transcription and/or translation.[48] As the molecular and enzymatic basis of HIV infection, replication, and pathogenicity become progressively better elucidated, additional targets for antiviral chemo- and immunotherapy will undoubtedly be explored both in the laboratory and then in the clinic.

CONCLUSION

At present, the medical management of patients with AIDS and related conditions is indeed complex. It consists for the most part of palliative therapies that may improve the quality of life but only temporarily delay the seemingly inevitable outcome—death. Looking to the future, it would appear that the only way to rid society of this disease is by preventing further spread of the virus to currently uninfected individuals, by means of education as to its modes of transmission and eventually by universal vaccination of the susceptible population. The prospects for actual cure of infected persons are dim, in my view. However, with patience, expanded research efforts in "drug discovery" programs, additional well-designed clinical investigations, and a lot of hard work, it may be possible to identify relatively safe antiretroviral agents which, when used alone or in some combination with immunorestorative therapy, will arrest the destructive disease process and improve the infected individual's ability to resist AIDS-related opportunistic infections and malignancies. If such a therapeutic regimen that can be tolerated on a long-term basis is devised, HIV-infected individuals may be able to anticipate a relatively normal life. The demonstration that an antiretroviral agent can delay death and the development of OIs in certain groups of ill patients is certainly an important step in the right direction. Partly because of this achievement, I believe that we can look forward to a rapid increase in the number of new therapies under investigation in HIV-infected individuals, as well as to the development of novel approaches to all aspects of the treatment of this disease and its associated conditions.

REFERENCES

1. Des Jarlais, D. C.; et al. "Kaposi's Sarcoma Among Four Different AIDS Risk Groups." *New England Journal of Medicine* 310:1119 (1984).

2. Rivin, B.; et al. "AIDS Outcome. A First Follow-up." *New England Journal of Medicine* 311:857 (1984).

2a. MMWR 36:15 (14 August 1987).

3. Shaw, G. M.; et al. "Molecular Characterization of Human T-Cell Leukemia (Lymphotropic) Virus Type III in the Acquired Immune Deficiency Syndrome." *Science* 226:1165–1171 (1984).

4. Lane, H. C.; Fanci, A. S. "Immunologic Abnormalities in the Acquired Immunodeficiency Syndrome." In *Annual Review of Immunology* Vol. 3, edited by William E. Rapul et al., 477–500 (1985).

5. Lane, H. C.; et al. "The Use of Interleukin-2 in Patients with the Acquired Immune Deficiency Syndrome (AIDS)." *Journal of Biological Response Modifiers* 3:512–516 (1984).

6. Lane, H. C.; et al. "A Phase I Trial of Recombinant Immune (Gamma) Interferon in Patients with AIDS." *Clinical Research* 33:408A (1985).

7. Barr-Sinoussi, F.; et al. "Isolation of Lymphadenopathy-Associated Virus (LAV) and Detection of LAV antibodies from U.S. Patients with AIDS." *JAMA* 253:1737–1739 (1985).

8. Mitsuyasu, R.; et al. "Treatment of Donor Bone Marrow with Monoclonal Anti-T-Cell Antibody and Complement for the Prevention of Graft-Versus-Host Disease." *Annals of Internal Medicine* 105:20–26 (1986).

9. Martin, P. J. "Effects of In Vitro Depletion of T-Cells in HLA-Identical Allogenic Marrow Grafts." *Blood* 66:664–672 (1985).

10. Rouse, B. T.; Horohov, D. W. "Immunosuppression in Viral Infections." *Reviews of Infectious Diseases* 8:850–873 (1986).

11. Whimbey, E.; et al. "Bacteremia and Fungemia in Patients with the Acquired Immunodeficiency Syndrome." *Annals of Internal Medicine* 104:511–514 (1986).

12. Fischl, M.; Dickinson, G. "Acquired Immunodeficiency Syndrome." In *Conn's Current Therapy 1986*, edited by Robert E. Rakel, 25–32. Philadelphia: W. B. Saunders Co., 1986.

13. Gordin, F.; et al. "Adverse Reactions to Trimethoprim-Sulfamethoxazole in Patients with Acquired Immunodeficiency Syndrome." *Annals of Internal Medicine* 100:495–499 (1984).

14. Castella, A.; et al. "The Bone Marrow in AIDS: A Histologic, Hematologic, and Microbiologic Study." *American Journal of Clinical Pathology* 84:425–432 (1985).

15. Gelmann, E. P.; Broder, S. "Kaposi's Sarcoma in the Setting of the AIDS Pandemic." In *AIDS: Modern Concepts and Therapeutic Challenges*, edited by Samuel Broder, 227–229. New York: Marcel Dekker, Inc., 1987.

16. Krown, S.; et al. "Kaposi's Sarcoma and the Acquired Immune Deficiency Syndrome: Treatment with Recombinant Interferon Alpha and Analysis of Prognostic Factors." *Cancer* 57:1662–1665 (1986).

17. Levine, A. M.; et al. "AIDS-Related Malignant B-Cell Lymphomas." In *AIDS: Modern Concepts and Therapeutic Challenges*, edited by Samuel Broder, 240–241. New York: Marcel Dekker, Inc., 1987.

18. Parks, W. P.; Scott, G. B. "An Overview of Pediatric AIDS: Approaches to Diagnosis and Outcome Assessment." In *AIDS: Modern Concepts and Therapeutic Challenges*, edited by Samuel Broder, 245–262, New York: Marcel Dekker, Inc., 1987.

19. Polk, B. F.; et al. "Predictors of the Acquired Immunodeficiency Syndrome Developing in a Cohort of Seropositive Homosexual Men." *New England Journal of Medicine* 316:61–66 (1987).

20. Francis, D. P.; et al. "The Natural History of Infection with the Lymphadenopathy-Associated Virus Human T-Lymphotropic Virus Type III." *Annals of Internal Medicine* 103:719–722 (1985).

21. Rutherford, G.; et al. "The Natural History of LAV/HTLV-III Infection and Viraemia in Homosexual and Bisexual Men: A 6-year Follow-up Study (Abstract)." In *Proceedings of the International Conference on AIDS*, Paris, 23–25 June 1986, 99.

22. Kaplan, J. E.; et al. "HTLV-III Viremia in Homosexual Men with Generalized Lymphadenopathy." *New England Journal of Medicine* 312:1572–1573 (1985).

23. Chaisson, R. E.; et al. "Significant Changes in HIV Antigen Level in the Serum of Patients Treated with Azidothymidine (Letter)." *New England Journal of Medicine* 315:1610–1611 (1986).

24. Goudsmit, J.; et al. "Expression of Human Immunodeficiency Virus Antigen (HIV-AG) in Serum and Cerebrospinal Fluid during Acute and Chronic Infection." *Lancet* ii:177–180 (1986).

25. Eysler, M. E.; et al. "Acid-Labile Alpha Interferon: A Possible Preclinical Marker for the Acquired Immunodeficiency Syndrome in Hemophilia." *New England Journal of Medicine* 309:583–586 (1983).

26. Metroka, C.; et al. "Acid-Labile Interferon Alpha in Homosexual Men: A Preclinical Marker for Opportunistic Infections (Abstract)." In *Proceedings of International Conference on AIDS*, Paris, 23–25 June 1986, 80.

27. Murray, H. W.; et al. "Impaired Production of Lymphokines and Immune Interferon in the Acquired Immunodeficiency Syndrome." *New England Journal of Medicine* 310:883–889 (1984).

28. Lange, M.; et al. "Prospective Study on a Homosexual Cohort: Significance of Persistant Acid Labile Alpha Interferon and Decreasing Erythrocyte Complement 3B Receptors (Abstract)." In *Proceedings of International Conference on AIDS*, Paris, 23–25 June 1986, 73.

29. Cronin, W.; et al. "Prognostic Significance of Antilymphocyte Antibodies in Serum of Patients with AIDS and ARC (Abstract)." In *Proceedings of International Conference on AIDS*, Paris, 23–25 June 1986, 80.

30. Sissons, J. G.; Oldstone, M. B. A. "Host Responses to Viral Infections." In *Virology*, edited by B. N. Fields et al., 266. New York: Raven Press (1985).

31. Lane, H. C.; Fanci, A. S. "Immunologic Reconstitution in the Acquired Immunodeficiency Syndrome." *Annals of Internal Medicine* 103:714–718 (1985).

32. Rubinstein, A.; et al. "Treatment of AIDS with Intravenous Gammaglobulin (Abstract)." *Pediatric Research* 17:263A (1984).

33. Lane, H. D.; et al. "Partial Immune Reconstitution in a Patient with the Acquired Immunodeficiency Syndrome." *New England Journal of Medicine* 311:1099 (1984).

34. Fischl, M. A.; et al. "Safety and Efficacy of Sulfamethoxazole and Trimethoprim Chemoprophylaxis for *Pneumocystis carinii* Pneumonia in AIDS." *Journal of the American Medical Association*, 259:1185–1189 (1988).

35. Hartshorn, K. L.; et al. "Synergistic Inhibition of Human T-Cell Lymphotropic Virus Type III Replication In Vitro by Phosphonoformate and Recombinant Alpha-A Interferon." *Antimicrobial Agents and Chemotherapy* 30:189–191 (1986).

36. Hartshorn, K. L.; et al. "Effects of Combination Antiviral Therapy on LAV/HTLV-III Replication In Vitro (Abstract)." In *Proceedings of International Conference on AIDS*, Paris, 23–25 June 1986, 69.

37. Lester, W. "Tuberculosis." In *Medical Microbiology and Infectious Disease*, edited by Abraham Brande et al., 977–978. Philadelphia: W. B. Saunders & Co., 1981.

38. Mitsuya, H.; et al. "3'-Azido-3'-Deoxythymidine (BWA509U): An Antiviral Agent That Inhibits the Infectivity and Cytopathic Effect of Human T-Lymphotropic Virus Type III/Lymphadenopathy-Associated Virus In Vitro. *Proceedings of National Academy of Sciences USA*, 821:7096–7100 (1985).

39. Yarchoan, R.; et al. "Administration of 3'-Azido-3'-Deoxythymidine, an Inhibitor of HTLV-III Replication, to Patients with AIDS and AIDS-Related Complex." *Lancet* i:575–580 (1986).

40. McCormick, J. B.; et al. "Ribavirin Suppresses Replication of Lymphadenopathy-Associated Virus in Cultures of Human Adult T Lymphocytes." *Lancet* ii:1367–1369 (1984).

41. Mitsuya, H.; et al. "Suramin Protection of T Cells In Vitro Against Infectivity and Cytopathic Effect of HTLV-III." *Science* 226:172–174 (1984).

42. Cheson, B. D.; et al. "Suramin Therapy in AIDS and Related Diseases. Initial Report of the U.S. Suramin Working Group (Abstract)." In *Proceedings of International Conference on AIDS*, Paris, 23–25 June 1986, 35.

43. Rozenbaum, W.; et al. "Antimoniotungstate (HPA 23) Treatment of Three Patients with AIDS and One with Prodrome (Letter)." *Lancet* i:450–451 (1985).

44. Dormont, E.; et al. "Virologic and Immunologic Follow-Up of 15 Patients with AIDS or AIDS Related Complex, and 4 LAV/HTLV-II Seropositive Patients Treated with Daily IV Doses of HPA 23 During 4 to 15 Months (Abstract)." In *Proceedings of International Conference on AIDS*, 23–25 June 1986, 34.

45. Sandstrom, E. G.; et al. "Inhibition of Human T-Cell Lymphotropic Virus Type III In Vitro by Phosphonoformate." *Lancet* i:1480–1482 (1985).

46. Maddon, P. J.; et al. "The T$_4$ Gene Encodes the AIDS Virus Receptor and Is Expressed in the Immune System and the Brain. *Cell* 47:333–348 (1986).

47. Sarin, P.; et al. "Effect of a Novel Compound (AL 721) on HTLV-III Infectivity In Vitro." *New England Journal of Medicine* 313:1289–1290 (1985).

48. Zamecnik, P. C.; et al. "Inhibition of Replication and Expression of Human T-Cell Lymphotropic Virus Type III in Cultured Cells by Exogenous Synthetic Oligonucleotides Complementary to Viral RNA." *Proceedings of the National Academy of Sciences USA* 83:4143–4146 (1986).

8

Care of the Patient with AIDS

Jerome Schofferman

The medical care of the person with AIDS (PWA), especially one who is dying, requires recognition and treatment of the biological, psychological, and social components of each person and his or her illness.[1] The specifics of treatment vary according to the stage of the illness, but at every stage the goal is to provide maximum function and comfort in spite of progressive physical deterioration. Care must be scientifically potent and at the same time humanely sensitive. The unit of care is the PWA as well as significant others. Each must be a part of the health care team included in the process of making decisions regarding evaluation and treatment.

The AIDS Home Care and Hospice Program of Hospice of San Francisco has provided care for more than 700 patients with AIDS. These patients are extremely complicated medically, socially, and psychologically, and they benefit enormously from a multidisciplinary team approach.

This paper describes the management of the PWA who is in the late phase of the illness. A scientific foundation is provided for the biological aspects of treatment with an emphasis on symptom management. Particular areas of psychological and social concern are addressed as well.

BIOLOGICAL ISSUES

The treatment of symptoms in the patient dying of AIDS must follow the same guidelines used for the care of any patient. Optimal treatment is based on accurate and specific diagnosis.[2] Appropriate treatment decisions can be made only when the specific cause of a symptom is known. This fact remains true in every stage of the illness. However, the extent of the evaluation and the intensity of treatment must be appropriate for each individual patient based on the stage of the illness and the wishes of that patient.

Pain

Many PWAs complain of generalized discomfort which may be due to muscle or joint aches, intermittent fevers, general debility, or just being bedbound. A comfortable mattress with foam pads or an alternating-pressure mattress may help. A hospital bed provides easier positioning for the patient. Firm foam wedges are an alternative. Gentle massage is very useful for superficial generalized aches and pains.

When general comfort measures are not sufficient, medications are indicated.[3] For mild or moderate pain, a peripherally acting medication such as acetaminophen (APAP) or a nonsteroidal antiinflammatory (NSAID) should be the first choice. Either can be used as needed, but if pain is persistent, time-contingent dosing is more effective.

APAP is often chosen first because it is very safe and has a low incidence of side effects.[4] The dose range is from 325 mg to 1.0 g every 4–6 h.

The NSAIDs appear to be more effective than APAP in our experience, although there is a higher incidence of side effects. Aspirin (ASA) is the prototype and remains an excellent and inexpensive choice. It is equianalgesic on a milligram-for-milligram basis with APAP, but ASA and other NSAIDs seem to be more effective for fever reduction in AIDS. When patients require frequent dosing, other NSAIDs are more convenient than ASA to use and have fewer side effects. It may be necessary to try several NSAIDs before the best one for an individual patient is found.

A useful method to choose the NSAID is based on whether the need is for intermittent treatment or continuous treatment, coupled with the knowledge of the half-life of the NSAID. Drugs are used on an as-needed basis when pain is infrequent and intermittent. In this situation an NSAID with a short half-life should be used. Analgesia will occur sooner but will be of shorter duration. Ibuprofen, tolmetin sodium, naproxen sodium, indomethacin, and others are available. It is often necessary to use the drug at the high end of the dose range.

When pain is persistent, it is more appropriate to use the NSAID in a time-contingent fashion, and drugs with a longer half-life are more convenient. These include naproxen, sulindac, piroxicam, slow-release indomethacin, and others.

Significant side effects occur in 6–10% of patients. The more common side effects are nausea, vomiting, dyspepsia, and fluid retention. Occasionally headaches are seen. There may be an increased risk of bleeding due to the antiplatelet effect, but this has not been a significant problem clinically.

If a peripherally acting analgesic is insufficient, a centrally acting narcotic analgesic is added to (not substituted for) the APAP or NSAID.[3] Narcotics are usually given on a regular schedule. However, extra doses should be given for breakthrough pain. If breakthrough pain occurs frequently, the regular dose should be increased.

Codeine or its equivalent is usually the first drug used. It may be started at 30 mg every 4 h and the dose adjusted upward as needed. If analgesia is not adequate at a dose of 120–180 mg, a more potent analgesic should be used.

Oral morphine is our drug of choice because of its reliability, low incidence of side effects, ease of dose adjustment and titration, and the low incidence of abuse by the PWA or care givers. Morphine provides about 4 h of analgesia. This short duration may be particularly beneficial in the PWA who is demented because of the decreased incidence of significant deterioration of mental status.

The dose of morphine must be adjusted to the needs of the patient. In the patient who is on high doses of codeine, a starting dose of 20–30 mg oral morphine is given, and the dose is titrated upward in increments of about 25% until pain is significantly relieved. Many dosing forms of oral morphine are available. We have found the 20 mg/ml form particularly useful and well tolerated. Morphine is also available as tablets or suppositories (which are equianalgesic to oral solution).

Many other effective narcotics are available. When used in equianalgesic doses, they also provide effective analgesia. Longer-acting forms of morphine such as MS Contin or Roxinol SR may provide 6–12 h of analgesia. They are only available as 30-mg tablets, which restricts flexibility. Extra doses of short-acting morphine must be available for breakthrough pain. Methadone is an effective analgesic and is inexpensive. However, it is much more difficult to use. Its major advantage, high lipid solubility, is also its major drawback in that when side effects occur, they frequently last 3–5 days. I feel it should be avoided in demented patients, and I rarely use it in AIDS.

Hydromorphone is frequently prescribed and is quite effective. However, in my experience it often has a very short half-life of analgesia, which makes it inconvenient to use.

The specific choice of narcotic analgesic is less important than the proper use of the narcotic chosen. The correct dose is the dose that provides effective analgesia. Often this dose is much higher than the doses necessary to treat acute pain.[5] Loss of pain control may be due to tolerance or disease progression. Tolerance is relative, and increasing the dose of narcotics usually suffices to reestablish analgesia.

There are specific pain problems in AIDS that are not well managed by analgesics alone and that require additional forms of therapy.[6] The pains of peripheral neuropathy or postherpetic neuralgia respond poorly to narcotics alone. However, we had gratifying results with amitriptyline. Amitriptyline is started at 10 mg orally at bedtime and increased every 2 or 3 days in 10-mg increments to 75–100 mg. If there is no appreciable benefit by 75–100 mg, haloperidol may be added at a dose of 1 mg orally every 8 h.

Pain with swallowing may be due to esophagitis caused by *Candida albicans* or herpes simplex virus (HSV). *Candida* esophagitis often responds to oral ketoconazole 200 mg twice daily.[2] Rarely, low-dose intravenous amphotericin B may be needed. HSV esophagitis may respond to oral acyclovir 200 mg given five times per day. Higher or intravenous doses are occasionally necessary.

Headaches are common and may be due to acute or subacute viral (HIV, CMV, HSV, PML) meningoencephalitis, toxoplasmosis, or cryptococcal meningitis, or they may be nonspecific. Definitive therapy is indicated when a treatable pathogen can be identified. Once again, the degree of evaluation depends on the particulars of the individual patient. Most often, whether or not a treatable lesion is found, symptomatic pain control as discussed previously is indicated. Some patients do better with the addition of oral steroids such as dexamethasone 1–4 mg every 6 h. However, steroids pose the theoretical risk of even further increased susceptibility to infection and must not be used capriciously.

Mucocutaneous HSV infection is often painful, particularly if it occurs in the perirectal area. Topical acyclovir may help, but oral therapy is usually required.

Pulmonary Problems

Most PWAs have some form of pulmonary problem. Frequently there is a specific etiology that can be identified, but again, the evaluation must be appropriate for the individual patient. Commonly seen problems include *Pneumocystis carinii* pneumonia (PCP), bacterial pneumonia or bronchitis, bronchospasm, viral pneumonia, pulmonary tuberculosis (*M. tuberculosis* or *M. avium intracellulare*), or Kaposi's sarcoma.[2,7] Multiple problems may exist simultaneously.

In the terminally ill patient, we have found it useful to institute therapy based on clinical suspicion. Small infectious insults to previously damaged lungs can result in significant deterioration. Treatment can often return the patient to a more comfortable situation.

In a patient with deterioration of respiratory status, nonproductive cough, dyspnea, tachypnea, and nonspecific findings on pulmonary exam, PCP may be present. This is particularly true in the patient with prior PCP. Treatment can be instituted with trimethaprim sulfamethoxazole if the patient has not had previous adverse reaction. Alternatively, pentamidine can be used intravenously. Recent treatment results with nebulized pentamidine are encouraging and may provide a convenient and less expensive alternative. On the other hand, the patient with purulent sputum especially in the presence of localized findings of rales or pulmonary consolidation on exam, can be treated with oral antibiotics such as erythromycin or amoxicillin.

Bronchospasm can be treated with nebulized beta agonists via metered dose inhalers, oral theophylline, or, on occasion, oral steroids. Cough can be suppressed with low-dose oral narcotics, although some patients require up to 90 mg codeine to suppress cough. Energy conservation should be encouraged. Oxygen should be used liberally without fear of worsening mental status.

The use of oral narcotics to ease dyspnea has been especially gratifying. We have had success with no serious consequences. In the PWA who is narcotic naive, a starting dose of 5–10 mg oral morphine sulfate every 4 h is generally sufficient. The dose is titrated upward as needed. In the patient already on narcotics who develops dyspnea, higher doses are required.

Gastrointestinal Problems

AIDS can involve any part of the GI tract from the mouth to the anus. *Candida* oropharyngitis can appear in its classical pseudomembranous form (thrush) with creamy white plaques on an erythematous base or as an atrophic form with smooth, red, flat lesions. Oral candidiasis can be painful, cause an unpleasant taste, and interfere with oral intake. Multiple treatments are available. Nystatin can be given orally as the liquid (swish and swallow), 100,000 units 3–4 times per day, or by allowing nystatin vaginal tablets (100,000 units) to dissolve in the mouth three times a day. Clotrimazole 10 mg oral tablets dissolved in the mouth five times per day may be more effective and convenient. In unresponsive cases, ketoconazole 200 mg orally once per day usually will suffice. A few patients require higher doses.

Lesions of Kaposi's sarcoma (KS) can involve the mouth and oropharynx. Infection or ulceration may occur. However, obstruction of the airway or esophagus is the most significant complication. Radiation therapy is indicated to shrink obstructive lesions.

Other oral lesions include herpetic stomatitis, intraoral HSV lesions, herpes zoster, severe periodontal disease, and hairy leukoplakia. Esophageal lesions have been discussed. The most common are HSV and *Candida* esophagitis.

Diarrhea is a major problem in AIDS and may be particularly troublesome in the bedbound patient. We have found it helpful to divide the causes of diarrhea into infectious and noninfectious etiologies with a subdivision of each of these into those for which specific treatment is available and those for which it is not.[1] Stool specimen for white blood cells, culture for bacterial pathogens, *Mycobac-*

terium avium intracellular (MAI), and examination for ova and parasites, including *Cryptosporidium* and *Isospora*, will usually suffice to separate the etiologies. Evaluation is appropriate for the patient with persistent or severe diarrhea of recent onset.

Treatable infections include *Shigella, Salmonella, Campylobacter, Giardia lamblia,* and *E. histolytica.* Infections that do not respond to specific treatment are *Cryptosporidium, Isospora,* and MAI. These are treated symptomatically.

Noninfectious causes of diarrhea include medication side effects including antibiotic associated colitis, KS or lymphoma involving the small intestine, AIDS enteropathy, fecal impaction, and osmotic diarrhea due to lactose intolerance or certain nutritional supplements.

Symptomatic treatment of diarrhea proceeds in a stepwise fashion. Unfortunately regimens such as Kaopectate, Peptobismol, or bulk are rarely effective, and stronger agents are required. Diphenoxylate hydrochloride tablets (2 tablets four times daily) or liquid (10 ml four times daily) may control diarrhea. Loperamide 2 mg (1 tablet or 10 ml) four times daily may be better tolerated. If these drugs are not successful, oral narcotics are necessary. Oral morphine, deodorized tincture of opium, or others are equally efficacious when the dose is titrated to the desired effect.

Nausea and/or vomiting is a common problem. Again treatment success is enhanced if there is an accurate diagnosis. Many medications can cause nausea, and it is fruitful to review current medications and discontinue those that are no longer necessary or are only marginally beneficial. Consider an evaluation for systemic infection, adrenal insufficiency, hypercalcemia, renal or hepatic insufficiency, or esophagitis, and check for fecal impaction.

In the absence of a specific treatable etiology, symptomatic treatment is necessary. Prochlorperazine is the drug used by most clinicians and is usually effective. However, when prochlorperazine fails, the change in medications should be based on receptor site theory, selecting the drugs according to the receptors that need to be blocked.[8] Most often nausea and/or vomiting is due to the stimulation of the chemoreceptor trigger zone, which contains dopamine receptors. Haloperidol is the most useful drug in this clinical setting at doses of 0.5–1.0 mg every 8–12 h. If not successful, drugs that block H1 and others that block anticholinergic receptors in the vestibular center and vomiting center are added to haloperidol. Meclizine at 12.5–25 mg every 6–8 h, diphenhydramine at 25 mg every 6–8 h, or promethazine at 12.5–25 mg every 6–8 h block H1 receptors. Transdermal scopolamine patches block the anticholinergic sites. If side effects occur, patches can be cut in half. If this regimen fails, some patients respond to oral steroids, metoclopramide in high doses, or lorazepam at 1.0–2.0 mg every 6 h.

Urinary Tract

Urinary incontinence or retention occurs fairly frequently. Both are usually of neurological origin but may be due to medication side effects or infection. Treatment of retention usually requires an indwelling catheter or an intermittent straight catheterization program. Incontinence requires evaluation for overflow secondary to retention and then either a condom catheter, indwelling catheter, or intermittent catheterization program.

NEUROPSYCHOLOGICAL PROBLEMS

Neuropsychological problems have become the most difficult area in the management of the late stages of AIDS. Patients may suffer from an organic mental disorder (dementia, delirium, or endogenous depression) or an affective disturbance (reactive depression (adjustment disorder with depressed mood), anxiety, or grief reaction).

AIDS Dementia Syndrome

Dementia is a loss of intellectual capabilities associated with memory impairment and impairment of some aspects of higher cortical function occurring in the presence of an unclouded sensorium. Dementia occurs in as many as 65% of PWAs.[10] Early in dementia the symptoms may be very mild, with only small changes in personality. These early changes may initially be attributed to anxiety or depression or to the fact that the patient is physically deteriorating. There may be forgetfulness, inability to concentrate, loss of impulse control, or irritability as well. At this stage diagnosis may be difficult, but careful mental-status testing will usually reveal the cognitive deficits. Because the personality changes may be misunderstood by the patient and care givers, early diagnosis is extremely important to put changes in perspective and to prepare for future needs.

Distinguishing dementia from other causes of change in personality is often difficult.[11] Functional psychological problems such as depression can present as dementia, and dementia can initially appear as a functional psychological disorder such as generalized anxiety disorder, panic attacks, depression, paranoia, bipolar episodes, or even schizophrenia.

The time course of dementia is variable.[10] A few patients remain stable or progress slowly. However, in many patients, there is significant deterioration in mental status over a period of months. Patients usually become incapable of caring for themselves and require 24-h care and supervision.

There are many cases of AIDS dementia, and several may coexist in an individual patient.[9] Some causes are treatable, but most are not. The most common cause of AIDS dementia is presumed to be direct involvement of the brain by the neurotropic human immunodeficiency virus (HIV). HIV dementia is also known as diffuse subacute encephalitis or subacute encephalopathy. Patients may also have focal neurological deficits, seizures, myoclonus, or peripheral neuropathy. There are no clinically useful means for diagnosis and no specific therapy. Other virus infections can cause dementia and require brain biopsy for treatment. Of course this is not appropriate at this stage of illness.

Toxoplasmosis can cause dementia, and treatment is helpful. Diagnosis requires magnetic resonance imaging of the brain and the demonstration of a mass lesion. Empiric therapy with sulfadiazine and pyrimethamine and leucovorin can often result in shrinkage of lesions.

Other causes of dementia in AIDS include lymphoma of the brain, cryptococcosis, cerebral hemorrhage or infarction, and rarely *Candida*, aspergillosis, histoplasmosis, or severe deficiency.

Dementia can be caused by, or accelerated by, medications such as narcotics, sedative-hypnotics, or antidepressants. Concurrent physical problems such as systemic infection, hypoxia, fluid or electrolyte disturbances, or anemia may accelerate dementia.

Treatment of dementia requires a multidimensional approach using medical, psychological, and social resources. The family and other care givers must be part of the unit of care.

Psychosocial and environmental approaches are the mainstays of treatment. Orienting cues such as a large calendar and clock in conspicuous places help. All appointments and scheduled visitors should be indicated. Important phone numbers and names of care givers should be easily accessible to the patient. For reasons of safety, the PWA may need restrictions. The patient will need to be accompanied for any travel outside the home. Smoking or cooking must be supervised. Care givers must be instructed in the need to set limits that are clear and simple.

When environmental modifications are not sufficient to help the patient, medications may be necessary to provide a comfortable and manageable patient who then responds to the improved psychosocial milieu. Behaviors such as sleeplessness, emotional lability, hallucinations, suspiciousness, and agitation are likely to respond to medications. Memory loss, apathy, and unsociability are not likely to respond.

Haloperidol may be useful to control anxiety, sleep disturbance, emotional lability, hallucinations, and agitation. Doses of 0.5–1.0 mg 2–3 times a day can be used when behavioral methods fail or the patient is very uncomfortable. Lorazepam at 0.5–1.0 mg every 6 h may help and can allow lower doses of haloperidol.

Medications that are not essential should be eliminated. Drugs that affect the CNS should be used at the lowest possible dose. Long-acting sedative-hypnotics or narcotics should be avoided.

Depression

Depression in the late stages of illness of the PWA is a complex problem. It is incorrect and does the patient a major disservice to assume that the depression is expected because the patient is dying and "has a right to be depressed." Accurate diagnosis is not just a futile exercise, because proper treatment with antidepressants and/or psychotherapy may greatly improve the patient's quality of life.

The usual criteria for diagnosis of major depression are not very useful in the presence of a severely debilitating physical process such as AIDS. The vegetative somatic signs of depression cannot be distinguished from the symptoms and signs of the physical deterioration and are therefore not useful diagnostically. Diagnostic emphasis must be placed on the cognitive and affective symptoms instead. Loss of self-esteem, feeling like a failure, loss of interest in people, intense feelings of guilt, suicidal ideation, or frequent unprovoked crying spells may suggest depression.[13,14] A past history of major depression or response to treatment with antidepressants may be helpful clues. Patients who seem depressed far out of proportion to the degree of physical illness may have an underlying major depression as well.

Pharmacological treatment of depression is somewhat controversial, particularly with regard to the choice of antidepressants and their effects on other aspects of the AIDS complex. Some psychiatrists feel that drugs with the least anticholinergic effects should be chosen and prefer alprazolam or desipramine.

On the other hand, we have had very few problems with the use of low doses of amitriptyline or doxepin, starting with 10 mg orally at bedtime and increasing the doses of either in 10-mg increments every 2–3 days.

The side effects of these drugs may be useful to manage other symptoms. The H1 blocking (antihistamine) action causes sedation, which proves beneficial for sleep disturbance and decreases nausea. The anticholinergic side effects of drying airway secretions, decreasing bowel motility, and alleviating nausea are often desirable. The H2 blocking effect of decreasing gastric acidity may alleviate dyspepsia from NSAID. When using any psychoactive medication in a patient with altered mental status, careful attention to adverse changes in mental status is essential.

Many dying patients develop a "reactive depression" in response to the diagnosis of terminal disease, progressive physical deterioration, psychosocial changes, or progressive losses. Dr. Mary Baines has discussed depression in the dying patient from a very practical and functional perspective.[15] She categorizes depression according to past memories, present worries, future fears, and existential dilemmas. Past memories include unresolved grief which may be rekindled by the present illness, unsettled relationships, and guilt from "unfinished personal business." Present worries revolve around physical symptoms and, even more so, the meaning of symptoms, the fear of becoming a burden to others, changes in body image, boredom, financial problems and concerns, fears of isolation, and loss of identity. Future fears include fear of pain or other symptoms, fear and concern about the dying process itself, and fears of the afterlife. It is at this stage of life that one evaluates what has and what has not happened and evaluates his or her life as having been a success or a failure. Awareness and anticipation of these areas of concern may allow prompt intervention.

Delirium

Delirium in AIDS is usually of multifactorial origin. Infection, hypoxia, or electrolyte imbalance coupled with psychological distress, isolation, sleep disturbance, and sensory deprivation may precipitate delirium.[11,14] The hallmark of delirium that helps to differentiate it from other organic mental disorders is the fluctuating clouding of consciousness coupled with cognitive dysfunction. There are often associated emotional changes.

Treatment of delirium usually involves a search for and treatment of the underlying precipitant. Medications are often necessary. Haloperidol and/or lorazepam is useful, but doses may need to be higher than those previously discussed.

PSYCHOSOCIAL ISSUES

In our experience, psychosocial issues are so complex that they often dominate the clinical picture of the person dying of AIDS. Some issues are common to any dying patient, whereas others are unique to AIDS.[1,16,17]

Isolation is common and takes many forms. Patients dying of AIDS in some communities are even more isolated than persons dying of cancer. AIDS may be considered a socially unacceptable disease, because the common routes of infection are homosexual transmission or intravenous drug use. In some communities health professionals, politicians, and members of the community are uninformed about the risk of infection and recommend inappropriate isolation precautions or even quarantine. Even in more enlightened communities, visits by friends and family decrease as the disease progresses.

Homophobia may be present in the community. Even the patient himself may turn against his own sexuality and feel extreme guilt or shame for being ill. Patients may be blamed or blame themselves for "getting what they deserve."

The PWA who is or has been an intravenous drug user has many unique problems. There is prejudice against drug users. They are often considered to be undesirable patients who caused their own problem. They frequently have inadequate housing, nobody to care for them, poor baseline health, lack of health insurance, and inadequate financial resources. These patients are often preoccupied with medications and display a high degree of drug-seeking behavior. There is frequently poor compliance with prescribed medications and treatment regimens.

Early onset of dementia creates special problems.[4] Treatment choices must be considered and discussed with patient and partners while there is still a clear mental status. Decisions regarding blood transfusion, degree of aggressiveness of treatment of infections, and whether the patient wishes to be hospitalized or remain at home when deterioration occurs must all be addressed.

The dying process itself can be quite frightening.[5] Certain fears are common. Patients fear the indignity of the process, especially loss of bowel control, bad bodily smells, disfiguring lesions, and their near total reliance on others. They fear pain, suffocation, and losing their minds. They fear abandonment. They fear their own nonexistence.

Dr. Baines further clarifies these fears and reiterates the need to be open, to explain things clearly, and to anticipate the problems to allow for early intervention. Patients fear not only their symptoms but also the meaning of the symptom. Each new symptom or recurrence of old symptoms must be evaluated, interpreted, and explained to the patient. Simple problems often create significant anxiety which dramatically decreases when explained.

Loss of control becomes a major although often subtle issue. When healthy, these PWAs may have been active, functional, bright, productive people. Now when ill, they lose control of bodily functions, finances, job, their environment, and their future. We must give back as much control and decision making as possible. When feasible, patients can give themselves their own medications, make their own appointments, and remain in charge of their own health.

Patients fear their doctors or nurses will not have the necessary skills to care for them properly, especially as the disease progresses. Dr. Solomon Papper elaborated on some of these issues based on his own experience as a chronically ill and dying patient.[17] He feels health care providers must be skilled and informed and must be able to convey the facts implicitly and explicitly to the patient. Care givers must be clinically creative and flexible. Therapeutic goals and treatment must be appropriate for the individual patient according to his needs and the stage of the illness. Dr. Papper stresses how important it is to develop a trusting and meaningful relationship with open and honest communication. Be aware of the subtleties of tone of voice and body language. It is appropriate for care givers to share their own feelings with the patient.

Pay attention to details. Return phone calls. Try to be on time for appointments. Include the partner, family, and friends in the communication when appropriate and when the patient wishes.

A neglected area in the health care of the PWA is the support of other professional care givers. For many health care providers, working with AIDS patients who are dying is even more stressful than traditional hospice work, because patients are more likely to be of similar age, background, or social set. In addition, gay male health care providers are themselves in a high-risk group for AIDS, which furthers identification. The similarities accentuate anxieties and fears about sexuality, chronic illness, physical deterioration, and death at a young age. Intense relationships between the care giver and client may develop, making the inevitable deterioration and death of the PWA extraordinarily painful and the grief of the care giver especially profound.

Over time, the effects of multiple losses accumulate and can lead to a high level of stress and anxiety with somatization, physical illness, and eventual burnout. Health care providers caring for PWAs must be given adequate opportunity to manage these stresses and to grieve.

The support of health care professionals must be done in an anticipatory fashion. There should be time set aside at regular patient care conferences to discuss deaths and to share personal feelings. There should be a regularly scheduled and professionally led support group for professional staff. Time should be available despite busy schedules for care givers to attend memorial services or funerals or to meet with survivors. A staff that feels supported will be best equipped to support others.

REFERENCES

1. Schofferman, J. Hospice care of the patient with AIDS. *Hospice J.* 1987; 3(4):51–74.

2. Kaplan, L. D.; Wofsy, C. B.; Volberding, P. A. Treatment of patients with acquired immunodeficiency syndrome and associated manifestations. *JAMA* 1987; 257:1367–1374.

3. Schofferman, J. Medical management of the dying patient. *Front. Radiat. Ther. Oncol.* 1986; 20:178–181.

4. Amadeo, P. Peripherally acting analgesics. *Am. J. Med.* 1984; 77:17–26.

5. Newman, P. B.; et al. Plasma morphine concentrations during chronic oral administration in patients with cancer pain. *Pain* 1982; 13:247–252.

6. Twycross, R. G. Narcotic analgesics in clincial practice. In Bonica, J. (ed.): *Advances in Pain Research and Therapy*. Raven Press, New York, 1983; pp. 435–458.

7. Stover, D. E.; White, D. A.; Romano, P. A; et al. Spectrum of pulmonary diseases associated with the acquired immune deficiency syndrome. *Am. J. Med.* 1985; 78:429–437.

8. Peroutka, S. J.; Snyder, S. Antiemetics: Neurotransmitter receptors predict therapeutic actions. *Lancet* 1982; i:658–659.

9. Schofferman, J.; Schoen, K. AIDS dementia syndrome. *Medical Aspects of Human Sexuality* 1987; 21:58–70.

10. Navia, B. A.; Jordan, B. D.; Price, R. W. The AIDS dementia complex. I. Clinical features. *Ann. Neurol.* 1986; 19:517–524.

11. Wolcott, D. L. Neuropsychiatric syndromes in AIDS and AIDS related illnesses. In McKusick, L. (ed.): *What to Do about AIDS*. University of California Press, Berkeley, 1986, pp. 32–44.

12. Risse, S. C.; Barnes, R. Pharmacologic treatment of agitation associated with dementia. *J. Am. Geriatr. Soc.* 1986; 34:368–376.

13. Plum, M.; Holland, J. Comparative studies of psychological function in patients with advanced cancer. *Psychosom. Med.* 1977; 39:264–276.

14. Ochitill, H. N. The neuropsychiatry of AIDS. Presented at *AIDS and the Nervous System*, University of California, San Francisco, Dec. 11–12, 1986.

15. Baines, M. The treatment of symptoms in the dying patient. Presented at the 4th International Seminar on Terminal Care, Montreal, Oct. 4–6, 1982.

16. Schofferman, J. Medicine and the psychology of treating the terminally ill. In McKusick, L. (ed.): *What to Do about AIDS*. University of California Press, Berkeley, 1986, pp. 51–60.

17. Schoen, K. Psychosocial aspects of hospice care for AIDS patients. *Am. J. Hospice Care*, 1986; 3(2):32–34.

18. Papper, S. Care of patients with insurable, chronic neoplasm. One patient's perspective. *Am. J. Med.* 1985; 78:271–276.

9

Therapeutic Apheresis as a Treatment Modality in AIDS and AIDS-Related Conditions

Dobri Kiprov, Marcus A. Conant, Randolph Lippert, Wolfgang Pfaeffl, Robert Miller, and Donald Abrams

The basic immunologic abnormality in the acquired immune deficiency syndrome (AIDS) and AIDS-related complex (ARC) is the selective depletion of the helper/inducer (CD4) subpopulation of T lymphocytes. The CD4 surface antigen is the receptor for the human immunodeficiency virus (HIV); the virus replicates in activated CD4 cells and is eventually cytotoxic to them. However, there is strong evidence that the direct cytopathic effects of the virus cannot, by themselves, account for the overall T-cell depletion, since the virus infects less than 1 per 10,000 CD4 cells at any time.[1-3] Therefore, additional factors may contribute to the loss of CD4 cells in AIDS. Autoimmune responses are believed to play an important role.[3-5] Patients with ARC or AIDS often display an array of autoimmune phenomena, including cytotoxic antilymphocyte autoantibodies with preferential affinity for CD4 cells, circulating immune complexes, and suppressor factors for lymphoproliferation.[6-11] These could play an important role in the induction and maintenance of cellular immune deficiency in this disease. Autoantibodies and immune complexes are believed to be responsible for the clinical manifestations of at least two ARC/AIDS-related syndromes, peripheral neuropathy and immune thrombocytopenia.[4,12-14] The presence of abnormal circulating soluble factors and autoantibodies has provided a rationale for the treatment of patients with AIDS and AIDS-related conditions by plasma exchange and other apheresis-related procedures.

PLASMAPHERESIS IN ADVANCED AIDS

Several attempts have been made to use plasmapheresis for the treatment of full-blown AIDS. A modest increase of CD4 lymphocytes was observed in a single patient with AIDS treated with partial plasma exchange.[15] The investigators were unable to demonstrate a decrease in antilymphocyte antibodies. The immunologic changes were not associated with significant clinical improvement. In another study, five patients with AIDS and opportunistic infections but without Kaposi's sarcoma underwent intensive plasmapheresis every other day for 3 weeks.[16] Removal of immune complexes, suppressor factors, and antilymphocyte antibodies was successfully accomplished. No significant changes in cellular

This work was supported in part by Dr. Victor Richards' Chair of Surgical Education and Research. The authors thank Ms. Mary Sorensen for typing the manuscript.

immunity occurred. Although all patients reported some improvement of constitutional symptoms during the first week of treatment, no objective improvement could be documented in any of the patients, and the course of the disease was not changed by the plasmapheresis treatments. Three of the patients died several months following the completion of treatment from overwhelming opportunistic infections. Although two patients survived for 1 and 2 years, respectively, after the last treatment, their longer survival could not be attributed to this form of therapy.

More recently, seven patients with AIDS-related Kaposi's sarcoma without opportunistic infections were treated with plasmapheresis.[17] In none of the cases was regression of the Kaposi's sarcoma lesions observed. No significant changes were observed in a number of immunologic parameters investigated.

The above studies indicate that plasmapheresis alone is not associated with clinical improvement and does not change the natural course of the disease in patients with full-blown AIDS having either opportunistic infections or Kaposi's sarcoma.

TREATMENT WITH STAPH PROTEIN A COLUMN

Kaposi's Sarcoma

Purified staphylococcal protein A has the ability to adsorb most subclasses or immunoglobulin G and immune complexes containing IgG. Immunoadsorbent columns containing purified protein A have been associated with variable response rates in the treatment of both animal and human malignancies.[18] The exact mechanism by which the tumoricidal effect is produced in some animal and human cancers by protein A plasma perfusion is not fully understood. However, it appears that besides the removal of antibodies and immune complexes, other events such as complement activation may play an important role.[18,19]

Treatment of a retroviral animal disease with protein A has also been demonstrated. Feline leukemia retrovirus (FeLV) causes profound immune deficiency and is associated with the development of leukemias and lymphosarcomas in cats. Rewarding results have been observed using ex vivo immunoadsorption with purified protein A columns.[20]

An immunoadsorbent column containing 200 mg of purified protein A bound to silica (Prosorba, IMRE Corporation, Seattle, WA) was used to treat a group of patients with AIDS-related Kaposi's sarcoma.[16] A phase I study revealed minimal toxicity characterized by self-limited chills and fever. Partial responses were observed in 60% of the patients involved in the phase I study. The phase II study is near completion at the present time. The response rate is over 50%. In addition to an arrest in the progression of the Kaposi's sarcoma lesions and a regression of some of the lesions, patients experienced increased energy levels and decreased constitutional symptoms. White blood cell counts and lymphocyte counts were increased. The survival rate of the responders has exceeded 14 months (the time of last follow-up evaluation).

Further studies are necessary to evaluate the role of protein A immunoadsorption as a treatment modality in AIDS-related Kaposi's sarcoma. Protocols combining protein A immunoadsorption with other treatment modalities (AZT, interferon) are being developed at the present time.

HIV-Associated Immune Thrombocytopenia

Immune thrombocytopenia (ITP) is a recognized clinical entity in HIV-infected homosexual men.[21,22] There is strong evidence that antiplatelet antibodies and immune complexes contribute to the destruction of platelets in this disorder.[12,13] Conventional modes of therapy for autoimmune thrombocytopenia such as immunosuppressive drugs and splenectomy may be hazardous in HIV-infected patients, who are already severely immunocompromised. Intravenous immunoglobulin does not appear to be as effective as in conventional ITP and may be associated with serious side effects.[23] Removal of antiplatelet antibodies and immune complexes by conventional plasmapheresis achieves a rapid but temporary increase in platelet counts (Kiprov D, Abrams D, unpublished observations). Protein A immunoadsorption has been evaluated in two studies using Prosorba protein A columns. In one study, six of nine patients responded to treatment with a mean increase in platelet count of 95,000 mm³.[24] In another study, four of six patients had favorable responses, with three patients reaching platelet levels above 150,000 mm³.[4]

A small number of HIV-infected patients with thrombocytopenia also have associated neutropenia and/or hemolytic anemia. These appear to be antibody-mediated. Either may be present without thrombocytopenia. We have treated one patient manifesting both autoimmune neutropenia and immune thrombocytopenia who responded favorably to treatment with protein A plasma perfusion with normalization of platelet and granulocyte counts.

PLASMAPHERESIS IN ARC/AIDS–RELATED PERIPHERAL NEUROPATHY

Neurologic symptoms are common in patients with AIDS and ARC.[25] Some of the neurologic abnormalities are due to opportunistic infection or neoplasms, whereas others remain unexplained. Peripheral neuropathy is a distinct neurologic syndrome seen in patients with ARC and AIDS.[26] The clinical presentation and the histologic and electrophysiologic findings may be similar to chronic progressive inflammatory demyelinating polyradiculoneuropathy (CIDP) or, more commonly, as a distal symmetric polyradiculoneuropathy (DSPN). Mononeuropathy multiplex is less frequently seen. A clinical syndrome resembling acute Guillain-Barré syndrome has also been described.[27]

In one study, autoantibodies to peripheral nerve tissue were identified in all patients suffering from ARC/AIDS-related peripheral neuropathy.[4,14] It has been demonstrated that corticosteroids are not effective in this condition and may be hazardous to use in immunocompromised patients.[26] Plasmapheresis has been successful in controlling clinical symptoms in several independent studies.[14,26-28] Electrophysiologic studies suggest that patients having the demyelinating inflammatory form of peripheral neuropathy are more likely to respond to treatment than patients with axonal damage.[29]

Protein A immunoadsorption has been used in one patient with AIDS-related peripheral neuropathy, resulting in a complete clinical remission (D. Henry, personal communication). In some of the patients, the antiperipheral nerve antibodies are of IgG class, in which case one might expect a beneficial effect from protein A immunoadsorption. In others, however, where the antibodies are of the IgM class, protein A immunoadsorption would not be expected to be as effective.

IS THERE A RISK OF HIV TRANSMISSION DURING THERAPEUTIC APHERESIS?

Much concern has been raised regarding the safety of health care workers exposed to blood or other body fluids from patients infected with HIV. Previous studies have suggested that health care workers exposed to blood or other body fluids from infected patients are not at high risk for acquiring HIV with the possible exception of accidental needlestick exposure.[30-32] We studied seven health professionals involved with the routine work in our plasmapheresis unit in a prospective study evaluating immunologic parameters and HIV antibody status over a period of 3 years. These individuals were exposed on a daily basis to blood and body fluids from patients diagnosed with AIDS or ARC. None belonged to any of the known high-risk groups for the development of AIDS. At the end of 3 years, all participants of this study remained HIV-seronegative and had normal immune function.[33]

Blood products are routinely used during plasma exchange procedures.[34] The most commonly used replacement fluids are 5% human albumin, plasma protein fraction (PPF), and fresh frozen plasma (FFP). Less frequently, immunoglobulin preparations are used both intramuscularly and intravenously for severely immunocompromised patients. To investigate the possible transmission of HIV or HIV antibodies during therapeutic apheresis, we studied serum samples for the presence of antibodies to HIV in 110 patients undergoing therapeutic plasmapheresis for a variety of diseases not related to AIDS.[33,35] The majority of patients received 5% human albumin as the replacement fluid. Four patients received FFP. Fifty-five patients received intravenous immune globulin in addition to the above-mentioned replacement fluids. Seven of the patients were homosexual men. The remaining patients did not belong to any known high-risk group for the development of AIDS.

Blood samples were tested before the beginning of therapeutic plasmapheresis and at the last follow-up visit. The mean follow-up period exceeded 24 months. The seven homosexual males started the study HIV-seropositive and remained so throughout the study period. None of the patients who did not belong to a high-risk group for AIDS were seropositive at the beginning of the study and none had seroconverted upon follow-up. None of the patients who received intravenous gammaglobulin developed HIV antibodies. One of the patients receiving FFP did seroconvert to an HIV antibody-positive state after a single plasma exchange where FFP was used as a replacement fluid. The patient reconverted to a seronegative state 2 days later following the next plasma exchange procedure also using FFP. This patient remained seronegative until she died 6 months later from metastatic carcinoma. This case illustrates the possibility of passive transfer of HIV antibodies occurring when using FFP and commercially available immune globulin products.[36]

COMMENT

The above-mentioned studies indicate that therapeutic apheresis has a limited application in the treatment of AIDS and AIDS-related conditions. Plasmapheresis appears to be effective in temporarily alleviating the neurologic symptoms in selected patients with AIDS/ARC-related peripheral neuropathy. Protein A immunoadsorption may play a role in the treatment of the immune thrombocytopenia associated with ARC/AIDS and also shows some activity against Kaposi's sarcoma. Further studies are required to investigate the possible application of therapeutic apheresis in conjunction with other treatment modalities in AIDS and AIDS-related conditions.

REFERENCES

1. Shaw, G. M.; Hahn, B. H.; Arya, S. K.; Groopman, J. E.; Gallo, R. C.; Wongstaal, F. Molecular characterization of human T-cell leukemia (lymphotropic) virus type III in the acquired immune deficiency syndrome. *Science* 1984; 226:1165.

2. Klatzmann, D.; Montagnier, L. Approaches to AIDS therapy. *Nature* 1986; 319:10–11.

3. Andrieu, J. M.; Even, P.; Venet, A. AIDS and related syndromes as a viral-induced autoimmune disease of the immune system: An anti-MHC II disorder. Therapeutic implications. *AIDS Res.* 1986; 2:163–174.

4. Kiprov, D. D.; Abrams, D.; Pfaeffl, W.; Jones, F.; Miller, R. G. ARC/AIDS-related autoimmune syndromes and their treatment. (Abstract.) *International Conference on AIDS*, Paris, 1986, p 32.

5. Ziegler, J. L.; Stites, D. P. Hypothesis: AIDS is an autoimmune disease directed at the immune system and triggered by a lymphotropic retrovirus. *Clin. Immunol. Immunopathol.* 1986; 41:305–313.

6. Cunningham-Rundles, S.; Michelis, M. A.; Masur, H. Serum suppression of lymphocyte activation in vitro in acquired immunodeficiency disease. *J. Clin. Immunol.* 1983; 3:156–165.

7. Laurence, J.; Gottlieb, A. B.; Kunkel, H. G. Soluble suppressor factors in patients with acquired immune deficiency and its prodrome. *J. Clin. Invest.* 1983; 72:2072–2081.

8. Siegal, J. P.; Djeu, J. Y.; Stocks, N. I.; Masur, H.; Gelmann, E. P.; Quinnan, G. V. Sera from patients with the acquired immunodeficiency syndrome inhibit production of interleukin 2 by normal lymphocytes. *J. Clin. Invest.* 1985; 75:1957–1964.

9. Kiprov, D. D.; Busch, D. F.; Simpson, D. M.; et al. Antilymphocyte serum factors in patients with acquired immunodeficiency syndrome. In Gottlieb, M.; Groopman, J. (eds.): *Acquired Immune Deficiency Syndrome*. New York: Alan R. Liss, 1984, pp. 299–308.

10. Kiprov, D. D.; Anderson, R. E.; Morand, P.; et al. Antilymphocyte antibodies and seropositivity for retroviruses in groups at high risk for AIDS. *N. Engl. J. Med.* 1985; 312:1517.

11. Kloster, B. E.; Tomar, R. H.; Spira, T. J. Lymphocytotoxic antibodies in the acquired immune deficiency syndrome (AIDS). *Clin. Immunol. Immunopathol.* 1984; 30:330–335.

12. Walsh, C. M.; Nardi, M. A.; Karpatkin, S. On the mechanism of thrombocytopenic purpura in sexually active homosexual men. *N. Engl. J. Med.* 1984; 311:635–639.

13. Stricker, R. B.; Abrams, D. I.; Corash, L.; Shuman, M. A. Target platelet antigen in homosexual men with immune thrombocytopenia. *N. Engl. J. Med.* 1985; 313:1375–1380.

14. Miller, R. G.; Parry, G.; Pfaeffl, W.; Lang, W.; Lippert, R.; Kiprov, D. D. Successful treatment with plasma exchange of peripheral neuropathies associated with ARC and AIDS. *J. Clin. Apheresis* 1988; 4:3–7.

15. Tomar, R. H.; Kloster, B. E.; Lamberson, H. V. Plasmapheresis increases T_4 lymphocytes in a patient with AIDS. *Am. J. Clin. Pathol.* 1984; 81:518–521.

16. Kiprov, D. D.; Lippert, R.; Miller, R. G.; et al. The use of plasmapheresis, lymphocytapheresis, and staph protein-A immunoadsorption as an immunomodulatory therapy in patients with AIDS and AIDS-related conditions. *J. Clin. Apheresis* 1986; 3:133–139.

17. Reiss, R. F.; Rubinstein, R.; Freidman-Kien, A.; et al. Partial plasma exchange in patients with AIDS and Kaposi's sarcoma. Plasmapheresis in AIDS. *AIDS Res.* 1986; 2:183–190.

18. Terman, D. S. Immunoadsorbents in autoimmune and neoplastic diseases. *Plasma Ther. Transfus. Technol.* 1983; 4:415–433.

19. Kiprov, D. D.; Lippert, R.; Jones, F. R.; Lagios, M. D.; Balint, J. P.; Cohen, R. J. Extracorporeal perfusion of plasma over immobilized protein A in a patient with Kaposi's sarcoma and acquired immunodeficiency. *J. Biol. Response Mod.* 1984; 3:341–346.

20. Jones, F. R.; Yoshida, L. H.; Ladiges, W. C.; Kenny, M. A. Treatment of feline leukemia and reversal of FeLV by ex vivo removal of IgG: A preliminary report. *Cancer* 1980: 46:675–684.

21. Morris, L.; Distenfeld, A.; Amorosi, E.; Karpatkin, S. Autoimmune thrombocytopenic purpura in homosexual men. *Ann. Intern. Med.* 1982; 96:714–717.

22. Abrams, D. I.; Kiprov, D. D.; Goedert, J. J.; Sarngadharan, M. G.; Gallo, R. C.; Volberding, P. A. Antibodies to human T-lymphotropic virus type III and development of the acquired immunodeficiency syndrome in homosexual men presenting with immune thrombocytopenia. *Ann. Intern. Med.* 1986; 104:47–50.

23. Biniek, R.; Malessa, R.; Brockmeyer, N. H.; Luboldt, W. Anti-Rh(D) immunoglobulin for AIDS-related thrombocytopenia. *Lancet* 1986; ii (Sept.):627.

24. Bertram, J.; Gill, P.; Henry, D.; Mittelman, A.; Kiprov, D. D.; Volberding, P. Protein-A therapy with the prosorba column in homosexual patients with ITP (abstract). *International Conference on AIDS*, Paris, 1986, p. 46.

25. Levy, R. M.; Bredsen, D. E.; Rosenblum, M. L. Neurological manifestations of the acquired immunodeficiency syndrome (AIDS): Experience at UCSF and review of the literature. *J. Neurosurg.* 1985; 62:475–495.

26. Lipkin, W. I.; Parry, G.; Kiprov, D. D.; Abrams, D. Inflammatory neuropathy in homosexual men with lymphadenopathy. *Neurology* 1985; 35:1479–1483.

27. Cornblath, D. R.; McArthur, J. C.; Griffin, J. W. Inflammatory demyelinating polyneuropathies associated with AIDS-related virus (ARV) infections. *Neurology* 1986; Suppl 1:206.

28. Miller, R. G.; Parry, G.; Lang, W.; Lippert, R.; Kiprov, D. D. AIDS-related inflammatory polyradiculoneuropathy: Successful treatment with plasma exchange. *Neurology* 1986; 36 (Suppl):206 (abstract).

29. Miller, R. G.; Parry, G.; Lang, W.; Lippert, R.; Kiprov, D. D. AIDS-related inflammatory polyradiculoneuropathy: Prediction of response to plasma exchange with electrophysiologic testing. *Muscle Nerve* 1985; 8:626 (abstract).

30. Hirsch, M. S. Risk of nosocomial infection with human T-cell lymphotropic virus III (HTLV-III). *N. Engl. J. Med.* 1985; 312:1–4.

31. McCray, E. Occupational risk of the acquired immunodeficiency syndrome among health care workers. *N. Engl. J. Med.* 1986; 314:1127–1132.

32. Stricof, R. L.; Morse, D. L. HTLV-III/LAV seroconversion following a deep intramuscular needlestick injury. (Letter.) *N. Engl. J. Med.* 1986; 314:1115.

33. Kiprov, D. D.; Simpson, D.; Romanick-Schmiedl, S.; Lippert, R.; Spira, T.; Busch, D. The risk of AIDS-related virus (HIV) transmission through apheresis procedures. *J. Clin. Apheresis* 1987; 3: 143–146.

34. Kiprov, D. D. An overview of therapeutic apheresis. *Dialysis Transplant* 1985; 14:195–200.

35. Kiprov, D. D.; Simpson, D.; Pfaeffl, W.; Romanick-Schmiedl, S.; Abrams, D.; Miller, R. G. AIDS and apheresis procedures—therapeutic and safety considerations. *Blood Purification* 1987; 5:51–56.

36. Gocke, D. J.; Raska, K.; Pollack, W.; Schwartzer, T. HTLV-III antibody in commercial immunoglobulin. *Lancet* 1986; i:37–38.

10

The Patient with AIDS: Care and Concerns

Patrice Murphy, Graham Bass, Carole Donovan, and Betsy Selman

INTRODUCTION

Where can a person afflicted with acquired immune deficiency syndrome (AIDS) turn for care? There is no easy answer to this question. Terminally ill persons are frequently spurned by traditional medical care, and this is all the more likely to occur when the person has AIDS. Currently 90% of persons with AIDS are homosexual or bisexual men, or intravenous drug users. Homosexuals and drug abusers have often been rejected by their biological families. The tendency toward homophobia in our society, intensified by a fear of death, has caused many social institutions as well to reject homosexuals, particularly those with AIDS. In some cases, lovers, friends, health care practitioners, and clergy abandon persons with AIDS due to the fear of contagion. Indeed, where can a person with AIDS turn for care?

To whom can persons suffering from AIDS turn if not to nurses, social workers, physicians, therapists, clergy, and volunteers who have been educated to confront the innumerable complexities of caring for the terminally ill patient with cancer, renal failure, pulmonary disease, and other dreadful illnesses? As hospice caregivers we have learned that symptoms of these diseases can be managed. So, too, can AIDS! We have seen miracles in our work; we are seeing them with AIDS patients and their families and friends. The work of the Supportive Care Program of St. Vincent's Hospital and Medical Center in New York City illustrates a hospice-related program which helps to care for those with AIDS.

The mission of St. Vincent's Hospital from its earliest days has been to serve the sick and poor of New York City. When St. Vincent's Hospital opened its doors in 1850, it was to provide care for the very poor, and often seriously ill, immigrant populations pouring into New York City. Today the mission remains the same, only the population using its services has changed, reflecting the changing demographics of the area and the needs of the times. Currently the issues of AIDS, the homeless, and the underserved are foremost in the Medical Center's concerns.

Located in the heart of Greenwich Village, St. Vincent's Hospital and Medical Center, with a bed capacity of 813, is the oldest community hospital in lower Manhattan, an area which continues to report the greatest incidence of AIDS in the nation. Although patients come from all five boroughs as well as New Jersey, St. Vincent's is the primary provider of acute medical care to residents of the area that immediately surrounds the hospital, commonly known as Chelsea and Greenwich Village. These two communities alone comprise half of the residential population of lower Manhattan and are home to a significant homosexual population. Almost 30% of the homosexual population are men between the ages of 18 and 44, and nearly half of the households are single persons living alone or together with a non-relative.

St. Vincent's has long been active in providing for the gay community's medical needs. Consequently, the staff are particularly aware of the special health care needs of this population. Since 1981 St. Vincent's Hospital has treated over 700 patients with AIDS. Eighty percent of the individuals live in Manhattan; 50% live within the hospital's immediate geographic area. The number of AIDS admissions has increased from a total of 20 in 1982 to nearly 500 in 1987. In late 1983, staff of the Supportive Care Program with expertise in caring for the terminally ill felt that this Program could provide care to AIDS patients. And so the staff began—slowly but determinedly—to incorporate AIDS patients into the Program. Currently patients with AIDS comprise approximately 70% of the Program's participants. The goal of the Program is to provide coordinated comprehensive services and caring through a multidisciplinary approach which enables patients to return to, and remain in, the familiar surroundings of the home environment and, when desired, to die at home.

The team at St. Vincent's Supportive Care Program includes physicians, nurses, social workers, pastoral counselors, and trained community volunteers. Because of the nature of the work, all are invited to explore the pastoral dimension, no matter what their official professional capacity. "Pastoral" here is defined in a broad sense, as distinct from the professional role of the pastoral counselor which often (but not always) applies to the clergy and religious from many faiths who are specifically trained to help people cope with existential and transcendent issues. In this broad definition, the pastoral dimension is the aspect within each human being which recognizes the intrinsic value of each other being and understands the very real connection existing among all people. This dimension needs to be encouraged in anyone who wishes to be of genuine service to a person with AIDS or to the patient's loved ones. In such a capacity we are constantly confronted by our own limitations. Are our unexamined biases regarding homosexuality or drug abuse obstacles to seeing the patient's inherent worth? Are we willing to accept the real human relationship we have to the addict with AIDS who perhaps is still abusing drugs, or to the young gay man denying his diagnosis (and mortality) who continues to be active sexually? How do we relate to the parents who disown their dying child because of his sexuality or abuse of drugs or to the despairing patient contemplating suicide because he has lost hope? These questions continually challenge our attitudes and judgments.

A nurse in the Program quickly realizes that the physical care which he or she extends to his or her patient, as taxing and complicated as it becomes due to the complex symptomatology of AIDS, is only part of the total picture. The emotional, psychosocial, and spiritual aspects are all intertwined. With the diagnosis of AIDS, the physical and the metaphysical come crashing together. There are the physical agonies of Kaposi's sarcoma (KS) lesions, *Pneumocystis carinii* pneumonia (PCP), intractable diarrhea, encephalopathy, neurological impairment, fevers and sweats, blindness, and exhaustion. Among with these physical ailments are the agonizing metaphysical questions for the patient and the caregiver: "Why me?" "Am I being punished?" "Did God make a mistake when he created me?" "Am I to blame for my illness?" "What was the meaning and purpose of my life?"

These questions form an important component of the care of AIDS patients. However, the purpose of the following anecdotes is to illustrate primarily the medical aspects of care, in particular the treatment of opportunistic infections which are often fatal to persons with AIDS.

JAMES

James was a 54-year-old gay male whom the Supportive Care nurse visited at his home for five weeks. Although there had been other opportunistic infections, his main problem at that time was a *Cryptosporidium* infection. This is a protozoan gastrointestinal illness which, in those with normally functioning immune systems, produces what is sometimes known as "travelers' diarrhea," a bothersome but usually self-limiting condition which "runs" its course and, perhaps with some symptomatic treatment, departs. In AIDS patients, however, it can become an intractable diarrhea, with continuous watery stools, incurable and often unimprovable, leading to physical exhaustion, dehydration, electrolyte imbalance, and eventually death. The latter is often welcomed as an end to an existence which many patients consider to be not worth living.

Such a patient was James. Fiercely independent during his adult years, he was a renowned collector of fine antiques and furniture, and his refined taste and artistic sensibility extended to all areas of his life. This man was found in bed lying in his stool on the nurse's first visit. Having been cleaned only 15 minutes previously in the ongoing, losing battle to keep dry, clean, and comfortable, he was once again wet, soiled, and most uncomfortable. Lomotil had been tried, but it literally failed to stem the flow, followed, equally unsuccessfully, by Imodium. James felt hopeless about any other possibilities. Both he and the young relative who was helping to care for him were exhausted by his constant diarrhea and the efforts involved in trying to keep him comfortable.

After evaluating the situation, the nurse suggested that a rectal tube might provide some immediate relief, if not from the diarrhea itself then at least from the incessant discomfort. James and his relative expressed interest, and the nurse inserted a large, #20 2-way Foley catheter with a 5-cc balloon, lubricated with KY jelly, with the distal end attached to a 2000-cc bedside drainage bag. The insertion itself was the occasion for some humor on the part of James, who commented acerbically that it was an attempt to relate sexually to him. This was the first glimpse of anything other than hopelessness and depression that had been seen in him on that visit. The balloon was inflated with 5 cc of air; immediately, watery stool proceeded to flow through the tube into the drainage bag. Determining that his caregiver felt able to assume the task of removing and reinserting the tube periodically to give the rectal mucosa a rest, the nurse instructed him in the technique of doing so and found him an apt pupil. The caregiver knew that the nurse would be available by phone or in person as necessary to deal with any problems that might arise. Due to the excellent care he had been receiving, James's skin was still in good condition despite the difficulty in keeping him clean. The nurse reinforced the principles and techniques of good skin care, however, to avoid additional problems.

That night, for the first time in many days, James and his caregiver were able to get uninterrupted sleep. And for the first time in weeks, James could lie on a dry, clean sheet with some degree of comfort.

The next step was to see if there could be any success in actually stemming the tide. The nurse spoke with James's physician, who ordered Paregoric. Although the diarrhea did not cease, it did slow down somewhat, so that the 2000-cc bedside drainage bag needed to be emptied only once every 24 hours rather than every 12 hours or less.

James was receiving home Total Parenteral Nutrition (TPN) at night through a Hickman catheter. TPN is a solution of protein and other nutritional elements to compensate for reduced food intake. His latest blood tests, however, had shown a rising blood urea nitrogen (BUN) and troublesome serum electrolyte changes. His physician ordered certain changes in the TPN formula and extra intravenous replacement fluids to correct the imbalances as much as possible. All of this was done at home, since James was adamant about not wanting to return to the hospital. However, at this point, he became adamant about something else as well—he had had enough. Weak, dependent, unable to pursue his interests, vocational or avocational, that made life worth living, he was ready to die. While his own religious beliefs did not permit suicide, he was not willing to do anything to prolong life. The nurse and James talked about this at length, including his caregiver, who had the most difficulty with the idea of not continuing the fight for life, in the discussions. Eventually the caregiver came to understand and respect James's decision to refuse any further TPN or IV fluids. Over the next week, James became progressively weaker, slipped into a coma, and died peacefully.

THOMAS, STEVE, AND JACKIE

Thomas was an actor and a dancer—one of the best! He had been on Broadway and in major films. At the age of 26 he was one of the few who was always working. His physical grace, skill, and appearance were central to his work and to his sense of self. And he had a large, dark purple lesion right on the tip of his nose.

Steve had similar lesions all over his face and body. His eyes were swollen shut, and large, angry, purple weltlike marks adorned his body.

Jackie had only a few lesions. But they were on his legs and the bottoms of his feet, and caused him excruciating pain when he tried to walk or even stand. He spent almost all of his time in bed.

All three patients had Kaposi's sarcoma, a normally rather innocuous form of cancer appearing as dark patches on the skin and usually affecting elderly men of Mediterranean or Middle Eastern descent. As manifested in AIDS, Kaposi's sarcoma (KS) knows no limitations, neither of age nor ethnic descent or extent of dissemination. Thus far it is not curable. Various chemotherapeutic treatments such as bleomycin or vincristine seem to help for a while. Indeed, the lesions and swelling can change dramatically, with lesions becoming smaller and lighter-colored. But upon completion of the chemotherapeutic regimens, the lesions seem to return within weeks, redoubled, almost as if the chemotherapy itself had provided renewed vigor. This was the case time after time.

KS does not always appear in such virulent fashion. Many patients have only a few rather unobtrusive lesions and remain in that condition for long periods of time. Others, like Steve and Jackie, seem to be completely overwhelmed by KS, internally as well as externally. Although the lesions themselves are not usually painful, they can be agonizing if, as in Jackie's case, they are on a part of the body that must bear weight or pressure.

The nurse noted an ironic phenomenon—many of these young men, often involved in professional theater, dance, fashion, or some other pursuit that involved their physical appearance professionally or socially, would, like Thomas, get a KS lesion in the worst of all places—right on the tip of their nose, resulting in an often grotesque, clownlike appearance. This phenomenon becomes understandable when one realizes that KS is actually a sarcoma of the capillary lining, and therefore an area of the body particularly well endowed with capillaries—such as the nose—would be a likely site for the appearance of the lesions. Unfortunately, the only current alternative to chemotherapy—radiation therapy—does not do much to improve their appearance. For Thomas, cosmetics helped. A young makeup artist for a TV soap opera volunteered her expertise to develop a makeup that could be matched to the individual patient's skin tone to cover the most blatant facial lesions. This allowed Thomas and Steve, with lesions on their faces, to go out in public with less self-consciousness.

A combination of narcotics, chemotherapy, and radiation therapy to his feet allowed Jackie to have increased comfort for a few weeks. However, the KS lesions on his feet were so abundant, interfering with his blood circulation, that his feet became gangrenous. Before a decision could be made on this latest development, Jackie went into respiratory failure due to KS lesions in his lung. He was intubated, and a few days later, despite all efforts, he died.

Steve's KS led to such facial swelling that his eyes could not open. For a patient whose main pleasure in life at this terrible time was to watch videos on a VCR that he had bought with his remaining money, until the death that he knew was approaching would overtake him, the loss of his vision was torturous. Maintaining a semi-Fowler's or Fowler's position (the head of the bed elevated from one to two feet) in bed, and using cold packs on his eyes, helped reduce the swelling somewhat. But it was ultimately the use of steriods that proved most successful. These drugs are generally contraindicated for AIDS patients, for they may mask infection, cause immunosuppression, and delay healing. But in Steve's case, they allowed him weeks of life that were meaningful to him. Shortly thereafter, the KS lesions affected his lungs, causing eventual respiratory failure.

Thomas's case of Kaposi's sarcoma never became a life-threatening problem, aside from the extent to which its appearance made him feel that his life was not worth living. Psychological counseling and support, giving him opportunities and the encouragement to express his feelings of loss and anger, were vital. During his last months he was able to come to terms with much that had at first seemed completely and incomprehensibly overwhelming. His death a few weeks later was due to a cytomegalovirus (CMV) infection which impaired his pulmonary and gastrointestinal functioning.

RODNEY

Rodney had been diagnosed with AIDS for several months. He had herpes on the whole left side of his face, but it was not the herpes simplex of the cold sore, it was herpes zoster ophthalmicus. The virus had affected the left eye, producing blindness. Torturously painful and itchy, it looked as if some blistering scalding process had attacked the whole left side of his face from jaw to temple. Herpes zoster is caused by the varicella zoster virus—the same virus which causes chickenpox. The first exposure to this virus causes chickenpox and usually the virus is subsequently destroyed. However, it is possible that some viruses lodge in nerve ganglia and remain dormant until reactivation by an unknown mechanism. If the body is unable to fight because its immune system is unable to initiate and maintain the effective response to destroy the varicella zoster viruses, the viruses will continue to multiply, spreading down the sensory nerves to the skin and causing the infection herpes zoster. Rodney's depressed immune system was unable to respond adequately to these viruses. The intense pain of his left eye and surrounding facial area was due to the virus having attacked the ophthalmic branch of the trigeminal nerve.

It is necessary to be on a constant "herpes watch" with AIDS patients, for the herpes simplex virus can strike almost anywhere—face, eyes, mouth, genitals, rectum, or other areas of the body. It can present as an innocuous-appearing sore, or, as in the case of Rodney's herpes zoster ophthalmicus, as an overwhelming catastrophe. Acyclovir is the treatment of choice, used either topically or systemically, and although it does not "cure" the patient of the virus, it can drive the infection into remission. Sight once lost does not return and the scars in cases such as Rodney's remain. But the acute intense discomfort, the severe burning pain, the open weeping sores, can be resolved with treatment. However, chronic, less intense pain may persist.

Rodney suffered bravely and at length; healing was a slow process because of the immunosuppression of AIDS. Suddenly, one evening during the healing period, Rodney became confused and disoriented as to time, person, and place; he was threatening and abusive to nurses, angry at anyone who approached him. Always gentlemanly and thoughtful in the past, this behavior took everyone by surprise, and a number of consultations were arranged immediately. The consensus of the professionals called to evaluate Rodney's sudden eruptive behavior and disturbed mental activity was that he was suffering from herpes encephalitis. Encephalitis is a severe inflammation of the brain which can be caused by a virus such as herpes. Intense lymphocytic infiltration of brain tissue and the leptomeninges (soft cerebral and spinal membranes) can cause cerebral edema, degeneration of the brain's ganglion cells, and diffuse nerve cell destruction. Herpes encephalitis also produces symptoms that vary from subclinical to acute and often fulminating disease.

It was at least 72 hours before Rodney became more subdued. Decadron to reduce cerebral edema, sedatives for restlessness, Dilantin to prevent convulsions, and aspirin or Tylenol for headaches and fever were administered; he responded eventually. But Rodney has never been fully himself again. Once eager to share thoughts and feelings, intellectually curious, loving to read, listen to music, watch TV, and just enjoy being with and socializing with others, he is now considerably less energetic, more passive and quiet—even listless. While the headaches associated with the herpes infection are long gone, new physical discomforts have replaced them—paresthesias (pricking sensations) of feet, legs and sometimes parts of this trunk, and varying degrees of foot pain. Weight loss is also apparent, although Rodney's home health aide prepares meals and in-between snacks which he continues to eat adequately. The greatest loss to Rodney seems to be that of the sight in his left eye. Deprivation of the ability to read has been an influence in his increasing apathy and listlessness. What is saddest for those caring for Rodney over many months is the gradual physical, emotional, and mental deterioration that is so much part of this disease.

BOB AND MIGUEL

Words were Bob's life. His job was tracing certain words back to biblical times to see how usage had changed. It was exacting, painstaking work. How cruel then that Bob's illness caused progressive loss of speech until he was mute, a left-sided paralysis, and a partial loss of vision. Bob seemed like a person who had suffered a stroke. He also had hallucinations and paranoid ideas. A psychiatrist worked with him during the months he was hospitalized, but it was not clear whether Bob had become acutely psychotic or had lost his ability to communicate from some destruction of his brain. Because of his helpless condition, an aide was hired to be with Bob 12 hours each day. Tommy—the aide—arrived, a gift from the gods.

Tommy helped Bob move from bed to chair, played tapes of Bob's favorite music, and encouraged him to eat his meals sitting up in a chair. After weeks of making no sounds, Bob suddenly called out one morning to the floor nurse, "MacGregor, get in here!" From that point on, Bob began to speak again. No one understood what had caused him to stop talking or to start again. Bob could now respond to questions but could not initiate conversation. Finally, he was discharged and Tommy continued to care for him Monday through Friday. Tommy carried out a passive range of motion exercises with him, kept the radio tuned to a classical music station, and read aloud concert reviews as ways of providing various forms of stimulation. Any mispronunciation of a composer's name prompted a correction from Bob. In talking with Bob it was clear that his recent memory was intact and, occasionally, that he could recall past information. Once when Tommy and the Supportive Care nurse were talking about an old Abbott and Costello movie, Bob suddenly interjected "Hey, Abbott!" Costello's frequent cry. At times Bob would become fixated on an idea and pursue it over and over. "Tommy, I won't have to have exercises anymore, will I?" he would ask and then repeat the question again in 15 minutes. Tommy patiently reassured him each time.

Bob's physicians believed that he suffered from progressive multifocal leukoencephalopathy (PML). PML is a demyelinating disease caused by a papovavirus that produces blindness, aphasia, hemiparesis (paralysis of one side of the body), and ataxia (impaired ability to coordinate muscular movement).[1] But any number of other neurological changes can occur in these patients and can be caused by viral as well as nonviral organisms.

Loss of recent memory is often the prelude to further neurological problems. Miguel, for example, would report that he could not remember simple things. He had no other neurological changes at the time and no such changes were being reported in the literature. Miguel became progressively more ill with fevers and diarrhea. Simultaneously, he became more and more noncommunicative and withdrawn until he could no longer speak. He would look at whomever was speaking to him but staff members had the impression that there no longer existed a person who could understand or respond on any level.

Some patients with neurological changes complain of numbness and tingling of their fingers, toes, and balls of their feet. It is not known what causes these sensations nor how to relieve them. Occasionally patients with Kaposi's sarcoma, that may or may not be visible, find walking extremely painful. Thick, rubber-soled shoes or slippers may offer some relief. Pain medication such as MS Contin seems to take the edge off the pain but offers no lasting relief. Some patients are put on Tegretol, others on Dilantin, in an effort to alleviate the neurological discomfort. Again results are disappointing.

What seems to help these patients most is allowing them to talk freely about the changes they are experiencing and then make practical suggestions to help them maintain certain functions. For example, if a patient is having difficulty walking, perhaps a walker or wheelchair is in order. Passive or active range of motion exercises may do more for morale than for muscle tone, but may be worth trying. Either heat or cold may reduce the intensity of pain. Often it is reassuring to the patient to know that what he is experiencing is part of the physical manifestations of the disease, not something that is psychological.

MARTIN AND ALAN

Martin had been diagnosed as having AIDS for about eight months. He had a number of medical problems—Kaposi's sarcoma and a cytomegalovirus infection among them. He complained of joint pain in his right wrist—an achiness and difficulty flexing it. There was no sign of inflammation or swelling, but eventually a great red lump developed on the outer aspect of his wrist. Soon similar lumps appeared on his thighs. His right ankle became so painful that he could not bear to have even the weight of a sheet on it. Martin always had an elevated temperature and so it was difficult to determine if his usual rise to 100 degrees or more was a signal for some new infectious process.

Martin was admitted to the hospital, his ankle was opened and cultured. The report read *Mycobacterium avium intracellulare* (MAI). A regimen of antituberculosis drugs were now added to his growing list of medications. MAI is one of a group of atypical mycobacteria. These organisms are not transmitted person-to-person but, rather, are acquired from the environment—for example, from soil or dust. The organism can cause a variety of reactions—lymphadenitis, pulmonary infections, cutaneous infections.[2] The organs commonly infected are bone marrow, liver, spleen, gastrointestinal tract, and lymph nodes.[3] Thus, anemia and pancytopenia (marked reduction of blood components) can occur; liver function tests can be abnormal; malabsorption and weight loss can result.[4]

Hot soaks to Martin's wrist helped ease his discomfort as did a footboard to lift the covers from his feet. Tylenol and codeine were the drugs of choice for pain because other analgesics upset his stomach. But knowing the cause of an infection and administering the drugs which resolve the illness in others does not necessarily change the course of illness for a person with AIDS. Martin continued on a downhill course and finally wished only to be kept comfortable. He wanted what he perceived to be his non-life to end.

Martin had been a fashion designer. When he knew he could no longer work 16 hours a day, he closed his business. Despite his difficulties, Martin maintained his sense of humor and kept a twinkle in his eyes. During the last days, he spoke often about his wish to die and to be with God. One of the Supportive Care Program's volunteer clergy visited regularly with Martin and reassured him, "We're praying for you." Martin rolled his eyes and said, "I know. That's the problem. It's working and I'm still here."

Alan was the director of an elementary school that he had established. He was an exacting person; he would call the manufacturer of the drug he was receiving to check the protocol he was on and to learn more about the drug's side effects. When he was assessed for acceptance in the Supportive Care Program, Alan expressed his concern about his diminished vision. He said that it seemed as though he had a veil over his left eye. The nurse encouraged him to visit an ophthalmologist who found that a wooly exudate on the retina represented a cytomegalovirus infection of the right eye.

Cytomegalovirus (CMV) is classified as a herpes virus and an infection resulting from it is considered to be a sexually transmitted disease.[5] Alan's visual changes are typical of those in patients who have CMV retinitis. The changes usually progress and are irreversible. Often retinitis signals active systemic CMV infection. CMV can be isolated from a number of body secretions and excretions—saliva, blood, urine, stool, secretions of the uterine cervix, semen, and breast milk[6]—and in the immunosuppressed patients can cause "hepatitis, pneumonitis, arthralgias, retinitis, and signs of disseminated disease.[7] Pneumonitis is generally the most common outcome of CMV infection, after fever and mononucleosis. Patients report fever, nonproductive cough, and dyspnea (shortness of breath), often associated with hypoxia (a deficiency of oxygen). The liver and gastrointestinal tract may also be affected by CMV.[8]

To slow the retinal destruction by the virus, Alan was admitted to the hospital for drug therapy. A Hickman catheter was inserted to begin treatment with an experimental drug, DHPG, which he then continued to receive at home.

During the Supportive Care nurse's visits to Alan, he would often evaluate whether or not his vision was changing by reading book titles from across the room, using only his affected eye. In general he found that the visual distortion made it impossible to engage in constructive activities, which distressed him and was a frequent source of complaint to his nurse.

There are a number of ways to alleviate the distress caused by visual distortion. Wearing a patch over the affected eye may help eliminate the conflicting images. Alan found it helpful to wear dark glasses both indoors and out. Safety must be stressed, however. The patient should be reminded to turn his head to check traffic when crossing streets to compensate for the loss of peripheral vision. Using recorded books may relieve the patient's frustration in attempting to read. Patients usually do eventually accommodate to their diminished vision but they need ample opportunities to express their sorrow and anger over the loss of yet another function that compromises self-image and independence.

TOM AND ROY

On a home visit, Tom's lungs were clear to auscultation (listening with a stethoscope). His respiratory rate was 24, his pulse was 84. Yet Tom reported that walking across the room—a small room at that—made him short of breath. He had no fever, but did have a persistent nonproductive cough. A call to his doctor resulted in Tom being placed on the list for hospital admission. Various tests were then carried out in the hospital and it appeared that Tom most likely had *Pneumocystis carinii* pneumonia (PCP). Once hospitalized, Tom was placed on intravenous pentamidine because of a previously established allergy to Septra, the medication of choice. His respiratory condition worsened. He was asked if he wished to be placed on a respirator if it became necessary and he replied, "Yes." Within four days of admission, Tom was intubated, placed on a respirator, and transferred to the medical intensive care unit.

PCP is one of the more common infections to occur in patients who have AIDS.[9] Its course is difficult to predict: it can rapidly cause death within days or it can progress slowly and resolve itself. Even a chest X ray can be difficult to interpret. The typical X ray of a patient with PCP shows bilateral interstitial and alveolar infiltrates. It can, however, also appear normal.[10] Septra is the drug of choice, but for those who develop a sensitivity to it, pentamidine is given. Pentamidine can, however, cause either hypoglycemia or hyperglycemia for which insulin may be required. It can also cause renal dysfunction, requiring dietary restrictions of potassium and protein.

Tom remained in the intensive care unit until he could be weaned from the respirator, which happened about one week following his admission. He was then discharged home one week later. His kidneys had been mildly damaged by the pentamidine therapy. With help from a dietician, Tom worked out a diet that was low in potassium and protein. Six weeks later his renal function studies returned to normal.

Roy's bout with PCP also began insiduously. He ran slight fevers and developed a persistent nonproductive cough. Initially his X ray demonstrated no abnormalities. He was placed on a course of erythromycin because of his cough and fevers. Within ten days, however, Roy began to complain of shortness of breath. Testing now revealed what seemed to be a PCP infection. Roy was admitted to the hospital and Septra therapy was begun. Four days after admission, he spiked fevers to 105 degrees which were followed by drenching sweats and chills. By the second week, his temperature had dropped to 99 degrees and he was ambulatory. By the third week, Roy was home again.

What is so difficult with the respiratory infections these patients experience is accurately determining what is going on in the patients' chests. Respiratory infections in some patients result in permanent changes in auscultory sounds — wheezes for some, diminished breath sounds for others, depending on what residual damage has occurred in the lung tissue. The type of cough also varies from patient to patient. The dry persistent cough seems to be the most annoying and difficult to control. Robitussin is usually the first line of defense moving to elixir of terpin hydrate with codeine for more disruptive coughs.

What seems to be a consistent finding, however, is the unpredictability of AIDS and its manifestations. A careful history needs to be elicited and recorded each week. Clues need to be pieced together to make some sense out of the many symptoms that result from the alterations of many systems. And, as always, the patient needs to be heard, to be comforted, to be reassured. Clearly he knows that little is really known about this disease and that not much is available to combat it.

Despite the uncertainty, despite the despair that comes from knowing friends who have died from this disease, the patient most often remains clearheaded about what is to come and prepares for his death by having his will drawn up and power of attorney assigned. Some patients are able to work on fragmented relationships with family and friends, repairing them where possible and, if not, at least acknowledging the relationship. The courage of each patient throughout the illness is awesome.

CAREGIVERS AND THE EXISTENTIAL

In their psychic pain—helpless and often hopeless—patients with AIDS pose thought-provoking, sometimes threatening, questions and reflections to their caregivers, particularly to nurses. How do we respond to the questions of a 35-year-old, "Will I be brave enough?", or a 23-year-old, "What will it be like—the end I mean?"

There is no single answer to such questions. The responses come from deep within each one of us—unique, as each of us is unique, issuing from levels that are deep and personal and spiritual. Levels where each of us communes with our God.

It is vital—possibly more vital than the medical treatment we administer—that we caregivers really be in touch with our innermost selves, with the essence of our spirit of caring, which is love. The following reflections provide us food for thought.

> . . .*And fear ruled.*
> *At first a lump appeared.*
> *On the body, the size of an egg.*
> *Then did spots cover the body.*
> *Then came the fever*
> *With vomiting,*
> *With coughing,*
> *Then swiftly—death.*
> *And despair ruled.*
> *Mothers abandoned their*
> *Children lest they themselves*
> *Be contaminated*
> *The young in fear*
> *Abandoned the aged, ...*
> *Fathers barred the door to sons*
> *And sons cast out infected fathers,*
> *Priests abandoned the infected*
> *And physicians, the dying.*
> *And the Death spared none:*
> *Neither bishop nor priest,*
> *Neither lad nor lass,*
> *Neither scholar nor student,*
> *Master nor journeyman,*
> *Neither merchant nor sailor*
> *Neither artisan nor smith; . . .*
> *Then did despair reign:*
> *There was no herb, no poultice,*
> *Neither cordial nor gold,*
> *No balm nor drink*
> *Nothing could prevent the Death.*

Then did anger reign:
There was the howling
And cursing,
Many shouted blasphemies
And cursed the day their
Mothers bore them,
Then did many curse God,
Then all gave way to silence.

This bleak description is taken from a monologue in a play written about Julian of Norwich, a fourteenth-century writer, mystic, and spiritual guide.[11] Julian survived two epidemics of the Black Plague. The fear, despair, and anger of which she speaks is easily applicable to the contemporary tragedy of AIDS. We twentieth-century humans respond in a similar way to our ancestors from the Middle Ages when dealing with a major catastrophe. The fear (however irrational) of contracting a terrifying illness, the despair of a terminal prognosis, the resulting anger at oneself, someone else, or God, are some of the compelling pastoral issues that confront the person caring for AIDS patients and their loved ones. The pastoral person doesn't presume to answer these questions but, rather, searches with the patient through the maze of pain and confusion. The path through this suffering may sometimes lead to vast unexplored places in the heart, or to stony walls that seem inpenetrable. The key throughout this cooperative journey is trust—trust that must be placed in the healer within the patient and in the covenant between this inner healer and the very heart of God. The pastoral person must be comfortable working within "kairos," God's time, and using a new language that emphasizes the interrogative form more than the declarative.

There are so many times with AIDS patients when their experience and our response transcends words. The power of communicating our care and acceptance nonverbally to our patients cannot be stressed enough. Nurses, volunteers, and pastoral counselors can say so much with a simple touch. One of our Program's pastoral counselors describes her experiences with a patient with AIDS.

> I remember visiting one of our first patients with AIDS in 1983. He was a young, extremely talented, and handsome man at the height of his career as a college professor when he was diagnosed. He was very angry and had alienated several of his caregivers. I listened and I listened to his anger and fear and to my anger and fear. Eventually the trust began to grow between us. During one visit, the frustration and pain spilled out in tears. He cried, "No one has touched me in months." Procedures had been done to him, he had been jostled, poked, and prodded, but the most basic human contact of a warm reassuring touch had been absent. Although my presence was helpful, it was ambiguous. I was contributing to the mixed message, "I really care about you and accept you, but you are an untouchable." "Being with" Joseph had to move from empathic conversation, to a more totally empathic presence, to a more primary physical level. It meant working through my own fears of contagion and intimacy. It meant putting my hands where I said my heart was. After this revelation, with his permission, I began to do body work with him. I used techniques gleaned from massage, polarity, therapeutic touch, visualization, and meditation. Almost every time I visited, he would ask with a shy grin, "Are you going to do that relaxing spiritual stuff today?" I'd say, "Sure, if that's what you'd like," after which, we would do little or no talking. I could see the tension leave his face and body as he relaxed. Usually he would drop off

to sleep, a wonderful result because his anxiety prevented him from getting the rest he so badly needed. These quiet sessions together did so much to deepen the trust between us. Ironically, the traditional pastoral issues and questions emerged as a result of this silent time together. I would urge caretakers to become proficient in some form of body work and meditation. It is an invaluable tool in working with AIDS patients.

As Supportive Care workers, we are truly connected to our patients and to each other. We teach each other and we minister to each other. It is a constant mystery in the healing arts—who is healing whom? What broken part of ourselves is being healed as we extend ourselves to another? Recently, on a particularly gray, muggy August afternoon, I (Betsy Selman) sat in my office, damp and miserable, complaining about life in general. There was suddenly a small commotion in the doorway. I went to see who had arrived. Paulette, our secretary, had gone over to the hospital to help one of our AIDS patients make the block-long trip to our office for the weekly AIDS support group. There sat Charles (a young man whose sweet and gentle disposition was reflected in his face) in his wheelchair. He had been attached to a dialysis machine for several days and there had been moments during this last hospital stay when we thought that we would lose him. He sat in his wheelchair and wept (exhausted, but exhilarated to have made it)—not because of his life-threatening illness, but because it was the first time in a month that he had been outside. His tears of gratitude at simply feeling the hot, humid air stunned me. That part of me that complains and takes so much for granted was stilled for a moment, and was given gentle instruction in gratitude and humility. Understanding that we are the patients, even as we are the caregivers, expands the pastoral dimension and improves the quality of our caring.

CONCLUSION

We know with certainty from experiences in the Supportive Care Program that hospice, palliative care, and supportive care programs are viable options and invaluable resources for patients with AIDS and their families, particularly as alternatives to hospitalization and routine home care.

Hospices have been affirmed and further challenged in their efforts by Elisabeth Kübler-Ross, who in her keynote presentation at the First Annual American Conference on Hospice Care in June 1985, said, "A hospice that doesn't accept AIDS patients should not be called a hospice." She stated that the special mission of hospice practitioners was to care for all dying patients with unconditional love; that is, love under any condition.

For all hospice practitioners facing the complex issues surrounding the AIDS crisis, the policy adopted by the National Hospice Organization in November 1985 provides guidance, inspiration, and challenge.[12]

The National Hospice Organization believes that the care of AIDS patients is as important as the cure of the AIDS disease. NHO affirms the pioneering work of our members in making hospice care accessible to AIDS sufferers and responsive to their needs. Those hospices which have pioneered palliative care for AIDS patients symbolize what hospices ought to do in fulfilling the standards and principles of the National Hospice Organization. NHO encourages all hospices to serve AIDS patients.

NHO understands that fear, stress, confusion, and lack of experience and resources may be obstacles to the care of AIDS patients in hospices just as in the rest of our society. The special needs of the AIDS patient and family should not be understated, but should be understood.

The significant issues posed by AIDS and the access of AIDS patients to hospice care must not result in avoidance, denial, or desertion by those to whom these patients can turn for help. The special needs of the AIDS patient call for the best in us as hospices and as hospice people.

We can only agree with this statement.

REFERENCES

1. Levy, Robert M.; et al. Neurological manifestations of the Acquired Immunodeficiency Syndrome (AIDS): Experience at USCF and review of the literature. *Journal of Neurosurgery* 62:482 (April 1985).

2. Reese, Richard E.; Douglas, R. Gordon, Jr. *A Practical Approach to Infectious Diseases.* Boston, Toronto: Little Brown and Company, 1983, p. 405.

3. Holmes, King K.; et al. *Sexually Transmitted Diseases.* New York: McGraw-Hill, 1984, p. 699.

4. Ibid., p. 699.

5. Ibid., pp. 474, 477.

6. Ibid., p. 475.

7. Mandell, Gerald L., et al. *Principles and Practice of Infectious Disease.* New York: John Wiley, 1979, p. 1317.

8. Ibid., pp. 1308–1319.

9. Holmes, King K. *Sexually Transmitted Diseases,* p. 695.

10. Ibid., pp. 695–696.

11. Janda, Julian J. *A Play Based On The Life of Julian of Norwich.* New York: The Seabury Press, 1984, p. 40, Reprinted with permission. Copyright © 1984 by Winston/Seabury and Harper and Row, Publishers, Inc.

12. *News Briefs:* NHO adopts policy on AIDS patients. *American Journal of Hospice Care:* 8–9 (March/April 1986).

11

Choosing Therapies

Chuck Frutchey

MEDICAL TREATMENTS

The decisions involved in choosing treatments are difficult for people with AIDS and ARC. For many, the decisions require both information and analytical skills that they may not have.

A physician should be consulted before pursuing any treatment plan; however, all decision-making authority should not be surrendered. The decisions ultimately remain the patient's and preparation is necessary to make them intelligently. A person with AIDS should use doctors, friends, and other people with AIDS/ARC as resources, but should retain and exercise the right to make choices about his or her own health.

Unlike many alternative therapies, where the effectiveness of the treatment is not certain, with medically supervised therapies there is usually a great deal known about the treatment process—its benefits and possible negative side effects. The patient should find out all pertinent information, investigating even those therapies not likely to be chosen, to understand why they may or may not be appropriate. The clinician should encourage the patient to ask lots of questions, and to keep asking if something is explained and is still not understood. Many patients will probably have to learn new things about how the human body functions in order to increase their knowledge to make appropriate decisions. Health care providers should be prepared to refer the patient to other resources for information they cannot provide.

The patient should also be made aware that in some cases no therapy at all may be an option. Some people, such as those with early and nonaggressive Kaposi's sarcoma, do not always need treatment. For other people, there may only be one type of medication to treat a particular infection which requires immediate attention. After the infection has been eliminated, however, patients may be able to "safely" stop treatment, or take some time to consider which treatment is best.

Since the treatment of most opportunistic infections in AIDS is fairly straightforward, the most difficult decisions will involve investigational drugs. In order to make an intelligent choice about a drug program, it is first necessary to understand how these programs are run and what are the possible side effects of the drugs.

Every drug trial involving humans is divided into four phases after first testing the drug in animal studies. During Phase 1, the drug is monitored for toxicity (harmfulness) and tested to see how the body processes or metabolizes it. In Phase 2, the test moves on to find out how effective the drug is in controlling the disease or its symptoms. Phase 3 introduces many of the elements we normally think of for "controlled" studies. In this stage, the study participants are randomly divided into two or more groups. One group receives the investigational drug at a dosage that is based on Phase 2 results. The other group will get a harmless, inactive compound, usually a sugar pill or equivalent, known as a placebo. Neither the researchers nor the participants know who is getting the drug and who is getting the placebo. This is called a "double-blind" study. Phase 4 studies are ongoing studies of the drug's effects and usefulness in clinical practice.

Double-blind studies are extremely important in proving whether or not a new drug is worthwhile. It is important for the participants not to know what they are receiving because it is very common for people taking placebos to show some improvement, simply because they *think* they are taking an effective medicine. At the same time, it is important for the researchers not to know which patients are receiving the placebo so that they are not prejudiced when evaluating the participants.

There has been a lot of criticism lately about the "immorality" of giving people placebos when they are very sick. But without placebo-controlled studies, it would be impossible to know if any observed benefits were the result of the drug or merely the participants' desire to get well. The mind can be a very powerful tool in healing and designing experiments that take this into account is necessary to evaluate the real cause behind a drug's apparent success. Even with the drug AZT, which has become more widely available though all of the effects are not fully understood, the initial evidence that it was useful came from double-blind, placebo-controlled studies. Only when the results are dramatically successful or unsuccessful can a solid determination of efficacy without placebo controls be made. (As we progress in our study of drugs to treat AIDS, it will become possible to replace the placebo with a drug whose effectiveness is known and measure the new drug's effectiveness against it. This is a variation of placebo-controlled studies and satisfies the same requirements.)

In the long run, the method of controlled trials benefits more people than uncontrolled drug testing ever would. But it is important for the patient participating in one of these studies to understand that it may or may not be beneficial. Investigational drug protocols are not the same as a proven, effective treatment or cure. The drug may be a failure or cause adverse side effects which could make the condition of the participant worse.

When considering whether to be a participant in a study, the patient should discuss the pros and cons of the experimental drug with a doctor. Important questions for the patient to ask him- or herself and the doctor include: How sick am I? Will this new drug interrupt another treatment that I am already receiving that is effective? How do I feel about entering the study? What are the existing statistics on the efficacy of the drug?

If the patient is not fully committed to participating, he or she should not do so. If the patient is not very sick, he or she may not want to participate in a study which may have serious side effects that worsen the current status of the disease. On the other hand, the patient may decide that intervention at an early stage—while he or she still feels well and strong—is the most promising course to take.

AZT provides a good illustration of this situation. AZT is now available to certain people with AIDS (those who have had *Pneumocystis carinii* pneumonia or who have a helper T-cell count less than 200). It is being tested on other AIDS and ARC patients, as well as on some asymptomatic seropositive individuals. Some people in the latter group may want to take a conservative approach and not take the drug. Since the drug does have several adverse side effects, most notably a depression of bone marrow function, a healthy asymptomatic seropositive person may choose to wait and see if the benefits outweigh the risks. Others, who may be more anxious about their future, may decide that enrolling in an experimental program with AZT is a reasonable bet, hoping that an early intervention might prevent the disease from progressing. At present, there is no scientific basis on which to make this decision. Personal feelings are the best guidelines.

The patient who decides to participate in a drug study must be reminded that he or she has the right to withdraw at any time. If the patient feels, for whatever reason, that the study is harmful, he or she can drop out of the investigational program. Whether the individual has AIDS, ARC, or is asymptomatic seropositive, the decision to enter an experimental drug program should be made with great care and consideration.

ALTERNATIVE THERAPIES

The term "alternative therapies" is defined here as all types of intervention against disease that are not part of the Western medical tradition. This covers a wide range of treatments—everything from acupuncture, yoga, and other non-Western traditional practices, to visualization, mega-vitamins, light therapy, and swallowing crushed gem stones. Many alternative therapies have much documented success and some have theoretical frameworks to explain how they work. Others are newer and although they seem to have some benefit, it is difficult to identify what is actually causing the effect—the patients' expectations, the therapy, or mere chance. There are also alternative treatments that are suspect or have clearly been discredited. If a person is considering using one of these therapies, it is helpful to be able to distinguish those that may work from those that probably won't.

A major problem in evaluating alternative therapies for AIDS/ARC is the lack of hard data. While many of these therapies seem promising, very few have been rigorously tested in controlled experiments. Without such testing, as mentioned previously, it is impossible to be sure how much healing is due to the therapy, how much is due to the placebo effect, and how much is due to chance. A group of people must be carefully followed through a particular therapy and its impact measured in order to determine what percent of people have benefited from utilizing the therapy. Some therapies, such as acupuncture, have a proven effect in one area (painkilling), but not in others (immune boosting).* Other therapies, such as visualization, seem to work well in some situations but have yet to be studied to understand their applications and their limitations.

There are many alternative therapies that deserve more careful study, but at this time very few are being examined. This is due not only to a preference for traditional Western medicine on the part of the doctors and financial sponsors,

---

*G. Chen, S. Li, and C. Jiang. Clinical studies on neuropsychological and biochemical bases of acupuncture analgesia. *Am. J. Clin. Medicine* 14(1 and 2):84–95 (1986).

but also to the suspicion or fear of being tested on the part of many alternative practitioners. Many alternative therapists feel it is unfair to give some patients a placebo in a controlled study. Yet, little concern is expressed for the much larger number of people who must, therefore, choose a therapy without knowing whether it is helpful or useless.

It's nearly impossible for an individual to be aware of all of the therapies, what they purport to do, and how effective they are, especially with the rapidly changing AIDS/ARC therapies. A practical solution is to have certain guidelines and questions that can be used for any therapy being considered. The following guidelines were developed mainly for evaluating alternative, nonmedical therapies, but most can be applied to discussions with a medical doctor about drug therapies as well.

The first step for the patient to take is to identify a primary care physician. Even if a patient decides to pursue an alternative therapy, there is no substitute for being followed by a doctor who can monitor vital signs, blood work, and so on. Any alternative practitioner who advises staying away from physicians should not be trusted. Likewise, using a doctor who warns people against considering any alternative therapy is not a wise choice.

It is also important for different caregivers to communicate with one another so they do not say or do things that will contradict each other or the therapy being followed. For example, a doctor and an herbalist may be prescribing medications which can react adversely with each other and endanger the patient. If each practitioner knows what the other is doing, dangerous situations can be avoided. The patient's medical record is usually the most complete description of health and disease history, so it is useful to have traditional as well as alternative treatments recorded there. However, this again points to the necessity of having clear communications among all caregivers.

If a patient decides to pursue an alternative therapy, it is advisable that careful research be done. There are various means for gathering information, such as asking friends or acquaintances for recommendations or asking at health education centers and/or public agencies for referrals. The patient should collect as much information as possible before making a choice of therapy. He or she may decide to pursue more than one therapy but, again, the different practitioners must be advised to talk with each other.

After deciding on a therapy, there are several important considerations in choosing a caregiver. First, who is the caregiver and what is his or her reputation? Are there any colleagues with the same specialty who will provide a reference? Is it possible for the patient to talk with previous patients? If the therapist is not known in the community or can provide no references, look for another one. Also ascertain whether the therapist has done any previous work with persons with AIDS/ARC and how long the therapy has been practiced.

Another consideration is whether the caregiver can explain the therapy in a way that makes sense to the patient. Is the alternative practitioner eager to answer questions? Is he or she willing to talk to a doctor or other caregivers? What is the underlying philosophy from which the therapist operates? Therapists who insist solely on faith and spurn hard data are likely candidates for quackery. If the patient gets explanations that sound more like gibberish than reasoned thought, he or she should think twice about whether to trust this person with his or her health.

The relevance of the therapy to the individual's condition is also a concern. Does the therapy seem to make sense and is it consistent with the patient's own philosophy? Can the patient believe in it or does it seem more like hype than healing? Is it affordable? Some alternative therapists maintain that belief in the effectiveness of the therapy is crucial to its efficacy. If the patient doesn't believe in the therapy, he may be wasting his time and resources.

Other questions that the patient should ask when evaluating the available therapies include: have the number of people who have utilized the therapy, the number who have improved, the extent of improvement, any potential side effects, and possible cross reactions with other drugs or conditions been documented? Has this therapy ever been used to treat AIDS/ARC? Does the therapist take a complete case history before and after therapy? Are adequate records being kept? How is confidentiality maintained?

There are a number of actions the patient should take while receiving therapy. He or she should monitor him- or herself by keeping a log or notes. The therapist should, of course, also be doing this, but it can be useful for the patient to have personal records to compare and to be able to provide accurate information to the practitioner. If there is no improvement after what seems like a reasonable amount of time, then further questions should be asked. Above all, the patient should continue to ask questions and be a part of the therapy, not just a passive recipient. The therapy should not be continued if the patient feels it is useless or harmful. The patient should also make sure that financial considerations are taken into account. Rent, food, and other necessities should not be sacrificed for the treatment. Most practitioners are willing to make some financial arrangement that is workable.

These questions and considerations can help the patient carefully explore alternatives. Although the benefits of some alternative therapies cannot be currently explained, neither can they be denied. Having an open mind about treatments is good, but chasing after cures without a critical eye may result in financial losses or, worse, physical harm. The patient should understand at the outset what he or she expects to gain, and how to know when that has been achieved. Perhaps the most vital factor in gaining or maintaining wellness is concentrating on being well, rather than spending enormous amounts of time or energy on sickness. It is possible to get well with AIDS/ARC, and it is important to know this fact. But the old adage still applies: Buyer beware!

The testing of experimental drugs or alternative treatments is a very important part of the ongoing attempt to control AIDS/ARC. People who participate in these studies are performing a valuable service which will help many people. But it is important to evaluate any treatment realistically. A hopeful attitude is essential; blind faith can have disastrous effects.

The best advice to a patient: Be an expert on your condition and know what is being done to and for you.

IV

EPIDEMIOLOGY

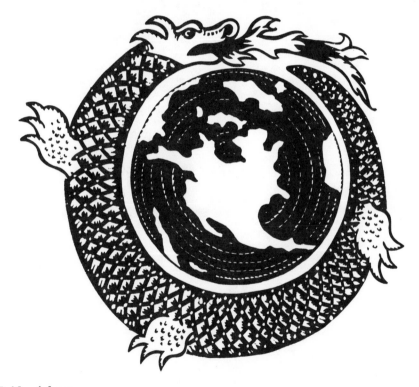

Epidemiology
The world is encircled by the dragon. No continent is exempt from the AIDS virus.

12

AIDS in Africa

Michael A. Simpson

No one knows how serious the problem of AIDS in Africa is, chiefly for reasons of unavoidable, inadvertent, and deliberate underreporting. A somber conference has concluded that Africa is currently the world center of AIDS problems, and a prediction has been made that at least 1 million Africans will die of the disease in the next 10 years. "We are witnessing the death of a continent," said one of the more alarmed speakers,[1] claiming AIDS is now a greater threat to human life in Africa than famine. A WHO report of cases reported to its agencies in the first 9 months of 1986[2] found cases in 74 of 100 countries reporting—31,646 cases worldwide (compared to 20,476 at the start of the year). Though the majority of present cases were in the United States, the most striking increase was shown in Africa, where 10 countries reported 1003 cases compared with 31 nine months earlier. In South Africa, the Chairman of the South African Medical Research Council predicted 31,232 cases by the end of 1996 in that country alone.

In New York, maybe one in 250 of the population shows infection, according to some estimates; but in Central Africa, perhaps one in five. Other estimates[1] put the percentage of the population infected with AIDS as 15% in Zambia and 10% in Uganda. There are also reports of a very high incidence in Tanzania, Rwanda, Zaire, and elsewhere. While one wishes to avoid alarmist overreactions and excessive estimates, the likelihood in Africa is that the scale of the problem is still being underrecognized. There are many reasons for this. Health services are feebly developed in many areas, for many reasons, and sophisticated diagnostic facilities are barely available. There is little capacity to study properly the incidence in the vast, isolated, rural areas. The best estimates have come from university teaching hospitals in those centers that have them. There has been marked political reluctance to admit the extent of the problem, pressure to suppress the publication of data coming from certain countries, and the withdrawal of papers documenting the epidemic from at least one international symposium due to such pressure. Other governments, like that of Rwanda, have been notably encouraging. There is an enormous potential for spread, not only by regular tourists, but by the very large numbers of formal and informal migrant workers, refugees, and illegal immigrants that move across African borders. In many areas, health services are not yet developed to the point of being able to cope with Africa's traditional burden of tropical disease and because of warfare, rebellion, and economic crisis in some areas, even such health services as did exist have virtually collapsed. In Mozambique, for example, health services are especially seriously affected. Clinical recordkeeping is of low priority in many areas, and facilities for laboratory confirmation of diagnosis are severely limited.

In this chapter, I will review the available information on the situation in Africa and how it has developed. As will be seen, there seem to be two contrasting forms of the problem. In South Africa, with the most highly developed health care and most Westernized society, the AIDS problem, contrary to some muddled U.S. reports,[3] has been predominantly among homosexual or bisexual men, often with U.S. connections, and similar generally to the situation seen in the United States. In the rest of Africa, the primary problem is heterosexually spread AIDS, affecting a substantial and growing proportion of the population.

EX AFRICA SEMPER ALIQUID MORI?

It remains unclear when the problem first arose in Africa. The first fully authenticated cases seem to have arisen at about the same time as the early European and U.S. cases. But whether AIDS originated in Africa at an earlier date is not clear. De Cock[4] doubted that the recently described infection is caused by a genuinely new agent, and proposed that AIDS originated in rural equatorial Africa. Williams et al.[5] have raised the possibility of an early case in 1959. Jenkins et al.[6] reported AIDS in an Englishwoman who developed the disease while living in the U.K., while "the only risk factor appeared to be sexual contact with her Ghanaian ex-husband prior to December 1979." He was believed to be an asymptomatic HTLV-III carrier infected in Zaire. This would imply an early pool of infection in Zaire and a latent period of at least 4½ years, but relies on the unsubstantiated veracity of the patient's history. Jenkins et al. suggested that HTLV may have existed in stable equilibrium in the African environment. There is an Italian report[7] of AIDS in an African woman from Gabon, living in Milan since 1978 (like Siegal and Siegal[8] in New York, who reported a woman from the Dominican Republic seen in 1979 with what, in retrospect, may have been AIDS). A Swiss journal[9] reported the death from AIDS of a young couple from Zaire who had arrived in Switzerland in 1981 in apparent good health and admitting to no risk factors. Bygbjerg[10] reported a case of AIDS in a Danish woman surgeon who had worked in Zaire from 1972 to 1975. Clumeck et al.[11] reported 17 cases (five previously described) in Zaire, commenting that although it was possible that AIDS had always been present but unrecognized in equatorial Africa, the increasing number of patients from the region seeking care in Belgium since 1980 suggested that this was a new disease spreading in central Africa. The cases suggestive of earlier African infection require the assumption that there was absolutely no exposure to any risk after they left Africa, and it is hard to be certain of that.

KAPOSI'S SARCOMA

There was also controversy over the relation between African Kaposi's sarcoma and AIDS. Kaposi described a rare disease in 1872, a sarcoma typified by painless, raised, multiple, bluish-red skin nodules or plaques. It used to be seen mainly in elderly immunocompromised black males in central and southern Africa, though it could occur in any race, age, or sex. It was a slow, chronic disease, lasting from 1 to 25 years.[12,13] In a study of malignant neoplasms in northeastern Zaire, 1971–1983,[14] Kaposi's sarcoma was the most commonly biopsied neoplasm in men (16.5%) but showed no change in frequency during those 13 years. McHardy et al.[15] described 72 cases diagnosed in Uganda, 1951–1976. Noting that cases tended to be postpubertal males, many of whom had been bitten by bloodsucking insects identified as similar to Haematopota, the question of insect-borne transmission was raised from time to time but with no consistent support. The fact that sex was another common occupation of postpubertal males does not seem to have led to a theory of sexual transmission at this stage.

During 1983 the number of cases of Kaposi's sarcoma more or less doubled in Zambia, and changes in the clinical presentation were noticed with a rapidly progressing, aggressive variant similar to that which had been described in the United States.[16] Later, Bayley et al.[17] showed that nearly 90% of patients with this new atypically aggressive Kaposi's sarcoma were seropositive for HTLV-III in Zambia and Uganda, whereas only 17% of patients with the classic form of Kaposi's were seropositive. At that time, 20% of the controls in Uganda, but only 2% in Zambia, were seropositive. The implication was that the virus was associated with the form of tumor and that the virus was relatively new in Zambia but may have been in Uganda for longer—perhaps for 10 years, atypical Kaposi's having been seen in Kampala earlier (where Kaposi's was the third commonest tumor).

Downing et al.[18] reported that Zambian patients with this aggressive form of the sarcoma showed similar changes in lymphocyte function and immunological profile to that seen in U.S. AIDS patients (though some[19] challenged this). Edwards et al.[20] reported a fatal case of AIDS in a woman from Uganda with aggressive Kaposi's sarcoma and no history of other risk factors, and suggested a common etiology for the conditions. Weber[21] now proposed that Kaposi's sarcoma in Africa is a sexually transmitted disease, spread predominantly by male homosexual intercourse, and that AIDS was caused by the same agent.

It is now clear that the endemic Kaposi's sarcoma of Africa is not related to HTLV-III infection and must not be confused with the Kaposi's sarcoma found complicating AIDS. The aggressive form appears more often in individuals from higher socioeconomic groups and reporting more promiscuity.

AIDS IN AFRICA

The first general report of AIDS in Africa appeared in 1983, including seven cases with viruslike particles in lymphocytes[22] and a case in a black Malian in France who had never been to central Africa.[23] Van de Pitte et al.[24] reported that at least a dozen Zairian patients with AIDS had been admitted to hospitals in Belgium in the previous 2 years and described a Zairian woman with probable AIDS seen in 1977, some 4 years before the syndrome was described in the United States. Taelman et al.[25] reported three patients who died of what appeared to have been AIDS during 1981–82. They suggested that 15 cases of crypotococcal meningitis (reported earlier) probably also had AIDS. In this series, one was a woman, and the men were heterosexual—an early indicator of the importance of heterosexual spread, since clearly recognized. In 1983, too, Ras et al.[26] reported the first two cases from South Africa.

By 1984, rather more structured reports from Africa appeared in the journals. Van de Perre et al.[27] described a study in Rwanda, where Kaposi's sarcoma is endemic. In a 4-week period, 26 new cases of AIDS were diagnosed, 17 males and 9 females. Most of the men were promiscuous heterosexuals, and 43% of the females were prostitutes. Only two had Kaposi's sarcoma. The risk factors appeared to be an urban environment, a relatively high income, and heterosexual promiscuity, especially with prostitutes. Piot et al.[28] wrote of 38 patients with AIDS, identified in Kinshasa during a 3-week period in 1983. The male:female ratio was 1.1:1. The annual case rate for Kinshasa (an underestimate) was considered to be at least 12 per 100,000. The predominantly heterosexual transmission in Africa was becoming obvious.

The onset of AIDS in Kinshasa cannot be dated, though it is notable that cases of cryptococcal meningitis averaged one per year in the two major hospitals from the mid-1950s to late 1979, whereas over 35 cases were seen from 1981 to 1983.[24]

A further study[29] showed a relation between sexual lifestyle and HTLV seropositivity in 58 African men from Rwanda with AIDS or AIDS-related complex (ARC). They had significantly more heterosexual partners per year and more contact with prostitutes than control subjects. Of 42 similarly affected African women, 24% were prostitutes. Brun-Vezinet et al.[30] reported antibodies to lymphadenopathy-associated virus (LAV) in about 90% of patients with AIDS in Zaire and in about 5% of control patients whose sera had been obtained in 1980 and 1983. One patient was retrospectively diagnosed as having had AIDS in 1977, with LAV antibodies at that time, though the blood tests may not have been free from false positives at that stage. Biggar et al.[31] surveyed 250 outpatients at a remote hospital in Zaire. They found no clinical cases of AIDS. HTLV-III antibodies were clearly positive in 12.4% and borderline positive in a further 12%, with a high occurrence in childhood and a relatively high prevalence among the rural poor.

In South Africa, Lyons et al.[32] reported on seroepidemiology of HTLV-III in that country. On screening they found no such antibodies in low-risk populations and stated that the virus is not endemic in southern Africa. Opperman et al.[33] had tested 922 sera, 883 with no known risk factors. There were no antibodies in low-risk individuals, but 23 of 27 male homosexuals with chronic lymphadenopathy had antibodies to HTLV-III, as had 12 out of 12 cases of AIDS. A red herring arose with a report[34] of reactivity of Bushman sera with HTLV-III; nine of 22 samples from these remote, desert-living people showing low positive reactions with ELISA testing. When retested with Western blot techniques,[35] none proved to have specific antibodies.

Sher and Santos,[36] in a survey of the sera of 375 homosexual men examined in Johannesburg 1983–85, found HTLV-III testing positive in all of 13 with AIDS, 7.8% of 46 with chronic lymphadenopathy, 67% of a group with decreased cell-mediated immunity (CMI), and 15% of a group with normal CMI.

They considered 15% as the likely proportion of the male homosexual population of Johannesburg that had been exposed to HTLV-III.

Other studies of sera also raised the question of how early AIDS had occurred in Africa. A cluster of HTLV-III infection was reported[37] in a Rwandese family, beginning with the mother in 1977. Another study[38] found that 50 of 75 serum samples collected in the West Nile district of Uganda between 1972 and 1973 contained HTLV-III antibodies, with 12 also positive for HTLV-I. The high prevalence and relatively low titers (compared to those in patients with AIDS) in sera "from this population at a time that may predate or coincide with the appearance or spread of the AIDS agent (HTLV-III) suggest," concluded the authors, "that the virus detected may have been a predecessor of HTLV-III or is HTLV-III itself but existing in a population acclimated to its presence." They felt this further supported the suggested African origin of HTLV-III.

Other such studies, raiding stored serum in African deep-freezers, led to claims, for instance, that 80% of Ugandan children in 1969 were seropositive for HIV. But such studies used earlier, far less specific tests for the antibodies, with a far greater chance of false-positive results, especially in the immunologic miasma of stored sera of African patients who had been exposed to multiple parasites. The studies seem to have been less eagerly repeated using the better tests now available, and less eagerly reported. Reactivity is altered in people who have had recurrent malaria and other parasitic diseases,[39] or who have had previous pregnancies.[40–42] ELISA seropositivity is not necessarily confirmed by Western blot techniques. The early reactivity could, conceivably, be related to antibodies against an unrecognized, cross-reacting virus, but the test results imply that the antibodies are not directed against common antigens.[43]

A crucial question is what will be the fate of the seropositive people. The experience in the United States and Europe has been that a slow decline in cell-mediated immune function follows HIV infection, usually taking several years before it is clinically apparent.[44] Within 3 years of being found to have HIV antibodies, AIDS has occurred in 15–30% of Americans in high-risk groups, and the proportion that is seen to develop AIDS later seems to increase with time.[45] So it is still not sure what proportion of infected people will develop AIDS, but the proportion seems likely to be high. Only one study has looked at the risk of AIDS in healthy seropositive Africans,[46] finding a 1% risk after 1 year, which obviously underestimates the long-term risk.

RETROVIRUSES IN AFRICA

There is a literature on the retroviruses themselves in Africa. Fleming[47] argued that HTLV was introduced to Japan via Portuguese ships from Africa and that the highest incidence of HTLV in Japan is in communities that had the closest contact with the Portuguese missionaries and African slave crews. ATLV/HTLV-I is widely distributed in an endemic pattern in Africa,[48] with an estimated 10 million people infected. Variant strains have been reported.[49] Prevalences reported among African countries range from 1% to 8% of those tested, being around 4% in Ghana.[50] HTLV-I-positive leukemia/lymphoma cases in Africans have been reported.[51,52]

A persistent issue has been the possibility of a simian (monkey) pool of such viruses, as has been operative in the case of some other lethal virus diseases. ATLV/HTLV-I virus antibodies are present in various primate species, mainly in African green monkeys, and less often in chimpanzees and crab-eating monkeys,[53] and in southern Africa, in indigenous vervet monkeys and baboons[54] but not in other primates.[55]

Such antibodies were found[53] in 1–2% of people from Kenya, compared to well under 0.1% of the West German population. Another study[55] confirmed the incidence of HTLV antibodies in some but not all primate species, and in nearly 4% of blood donors in Nigeria. A later South African report[54] found HTLV-I antibodies in 3.5% of a group of Asian South Africans, 3.5% of black South Africans, 4.1% of so-called "coloureds," and in only 0.3% of whites. In a primate study, the same researchers found antibodies in 29% of vervet monkeys and 33% of baboons. HTLV and related viruses seem to cause widespread infection in nonhuman primates in southern Africa. Yet another study[56] described an absence of antibodies reactive with simian AIDS virus surface antigens in the sera of the same species of vervet monkeys and baboons in southern Africa. A survey[57] of sera from hospital staff and patients, baboons and vervets, and some adults from Namibia and Kenya were all negative for HTLV-III antibodies, suggesting further that *this* infection is not endemic in southern Africa, where only homosexual men with AIDS or related disorders were positive, most having visited the United States or having had sexual contact with others who had visited the United States.

More recently,[58,59] a new retrovirus has been isolated from AIDS patients in West Africa (Cape Verde and Guinea Bissau), called human immunodeficiency virus type II. Within the HIV family by many properties, it shows cross-reactivity with a simian retrovirus (STLV-III mac), isolated from captive macaques presenting with disease very similar to human AIDS.[60] HIV-I is evident in Central Africa (e.g., Zaire and the Central African Republic),[61] but HIV-II has not yet been described there. Positivity to HIV-I and II seems to occur in varying proportions in African patients and in symptomless mothers of undernourished children, according to these reports. One woman who died of suspected AIDS was positive to both, and her 6-year-old son was seropositive to both.

Monkeys with simian AIDS either have been experimentally inoculated with malaria, harbor nonopportunistic parasites, or have been experimentally exposed to alloantigens. This is reminiscent of the earlier theories explaining western AIDS on the basis of extraneous immunosuppression or immune system "overload" by multiple parasites. Parasites are both immunosuppressive and mutagenic for T cells, so retroviruses might well prefer primates and humans loaded with parasites, such as American promiscuous homosexuals and many people living in the tropics.

The simian AIDS virus (STLV-III) also occurs in about 50% of healthy African green monkeys living in the wild.[62] It has been hypothesized that there might be a spectrum of related viruses, infecting different primate hosts, and with a range of pathogenic effects ranging from none to full-scale AIDS. Healthy prostitutes in Dakar, Senegal, where AIDS is still rare, carry antibodies suggesting infection with a virus closely related to STLV-III. With the advent of these new viruses and the multiple nomenclatures in use, the situation is becoming confusing. Kanki et al.[60] have called their new virus HTLV-IV. It does not kill the cells it infects, as HTLV-III and STLV-III do. According to early reports, HTLV-IV may not be associated with any illness. If so, this may be very important, as comparative studies of HTLV-III and IV may help identify the source of the lethal effects of the AIDS virus, and understanding how and why the two viruses are treated differently by the immune system may help choose strategies to deal with AIDS (see also [63]).

But just as both American and French teams identified HTLV-III/LAV, so now, as the Harvard group announced HTLV-IV, Montagnier and his group in Paris have described a new related virus, which they call LAV-II. Like HTLV-IV, this also is more closely related to STLV-III than to the AIDS virus, but it was isolated from AIDS patients and does kill all the helper cells it infects (see also [59]).

Biberfeld et al.,[64] in December 1986, describe the sera of four African women living in Sweden (from Gambia and the Ivory Coast) who are HTLV-IV-positive and have signs of immune deficiency as well as a woman from Guinea Bissau with HTLV-IV antibodies who died of an illness similar to the "slim disease" form of AIDS typically described in Uganda. LAV-II certainly seems as deadly as HTLV-III/HIV;[65] Montagnier told a recent conference that 11 of 63 people infected with LAV-II—all heterosexuals—have developed AIDS, and 10 have AIDS-related conditions. A real problem is that antibodies to LAV-II are not always recognized by the ELISA used to detect HIV antibodies. Though first reported in West Africa, LAV-II infection has now been found in Western Europe, too.

Questions relating to the origins of the AIDS virus are of far more than academic interest. It is a very complex organism, which could not have arisen de novo. If its ancestral agent, from which it evolved, by mutation or recombination, could be discovered, it could provide valuable information, for instance, on which portion of the genome confers its malicious pathogenicity, which would greatly assist the search for rationally effective treatments. Also, the ancestor, if not itself pathogenic, and if there is any neutralizing cross-reactivity between the two viruses, could provide a safe source of immunizing material in vaccine development, as Biggar[43] has emphasized.

Such an ancestral virus would probably be either a human virus with different pathogenicity or a virus in some animal reservoir. Some virologists feel it most likely that the transformation to AIDS perhaps occurred in some isolated primate stock in an isolated area where animal and human populations are scattered and remote—central South America, central Africa, Asia, and the Pacific islands are possible areas of such origin. Its arrival via a primate species seems a popular concept, though rural peoples usually have little contact with primates and far more with cattle, goats, sheep, and similar domestic animals.

A plausible hypothesis is that from the seemingly harmless monkey virus STLV-3 developed a similarly harmless human virus, HTLV-4, evolving into the damaging HIV-2, from which developed HIV-1.

EXTENT AND RISK FACTORS

AIDS has so far been reported in patients in 23 African countries including Zaire, Congo, Rwanda, Kenya, Angola, Burundi, Mali, Central African Republic, Gabon, Cameroon, Zimbabwe, Botswana, Caprivi, Ghana, Ivory Coast, Burkina Faso, Senegal, Zambia, Guinea-Bissau, Cape Verde, South Africa, and possibly in Swaziland and Namibia. A lack of reports, however, does not mean a lack of cases.

There are many loose ends in the African literature. For example, Hayes et al.[66] published a report of a case of Kaposi's sarcoma which they felt might represent AIDS in a black South African male, yet no follow-up report is apparent, and more recent surveys insist that no case of AIDS has yet been confirmed in a black South African. The pattern of the disease in South Africa has been anomalous, following the U.S. rather than the African pattern. The first case was diagnosed in 1982, and the first two deaths occurred in that year.[67] One more case was diagnosed in 1983, and eight in 1984. By May 1985, nine more had been seen. Of the 19 patients thus far, 11 had died. Eighteen were white; one was a black man from Zaire. All were male. Sixteen were known to be homosexual, the age range 30–40 years. Three were heterosexuals—one from Zaire, and two who had had sexual relations with Zairians. A voluntary blood donor exclusion program had begun. By mid-1986, 32 patients had been seen—28 South Africans and 4 referred from countries to the north. There had been one case in a child with hemophilia. Of 27 adults, 25 were homosexual or bisexual males, and 1 appeared to have been infected from a blood transfusion. Of the 28 South African patients, 23 (82%) died. By 1985 there were 12 new cases, and a doubling time of 6–12 months was projected, expecting 24–48 new cases in 1986. But by the end of June 1986, only eight new cases had been diagnosed. By August 1986,[68] the total was 36 cases, 24 dead, with one further case in a hemophiliac; there were only 12 new cases by that date. Of the six non-South African residents seen, two each were from Malawi and Zambia, and one each from Zaire and Haiti. The predominance of homosexual patients followed the U.S. pattern. One had fallen ill with AIDS while living in Boston; one was an airline flight steward who had lived in New York. Initially most cases seemed to have had direct or indirect contacts with North American homosexual men, usually as the passive partner.[69] But more recent cases have acquired the infection from other infected South Africans. Heterosexual spread has yet to be seen in South Africa, but it is expected to occur. One bisexual patient has died of AIDS, and his spouse has seroconverted. A further seropositive bisexual has been identified.

In South Africa, by late January 1987, 50 cases had been seen (41 in local citizens). The government, after their Advisory Group on AIDS' booklet "What You Should Know About AIDS" (Department of National Health and Population Development, October 1986) opened a formal research unit and began planning realistically for the care of AIDS patients. British health authorities have revised their warning about who should not give blood donations to include anyone "who has had sexual intercourse with anyone from Africa south of the Sahara."

Studies of the prevalence of HTLV-III antibodies in homosexual men in Johannesburg[36,70] estimated that 10–15% had been exposed to HTLV-III. Of 375 homosexual men, 13 had AIDS, 46 had chronic lymphadenopathy, and 316 were healthy. Anderson et al.[71] had reported finding acquired immunosuppression in 80% of a smaller group of homosexual men, so the later, smaller incidence reported was less alarming.

Epidemiological studies have been largely absent or poor. AIDS in Africa seems to occur[72] mainly in young to middle-aged men and women, with nearly equal frequency in the two sexes (unlike the U.S. reports of 93% male victims). Most African AIDS patients do not seem to belong to the major high-risk groups recognized in the United States. Infection rates of 10–20% among blood donors and in antenatal clinics are worrying. Are these data typical of population incidence, or may donors in Africa have been infected during previous blood donations? Similarly, do other sexually transmitted diseases, by their genital lesions, make it easier to become infected with AIDS, increasing the incidence seen in STD clinics?

There have never been any competently conducted surveys of sexual behavior in Africa. Although a similar incidence of homosexual and bisexual behavior is likely, surveys of risk factors so far conducted have never yet used interviewers with the language and communication skills needed to elicit such a history reliably. In Africa, the frequency of heterosexual anal intercourse and orogenital and oral-anal contact are unknown. They tend to be denied in informal and inexpert interviews.

One case has been reported in a woman in Rwanda who had received a blood transfusion[73] raising the issue of the status of African blood donors. In South Africa there has been one case of AIDS in a child who received blood products. The South African Blood Transfusion Service, which has adopted screening, has identified 45 seropositive carriers so far, a rate of about 1 person in 10,000 among South African blood donors. In South Africa, there has been a marked difference in the prevalence of HTLV-III/LAV antibodies in hemophiliacs between those receiving large donor-pool products from the United States and those receiving small donor-pool local cryoprecipitates. Eighty-three percent of a group of hemophiliacs who had received U.S. factor VIII were seropositive, but none of those who had received local small-pool products were seropositive. A small number of hemophiliacs in South Africa have been classified as having the ARC syndrome.[74] A study[75] of pediatric patients with bleeding disorders revealed 88% seropositive among those treated with imported blood products, compared with only one out of 29 who had received local products.

Transfusion has been implicated in some African cases in Africa and Europe,[31,76] though the great majority of African patients with AIDS deny exposure to blood or blood products. In some areas it has been reported that donated blood is frequently seropositive.[73] A Rwandan study found HTLV antibodies in 35.6% of blood donors, as compared to less than 1% in the United States. The issue is not clear, since the reliability of the ELISA test in African sera has been questioned. One British case of a nurse showing seroconversion occurred after a needle-stick transmission from an African AIDS patient.[77]

Izzia et al.[78] described AIDS in a young man with sickle cell anemia and suggested that such patients in Africa should be considered a risk group for AIDS because of their need for blood transfusions and their functional asplenia or hyposplenia. They might be the African equivalent to the hemophiliac risk group in the West. But there seem to have been no further reports of this association or risk.

Insect transmission has been proposed.[79] There are some similarities between HIV and the hepatitis B virus, for which there is strong evidence of transmission by the common bedbug. Children, according to several reports, may comprise

15–22% of AIDS cased in Africa (compared with only 1–4% in the United States). Bedbug and similar insect infestation is common throughout Africa, and children may be continually exposed to the bites of such insects. Tests in Johannesburg allowed adult bedbugs (*Cimex lectularius*) and *Aedes aegypti* mosquitoes to gorge themselves on defibrinated blood infected with HIV. An hour later they were killed, homogenized, and tested for HIV presence. The ground mousse of bedbug proved highly positive, though cultures inoculated with ground mosquitoes remained negative. The authors suggested that mechanical transmission of the virus between humans by bedbugs was possible.

Other risk factors suggested have included ritual exposure to human or animal blood during religious activities or blood exchange in "blood brotherhood" ceremonies. One case,[80] reported earlier as having "no known risk factors," occurred in a white Scottish heterosexual male who worked for 3 years in Kenya and Tanzania and died of AIDS in Glasgow in 1982. No history of recognized risk factors was obtained. But he had been interested in anthropology and had taken part in ritual interchange of blood with people in remote tribes in East Africa in "blood brotherhood" rituals. He had also had a Tanzanian girl friend during this time, and heterosexual spread had not been taken seriously at the time of his death.

Wyatt[81] has stressed the risk of spread by needle and syringe, in injections. Injections are very popular in central Africa, mostly given with unsterile needles, syringes, and contents.[82] Most injections are given by traditional healers with no concept of sterile technique; some are given by health workers who take syringes from clinics to use in "private practice." Lack of supplies may mean that many doctors give multiple injections with the same syringe and needles. Transmission by accidental needle-stick injection has occurred in the West; multiple reuse of needles in Africa may at times approximate the situation of intravenous drug users in the West. Some traditional healers specialize, for instance, in venereal diseases and could be visited by a high proportion of infected prostitutes, receiving injections from the same needle used on other clients. As an example of the scale of the potential risk, one study[83] found that in just 1 month in the Cameroon, one in 10 children received an injection at a health clinic.

The prevalence of HIV infection in drug abusers in Africa is not known. Even in South Africa, with the most westernized society, intravenous drug abuse is not uncommon. In a study of a group of addicts in Johannesburg, De Miranda et al.[84] reported that of 176, 11 used intravenous drugs only, 105 used oral only, and 60 used both. One hundred forty-nine were heterosexual, 18 bisexual, and 9 homosexual. On blood testing, only one drug addict had HIV antibodies and lymphadenopathy, and he was a practicing homosexual. The incidence would therefore seem low in South African addicts. One is reminded that risk factors overlap—sexuality, drug abuse, and prostitution, for example.

Homosexuality is definitely present in Africa—probably as commonly as anywhere else—but so far no case of AIDS has been described in a black African homosexual. Colebunders et al.[72] describes a case of Belgian homosexual AIDS patient who had lived for over 20 years in Zaire, highly sexually active with multiple African, often bisexual, partners. But, as he had also had multiple partners in Europe and Brazil, it is unclear where he acquired the disease.

To what extent can AIDS be transmitted between members of a family? Mann et al.[85] conducted a useful study in Kinshasa, Zaire, of household members of patients with confirmed AIDS and seronegative controls; 9.8% of members of the AIDS patients households were HTLV-III/LAV seropositive, compared with 1.9% of control household members (relative risk = 5.1; 95% confidence interval 1.7–15.2). Of the spouses of AIDS patients, 61.1% were seropositive, compared to one (3.7%) of control spouses (relative risk = 16.5; 95% confidence interval 3.7–75.0). Except for spouses, there was not a significant difference in rate of seropositivity between the households. The data of this and other studies suggest transmission heterosexually and perinatally but do not support the idea of nonsexual transmission in households, even in those as crowded and often unsanitary and infested as those involved in this study, except with the possible transmission by bedbugs.

There is, of course, more contact between Africa and the Caribbean than many people realize—from Cuban troops in Angola and elsewhere to the fact that thousands of Haitians went to Zaire in the 1960s to become teachers and other professionals (having the advantage of being both black and French-speaking), and many Haitians are still there, especially in Kinshasa.[86]

There are several reported cases (including those already cited) of Europeans who seem to have contacted AIDS while living in central Africa or with natives of central Africa.[87–90] Yet many of the earliest African cases reported had traveled frequently to Europe and might have acquired the infection there.

African AIDS patients tend, according to several studies,[72] to have had multiple sexual partners (though fewer than American homosexual cases); to be better educated and with more time spent in urban areas;[85] to have travelled a lot, with sexual contacts during these travels; and often to have a history of other sexually transmitted diseases.

CLINICAL FEATURES

The basic clinical features of AIDS in African patients are very similar to those described in Haitian patients, and a little different from the typical U.S. cases. Profound weight loss; severe chronic, watery diarrhea; and fever of unknown origin are common and striking features. Diarrhea is the predominant and often the presenting complaint in 90–95% of African cases, compared to about 50% of American cases during the prodromal period.[86] Indeed, this severe enteropathic form has been called "slim disease" in Uganda because of the major weight loss. Generalized lymphadenopathy was found in 50% of the Zairian patients Piot et al. reported[28] and in 76% of the Rwandians in Van de Perre's series.[27] Pruritic maculopapular or pustular skin lesions on the extremities are often seen.

Of course, opportunistic infections are common, with prevalence rates slightly different from those seen in the United States and Europe. Thrush is frequent; candida esophagitis common. Cryptococcosis seems more common in Africa than in the United States, especially CNS infections. Cryptosporidiosis, *Isospora belli* infection, strongyloidiasis, and herpes simplex infections occur; cytomegalovirus infections are very frequent. *Pneumocystis carinii* pneumonia seems less frequent than in the United States, though accurate diagnosis is often very difficult in the African context. In South Africa, it has been the most commonly diagnosed opportunistic infection. Cerebral toxoplasmosis and lymphoma are also difficult to diagnose under these circumstances. Tuberculosis is a common infection, sometimes infection with aptypical mycobacteria. Other infections are seen—*Salmonella, Pseudomonas, Entamoeba histolytica* liver abscess, and others. Considering the frequent incidence of multiple parasitic infections in the general population of many areas in Africa, one might expect the deficient cellular immunity to have an effect on these parasitic diseases and malaria, but no effect has yet been reported. Aggressive Kaposi's sarcoma is seen in 17% of African AIDS patients, a similar rate as in Haitian and nonhomosexual American cases.[72,87-90]

There have been reports from the United States suggesting an association between AIDS and B-cell non-Hodgkin's lymphomas, including Burkitt-like lymphomas.[91] Yet no such association has been reported in Africa, although Burkitt's lymphoma is quite common in some areas. Perhaps, as Biggar[43] suggests, this may be because Burkitt's lymphoma is, in Africa, a disease of mid-childhood, when HIV infection is still uncommon.

According to Schoub,[92] summarizing the Brussels International Symposium on African AIDS, three particular presentations—profound weight loss, diarrhea, and itchy dermatosis—were statistically highly significantly more common in African than in U.S. AIDS patients. Local doctors in some parts of Africa recognize these as three types: "hot AIDS," where the predominant symptom is fever; "wet AIDS," when diarrhea dominates the picture; and "slim disease," the diarrhea/wasting syndrome or enteropathic form. The last form, "slim," usually begins with malaise, intermittent fever, and chronic diarrhea lasting for some 6 months before the patient comes to medical attention.

The chronic dermatitis is especially prominent in African AIDS—an initially itchy maculopapular rash, later becoming hyperpigmented and scarred. It can be a significant prodromal sign, which may be referred to a determatologist before other signs of AIDS are apparent.

An unusually common presentation in African AIDS, especially in the pediatric cases (15–22% of African cases occur in children, compared to under 2% in the United States), is diffuse lymphoid infiltration of various organs, notably lymphoid interstitial pneumonia. This variety seems to run a more prolonged, stable course than others.

African AIDS cases may present with CNS signs—lethargy and mental dullness. But whereas most U.S. cases with a neurological involvement present with viral encephalitis or cerebral lymphoma, most such African cases present with cryptococcal or toxoplasmosis CNS infections. Exposure to *Cryptococcus neoformans* in the home environment is common in Africa, in house dust, in chicken and pigeon droppings, and in the droppings of cockroaches (*Periplaneta americana*).

Infectious or malignant eye involvement is rare in African AIDS patients, unlike U.S. cases. No cases of CMV retinitis have been reported, and only three cases of conjunctival Kaposi's sarcoma. But ocular involvement with an "AIDS retinopathy" has been reported in around half of the adult African cases, with sheathing of peripheral vessels, cotton-wool spots, Roth spots, and hemorrhages.

HETEROSEXUAL TRANSMISSION OF AIDS

There seems to have been a strange reluctance in some quarters to accept the evidence supporting the importance of heterosexual transmission of AIDS, though the African data have consistently supported this hypothesis. In the United States, male:female case ratios of around 13:1 have been reported from the early days of the epidemic. In Africa it has generally been 1:1 (occasional reports of 1.1:1[28] and at most 2:1[27]). Some workers, like Padian and Pickering,[93] have shown great ingenuity in trying to challenge the figures and the inferences. They claim to be able to explain the 1:1 incidence without involving female-to-male transmission. Their arguments fail the test of Occam's razor and raise intriguing psychodynamic doubts. They suggest that there could be a far higher proportion of bisexual rather than homosexual men in Africa than in the United States, with most homosexual behavior occurring between bisexual men, who could in turn be responsible for male-to-female transmission. The actual case ratio will of course depend on frequencies of sexual behavior and relative transmission efficiencies between man to man, man to woman, and woman to man.

Redfield et al.,[94-96] commenting on figures for incidence in U.S. soldiers, argue that there is no evidence that "soldiers are more likely to lie than civilians" (about homosexuality or intravenous drug abuse) and conclude that 10 married servicemen with AIDS were telling the truth when they claimed their only risk factor was contact with European prostitutes. Pearce[97] concluded, "It is *not* improbable, therefore, that a virus might infect *bidirectionally* in Africa, but does so only rarely in the United States." More recently, Melbye et al.,[98] in a careful study of patients in Lusaka, Zambia, found no significant difference in prevalence by sex after adjusting for age.

It appears that the incidence of AIDS among heterosexuals in regions like the United States (where it has hitherto been seen as a predominantly homosexual disease) may be increasing at a faster rate than among homosexuals. It appears that "normal" vaginal intercourse alone is enough to transmit the virus to around half of the spouses or sexual partners of patients with AIDS or ARC. It would seem that the African lesson as to heterosexual transmissability will be learned elsewhere, and there is no need for the excessive skepticism proposed by authors like Potterat et al.[99] as to the veracity of patients who claim not to fall into other risk groups and to have gained the virus heterosexually.

FEMALE PROSTITUTION AND THE
SPREADING OF AIDS

Kreiss et al.[100] found HTLV-III antibody in 42 of 64 prostitutes from a poor area of Nairobi, Kenya, and in 8 of 26 higher-socioeconomic-status Nairobi prostitutes. Their seropositivity was associated with contact with men from Rwanda, Uganda, and Burundi, implying that heterosexual men serve as vectors of infection between communities of prostitutes. Of three seropositive men with contacts with prostitutes, one was bisexual.

Neequaye et al.[101] reported that in a February 1986 survey of 98 Ghanaian prostitutes in Accra, only one was HTLV-III seropositive. Of 247 Ghanaian blood donors, none were seropositive. Up to March 1986, no clinical case of

AIDS had been seen in Accra. But there has been a rapid increase in the number of seropositive Ghanaians. Two were identified in March 1986, 72 in September, with 44 cases of AIDS or ARC. Sixty-three of the 72 were female. Most had come home from neighboring African countries, ill and in some cases dying soon after arrival—55 from Abidjan (Ivory Coast), two from Burkina Faso, one from Senegal, and two from West Germany. They emphasized the extent to which young women in conditions of severe economic hardship in Third World Africa may be driven to go to other countries as prostitutes to earn a living—this was the account many of their patients gave. The extent to which such prostitutes also serviced Japanese and Korean sailors can give rise to concern about the potential for spread of the African pattern of AIDS to Asia and elsewhere. This sex ratio, with 88% of the seropositive group female, is unusual.

There is a high prevalence of HIV antibodies in female prostitutes in central and East Africa.[29,100,102,103] Prostitutes in Africa seem to be less likely to use condoms (which can provide significant protection) and to have younger and more promiscuous clients. This is unlike the situation in Europe. Krogsgaard et al.,[104] for example, surveyed 101 prostitutes in Copenhagen, who averaged 20 encounters per week (range 4–100). Twenty-five suggested that up to one-fifth of their clients were homosexual or bisexual (albeit an unreliable estimate). Thirty-seven had occasional clients from the United States, Africa, or the Caribbean. But none had HTLV-III antibodies, and their incidence of hepatitis B, and of cytomegalovirus, was similar to that of Danish women who were not prostitutes. But they used condoms for most encounters. Similarly, Smith and Smith[105] report that licensed prostitutes in West Germany have a 1% prevalence rate of HIV antibody; whereas unlicensed prostitutes showed a 20% prevalence. Though active, the licensed prostitutes made substantial use of condoms. Barton et al.[103] state that preliminary observations from England, France, and Italy suggest a near nil prevalence of anti-HIV in prostitutes where condom use is widespread.

Another report,[106] from the second International Conference on AIDS, cites studies of the unequal distribution of the virus. Among prostitutes coming to STD clinics for treatment, 27% in Zaire carried antibodies, 59% in Kenya, and 88% in Rwanda. Urban/rural distribution also varies—in Rwanda, an antibody incidence of 18% in the capital city was quoted, but of only 3% in rural areas.

RESPONSES TO AIDS IN AFRICA

The means of attempting to deal with the AIDS epidemic has varied widely among African countries, and very little has been written about this. In South Africa, an Advisory Group on AIDS has been formed, but with very little effect as regards providing accessible advice and information to the public. Blood tests are available free under some circumstances (though not to reassure the worried at-risk individual). Some counseling and support have been made available through the gay organization—GASA, but expert psychosocial support has not been properly available to persons with AIDS. There has been much misery, and at least one patient has committed suicide. The Advisory Group has been cautious, relatively inactive, and not very effectively reassuring, inappropriately minimizing the very real risk of the epidemic. They have recently published a coy and inexplicit information pamphlet which is out of date and widely criticized. The

Medical Research Council's urgent support for a major education campaign has, so far, been unwisely ignored.

However, routine screening has been instituted of blood donors, STD clinic attenders, prostitutes, and other high-risk groups. It has been claimed that no evidence of AIDS infection has been found in black prostitutes servicing mining areas. An influx of AIDS with the migrant laborers from elsewhere in Africa who come to South Africa to work in the mines is of concern. For instance, some 30,000 Malawians come to South Africa each year to work (20,000 on the mines). All such legal migrant mine workers are carefully screened medically. A small percentage of seropositive migrants have been thus identified, but, despite some public debate as to whether they should be sent home, it is unclear how many there are and what has happened to them. The extent of infection in the tens of thousands of unscreened migrants is unknown, and the Advisory Committee claims that any risk is minimal.

In an unusual move,[107] a special meeting was held at the South African Institute of Medical Research between traditional African healers (sangomas) from all over the country and medical researchers. This was considered important, as about 80% of the black population consult sangomas before seeing physicians. It was hoped that they could advise people against promiscuity and encourage the use of condoms. A small proportion of sangomas expressed the belief that AIDS is caused by witchcraft and that they had ways of curing it.

It has been clear that there have been problems of underreporting of AIDS cases even in the United States. The U.S. Conference of Mayors is said to have found wide variance between local community figures of incidence and those of the CDC. The situation is far more shaky in Africa. There is no coherent infrastructure of health care and case reporting in many of the areas most severely affected. Where victims are illegal immigrants, fearing deportation and discrimination, they are disinclined to seek official help or to admit to risk factors. Yet, so far, the majority of cases are among heterosexuals rather than in stigmatized or marginal social minority groups. This is just as well in a continent where formal recognition and protection of such minority groups are rare.

Other political and economic factors may have induced a reluctance to admit the existence or the extent of the epidemic in many territories. With the world concern to "blame" some area as at fault for being the "origin" of the deadly virus, there is sensitivity over the theories that hold that the virus originally emerged from Africa. The case in Haiti has been cautionary in regard to the potential impact on the tourist industry. It has been reported[108, 109] that American tourists to Haiti dropped from 70,000 in the winter of 1981–82 to 10,000 the next year, after the first major report of AIDS and Haitians. Cruise ships stopped calling. There has even been speculation linking the economic impact of the drop in tourism with the food riots in spring 1984 and the ultimate ousting of Duvalier. Whatever the basis for such speculation, any such possibility is not appealing to many African governments. In 1987, there was concern over the possibility that British troops might have become infected with AIDS from local prostitutes after visiting Africa.

Zambian newspaper reports claim that at least 50 children under the age of 4 are suffering from AIDS: over 200 new cases overall in 1986, bringing the total since 1983 to over 1,000. It has been estimated that there could be some 6,000 babies with AIDS within a year or two—a study suggested that 9.6% of mothers attending antenatal clinics had AIDS-related symptoms. An "AIDS scare" has been reported with cases of teachers boycotting classes and some parents refusing to send their children to schools where they suspect that other pupils have the disease. There have been further reports of AIDS in children under the age of 2 years in Zaire.[110]

Ethiopia[111] is described as having accused some European countries of denying entry to Africans on suspicion of being carriers of AIDS without a medical examination. A health minister is quoted as denouncing what he called attempts to label AIDS as a black African disease. Ethiopia seems to have been one of the few African countries that had not yet reported any case of AIDS (though to what extent that reflects the incidence is unclear).

A major problem, not yet discussed in this paper, is the potential cost of treatment for AIDS. So far, except for some cases, the majority of African cases of AIDS are receiving at best low-level supportive care. Simple means of limiting spread are not in regular use in Africa, although educational campaigns are beginning in several countries. According to one estimate, between 1,000 and 1,500 new infections could be prevented in just one major hospital in Zaire if routine screening of blood donors for HIV were instituted. But each such test would cost between 3 and 30 times the average sum per person spent on health care in Africa. For just a few million dollars, blood screening could become routine throughout central Africa, but how could this be afforded? The cost of routine care for 10 American AIDS patients is more than the total budget of a large hospital in Zaire, yet 25% of their admissions, adult and pediatric, may be infected. Is foreign aid for AIDS really likely?

There are estimates that the first 10,000 confirmed cases in the United States cost $6.2 billion in medical expenses and in loss of manpower by premature death. Existing drug treatment alone for AIDS patients has been calculated as about 6½ times the average cost of all medications for other hospitalized patients. A Public Health Service projection[112] assumes the average cost per patient will be about $46,000. The United States has already spent more on its early AIDS cases than the total health budget of several African nations added together.

Ironically, recent American developments in product liability laws and actions could mean that even if effective vaccines or treatments for AIDS become available, no drug company may be able to afford the risk or product liability insurance to enable them to produce and market them. If this problem can be overcome, the cost of vaccine and treatment is likely to be extremely high. How will Africa be able to afford to treat or protect its populations?

There have been few accounts of how the AIDS epidemic is affecting life in central Africa. Hooper,[113] in the New York Times, has described the situation in rural Uganda. There are many deaths, and few families are unaffected. Some clergymen, it is said, avoid the many funerals, fearing the disease and considering its victims as sinners not deserving a final blessing. AIDS is known as "Slim."[114] Hooper reports that in Gwanda parish, for example, with a population of about 9000, 13 people had died in the previous week—12 of them of AIDS. At such a death rate, some 7% of the parish's citizens would be dead within the year, but they were sure the situation was worsening more rapidly. The reporter met a boy whose father, mother, sister, and four brothers had all died of AIDS within the preceding 2 years. Uganda's first death from Slim was in 1982 in the village of Kasensero. Since then, the village has seen 101 further deaths, and the population has fallen from around 500 to 176 as others flee the area. Earlier, Slim was believed to be due to witchcraft induced by disgruntled competitors in trading and smuggling; now it is accepted as being spread by sexual contact. A Ugandan Ministry of Health newsletter is quoted as reporting that Ugandan AIDS patients had an average lifetime total of 18 sexual partners each, compared to nine for other patients. A health education campaign is under way, warning of the risks of promiscuous sex, unsterile needles, and sharing razor blades or toothbrushes. Some have turned to cautious habits; others, fatalist, stubborn, or ill-informed, carry on despite the risk.

Africa has been accustomed to carrying a heavy burden of infectious disease through all ages. New diseases or epidemics are not unusual—Burkitt's lymphoma, kuru, endomyocardial fibrosis, Buruli ulcer, and other conditions were identified in the tropics in recent times. Deadly new disease like Lassa fever, Congo fever, and Marburg and green monkey virus diseases have occurred. The sudden or slow death of young people by famine or pestilence is nothing strange, as it may be for the *jeunesse dorée*, the gilded youth of the West. But the scale and ruthlessness of the new plague, the lack of effective intervention, the potential loss of human life, and the social disruption are awesome. There has been great alarm in the United States, the richest nation on earth, where around one in 100 of the population may be seropositive. When one in 10, one in five or more are affected in some of the poorest nations, the prospects are far more grim, and the alarms are less pronounced.

Outside of Africa, some[115] have argued that the view is not so gloomy—that in the United States some 90% of cases are still among "recognized high-risk groups" and that there has been little sign of major heterosexual involvement outside Africa (small comfort for members of high-risk groups). Several studies have found no increased risk from oral sex, and condoms seem surpisingly effective in reducing risk. Fultz[116] has even provided evidence that some component in saliva can inactivate the immunodeficiency virus. Bradbeer[115] comments on the "very low infectivity of the virus under normal circumstances," and on the many ways by which it cannot be spread. There is evidence of change of sexual life style[117] of the sort that would have wider benefits—it seems to be reducing the incidence of other sexually transmitted diseases and in the heterosexual context could help to reduce the incidence of tubal infertility, cervical cancer, and other far more common problems. It is hard to see any bright side to the picture, but at least one author managed to. In a most odd editorial in Tropical Doctor,[118] Hutt comments peculiarly on an article on AIDS in Africa that "for the average doctor working in the tropics these problems may seem remote," then adds approvingly, "but AIDS has done more than any other event since World War II to reawaken the interest of the medical establishment to the importance of infectious and parasitic diseases."

POSTSCRIPT

This chapter has reflected the position, viewed from within Africa, as of January 1987. This postscript, in January 1988, incorporates important new information. During this year, more data have confirmed the awful extent of the problem in central Africa. Also, the author's projections of likely developments in South Africa have proved tragically true.[119] This especially appalling example of politically perverse handling of the disease is discussed in some detail, as the lessons of this situation, where the "right-wing virus" met an especially susceptible right-wing host government, need to be learned.

> In 10 years' time more African people worldwide will be dead from AIDS than died in the Atlantic slave traffic over a period of 400 years. . . . Where are the demonstrations? Who is making an outcry? Where is our rage? Why are we not angry? Where are our leaders? Where the black media?"

These passionate words of the 1987 article "AIDS and the Conspiracy of Silence" in the black American paper *The City Sun* were later reprinted ominously in a major South African newspaper.[120] Within the United States it was becoming clear that AIDS was having a disproportionate impact among black and Hispanic people, and those communities had begun to mobilize responsibly to deal with the threat. As John E. Jacob, president of the National Urban League, pointed out, the fear of a racial backlash against minorities as they became identified with AIDS was "one of the reasons the black community has been slow to address this issue, to put it on our agenda." In Africa itself, it has become even more starkly clear during 1987 that the threat to the communities of Africa could be of genocidal proportions. This supplement to the chapter has become necessary to reflect these developments.

Thus far, there have been numerous reports[121] of how African governments have tried to minimize the risk of AIDS, for instance, by forbidding doctors in their employ from talking to Western media. This response, which has undoubtedly delayed the implementation of significant efforts to control the growing disaster, has been ascribed to "a natural aversion to bad news, coupled with bitterness over reports that the virus originated in Africa."[121] Some governments have required Western AIDS researchers working in Africa to sign formal agreements not to give press interviews. The official total of AIDS cases in Africa, including that reported through WHO, has, as a result, been absurdly low and grossly inaccurate. For example, in February 1987, the official total for Africa was 2627, when several individual countries had probably already exceeded that number of cases.

Conservative estimates suggest that 10–15% of the urban population of central Africa already carry the virus. In Kenya, for instance, Health Minister Kenneth Matiba stated in August that the number of AIDS cases reported in Kenya had more than doubled, to 625, in the preceding 4 months.[122] Those few of us involved with continuing screening programs note an ominous increase in the rate of increase of seropositives identified. Studies of Nairobi prostitutes showed 4% HIV-positive in 1981; by 1985, 59% were positive, and by 1987, 67%. Although earlier studies suggested that 10–30% of people infected with HIV develop AIDS within 5 years, and some have taken this to indicate that a high proportion may escape the eventual development of the disease, more recent studies suggest that 75% will develop AIDS within 15 years. The longer the period of follow-up, the larger the proportion of people eventually dying of the disease. The eventual mortality rate could be on the order of 90%.

The originally mystifying question of why AIDS seemed to be spreading so readily in Africa has begun to clarify. A range of cofactors seem to be involved.

The high incidence of other infectious diseases and malnutrition can reduce the efficacy of the immune system. The commonness of other sexually transmitted diseases can render the genital mucosa more vulnerable to viral entry. Frequent pregnancies, affecting the immune system, could also be relevant. Also, some have suggested that certain antigen types, common in Africa, may be associated with greater vulnerability to the virus. Ghendon (in ref.[123]) has suggested that hepatitis B may activate the AIDS virus in some way, which might help explain the rapid spread of AIDS in Africa where hepatitis is common.

Most affected seem to be sexually active urban adults aged 20–39. This group happens, according to many commentators, to disproportionally include the best and brightest products of decades of community development: educated, skilled, and desperately needed by their countries. Africa's small reservoir of trained teachers, health workers, administrators, professionals, and business entrepreneurs seem to be especially heavily affected, ensuring that the disease will have a far more damaging social impact than the mere numbers of victims would imply. When one of Africa's extremely few neurosurgeons died of AIDS, the impact was large. In areas with one doctor per 22,000 people, the death of even one clinic doctor can threaten the health of many thousands. Zambian figures[121] claim that two-thirds of HIV-positive men were skilled professionals.

The international Panos Institute, in their report on AIDS and the Third World, said: "The young elite represents Africa's first post-independence generation to come to power. In several capitals they are already heavily infected, and will die in increasing numbers. The political, social, economic and psychological impact of this gathering death-march cannot be under-estimated." The evolving effects on unstable regimes, complex societies, fragile institutions, and rare resources are likely to be devastating. They are persistently, dangerously, and deliberately underestimated and played down by politicians and leaders in many countries.

The economic impact has barely begun to be seriously assessed (publicly, at least). Economists are just beginning to calculate the effects of AIDS. A Shearson Lehman Brothers report is quoted[124] as saying that the epidemic in Zaire and Zambia could hit "Copperbelt" supplies, already insecure owing to infrastructure and transport problems, and representing 15% of the Western world's total supplies. The insurance industry in Africa has begun[125] to express extreme concern about the possible impact of AIDS.

Mother-child transmission is common. In some parts, already, 5% of newborns are HIV-infected; 6,000 children in Zambia have AIDS.[126] In Kinshasa, Zaire, Piot (in ref.[123]) has said, 7% of all pregnant women are infected with HIV; 9% in Lusaka, Zambia; 14% in Kampala, Uganda. Twenty percent to 50% of infants are infected by in utero transmission. Piot has also reported (in ref.[123]) that in central Africa, some 80% of adult cases are due to heterosexual spread, the rest being due to blood transfusions. In Rwanda, Uganda, and Zambia, 15–20% of blood donors are HIV-positive. It is economically impossible to institute full screening of all blood donation in Africa, at least if using currently accepted tests and methods. Conditions requiring frequent transfusions are common in Africa, such as sickle cell anemia, malaria, and major obstetric problems. Yet at one hospital in Kampala, Uganda, 14% of the stored blood was found to contain HIV antibodies.

The tragic ironies abound. Underdevelopment and poverty have damaged the previously stable family systems, increasing promiscuity, and have driven young women into prostitution, multiplying the spread of the AIDS epidemic, which will increase the poverty and underdevelopment. Complexities are added by ancient customs. In one area, for instance, it is believed to be essential that a widow should, after the burial of her husband, have sexual relations with older male cognates of her husband's lineage, to ritually remove highly dangerous influences from her. But if the husband died of AIDS, and she carries the virus, the custom can be deadly.

People in heavily affected areas of Uganda[127] say that they first began to see the disease after the 1979 invasion by Tanzanian troops and Ugandan guerrillas when Idi Amin was ousted. They blame Tanzanians for the epidemic, especially "the women of Bukoba," women reported to comprise a high proportion of prostitutes in that region. It is interesting that the African green monkey, which lives throughout those border regions and which has been found to carry the very similar simian virus, is a great delicacy to the people of Bukoba. There is also clear evidence that the disease has spread along major transport and trucking routes across Africa.

AIDS is still being dismissed in Africa as irrelevant, affecting only foreigners or other countries, and as less important than other national and regional priorities. But Africa has probably never faced a greater menace to its people and its fate. No loathsome disease—smallpox, apartheid, malaria—has had such a capacity to destroy on such a scale. There is an urgent need for help from the rest of the world for screening of blood supplies, population screening and counseling, major educational campaigns, and research. Pekkanen[121] quotes one African expert as saying: "We must do something now, because in 10 years there may not be enough of us to do anything."

The immune deficiencies related to AIDS (there has been little study of ARC and related states in Africa) may be playing a part in what appear to be (again, details are being suppressed and are not available) other significant and unusually severe outbreaks of other infectious diseases in the afflicted regions: cerebral malaria, sleeping sickness, and yellow fever. Piot (in ref.[123]) confirmed that even where full-blown AIDS does not develop, ARC and AIDS carrier states may affect susceptibility to important vaccines (e.g., measles) and affect the incidence and virulence of such infections.

Research regarding the control and prevention of the African expression of AIDS may be best conducted in regions like South Africa where it is still uncommon enough for interventions to demonstrate efficacy. It has been said that research on the possible protective value of spermicides, for example, has been difficult in central Africa because of the great difficulty in finding seronegative prostitutes to take part in such studies.

The story, so far, of the official South African response to AIDS has been deplorable, though hardly surprising from a country where sterile political ideology has led to the wastage of very scarce resources on a proliferation of more than a dozen different health administrations and "ministers."

As in other countries, it has been mainly Conservative politicians who have proposed unrealistically rabid responses to the prospect of AIDS. Typical of many responses is a letter to the editor[128] saying that "nature . . . with an exquisite sense of poetic justice, has chosen the most appropriate scourge with which to cleanse this continent from the blight of over-population." In South

Africa, a Conservative Member of Parliament has asked whether there should not be a screening of all people coming into the country.[129] Such proposals are, of course, unrealistic in that they are not only impractical but ineffective. A World Health Organization report concluded:[129] "No screening programme of international travellers can prevent the introduction and spread of HIV infection . . . at best and at great cost (it can) retard only briefly the dissemination of HIV both globally and with respect to any particular country."

It has been calculated, in the case of South Africa,[129] that the cost of attempting (ineffectually) to screen entrants to the country for AIDS for 1 year would buy at least 250 million condoms, which would, at present rates of use, be a 10-year national supply.

As of March 1987, 49 cases of AIDS had been officially recognized in South Africa. In July the Minister of National Health admitted to 2234 AIDS carriers in South Africa. Dissecting the numbers racially, he said 1,140 were white, 1,093 black (946 of them miners), 31 "Coloured," and 3 Indian.

A report in Epidemiological Comments, cited in the *South African Medical Journal*,[130] was adamant that the high-risk group was "homosexual and so-called bisexual white males" (the use of "so-called" represents a prime example of gross ignorance of human sexuality displayed by an epidemiologist pontificating on a subject he knows nothing about, a problem that has bedeviled action on AIDS in southern Africa). That "authority," in the same officially highly regarded report, goes on to say, "For all practical purposes it is reasonable to state that the other well-known high-risk groups are as yet uninfected: drug abusers, haemophiliacs, blood recipients and prostitutes. Also, the virus is not endemic."

Intravenous drug abuse is rare in southern Africa, but at that time it was already known that hemophiliacs and blood product recipients had been affected. South African cases have already included two infected by blood transfusions and two hemophiliacs. There is reason for serious concern about the 3000 hemophiliacs in South Africa, many of whom, as a result of poor planning, received U.S. blood products (not then screened for AIDS and with a significant risk of carrying the infection) between 1982 and 1984–85, after which screening and heat treatment were broadly introduced. Since 1985, far safer local blood products have been used. It is also known that local prostitutes are infected, but nothing is being done to deal with that risk.

There have been recurrent snide criticisms by the AIDS Advisory Committee of the news media for "overdramatizing" the issue of AIDS. Yet, the African media have in fact behaved highly responsibly and have given the public very accurate and useful information, in comparison with the misleading and irresponsibly inadequate information provided by that advisory committee.

Schoub[131] has usefully criticized the "smug complacency" in South Africa. Within the initially affected group of white men, mainly homosexual or bisexual, assuming that they number 25,000 in the population, with a seropositivity rate of 30% and a conversion to clinical AIDS of one-third of those affected over a 5-year period, he estimated that there will be around 2500 cases in South Africa by 1991. He also recognized the menace of AIDS within the black population but mistakenly states that "to date various serological studies have consistently failed to reveal evidence of significant infection in South African black populations." This was too strong a conclusion to draw, as the authorities had failed to conduct sufficient and suitable screening studies to warrant such an inference. As a professor of forensic medicine[132] has said: "We are part of Africa and we cannot hide behind the often-heard argument that African AIDS will never become a problem here, or that it is still a small problem."

Schoub[131] also called for a major educational/preventive campaign. Sadly, like other influential advisers to the South African authorities who wholly lack experience in interpreting psychosocial data within the medical and health context, he placed excessive weight on a single paper,[133] which questioned the efficacy of one of the British Department of Health's advertising campaigns. Other evidence of the value and impressive effects of other advertising, information, and educational efforts has been ignored by the South African authorities. Schoub's conclusion in early June 1987 was, "Now is the time to act— rationally and aggressively."

Evidence of the poor-quality, amateur, or nonexistent psychosocial care the South African AIDS patients receive is the high rate of suicide and suicide attempts among them. One leapt to his death from Chapman's Peak in Cape Town, but the only popular concern expressed was whether the paramedics who recovered his shattered body had been exposed to the virus. Later, when another AIDS sufferer jumped from the seventh floor of a city-center building, after running away from the hospital where he was supposedly receiving psychiatric treatment,[134] the same issue arose. No one asked why people under competent medical care should be so desperate.

Tragically, the Chairman of the Government Advisory Committee on AIDS has continued to insist that the pattern of AIDS in South Africa is similar to that of the United States and Europe, not that of the rest of Africa, and that it is not a major health problem for the country. Some experts now believe that this committee will prove to have made, to South African public health, as useful a contribution as did Typhoid Mary.

In South Africa it has also become tragically obvious that a government irretrievably committed to seeing only what it wishes to see and hearing only what fits its minutely narrow preconceptions has been dealing with the AIDS threat in a manner, the apotheosis of smug, that reinforces a Neanderthal world view and tragically magnifies the risk to the peoples of the subcontinent. Venter[135] states, as do others who have looked seriously at the situation, "South Africa is as guilty of a conspiracy of silence as Zambia, Tanzania, Mozambique, or Kenya."

A significant route of entry of the African pattern of heterosexually transmitted AIDS has been via migrant labor. Dr. Brian Brink of the South African Chamber of Mines reported to the third international AIDS conference in Washington in 1987[136] that miners migrating to South Africa from countries to its north, especially Malawi, are importing AIDS. In the study he reported, of 30,000 migrant miners, 4% of 3165 Malawians tested as HIV-positive, a rate of one in 25, and potentially 1000 of the 20,000 Malawian migrant workers in South Africa. There had been an 18% increase in the number of identified carriers from 1986 to 1987.[137]

There has been considerable haggling between the South African Government and the Chamber of Mines about what to do about migrant HIV carriers.[138] There were lengthy negotiations, delaying a fully effective response. The Chamber of Mines was adamant that the correct procedure with infected miners would be counseling and education, to treat such illnesses as developed within the mines' medical system, to allow them to continue to work as long as possible, enabling them to continue to earn funds to support their families and to repatriate them only when they became too ill or when the miners themselves requested this. The South African Government, on the other hand, wanted to have the men repatriated to their countries of origin promptly, once they were diagnosed. There was concern that the disease would spread, both through facultative homosexual relations between miners within the "hostel" system in "single" men's quarters, separated from wives and families) and via the prostitutes (mainly heterosexual) and girl friends who serve them.

The Department of Health is quoted[137] as demanding that the AIDS migration route, bringing 20,000 miners from Malawi to and from South Africa, be closed or curtailed. At least 940 HIV-positive miners were identified by early 1987. There was prolonged dithering about whether to start a national education campaign, especially among South African blacks.

In September 1987, the Minister of National Health, Dr. Willie van Niekerk, told Parliament that the Government had decided that all foreign AIDS carriers would be repatriated.[139] He said the danger of AIDS was alarming and measures to combat its spread therefore had a high priority at government level. Yet he failed, throughout 1987, to take any of the other steps which would have been more genuinely protective of the population, especially the black community.

Fears of "witch hunts" were widely expressed after the announcement.[140] According to some estimates, there are over a million registered foreign African workers in South Africa and many thousands more unregistered "illegal workers." The most conservative estimate, in another study, put the number of potentially affected migrant African workers at 378,000, rising to some 570,000 if illegal immigrants were included.[141] Trade union spokesmen condemned the decision, saying that the solution lay not in repatriating migrant workers but in providing proper counseling and medical facilities. "The question of whether a worker should return home should be decided by him and his family. Migrant workers are being used as scapegoats," said a National Union of Mineworkers spokesman. The General Secretary of the National Council of Trade Unions, Phiroshaw Camay, said the proposal would be discriminatory, as it seemed to be aimed only at workers from African countries, and "There is a responsibility on the Government to give affected people medical treatment, and not to send them to countries which have no facilities."

As an example of the potential economic, let alone human, impact of such repatriations, it was estimated that Malawi could lose up to 3 million rands a year in foreign exchange if 1000 of its migrant workers were sent home. Consider also the potential economic impact, locally and internationally, if AIDS has, as seems very possible, a substantial impact specifically on the workers in South Africa's gold and other strategic mineral mines.

Clear and compelling evidence that the incidence of seropositivity was far higher than suggested by official announcements has been ignored. Data presented by the South African Blood Transfusion Service showed a substantial incidence of HIV seropositivity among black women in Soweto (based on testing of antenatal clinic blood samples). They estimated an increase in seropositivity in these heterosexual black women at the rate of 300% a year.[119,141]

The AIDS Advisory Committee in South Africa, lamentably lacking in essential expertise, has persistently minimized the risk and seems to have allowed personality clashes and rivalries to influence decisions. For example, at the first National conference on AIDS, its chairman and other members persistently refused to allow the head of South African Blood Transfusion Service to present vital data or to discuss its significance. That expert, Dr. Shapiro, estimated in September 1987 that some 15,000 South African blacks were already infected. Successive samples in his ongoing study showed a 50% increase in the proportion of black women who were seropositive in the second 2-month period, compared with the first. Shapiro's figures were based on a sample of 13,500 women and provide far better data than any the so-called experts on the AIDS Advisory Committee have provided. Metz preferred his own figures, estimating only 3000 black AIDS carriers. Only very belatedly[142] has the AIDS Advisory Group reluctantly admitted that the African pattern of spread "will inevitably occur in the RSA [Republic of South Africa] in the future." Sadly, it was already occurring.

There was another report[141] that a wave of concerned individuals seeking blood tests in the Witwatersrand area was revealing some 30 new cases a week, mainly in white homosexual and bisexual men.

It has been reported[143] that 28 pregnant black women in Johannesburg have been advised to seek an abortion after being found to have been infected with HIV, but the majority have decided not to end the pregnancy, despite the risk of the baby developing AIDS. Earlier, amazingly, when doctors attempted, through Transvaal hospital authorities, to notify the seropositive women and the doctors treating them, hospital authorities refused to cooperate. A young doctor who had admitted a patient in Natal with a differential diagnosis including AIDS was hauled before his hospital superintendent, severely criticized, and warned not to mention AIDS in his recorded admission diagnosis again. A public health nurse in the Cape (personal communication) has said that her office was testing prostitutes and discovering an important incidence of HIV seropositivity, but that they were told to stop the testing, and their records were taken away.

Venter[135] has claimed that returning African National Congress refugees could be one of the routes by which AIDS will enter South Africa. He maintains, after traveling in Africa to make a TV documentary, that "Many of the young boys and girls who left South Africa in the seventies and early eighties for ANC holding camps in Tanzania, Angola and Zambia have been infected by AIDS in these countries. Some have already died." He further claims that the high incidence has affected some of the ANC command structure in Lusaka, and some ZAPU commanders.

Other reports[144] as early as July 1987 showed black women bearing HIV in all South African provinces and in both urban and rural areas. The Government and the Minister of Health failed to take appropriate action as early as it was urgently needed.

The urgent need for a massive public education campaign is very obvious. A pilot survey of the views of white South Africans[145] is of interest, reflecting the extent of the ignorance of these generally isolated and naive individuals at a time when the rest of the world was being inundated with the facts of AIDS. It found that more than half (53%) of the South Africans questioned believed you can catch AIDS from a lavatory seat; others thought you could catch it from holding hands (13.5%), from sharing a sauna, or from airline stewards (25%, compared with air hostesses—21.5%). Ninety-seven percent believed AIDS could be contracted through blood transfusions, and 64% believed it was transmitted by kissing.

Forty percent believed you could catch AIDS by sleeping in a hotel bed the night after it was occupied by a person with AIDS; 71.5%, by drinking from the same cup on the same occasion (43% even if the cup had only been used by the AIDS patient days before); 65.5% believed AIDS was spread by mosquitoes; 43% considered using a swimming pool a risk factor; 61% wanted AIDS sufferers to be isolated. Generally, the Afrikaans-speaking whites were more frightened and less well informed. The black population, with even less access to informed media, are likely to be even less well informed. In parts of Kwa-Natal, Zulu people have stopped smoking dagga (marijuana), as it is rumored to carry AIDS.

The authorities were very slow in deciding to act, however, and never made their plans adequately clear. By September 1987,[146] it was said that they had decided against an explicit and dramatic campaign such as the British had used. This seemed to have been decided on the basis of the persistently amateur advice of unsophisticated advisers devoid of relevant knowledge and skills in the behavioral sciences. They had apparently decided on a low-key campaign to give workshops to nurses and other health personnel. An AIDS Information and Training Center was set up at the Institute for Medical Research with a grant from the Chamber of Mines, but no serious attempt was made to seek appropriate expertise, and the center had zero impact throughout 1987. The reprehensible fact is that decisions about how to seek to change health and sexual behavior were being made by virologists and others totally lacking in any relevant training or experience.

Details of the planned national public anti-AIDS campaign due to be launched by the Department of National Health in 1988 were deliberately shrouded in maximum secrecy. No details would be revealed in advance, according to an official spokesman, "as it could be detrimental to the campaign."

Convincing reports late in 1987[147] suggested that the multi-million-rand anti-AIDS campaign due to be launched in 1988 by the South African government would be an irresponsibly ineffective waste of scarce public funds, as the content and impact of the campaign were to be diluted by the foolish extreme Calvinism of Government leaders. For fear of offending the cramped hypersensitivities of the tiny but overinfluential Afrikaner church hegemony, there was strong reason to believe that the need to promote the use of condoms would be ignored.

Senior Department of Health officials said that promoting condoms would cause problems "as far as morality was concerned." That men who do not consider the perversion of the provision of health care by doctrinaire apartheid to cause any problems "as far as morality is concerned" should tolerate a large easily avoidable increase in the risk of disease and eventual death of the people because of the dictates of an intensely politicized and isolated Church whose views were outdated in the 17th century is surely deplorable. They move from preconceived ideas to predetermined conclusions, unmoved by reality or the suffering of others.

Disgracefully, it appeared that condoms were regarded as a taboo subject by the Department of Health. Dr. Coen Slabber, newly appointed Director-General of the Department of Health, acknowledged to reporters that the condom was the most important method of preventing AIDS but said it was "very difficult" to include them in the proposed advertising campaign without alienating people.

In an astonishing statement, he said, "Homosexuality is not accepted by the majority of the population and certainly not by the Afrikaans-speaking part of the population. To advocate that homosexuals use the condom is therefore very difficult." This statement tragically reveals how the attitudes of the South African Government can constitute a major threat to public health (as has been seen in many other instances). The emotional needs of the Afrikaner minority are placed far above the life-and-death needs of the majority in policy planning. There is insufficient understanding of the facts of life: the heterosexual risk is ignored, and the problem is seen, instinctively, purely from the white point of view (as a disease of white homosexuals).

Dr. Slabber stated that the Minister of National Health himself has "thrashed out the contents of the campaign." It must be recognized that Dr. van Niekerk, that minister, has shown himself to be extremely resistant to criticism or to ideas not serving the needs of Afrikaner nationalism, and he is widely expected to attain still higher office.

A more sinister interpretation is tempting, tragically. Comments that "AIDS will solve the population problem in Africa" are all too common. There are those in South Africa to whom it would seem to be no great tragedy if AIDS decimated the black African population; it could weaken black resistance to apartheid and strengthen the position of the right-wing white minority. Some have suggested that the long delay in launching any noticeable effort to combat AIDS, and the deliberate emasculation of the essential needs of such an urgent education campaign, might be a deliberate policy rather than simply a series of naive errors. The insistence on ignoring highly relevant data and expertise is unlikely to be accidental.

Boekkooi[148] reports that South Africa's condom factories are gearing up to double production and to launch new marketing campaigns. Already, they have begun a far more imaginative, effective, and publicly beneficial campaign than the South African government's puny vision will allow, and long before the authorities could bring themselves to even try. Southern Africans are relatively low users of condoms, and much needs to be done to encourage their use. They are currently on sale only in a limited number and range of outlets. Vending-machine sales are very rare. In one typically ludicrous piece of official action, there was hysteria when a Transvaal bar installed a condom vending machine in the men's toilets. Within days, it was removed in a police raid, and the condoms were declared a threat to public morality! The Department of Health currently distributes 12–13 million condoms a year as part of family planning services (seeking to lower the high African birth rate) but is apparently too squeamish to propose the use of condoms too noisily or effectively.

Concern was expressed in 1988[149] about AIDS in South African prisons. The Minister of Justice in July 1987 admitted there were then two men suffering from clinical AIDS and eight others HIV-positive within the prisons. Homosexuality is illegal in South Africa and its prisons. A police spokesman said,[149] "Criminal or disciplinary steps are taken against anybody found engaging in homosexual activity. Members of the SAPD have been trained to identify active or latent homosexuals, and the necessary precautions are taken against the spread of these activities." There is no possibility of the issue of condoms within the prisons (as has occurred in other countries), as the spokesman stated, "Any provision of condoms to prisoners would in fact be a condonation of homosexual acts, which are prohibited."

Concern has been expressed[150] about warning other health professionals, such as dentists, of AIDS cases, but the soundest advice[151] has been that such patients need the same basic protective measures "appropriate in the care of all patients, regardless of the probability of HIV infection."[152]

In significant research, by August 1987, Shapiro et al.[153] identified nine confirmed HIV positives among the sera of 20,000 black women attending antenatal clinics in the Johannesburg area, a rate of one per 2300. This could, extrapolated nationally, mean 15,000 South African blacks already carrying HIV. (The Advisory Group on AIDS admitted a prevalence of 0.027% among South African blacks).

A national screening campaign in South Africa could be possible for a lower cost than the Government spent on the production of one propaganda song or the building of unneeded opera houses. The authorities have been dragging their heels, however, about taking serious initiative.

REFERENCES

1. Holtzhausen E. Now witness "the death of a continent." Sunday Times (Johannesburg), November 30, 1986.

2. Netter T. W. AIDS cases are said to rise sharply worldwide. New York Times, October 5, 1986, L9.

3. Wetzel J. Belli told South African AIDS problem heterosexual. Sentinal USA (San Francisco), 1985, April 25.

4. De Cock K. M. AIDS: An old disease from Africa? British Medical Journal, 1984, 189, 303–308.

5. Williams G., Stretton T. B., Leonard J. C. AIDS in 1959? Lancet, 1983, ii, 1136.

6. Jenkins P., Malthouse S. R., Banghan C. A., et al. AIDS: The African connection. British Medical Journal, 1985, 290, 1284–1285.

7. Suter F., Marchetti G., Caprioli S., et al. Su un caso di AIDS in una giovane africana residente in Italia. Giornale di Malattie Infettive e Parassitarie, 1984, 36, 8, 885–888.

8. Siegal F., Siegal M. AIDS: The Medical Mystery. New York: Grove Press, 1983, p 70.

9. Martin–Du Pan R. C., Roth A., Stamenkovic I., et al. Syndrome de deficit immunitaire acquis . . . chez un couple de zairois. Schweizerische Medizinische Wochenschrift, 1984, 114, 46, 1645–1650.

10. Bygbjerg I. C. AIDS in a Danish surgeon (Zaire 1976). Lancet, 1983, i, 925.

11. Clumeck N., Sonnet J., Taelman H., et al. Acquired immunodeficiency syndrome in African patients. New England Journal of Medicine, 1984, 310, 8, 492–497.

12. Fichardt T., Sandison A. G., Loock E. L. Radiotherapy for Kaposi's sarcoma: A review. South African Cancer Bulletin, 1984, 27, 3, 99–118.

13. Oettle A. G. Geographic and racial differences in the frequency of Kaposi's sarcoma as evidence of environmental or genetic causes. Acta Un. Int. Cancer, 1962, 18, 330–363.

14. Oates K., Dealler S., Dickey R., et al. Malignant neoplasms 1971–1983 in northeastern Zaire. Annales de la Societe Belge de Medecine Tropicale, 1984, 64, 4, 373–378.

15. McHardy J., Williams E. H., Geser A., et al. Endemic Kaposi's sarcoma: Incidence and risk factors in the West/Nile district of Uganda. International Journal of Cancer, 1984, 33, 2, 203–212.

16. Bayley A. C. Aggressive Kaposi's sarcoma in Zambia, 1983. Lancet, 1984, i, 1318–1320.

17. Bayley A. C., Downing R. G., Cheingsong-Popov R., et al. HTLV-III serology distinguishes atypical and endemic Kaposi's sarcoma in Africa. Lancet, 1985, i, 359–361.

18. Downing R. G., Eglin R. P., Bayley A. C. African Kaposi's sarcoma and AIDS. Lancet, 1984, i, 478–480.

19. Greenwood B. M., Whittle H. C. African Kaposi's sarcoma and AIDS. Lancet, 1984, i, 798.

20. Edwards D., Harper P. G., Pain A. K., et al. Kaposi's sarcoma associated with AIDS in a woman from Uganda. Lancet, 1984, i, 631–632.

21. Weber J. Is AIDS an epidemic form of African Kaposi's sarcoma? Discussion paper. Journal of the Royal Society of Medicine, 1984, 77, 7, 572–576.

22. Feremans W., Menu R., Dustin P., et al. Virus-like particles in lymphocytes of seven cases of AIDS in black Africans. Lancet, 1983, ii, 52–53.

23. Vittecoq D., Modai J. AIDS in a black Malian. Lancet, 1983, ii, 1023.

24. Van de Pitte J., Verwilghen R., Zachee P. AIDS and cryptococcosis. Lancet, 1983, i, 925–926.

25. Taelman H., Dasnoy J., Van Marck E., et al. Syndrome d' immunodeficience acquise chez trois patients du Zaire. Annales de la Societe Belge de Medecine Tropicale, 1983, 63, 1, 73–74.

26. Ras G. J., Simson I. W., Anderson R., et al. Acquired immunodeficiency syndrome: A report of 2 South African cases. South African Medical Journal, 1983, 64, 4, 140–142.

27. Van de Perre P., Rouvroy D., Lepage P., et al. Acquired immunodeficiency in Rwanda. Lancet, 1984, ii, 62–65.

28. Piot P., Quinn T. C., Taelman H., et al. Acquired immunodeficiency syndrome in African patients. New England Journal of Medicine, 1984, 310, 8, 492–497.

29. Clumeck N., Van de Perre P., Carael D., et al. Heterosexual promiscuity among African patients with AIDS. New England Journal of Medicine, 1985, 313, 3, 182.

30. Brun-Vezinet F., Rouzioux C., Montagnier L., et al. Prevalence of antibodies to lymphadenopathy-associated retroviruses in African patients with AIDS. Science, 1984, 226, 453–456.

31. Biggar R. J., Melbye M., Kestens L., et al. Seroepidemiology of HTLV-III antibodies in a remote population of eastern Zaire. British Medical Journal, 1985, 290, 808–810.

32. Lyons S. F., Schoub B. D., McGillivray G. M., et al. Sero-epidemiology of HTLV-III antibody in South Africa. South African Medical Journal, 1985, 67, 961–962.

33. Opperman J. C., Rubin D. M., Glocer J., et al. Prevalence of antibodies to human T-cell leukemia virus. South African Medical Journal, 1984, 66, 86.

34. Van der Riet F., Hesselring P. B. Reactivity of Bushman sera with HTLV-III—what does it mean? South African Medical Journal, 1985, 67, 617–618.

35. Van der Riet F., Hesselring P. B. Reactivity of Bushman sera with HTLV-III is not due to HTLV-III specific antibody. South African Medical Journal, 1985, 67, 1038.

36. Sher R., Dos Santos L. Prevalence of HTLV-III antibodies in homosexual men in Johannesburg. South African Medical Journal, 1985, 67, 13, 484.

37. Jonckheer T., Dab I., Van de Perre P., et al. Cluster of HTLV-III/LAV infection in an African family. Lancet, 1985, i, 400–401.

38. Saxinger W. C., Levine P. H., Dean A. G., et al. Evidence for exposure to HTLV-III in Uganda before 1973. Science, 1985, 227, 1036–1038.

39. Biggar R. J., Gigase P. L., Melbye M., et al. ELISA HTLV retrovirus antibody reactivity associated with malaria and immune complexes in healthy Africans. Lancet 1985, ii, 520–523.

40. Kuhul P., Seidl S., Holzberger G. HLA-DR4 antibodies cause positive HTLV-III antibody ELISA results. Lancet, 1985, i, 1222–1223.

41. Weiss S. H., Mann D. L., Murray C., et al. HLA-DR antibodies and HTLV-III antibody ELISA testing. Lancet, 1985, i, 157.

42. Hunter J. B., Menitove J. E. HLA antibodies detected by ELISA HTLV-III antibody kits. Lancet, 1985, ii, 397.

43. Biggar R. J. The AIDS problem in Africa. Lancet, 1986, i, 79–83.

44. Melbye M., Biggar R. J., Ebbeson P., et al. Long-term sero-positivity for human T-lymphotropic virus type III in homosexual men without the acquired immunodeficiency syndrome: Development of immunologic and clinical abnormalities. A longitudinal study. Annals of Internal Medicine, 1986, 104, 496–500.

45. Geodert J. J., Biggar R. J., Weiss S. H., et al. Three-year incidence of AIDS in five cohorts of HTLV-III-infected risk group members. Science, 1986, 231, 992–995.

46. Mann J. M., Bilak D. V., Colebunders R. R., et al. Natural history of human immunodeficiency virus infection in Zaire. Lancet, 1986, ii, 707–709.

47. Fleming A. F. HTLV from Africa to Japan. Lancet, 1984, i, 279.

48. Hunsmaun G., Bayer H., Schneider J., et al. Antibodies to ATLV/HTLV-I in Africa. Medical Microbiology and Immunology, 1984, 173, 3, 167–170.

49. Hahn B. H., Shaw G. M., Popovic M., et al. Molecular cloning and analysis of a new

variant of human T-cell leukemia virus (HTLV-Ib) from an African patient with adult T-cell leukemia-lymphoma. International Journal of Cancer, 1984, 34, 5, 613–618.

50. Biggar R. J., Saxinger C., Gardiner C., et al. Type-I HTLV antibody in urban and rural Ghana, West Africa. International Journal of Cancer, 1984, 34, 2, 215–219.

51. Stewart J. S. W., Matutes E., Lampert I. A., et al. HTLV-I-positive T-cell lymphoma/ leukemia in an African resident in UK. Lancet, 1984, ii, 984–985.

52. Oladipupo-Williams C. K., Alahi G. O., Junaid T. A., et al. Human T-cell leukemia virus associated lymphoproliferative disease: Report of two cases in Nigeria. British Medical Journal, 1984, 288, 1495–1496.

53. Hunsmann G., Schneider J., Schmitt J., et al. Detection of serum antibodies to adult T-cell leukemia virus in non-human primates and in people from Africa. International Journal of Cancer, 1983, 32, 3, 329–332.

54. Becker W. B., Becker M. L. B., Homma T., et al. Serum antibodies to human T-cell leukemia virus type I in different ethnic groups and in non-human primates in South Africa. South African Medical Journal, 1985, 67, 12, 445–449.

55. Fleming A. F., Yamamoto N., Bhusnurmath S. R., et al. Antibodies to ATLV (HTLV) in Nigerian blood donors and patients with chronic lymphatic leukemia or lymphoma. Lancet, 1983, ii, 334–335.

56. Van der Reit F., Fincham J. E., Seier J. V. Absence of antibodies reactive with simian AIDS virus surface antigens in sera of vervet monkeys and baboons. South African Medical Journal, 1985, 67, 17, 662–663.

57. Lyons S. F., Schoub B. D., McGillivray G. M., et al. Lack of evidence of HTLV-III endemicity in southern Africa. New England Journal of Medicine, 1985, 312, 19, 1257–1258.

58. Rey F., Salavin D., Lesbordes J. L. HIV-I and HIV-II double infection in Central African Republic. Lancet, 1986, ii, 1391–1392.

59. Clavel F., Guetard D., Brun-Vezinet F., et al. Isolation of a new human retrovirus from West African patients with AIDS. Science, 1986, 233, 343–346.

60. Kanki P. J., Alroy J., Essex M., et al. Isolation of T-lymphocytic retrovirus related to HTLV-III/LAV from wild caught African green monkeys. Science, 1985, 228, 951–954.

61. Georges A. J., Lesbordes J. L., Meunier D. M. Y., et al. Antibodies to LAV in various groups of the CAR. Ann. Virol. (Inst. Pasteur).

62. Marx J. L. New relatives of AIDS virus found. Science, 1986, 232, 157.

63. Kanki P. J., Barin F., M'Boup S., et al. New human T-Lymphotropic retrovirus related to simian T-Lymphotropic virus type III (STLV-III). Science, 1986, 232, 238.

64. Biberfeld G., Bottiger B., Bredberg-Raden U., et al. Findings in four HTLV-IV sero-positive women from West Africa. Lancet, 1986, ii, 1330–1331.

65. Anonymous. AIDS test can't detect LAV-II. Medical World News, 1986, December 8, 7.

66. Hayes M. M., Coghlan P. J., King H., et al. Kaposi's sarcoma, tuberculosis and Hodgkin's lymphoma in a lymph node—Possible acquired immunodeficiency syndrome: A case report. South African Medical Journal, 1984, 66, 6, 226, 229.

67. Sher B. AIDS in Johannesburg. South African Medical Journal, 1985, 68, 137–138.

68. Malan, M. AIDS in the USA and the RSA—an update. South Africa Medical Journal, 1986, 70, 119.

69. Sprackler, F. H. N., Whittaker R. G., Becker W. B., et al. The acquired immunodeficiency syndrome and related complex. South African Medical Journal, 1985, 68, 139–143.

70. McCarthy G. Prevalence of HTLV-III antibodies in homosexual men in Johannesburg. South African Medical Journal, 1985, 68, 6.

71. Anderson R., Prozesky O. W., Eftychis H. A., et al. Immunological abnormalities in South African homosexual men. South African Medical Journal, 1983, 64, 4, 119–122.

72. Colebunders R., Taelman H., Piot P. Acquired immunodeficiency syndrome (AIDS) in Africa: A review. Tropical Doctor, 1985, 15, 9–12.

73. Van de Perre P., Munyambuga D., Zizzis G., et al. Antibody to HTLV-III in blood donors in central Africa. Lancet, 1985, 1, 336–337.

74. Sher B. Acquired immune deficiency syndrome (AIDS) in the RSA. South African Medical Journal, Supplement, 1986, 11 October, 23–26.

75. Becker W. B. HTLV-III infection in the RSA. South African Medical Journal, Supplement, 1986, 11 October, 26–27.

76. Centers for Disease Control. Update: acquired immunodeficiency syndrome—Europe. Morbidity and Mortality Weekly Report (MMWR) 1985, 34, 583–589.

77. Editorial. Needlestick transmission of HTLV-III from a patient infected in Africa. Lancet, 1984, 2, 1376–1377.

78. Izzia K. W., Lepire B., Kayembe K., et al. Syndrome d' immunodeficience acquise et drepanocytose homozygote. A propos d'une observation Zairoise. Annales de la Societe Belge de Medicine Tropicale, 1984, 64, 4, 391–396.

79. Lyons S. F., Jupp P. G., Schoub B. D. Survival of HIV in the common bedbug. Lancet, 1986, ii, 45.

80. Morfeldt-Manson L., Lindquist K. Blood brotherhood: A risk factor for AIDS? Lancet, 1984, ii, 1346.

81. Wyatt H. V. Injections and AIDS. Tropical Doctor, 1986, 16, 97–98.

82. Wyatt H. V. The popularity of injections in the Third World: Origins and consequences for poliomyelitis. Social Science and Medicine, 1984, 19, 911–915.

83. Guyer B., Atemebakobisong A., Gould J., et al. Injections and paralytic poliomyelitis in tropical Africa. Bulletin of the W.H.O., 1980, 58, 285–291.

84. De Miranda S., Sher R., Metz J., et al. Lack of evidence of HIV infection in drug abusers at present. South African Medical Journal, 1986, 70, 776–777.

85. Mann J. M., Quinn T. C., Francis H., et al. Prevalence of HTLV-III/LAV in household contacts of patients with confirmed AIDS and controls in Kinshasa, Zaire. Journal of the American Medical Association, 1986, 256, 6, 721–724.

86. Melbye M., Biggar R. J., Ebbesen P. Epidemiology—Europe and Africa. In Ebbesen P., Biggar R. J., Melbye M., eds. AIDS: A Basic Guide for Clinicians. Copenhagen: Munksgaard/ Saunders, 1984, pp 29–42.

87. Brunet J. B., Bouvet E., Chaperon J., et al. Acquired immunodeficiency syndrome in France. Lancet, 1983, i, 700–701.

88. Biggar R. J., Bouvet E., Ebbesen P., et al. AIDS in Europe, status quo 1983. European Journal of Cancer and Clinical Oncology, 1984, 20, 155–173.

89. Glauser M. P., Francioli P. Clinical and epidemiological survey of acquired immune deficiency syndrome in Europe. European Journal of Clinical Microbiology, 1984, 3, 55–58.

90. Bygbjerg I. C., Nielsen J. O. AIDS from central Africa in a heterosexual Danish male, AIDS Memorandum, 1983, 1, 2, 9–10.

91. Biggar R. J., Horm J., Lubin J. H., et al. Cancer trends in a population at risk of AIDS. Journal of the National Cancer Institute, 1985, 74, 793–797.

92. Schoub B. D. Report back, International Symposium on African AIDS, Brussels, 22–23 November, 1985. Southern African Journal of Epidemiology and Infection, 1986, 1, 25–29.

93. Padian N., Pickering M. Female-to-male transmission of AIDS: A re-examination of the African sex-ratio of cases. Journal of the American Medical Association, 1986, 256, 590.

94. Redfield P. R., Markham P., Salahuddin S. Z., et al. Frequent transmission of HTLV-III among spouses of patients with AIDS-related complex and AIDS. Journal of the American Medical Association, 1985, 253, 1571–1573.

95. Redfield R. R., Markham P. D., Salahuddin S. Z., et al. Heterosexuality and HTLV-III/ LAV disease (AIDS related complex and AIDS): Epidemiologic evidence for female-to-male transmission. Journal of the American Medical Association, 1985, 254, 2094–2096.

96. Redfield R. R., Wright D. C., Markham P. D., et al. Female-to-male transmission of HTLV-III. Journal of the American Medical Association, 1986, 255, 1706–1707.

97. Pearce R. B. Heterosexual transmission of AIDS. Journal of the American Medical Association, 1986, 256, 590–591.

98. Melbye M., Njelesani E. K., Bayley A., et al. Evidence for heterosexual transmission and clinical manifestations of human immunodeficiency virus infection and related conditions in Lusaka, Zambia. Lancet, 1986, ii, 1113–1115.

99. Potterat J., Muth J., Markewich G. Serological markers as indicators of sexual orientation in AIDS virus-infection, Journal of the American Medical Association, 1986, 256, 6, 712.

100. Kreiss J. K., Koech D., Plummer F. A., et al. AIDS virus infection in Nairobi prostitutes: Spread of the epidemic to East Africa. New England Journal of Medicine, 1986, 314, 414–418.

101. Neequaye A. R., Neequaye J., Mingle J. A., et al. Preponderance of females with AIDS in Ghana. Lancet, 1986, ii, 978.

102. Van de Perre P., Clumeck N., Carael M., et al. Female prostitutes: A risk group for infection with human T-cell lymphotropic virus type III. Lancet, 1985, ii, 524–526.

103. Barton S. E., Underhill G. S., Gilchrist C., et al. HTLV-III antibody in prostitutes. Lancet, 1985, ii, 524–526.

104. Krogsgaard K., Gluud C., Pedersen C., et al. Widespread use of condoms and low prev-

alence of sexually transmitted diseases in Danish non-drug addict prostitutes. British Medical Journal, 1986, 293, 1473–1474.

105. Smith G. L., Smith K. F. Lack of HIV infection and condom use in licensed prostitutes. Lancet, 1986, ii, 1392.

106. Barnes D. M. AIDS research in new phase: Unsuspected prevalence of AIDS in Africa. Science, 1986, 233, 282–283.

107. Guy D. Sangomas drawn into battle against AIDS. Sunday Tribune (Durban), 1986, December 7.

108. Simons M. For Haiti's tourism, the stigma of AIDS is fatal. New York Times, 1983, November 29.

109. Treaster J. Haiti's hotels hit hard as tourists shun island. New York Times, 1984, October 11.

110. Mann N. M., Francis H., Davachi F., et al. Risk factors for human immunodeficiency virus seropositivity among children 1–24 months old in Kinshasa, Zaire. Lancet, ii, 654–657.

111. SAPA-Reuter. Ethiopia slams AIDS decision. Daily News (Durban), 1986, December 27.

112. Barnes D. M. Grim projections for AIDS epidemic. Science, 1986, 232, 1589–1590.

113. Hooper E. An African village staggers under the assault of AIDS. New York Times, 1986, September 30, C1.

114. Serwadda D., Mugerwa R. D., Sewankambo N., et al. Slim disease: a new disease in Uganda and its association with HTLV-III infection. Lancet, 1985, ii, 849–852.

115. Bradbeer C. HIV and sexual lifestyle. British Medical Journal, 1987, 294, 5–6.

116. Fultz P. N. Component of saliva inactivates human immunodeficiency virus. Lancet, 1986, ii, 1215.

117. Burton S. W., Burn S. B., Harvey D., et al. AIDS information. Lancet, 1986, ii, 1040–1041.

118. Hutt M. S. R. Acquired immunodeficiency syndrome (AIDS) Tropical Doctor, 1985, 15, 1.

119. Simpson M. A. AIDS and Africa. BBC World Service Broadcasts, November and December 1987.

120. Katzew H. Silence over AIDS among blacks is shattered. The Star, Johannesburg, August 27, 1987, p. 15A.

121. Pekkanen J. AIDS in Africa: A growing plague. Reader's Digest, June 1987, 130, 51–60.

122. Sapa-Reuter. Incidence of AIDS doubled in Kenya. The Star, Johannesburg, August 3, 1987, p. 3A.

123. Anonymous. Diagnosis, prevention and treatment of viral infections. News highlights from the Nijmegen, Netherlands, Symposium, 26–27 March, 1987. Organon Teknika, Belgium, 1987.

124. Behrmann N. AIDS seen coming to the rescue of copper prices. The Star, Johannesburg, October 16, 1987.

125. Shields M. AIDS biggest challenge to insurance industry? The Citizen, Johannesburg, December 11, 1987, p. 6.

126. Anonymous. AIDS becomes a threat to children. The Star, Johannesburg. December 10, 1987.

127. Anonymous. AIDS—the African horror. Inside South Africa, June 1987, Vol. 1, No. 6, 6–9.

128. Irwin W. Letter to the Editor. The Star, Johannesburg, November 25, 1987, p. 12M.

129. Boekkooi J. AIDS and the international traveller—a never-ending problem. Sunday Star Review, Johannesburg, September 13, 1987, p. 6.

130. Anonymous. AIDS and the RSA. South African Medical Journal, 1987, 71, xxi.

131. Schoub B. D. AIDS in South Africa—a time for action (editorial). South African Medical Journal, 1987, 71, 677–678.

132. Anonymous. SA cannot hide from African AIDS—warning. Pretoria News, Pretoria, June 11, 1987.

133. Mills S., Campbell M. J., Waters W. E. Public knowledge of AIDS and the DHSS advertisement campaign. British Medical Journal, 1986, 293, 1089–1090.

134. Abrahams E. Seven-floor jumper was AIDS victim on run from hospital. Sunday Times, Johannesburg, August 23, 1987.

135. Venter A. J. Conspiracy of silence in S. Africa about AIDS. The Star, Johannesburg, November 25, 1987, p. 12M.

136. Cheney P. AIDS epidemic spreading from North. Sunday Times, Johannesburg, June 7, 1987, p. 3.

137. Boekkooi J. Govt and mines set for clash over AIDS. Sunday Star, Johannesburg, June 28, 1987.

138. Vernon K. "AIDS" miners a timebomb for SA. Sunday Star, Johannesburg, July 5, 1987, p. 4.

139. Anonymous. Foreign AIDS carriers to be repatriated. The Star, Johannesburg, September 4, 1987, p. 4.

140. Anonymous. "Witch-hunts" feared after Govt says AIDS carriers to be deported. The Star, Johannesburg, September 4, 1987.

141. Boekkooi J. Experts in AIDS row: Doctor's figures show that African virus is increasing in SA. Sunday Star, Johannesburg, September 13, 1987, p. 9.

142. Advisory Group on AIDS. Update on AIDS: Number of cases in the RSA and abroad. South African Medical Journal, 1987, 72, 92.

143. Boekkooi J. AIDS carriers refuse abortion. Sunday Star, Johannesburg, December 20, 1987, p. 6.

144. Boekkooi J. Experts fear spread of African AIDS. The Star, Johannesburg, July 26, 1987, 2.

145. St Leger C. You can't get AIDS from loo seats, though most people think you can. Sunday Times, June 7, 1987, p. 18.

146. Boekkooi J. SA decides on low-key campaign against AIDS. Sunday Star, Johannesburg, September 6, 1987.

147. Anonymous. Fears of huge AIDS ads blunder. Sunday Star, Johannesburg, December 20, 1987, pp. 1-2.

148. Boekkooi J. Condom onslaught on SA to be total. Sunday Star, Johannesburg, June 21, 1987.

149. Burger M. AIDS prisoners freed. Sunday Times, January 3, 1988, p. 4.

150. Heydt H. Reporting AIDS to dental practitioners. South African Medical Journal, 1987, 71, 332.

151. Muller F. J. Reporting AIDS to dental practitioners. South African Medical Journal, 1987, 72, 90.

152. Gerberding J. L. University of California, San Francisco, Task Force on AIDS. Recommended infection-control policies for patients with human immunodeficiency virus infection: An update. New England Journal of Medicine, 1986, 315, 1562-1564.

153. Shapiro M., O'Sullivan E., Crookes R. Application of the anti-HIV pooling technique for blood donor screening and population studies. National Blood Transfusion Congress, Johannesburg, August 19, 1987.

ADDITIONAL BIBLIOGRAPHY

AIDS Action Group. Update: Medical Facts About AIDS. Capetown, GASA, 1986.

Altman L. AIDS in Africa. New York Times, 1984, April 17.

Becker M. L. B., Sprackler F. H. N., Becker W. B. Isolation of a lymphadenopathy-associated virus from a patient with the acquired immune deficiency syndrome. South African Medical Journal, 1985, 68, 144-147.

Biggar R. J. The clinical features of HIV infection in Africa. British Medical Journal, 1986, 293, 1453-1454.

Biggar R. J., Johnson B. K., Oster C., et al. Regional variation in prevalence of antibody against human T-lymphoxyte virus type I and III in Kenya, East Africa. International Journal of Cancer, 1985, 35, 763-767.

Brun-Vezinet F., Rouxioux C., Barre-Sinoussi F., et al. Detection of IgG antibodies to lymphadenopathy-associated virus in patients with AIDS or lymphadenopathy syndrome. Lancet, 1984, i, 1253-1256.

Cameron C. M. Serological tests for AIDS. South African Medical Journal, 1985, 68, 914.

Clarke E. Tell all about AIDS. Sunday Tribune (Durban), 1986, Dec. 21, p 7.

Clumeck N., Mascart-Lemone F., de Maulbeuge J., et al. Acquired immune deficiency syndrome in black Africans. Lancet, 1983, i, 642.

Editorial. Are we over-AIDed? South African Medical Journal, 1984, 66, 805.

Ellrodt A., Barre-Sinoussi F., Le Bras P., et al. Isolation of human T-lymphotropic retrovirus (LAV) from Zairian married couple, one with AIDS, one with prodrome. Lancet, 1984, i, 1383–1385.

Epstein J. S., Moffitt A. L., Mayner R. E., et al. Antibodies reactive with HTLV-III found in freezer-banked sera from children in West Africa. (Abstract 217). Twenty-fifth Interscience Conference on Antimicrobial Agents and Chemotherapy, Minneapolis, Sept. 29–Oct. 2, 1985.

Fettner A. The African connection. New York Native, 1984, Dec. 3, p 10.

Francis H., Mann J., Quinn T., et al. Immunologic profile of AIDS and other parasitic infections in Africa and their relationship to HTLV-III infection. Paper presented at the International Conference on Acquired Immunodeficiency Syndrome (AIDS) in Atlanta, April 14–17, 1985.

GASA. Safe sex for a safer community. Johannesburg, Gay Association of South Africa, March 1985.

Greenwood B. M. AIDS in Africa. Immunology Today, 1984, 5, 10, 293–294.

Isaacs G., Miller D. AIDS—its implications for SA homosexuals and the mediating role of the medical practitioner. South African Medical Journal, 1985, 68, 327–330.

Jonas C., Deprez C., De Maubeuge J., et al. Cryptosporidium in patient with acquired immunodeficiency syndrome. Lancet, 1983, ii, 964.

Kestens L., Biggar R. J., Melbye M., et al. Absence of immunosuppression in healthy subjects from eastern Zaire who are positive for HTLV-III antibodies. New England Journal of Medicine, 1985, 312, 1517–1518.

Kestens L., Melbye M., Biggar R. J., et al. Endemic African Kaposi's sarcoma is not associated with immunodeficiency. International Journal of Cancer, 1985, 36, 49–55.

Knoble G. J. AIDS—prevention through education. South African Medical Journal, 1986, 70, 119–120.

Kreiss J. K., Koech D. K., Plummer F., et al. HTLV-III infection in Kenyan prostitutes. (Abstract 277.) Twenty-fifth Interscience Conference on Antimicrobial Agents and Chemotherapy, Minneapolis, Sept. 29–Oct. 2, 1985.

Lamey B., Melameka N. Aspects cliniques et epidemiologiques de la cryptococcose a Kinshasa: A propos de 15 cas personnels. Medecine Tropicale, 1982, 42, 507–511.

Lyons S. F., McGillivary G. M., Coppin A. P., et al. Limitations of enzyme immunoassay tests for detection of HTLV-III/LAV antibodies. South African Medical Journal, 1985, 68, 575–576.

Mann J. M., Francis H., Quinn T., et al. Surveillance for acquired immune deficiency syndrome in a central African city: Kinshasa, Zaire. Journal of the American Medical Association, 1986, 255, 32, 55–59.

McHardy J., Williams E. H., Gesen A., et al. Endemic Kaposi's sarcoma: Incidence and risk factors in the West district of Uganda. International Journal of Cancer, 1984, 33, 203–212.

Menedez-Corrada R., Nettleship E., Santiago-Delpin E. A. HLA and tropical sprue. Lancet, 1986, ii, 1183–1184.

Milner L. V., Vorster B. J., Conradie J. D., et al. Anti-HTLV-III testing—a practical solution for blood transfusion services? South African Medical Journal, 1985, 68, 921–922.

Molbalk K., Lauritzen E., Fernandes D., et al. Antibodies to HTLV-I associated with chronic fatal illness resembling "slim" disease. Lancet, 1986, ii, 1214–1215.

Newmark P. AIDS in an African context. Nature, 1986, 324, 18/25, 611.

Offenstadt G., Pinta P., Hericord P., et al. Multiple opportunistic infection due to AIDS in a previously healthy black woman from Zaire. New England Journal of Medicine, 1983, 308, 775.

Panos Institute. Aids and the Third World. London, Panos Institute, 1986.

Piot P., Quinn T. C., Tallman H., et al. Acquired immunodeficiency syndrome in a heterosexual population in Zaire. Lancet, 1984, ii, 65–69.

Raine A. E. G., Ilgren E. B., Kurtz J. B., et al. HTLV-III infection and AIDS in a Zambian nurse resident in Britain. Lancet, 1984, ii, 985.

Ras G. J., Eftychis H. A., Anderson R., et al. Mononuclear and polymorphonuclear leucocyte dysfunction in male homosexuals with the acquired immunodeficiency syndrome (AIDS). South African Medical Journal, 1984, 66, 21, 806–809.

Sher D. AIDS and related conditions—infection control. South African Medical Journal, 1985, 68, 843–848.

Sher D., Lyons S., Dos Santos L., et al. An indirect fluorescent antibody test for antibodies against HTLV-III. South African Medical Journal, 1985, 67, 10, 357.

Sonnet J., De Brugere M. Syndrome de deficit acquis de l'immunite–acquired immunodeficiency syndrome (AIDS); etat de la question. Donnees personnelles de la pathologre observee chez de Zairois. Louvain Medicine, 1983, 102, 297–307.

Sterry W., Marmor M., Konrads A., et al. Kaposi's sarcoma, a plastic pancytopenia and multiple infection in homosexuals. Lancet, 1983, i, 924–925.

Teas J. Could AIDS agent be a new variant of ASFV? lancet, 1983, i, 923. Thomsen H. K., Jacobsen M., Malchow-Moller A. Kaposi's sarcoma among homosexual men in Europe. Lancet, 1981, ii, 1688.

Veitch A. The AIDS that Africa could do without. Guardian, 1984, October 31.

13

AIDS in Canada

Dorothy C. H. Ley

INTRODUCTION

In Canada as elsewhere, AIDS has become an increasingly important prob-lem, especially in health care. The rapid increase in patients with AIDS and AIDS-related disease states is placing a major burden on physical, financial, and human resources. Management of a catastrophic, fatal illness is compounded by the difficult psychosocial milieu in which it occurs and the associated ethical and legal problems that it poses. The Canadian health care delivery system is one in which the federal and provincial governments are the major (and fre-quently the only) funding sources. In some respects this has simplified the man-agement of this spectrum of diseases. In others, however, because of multitiered responsibility and restricted funds, it has inhibited the development of integrated models of care.

This paper will discuss the epidemiology of AIDS in Canada and the gov-ernmental response, provide an outline of management and care, and indicate future trends. It should be recognized that Canada is a large, diverse country, with many different approaches to the delivery of health care at different levels of government. The following information, therefore, only provides a broad outline of the Canadian response to AIDS.

EPIDEMIOLOGY

The first case of AIDS in Canada was diagnosed in February 1982. Since that time the number of persons diagnosed and reported as having AIDS has in-creased at an annual rate of approximately 2.5 times. As of February 1, 1988, a total of 1497 cases have been reported in Canada (1471 adult and 26 pediatric), 806 (53.8%) of whom had died (Table 1). Overall, the cumulative incidence was 59.0 per million population.[1] These figures compare with 496 cases in March 1986, with a cumulative incidence of 19 per million population.* Ninety percent of cases are from Ontario, Quebec, and British Columbia.

There was a decrease in the number of new cases of AIDS in 1986 from those projected. The doubling time in 1985 was 7.5 months, and in 1986 this increased to 13 months. The same phenomenon has been reported in the United States.[2] It should be emphasized that this reflects a *decrease in rate of notification*. However, there is some evidence that changing from a polynominal model (cur-rently in use internationally) to a logistic model for predictive purposes will provide figures that are closer to the reported incidence.[3]

* Comparable U.S. figures for November 1986 were 28,169 cases with an incidence of 118.4 per million population.

Table 1 Reported cases of AIDS in Canada

Age	Sex	Alive	Dead	Total
Adults	Males	654	746	1400
	Females	30	41	71
Children	Males	3	10	13
	Females	4	9	13
Total		691	806	1497

Homosexual and bisexual males continue to be the predominant group affected (81.8%). Unlike in the United States, only 0.6% of Canadian cases were classified as drug abusers, although approximately 2.9% of the homosexual/bisexual males also used intravenous drugs. Persons from an endemic area, usually Haiti, accounted for 5% of cases. It may be significant that 22 of the 26 pediatric cases occurred in children whose parents were at risk. The anticipated surge in the incidence of AIDS in heterosexual partners has not taken place, remaining stable at about 2.7% (Table 2).

The so-called hidden factor related to infection by means of blood and blood products is only now becoming overt, since the 2- to 3-year period before the "wash-through" of new cases is just commencing. The Canadian Red Cross, the supplier of all blood and all but a fraction of blood products in Canada, began testing all blood donations for HIV antibodies in November 1985. The incidence of serpositivity in Canada is low—0.018%. Therefore, the number of these cases is anticipated to be relatively small.

GOVERNMENT RESPONSE

The predominantly homosexual distribution of HIV infection in Canada has had significant implications for the prevention and management of the disease. The relatively low numbers and the absence of a large percentage of intravenous

Table 2 Classification of AIDS cases in Canada

Risk factors	No. of cases (%)	
Adult		
Homosexual/bisexual activity	1204	(81.8)
IV drug user	9	(0.6)
Both of the above	42	(2.9)
Recipient of blood/blood products	62	(4.2)
Heterosexual activity		
Origin in endemic area	73	(5.0)
Sexual contact with person at risk	39	(2.7)
No identified risk factors	42	(2.9)
Total	1471	(100.0)
Pediatric (12 mo to 14 yr)		
Perinatal transmission	22	(84.6)
Recipient of blood/blood products	4	(15.4)
Other	0	(0.0)
Total	26	(100.0)

drug abusers from reported cases have contributed to the restriction of AIDS to a relatively well-circumscribed population. These factors, combined with a year or more lag time behind the United States in the appearance of the disease, have given Canada the opportunity to proceed in a more orderly fashion in the development of public policy and management philosophy than otherwise might have been possible.

Federal

Since the first diagnosis of AIDS in Canada, a number of important initiatives have been taken by the Ministry of Health and Welfare. In September 1983, the federal government established the National Advisory Committee on AIDS (NAC-AIDS) to "recommend activities to control, prevent, and manage AIDS in Canada." Members were drawn from across Canada and from multiple disciplines. The committee functions in an advisory capacity to the federal Minister of Health and works closely with the Laboratory Centre for Disease Control. The latter is Canada's center for dealing with the complex issues of AIDS and is the national reference laboratory for blood testing. It works closely with its U.S. counterpart, the Centers for Disease Control (Atlanta), and with the World Health Organization.

In October 1985, the Standing Committee on National Health and Welfare of the House of Commons commenced hearings to assess the impact of AIDS on the health care and social fabric of Canada. Its report was published in May 1986.[4] As a response, the federal government established a National AIDS Centre to function as a national coordinating and facilitating unit and has strengthened (and funded) the advisory role of the National Advisory Committee. As well, consideration is being given to the establishment of a National AIDS Foundation to act as a fund-raising organization for AIDS support groups and a coordinating office and monitoring agency for community-based AIDS organizations across Canada.

Intensive educational activities directed at professionals and the public alike are being stimulated through funding of an education and awareness program directed by the Canadian Public Health Association and the establishment of a subcommittee on education of the National Advisory Committee on AIDS.

Other recommendations of the committee that are being implemented by the federal government are the provision of biocontainment laboratories in appropriate centers in Canada, the support of major AIDS-related research programs, and the funding of doctoral and postdoctoral fellowships in relevant fields. A study of the need for and development of suitable hospice programs for persons with AIDS has been initiated.

In November 1986, Health and Welfare Canada approved the use of azidothymidine (AZT) in AIDS patients with *Pneumocystis carinii* pneumonia (PCP).[5] It is estimated that 150–180 patients will be eligible for therapy in 1987. The drug will be administered by the patients' physicians, under strict medical conditions directed by selected coordinators in each province.

Provincial

The direct delivery of health care in Canada is the responsibility of the provinces. To coordinate care of patients with AIDS, a Federal-Provincial Ad Hoc

Committee on AIDS was established in 1983. This committee works closely with Health and Welfare Canada, Laboratory Centre for Disease Control, NAC-AIDS, and the newly established National AIDS Centre to coordinate education, management of patients, and research across Canada.

Two provinces, Ontario and Quebec, have established and funded multidisciplinary information bodies to develop and distribute material aimed at the education of at-risk groups and the public. In Ontario, for example, the Ontario Public Education Panel on AIDS (OPEPA) has produced a series of fact sheets and educational videos and has established a speakers' panel to disseminate accurate information about AIDS and its management. Other provinces, Alberta and British Columbia in particular, have less formalized educational programs usually originating in the provincial Ministry of Health.

It is within provincial jurisdiction to make AIDS a reportable disease. At present all but two provinces (Manitoba and Newfoundland) require reporting of persons with AIDS. Only two (Nova Scotia and New Brunswick) require that serologically positive blood tests be reported. To date, relative confidentiality has been guaranteed (i.e., results are known only to medical health authorities, patient, and doctor). There is a growing consensus that better documentation of the incidence and occurrence of AIDS, AIDS-related complex (ARC), and seropositivity must be developed to curtail the spread of HIV infection. It is felt to be essential that any such documentation be carried out in a manner that will maintain confidentiality and protect the individual's rights and freedoms. Finally, any system of reporting must be accompanied by effective counseling and appropriate contact tracing.[4]

LEGAL ISSUES

Although the Canadian Charter of Rights and Freedoms protects the individual's rights, it expressly approves of the setting aside of those rights for the "greater good of society." The Canadian Bar Association has set up a Special Committee on Legal Implications of AIDS to consider the problems of confidentiality, contact tracing, labor relations, informed consent, wills, and other issues. A number of provinces have human rights commissions that have ruled on problems related to AIDS. In Ontario, for example, the Human Rights Code forbids discrimination based on a disabling condition, including AIDS.[6] An employer cannot fire a person with AIDS, nor can a co-worker refuse to work with a person with AIDS. A health care worker cannot refuse to provide care for an AIDS patient, and no one can refuse to provide a personal service to someone with AIDS. Further, an employer does not have the right to know if an employee has AIDS or the right to insist on mandatory testing.[7] Despite such legal protection, there are many instances of flagrant discrimination reported in Ontario and elsewhere.

COMMUNITY SUPPORT GROUPS

Community support groups have developed in all the major centers in Canada. These groups, particularly AIDS Vancouver and the AIDS Committee of Toronto (ACT), have been particularly active in the development and distribution of materials aimed at the homosexual communities stressing "safe sex," prevention of infection, and safe management of AIDS patients in the communities. They have also provided invaluable counseling services for persons with AIDS, their friends, and their families, and they have worked unstintingly as volunteers with the care-giving teams in their communities. In the summer of 1986 a Canadian AIDS Society was formed to bring these groups together to share information and expertise and to coordinate their activities.

CARE FOR PERSONS WITH AIDS

At the present time the care for persons with AIDS (and with ARC) is being provided within the acute-care setting. This will be so for the foreseeable future. Over 90% of AIDS cases have occurred in Vancouver, Toronto, and Montreal, with significant numbers in Calgary and Halifax. These cities are sites of major medical schools, and most AIDS patients are cared for in teaching institutions. However, there is some movement of patients into the community (frequently as they return to their own homes), and smaller community hospitals now are having to provide care for people with AIDS.

It should be borne in mind that AIDS is a fatal disease and that the spectrum of care required ranges from the management of fulminating acute infections, rapidly spreading malignancy, and dementia, to intensive psychosocial counseling of patient, family, and friends, and bereavement support—the pillars of hospice or palliative care. It is unrealistic to expect any one institution or team of care givers to be able to provide all facets of care throughout the course of illness of a person with AIDS without a new approach to case management. This has led to the application of the concept of the multidisciplanry team and attempts to develop integrated systems of care in those cities where there is a high concentration of HIV infection. In Montreal, for example, consideration is being given to the establishment of a nuclear consultative team to work across hospital boundaries, particularly within the McGill teaching system, to assist in the care and management of the 18–24 persons with AIDS in those hospitals at any one time.

The pattern of care in the acute-care hospitals is relatively uniform, although the site of that care varies across hospitals. The complexity of the disease itself dictates the involvement of a multiplicity of specialists; however, primary responsibility for care is most frequently held by those with expertise in infectious diseases. In some hospitals, such as the Victoria General in Halifax, a special "unit" has been established—in this case a general-medical floor—with specially trained staff. In others, such as St. Paul's Hospital in Vancouver, a conscious decision has been taken to disperse AIDS patients throughout the hospital to avoid "ghettoizing" and to spread the burden of care more evenly. In most institutions, such as the major teaching hospitals in Toronto, the patients are clustered at various sites, usually general medicine, oncology, or infectious-disease units, depending on the patients' major problem and the admitting privileges of their attending physician.

Management of AIDS within the acute-care setting has produced a number of universal problems. Staff stress can become critical, particularly among nursing and medical staff unaccustomed to caring for young, dying patients. The disease itself, its relationship to homosexuality and drug abuse, and its inevitably fatal ending all contribute to stressing the health care team. All programs have implemented varying degrees of staff support. St. Paul's in Vancouver, caring for 75% of the persons with AIDS in British Columbia, has established a multidisciplinary AIDS Care Group to advise senior hospital executives and discuss policy matters. They have intensive in-service education, seminars for staff and their families, and a newly developed AIDS reference manual for each ward where AIDS patients are nursed. Most hospitals have initiated interdisciplinary team meetings and staff support groups, some with a psychologist as part of the team. It has been found that stress is particularly high in dedicated or high-use areas where staff turnover can become a problem.

FINANCING

The concentration of care in hospitals, particularly large teaching hospitals, has led to increasing concern about the financial impact of AIDS on the health care system as a whole in a country where its funding is the sole responsibility of government. In 1985 a study of AIDS patients in Canada found that a typical patient spent an average of 75 days in the hospital. The minimum estimate of cost was $37,000 and the maximum $42,000. The minimum estimate included 10 days in an intensive care unit, the maximum 20 days. Thirteen to 14 outpatient visits at $73 each accounted for an additional $1000.[8] Toronto General Hospital (a major teaching hospital) studied the cost of the care of persons with AIDS. They found, not surprisingly, that the cost of care depended on the complexity of the diagnosis at admission and the intensity of care required. The average was $15,691, approximately $5000 more per admission than allocated in the global budget by the Ministry of Health of the province. The per-diem cost ranged from $560 to $906, significantly more than the per-diem rate of $455 accepted by the Ministry for global funding. Although significant, the overall budget deficit was not as large as expected, and probably fell within the same range as highly specialized services such as dialysis and oncology.[9] The significant factors affecting future costs were identified as the rapidly increasing volume of patients and the increasing complexity of the disease states being referred to teaching hospitals. In fact, St. Paul's Hospital (Vancouver) has demonstrated that persons with AIDS now require up to three times the nursing care budgeted for the average medical/surgical patient and may need up to 20 h per day.

ISSUES AND TRENDS

The inability to discharge persons with AIDS from the hospital not only contributes to the high cost of their care but diminishes its quality overall and restricts their ability to live their lives as fully as possible for as long as possible. Among important factors contributing to prolonged inpatient care are the lack of comprehensive outpatient facilities, primary-care physicians, and home care, including palliative care. In this respect, the person with AIDS resembles both the elderly and the terminally ill with other diseases.

Although no hospital in Canada is anxious to be designated the "AIDS Centre" for an area or city, there are strong indications that in Toronto and Montreal at least, some consolidation and concentration of services in designated teaching hospitals will be necessary to provide a comprehensive range of medical and social services and expertise. To facilitate the shift from inpatient to outpatient care, and as part of the development of an integrated system of care, most major centers are planning the establishment of a central outpatient clinic in association with a teaching hospital. This would provide highly specialized, multidisciplinary care for both persons with AIDS and HIV-positive individuals and would be a link between the institutional and community settings.[9]

The availability of home care and community care in Canada varies from province to province, but in general it is limited. Ninety percent of the Canadian health care dollar is spent on institutional and medical services, and only 10% on community care.[10] There is a growing demand in all provinces and centers with a high incidence of AIDS for governments to shift their spending priorities and to alter their criteria for home care to allow improved accessibility to such care, including palliative or hospice care. Of major concern in all centers caring for persons with AIDS is the lack of community services such as nursing, home care, palliative care, suitable housing, social and psychological and bereavement support, and counseling for persons with AIDS and their families and friends. Only 53 of a total of 216 persons with AIDS in metropolitan Toronto have been able to obtain home care.[9] Almost all returned to the hospital to die. In Canada less than 10% of AIDS victims die outside the hospital compared with 90% in San Francisco.[11]

The care of the person with AIDS, because of its complexity, tends to become fragmented among a number of specialists. In some cities it is difficult to find a primary-care physician to take responsibility for a patient on discharge from the hospital. This is partly due to a lack of knowledge and experience in case management and partly due to reluctance by family physicians to become involved in caring for members of the homosexual community. However, across the country, homosexual physicians such as those associated with St. Paul's Hospital in Vancouver or the Hassle Free Clinic in Toronto have come forward to offer primary care. In Montreal, the regular staff physicians from some Local Community Service Centres (CLSCs) have taken responsibility for AIDS patients in their districts. As well, the home care and support services of these centers have been made available through the liaison nurse to the hospitals. This relationship, particularly the primary-care physician involvement, is proving of great value in maintaining AIDS patients in the community. It is being given educational support by the hospital-based care teams.

The roles played by the palliative care or hospice community in Canada to date have been more indirect than direct, although Hospice Victoria has provided full hospice care for persons with AIDS. Palliative care units in general are not suited to the care of the terminally ill AIDS patient. In most cities where palliative care programs exist (e.g., Montreal, Toronto, Hamilton, and Winnipeg), their involvement has been limited to consultations for pain control and limited psychosocial counseling and family bereavement support. Their most important function has been to provide staff education and support regarding issues related to grief and death. In Halifax, however, all AIDS patients admitted to Victoria General are introduced to the potential of hospice care. About one-half avail themselves of it, particularly for emotional support and counseling.

In Calgary, with a significant but relatively low incidence of AIDS, it has been possible to integrate the care of terminally ill patients into the Hospice Calgary consultation team program in most hospitals. The patients, although cared for by the appropriate medical specialty, are referred to the hospice team for the full spectrum of palliative care. As well, the staff of Hospice Calgary has conducted training sessions for counselors from the homosexual community in the specifics of AIDS and issues surrounding grief and death.

Although there is considerable controversy about their merits, there is growing agitation for the establishment of hospices for persons with AIDS, particularly in Vancouver and Toronto. Canada does not have a tradition of free-standing hospices. It has only one, the Hotel Michel Sarrazin in Quebec City, which is allied with Laval University and was established to care for cancer patients. In a government-funded health care system, any such development must obtain government approval and must be funded as part of that system. Such approval has not been forthcoming. It has been estimated in Toronto that capital expenditures for such a hospice would approximate $1.6 million and the annual operating costs $1.5 million.[9,12]

The long-term, fluctuating nature of the disease and the unique social problems created by its homosexual milieu produce major difficulties in management. These, coupled with a general lack of services for community care and an expressed desire by professional care givers to accentuate outpatient as opposed to institutional care contrive to make the establishment of AIDS hospices an attractive and functional option. In large cities, such as Vancouver, Toronto, Montreal, and Halifax, they could provide desperately needed residential and respite care and, for selected patients, palliative or hospice care. They could become important sites of counseling and support for persons with AIDS, those with AIDS-related complex, and seropositive individuals. They could be an important link in the development of an integrated system of care for AIDS. Community support groups have provided much of the impetus for the development of residential care and hospices. However, many health care professionals involved in the care of persons with AIDS have recently become advocates for their establishment, and there currently are proposals before two provincial governments (British Columbia and Ontario) for their funding.

Initially the care of the terminally ill person with AIDS was seen as a challenge to the hospice to move beyond care for cancer patients and reach out with psychosocial assistance and counseling and bereavement support to a group of people whose mores were alien and little understood. More recently, in many places in Canada, it has precipitated a reappraisal of the roles of nurses and physicians on the multidisciplinary team, a growing appreciation by AIDS professional care givers of the philosophy of the hospice, and growing participation by them in the practice of palliative care.

SUMMARY

AIDS in Canada has mirrored the pattern of the disease elsewhere in the world, although it lags about 1 year behind the United States in its development. Although the absolute number of cases is relatively small, it ranks third in incidence per million population, behind the United States and Haiti. AIDS occurs primarily (82.4%) in homosexual/bisexual males; there are only small numbers of drug abusers (0.4%), women (5.8%), and children (2.0%). It is concentrated in major cities, 90% of cases occurring in the provinces of Ontario, British Columbia, and Quebec.

Government response at all levels, but particularly federal, was swift and has continued. Emphasis was placed on epidemiology, dissemination of information, and education of professionals, high-risk groups, and the public. Cooperation with CDC (Atlanta) and WHO has been close and continuous in epidemiology and the sharing of research and treatment information and protocols.

The care of persons with AIDS in Canada has been confined to the acute-care institutions, mainly teaching hospitals, but with a growing spread into smaller communities. Home care has been inhibited by a general lack of community care services, including nursing, primary physician care, palliative care, and residential facilities. Community support groups have provided valuable support for persons with AIDS. They are growing in number and sophistication and have made a major contribution to the education of high-risk groups and the public. Educational activities from all sources are increasing. There is a move in some provinces to extend such education into the school system as soon as possible.

Future trends include concentration of institutional care in designated hospitals, the establishment of comprehensive outpatient facilities in major centers, and the development of an integrated system of care, including home care. Governments are being pressured to supply additional funds to the health care system for these purposes, including support for AIDS hospices within the system of care.

AUTHORS' NOTE

Since the completion of this article, several developments have taken place in the care for dying persons with AIDS in Canada. In March 1987 the government of the province of Ontario agreed to fund both capital and operating expenses of "Casey House," a 12-bed hospice for terminally ill AIDS patients in Toronto. It is affiliated with a major teaching hospital (St. Michael's) at the University of Toronto. It was officially opened on March 1, 1988, and received its first patients on March 9, 1988. It is the first such hospice in Canada. The new facilities for the McGill Palliative Care Unit at Royal Victoria Hospital in Montreal, to open in May 1987, will also have accommodations suitable for the care of AIDS patients.

In another development the national education program, directed by the Canadian Public Health Association, has produced a series of short videos aimed at the general public, stressing the prevention of AIDS. It is anticipated these will be aired nationally on television in 1987, although there has been some initial resistance from the broadcast media.

D. C. H. L., May 1987

ACKNOWLEDGMENTS

The author thanks all those who so unstintingly provided information about their programs and shared their expertise and their concepts of the future of AIDS in Canada, in particular: Dr. Alan Meltzer and Greg Smith of the National AIDS Centre; Dr. Norbert Gilmore, Chairman, National Advisory Committee on AIDS, and Royal Victoria Hospital, Montreal; Irene Gilmore and Dr. A. McLeod, St. Paul's Hospital, Vancouver; Bob Tivvey, AIDS Vancouver; Dr. R. Hatfield and staff, Hospice Calgary; Dr. E. Latimer, Palliative Care Program, Hamilton Civic Hospitals; Dr. Mary Fanning, Toronto General Hospital and University of Toronto; Marilyn Lundy and Pat Maynard, St. Elizabeth Visiting Nurses' Association, Toronto; members of the Hospice Committee of ACT, Toronto; Dr. Ina Ajemian, McGill Palliative Care Program, Montreal; Dr. Louis Dionne, Hotel Michel Sarrazin, Quebec City; Heather Rose, Palliative Care Program, Victoria General Hospital, Halifax; and unnamed but nonetheless valued for the insight they provided, two persons with AIDS.

REFERENCES

1. *Update on AIDS in Canada*. National AIDS Centre, Laboratory Centre for Disease Control, Health Protection Branch, Health and Welfare, Canada; Ottawa, February 1, 1988.

2. Meltzer, A., Medical Director, National AIDS Centre, Ottawa, Canada. Personal communication, 1987.

3. Wallace, E. The Epidemiology of AIDS in Ontario. Paper presented at the Ontario Hospital Association Conference "AIDS: A Clinical and Legal Update"; Toronto, January 1987.

4. *Report on AIDS in Canada*. House of Commons Standing Committee on Health and Welfare; Ottawa, Canada, May 1986.

5. Availability of azidothymidine (AZT). Bulletin, Health and Welfare Canada; November 1986.

6. Tremayne-Lloyd, T. Legal Issues in AIDS. Paper presented at the Ontario Hospital Association Conference "AIDS: The Hospital Perspective"; Toronto, January 1986.

7. AIDS and the workplace. Fact sheet, Ontario Education Panel on AIDS (OPEPA); Ministry of Health of the Province of Ontario, 1986.

8. *Canada Disease Weekly Report*; Health and Welfare Canada; Ottawa, July 1985.

9. *Report of the Working Group on the Co-ordination of Services to AIDS Patients*. Metropolitan Toronto District Health Council, Toronto; January 1987.

10. Marshall, S. Canada's Health Care Policy, Opportunities and Options for VON. Presented at the Annual Meeting of the Victorian Order of Nurses, Calgary, October 1986.

11. Gilmore, N. Chairman, National Advisory Committee on AIDS (Canada). Personal communication, 1987.

12. *Proposal to Establish Casey House Hospice—A Hospice for People With AIDS*. Hospice Steering Committee, AIDS Committee of Toronto; December 1986.

14

AIDS in Japan

Kazumi Wakabayashi

In 1986, there were 21 AIDS patients in Japan. Over half of them had hemophilia and blood transfusions from imported blood products, 90% of which came from the United States, where there are a large number of AIDS patients and HIV carriers. In Japan, doctors usually do not inform patients about the prognosis of a life-threatening disease such as cancer. So some doctors insist that AIDS patients and carriers should not be told. The reality remains that no one really knows who has been infected with the virus and how far the sickness will spread.

AIDS HISTORY

In Japan, the first patient was officially recognized by the government as having AIDS on May 22, 1985. Eighteen months later the number had reached 21. This number is far less than that reported in the United States, where the number as of Sept. 19, 1986, was 27,166. In Europe as of the same date, the number was 3127.

Because these numbers are large when compared with Japan, specialists in Japan have arrived at two interpretations in recognizing the severity of the AIDS problem in Japan. One group says that the low figure for AIDS in Japan represents "the calm before the storm," that the disease is latent and that there is a good chance that it could soon spread rapidly. The other is more optimistic, saying that there are few homosexuals in Japan so the chances of spread of the disease to the general population are slim. Since more than half of the AIDS cases in Japan occur among hemophiliacs, the further spread of the disease within this group can be easily controlled through tighter measures in checking the blood products used for these patients.

According to Dr. Kusuya Nishioka, director of an international medical research center, the Kitasato Institute, a study was done of the 21 AIDS cases that had appeared by July 1986 in Japan (Table 1 and Figure 1). Of these 21, 10 were homosexuals and 11 were hemophiliacs. Of the 10 who were homosexual, three are foreigners and seven are Japanese who report that they have often gone abroad and/or have had sexual relations with foreigners. Table 2 gives data on AIDS patients in Japan through May 1988.

These figures indicate that the outbreak of AIDS in Japan is different from that in the United States in that it seems to be occurring equally among hemophiliacs. Over half of the AIDS patients in Japan have hemophilia, whereas in the United States over two-thirds of the AIDS patients discovered so far are homosexual. Thus in Japan, hemophiliacs seem to constitute the high-risk group, and countermeasures to prevent the spread of the disease in Japan would have

185

Table 1   AIDS patients in Japan (26 Sept. 1986)

No.	Diagnosis date	Death	Risk group[a]	Age	Comment
1	Aug 1981	July 1983	HB	48	
2	May 1982	July 1983	Homo	30	Foreigner
3	Nov 1982	Sept 1985	Homo	50	
4	Jan 1983	(?)	HB	60	
5	Mar 1983	Apr 1985	Homo	36	
6	Oct 1983	Alive	HA	62	
7	Nov 1983	Nov 1984	HB	39	
8	Mar 1984	Feb 1985	HA	27	
9	Aug 1984	Alive	Homo	35	
10	Jan 1985	Feb 1986	Homo	33	Foreigner
11	Jan 1985	Alive	Homo	33	
12	Feb 1985	Sept 1985	HA	27	
13	June 1985	Aug 1985	Homo	44	
14	July 1985	Alive	HA	34	
15	Sept 1985	Alive	Homo	50	Foreigner
16	Dec 1985	Alive	HA	26	
17	Jan 1986	Alive	HA	24	
18	Jan 1986	May 1986	HA	44	
19	Feb 1986	March 1986	Homo	37	
20	July 1986	Alive	Homo	32	
21	July 1986	Sept 1986	HB	24	

[a]HB, hepatitis B; HA, hepatitis A; homo, homosexual.
Source: Courtesy of K. Nishioka.

to take this into account. The main thrust would be aimed at checking the quality of the blood products before they are transmitted to hemophiliac patients. This is important when one realizes that 90% of the blood products imported into Japan for hemophiliac patients come from the United States, where there are a large number of AIDS patients and AIDS virus (HIV) carriers. Since 1985, the Japanese Red Cross has begun to check blood coming into Japan.

In April 1986, a larger study was conducted throughout Japan by the Japanese Red Cross of the many people who had donated blood in Japan. Of the 900,000 people who were checked, six were found to be AIDS carriers. Of the six, two

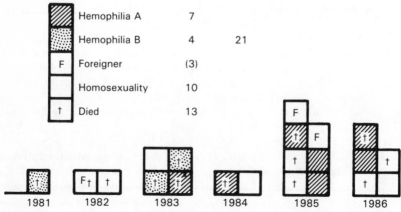

Figure 1   AIDS Patients in Japan. Source: Courtesy of N. Nishioka.

Table 2 AIDS patients in Japan

	Patients	Died	HIV-carrier
Homosexuality	20 (7)	8 (2)	32
Heterosexuality	10 (4)	5 (3)	25
Blood-product	46	30	966
Others	4	3	15
Total	80 (11)	46 (5)	1038

Note: Parentheses indicate foreigners.
Source: Data from the Ko Sei Sho (Health and Welfare Ministry of Japan), 18 May 1988, courtesy of K. Nishioka.

had been to Africa and were reported to have had sexual relations with women there.

Another check was made on the blood used in 23 national hospitals throughout Japan. This investigation was conducted under the auspices of the Osaka National Hospital by clinical researcher Nobuko Ikegami, and it was presented at the 27th Japanese Virus Clinical Conference and reported in the *New Medical World Weekly* (Sept. 1987, Vol. 1713, Igaku Shoin Pub. Ltd.).[1] According to this study, 1128 checks were made among people who received transfusions for any reason and those who received transfusions because they were hemophiliacs. People with various kinds of cancer of the blood were also checked along with people who have Epstein-Barr virus (EBV) deficiencies. People professing to have had homosexual experiences were also checked. And of course, the donated blood on hand was screened.

Of the 1128 checks made in these hospitals, 87 carriers (36.7%) were found to be hemophiliac. Two carriers had received injections of blood products, and inquiries about them constituted 13.3% of the checks made. Two were homosexual and made up 8% of the checks. All the rest were negative.

Another study was conducted in July 1986 by Dr. Takao Matsumoto, who does AIDS research at Juntendo University Medical School. He tested 113 homosexual men. Of these, five were determined to be seropositive. Two of the five were foreigners, and the other three were Japanese. Of the 113, there were 93 who were Japanese and 20 who were foreigners. (New Medical Weekly: Sept. 1987 Vol 1713, Igaku Shoin Pub Ltd.) Nobuko Ikegami

AIDS CLINIC

In October 1985, an AIDS clinic was opened at the Department of Infectious Diseases at Toritsukomagome Byoin, Tokyo Metropolitan Hospital, Komagome, Japan. The director, Dr. Mikio Minamitani, is a member of the AIDS Association, an organization headed by Professor Shiokawa set up to find countermeasures to fight the disease. Dr. Minamitani saw that AIDS was becoming a big social problem in the United States, and he thought that perhaps the same thing could occur in Japan. Therefore, in the spring of 1983, he joined other specialists, Dr. Nishioka and Dr. Matsumoto, to form the AIDS Association. This group is composed of 10 people from different fields—hemotology, virology, pharmacology, and clinical immunology. One of the members is a government spokesman.

In the 2 years since this association was started, it has organized eight study groups that have looked into three areas. First, the U.S. situation was examined. The second area considered was the reaction that ensued in the United States as a result of mass communication focusing on AIDS. Lastly, how AIDS patients were treated in U.S. hospitals and the attitude of hospital workers toward them were considered. The U.S. situation caused them to reflect on what they would do in Japan if the spread of the disease got to be as serious as it was in the United States. Would Japan respond in the same way as the United States?

The AIDS Association in its capacity as a private organization was asked by the Ko Sei Sho, the Health and Welfare Ministry, to prepare for any response that might be necessary should the disease spread in Japan. It also suggested that to avoid unnecessary public concern, information about AIDS come from the Ko Sei Sho.

Public response to news about the spread of AIDS followed the noted chronology. On March 22, 1985, it was announced that the first patient in Japan was found to have AIDS. No one paid much attention to this. The second case was announced 3 months later, in July. Up to this time Dr. Minamitani's office received only 20 telephone calls inquiring about AIDS spreading in Japan. But from summer to autumn 1985, the third and fourth cases of AIDS were announced. Then TV, newspapers, and magazines began to step in and give these announcements coverage. A lot of public attention began to focus on AIDS.

Because of this concern, it was decided to open an AIDS clinic in October. During the first week the clinic was open, fear of the disease was readily seen in the reactions of other patients who heard or saw people register at the clinic desk and request to be examined for AIDS.

By the second week, it was decided to have patients requesting exams for AIDS to make appointments and only come at specially designated times 1 h a day, 3 days a week to avoid the adverse reactions of other patients. This is now how the clinic is operating, and it shows the influence of the public's attitude.

Another way that public opinion is seen is in the policy by which Japanese medical insurance deals with AIDS patients. In Japan, medical insurance will cover just about anything, but it does not cover the cost of preventive medicine. The examination to determine whether one has AIDS is considered to be preventive medicine. It costs 8000 yen for one test, a fee that is considered high by most Japanese, who are not accustomed to paying exorbitant medical costs. The point is that medical insurance has decided to pay for this test, but not for homosexuals, the reason being that hemophiliacs did not bring on the disease by themselves and therefore should not have to pay. The implication is that homosexuals brought the disease upon themselves through their actions and should therefore have to pay.

On October 1, 1985, Dr. Minamitani did a study among 701 people to determine whether the AIDS virus found in that population was passed by homosexual contact or by other means. Of the 701 people tested, 17 were found to be carriers of the AIDS virus. Of these 17, 13 were hemophiliacs, three were homosexuals, and one was the wife of a hemophiliac. Of the 701 tested, 82% were between the ages of 20 and 50. Twelve people (children of hemophilia patients) were under 10 years old. Nineteen people were over the age of 60. Most of the testees were from the greater Tokyo area, although some came from Hokkaido and Kyushu. The breakdown of those tested was as follows: 255 were homosexuals; 250 were heterosexual; one was the wife of a hemophiliac; 13 had received blood transfusions; 16 were hemophiliacs; and one had received acupuncture. Sexual orientation and risk factors for the other 165 are unknown. These statistics again point to the probability that the AIDS virus has been spread mainly through contaminated blood products imported from the United States.

TO TELL OR NOT TO TELL

Doing this kind of general population screening raised some questions in regard to telling a person whether or not he or she is infected with the AIDS virus. In Japan, doctors usually do not inform patients about the prognosis of life-threatening diseases such as cancer. Because AIDS is not curable, doctors wonder if the patient should be told, and if told the result, whether the realization might be too much for the person. Even if a person is just a carrier of the disease, knowing this would be quite traumatic, it was thought.

Dr. Minamitani, after reflecting on these issues, decided that it would be better not to inform a person whether he or she was a carrier or a victim of the disease until he received a request from one of his hemophiliac patients to know the truth. This patient said he needed to know his situation so he could take measures to protect his family if need be. On hearing this, Dr. Minamitani decided that he himself from then on would tell the patients what their diagnosis was.

There are now 5000 hemophiliacs in Japan. Thirty percent of these have tested positive as having been exposed to AIDS. This means that at least 1500 are carriers of the disease, and of these it is estimated that 150 may come down with the disease. The overall homosexual population in Japan is thought to be somewhere around 200,000–300,000. At the present time the AIDS clinic receives about 20–30 phone calls a day. Most of these calls are made by people who wonder if they have been exposed to AIDS through homosexual contact.

In these screenings, the issues of telling a person he is a carrier and who should be the one to do this again arose. It was wondered what the merit would be for a carrier to know that he has been infected with the AIDS virus. Also, if a person has been part of a general screening, he was not reached through his own physician. It was thought that only the primary-care physician should do something like tell a patient about a potentially life-threatening illness.

PROBLEMS IN JAPAN

It appears the doctors are dealing with AIDS patients very much as they would with a cancer patient. Certainly, the disease evokes strong emotions, because it has a high death rate and spreads easily through blood products or sexual transmission. But whether it should be kept secret is another matter. Not telling could give rise to many other social problems. For example, if a person does not know he is a carrier, he could pass the virus on to many people without realizing that he needs to take preventive measures to keep from infecting others.

Another example would be that a person could come down with AIDS and suspect that he has the disease, despite not being told. His worry and concern over his health could cause mental problems without benefit of someone to talk to about the illness. On the other hand, the person might not have the disease but show similar symptoms. Because he does not trust the doctor's report to him, he may think he has some serious disease like AIDS when in fact he has psychosomatic or other medical problems.

It is true that with regard to cancer many people end up going to a clinic specializing in psychosomatic medicine because they think they have cancer but they don't. Of course, every now and then someone who really does have cancer shows up at these clinics. It could be the same for AIDS.

We have to start being aware how such attitudes could affect the spread of AIDS. The ostrich with its head in the sand could be bringing on its own disaster by avoiding dealing with the problem.

The AIDS Association met to figure out ways to deal with AIDS in Japan. The three main topics they covered were (1) how to diagnose AIDS, (2) how the disease develops, and (3) research on high-risk groups. They received 13 million yen in a grant from the government to research these three areas more deeply. This may sound like a lot of money, but when compared to amounts given to other medical projects, it is really not so much. It makes one wonder whether the government considers the AIDS problem to be not so serious because now there are only a few affected with the disease and the general population is not overly concerned.

In September 1986, the Japanese government decided that all blood donated for transfusion in Japan will be checked for HIV antibody and HTLV-I antibody, another blood-borne viral infection associated with adult T-cell leukemia (ATL). The budget for the screening program is 5000 million yen.

This is a critical breakthrough for the prevention of blood transfusion-associated infection, since hepatitis B virus is already established in Japan. Primary care for HIV carriers is a serious problem for Japanese society. The prevention of the development of AIDS from carrier states to full symptomatic AIDS is an urgent research project, since it is estimated that more than 1000 cases of hemophilia patients who are HIV carriers exist in Japan.

How many of those infected will go on to develop the disease is uncertain, but the PHS report indicates that the conversion rate from being infected with HIV to having the disease is between 20% and 30%. Who does care when someone is found to be infected with HIV virus?

We really need educational programs targeted at special populations, including homosexual and hemophiliac patients and those infected with the HIV virus, and the general population. The reality remains that no one really knows who has been infected with the virus or how far the sickness will spread in Japan.

ADDENDUM

After this article was written, the attitudes of the Japanese people toward AIDS changed, and the Japanese government made up new counterplans for AIDS. We were forced to face the fact that AIDS is not a special person's disease, but everyone's.

From the end of 1986 to the beginning of 1987, AIDS caused panic among the Japanese people. New patients were found, and they were not men, but women. One case was in Kobe; she was a foreigner and has already died. Another case happened in Matsumoto (Nagano Prefecture). One day a short article in the newspaper began: "Manila Government asked that the Japanese Embassy repatriate the Philippine woman working in Japan to her own country, because she was infected with AIDS." It also said, "She may work at the nightclub in Nagano Prefecture as a 'Japayuki-san' (prostitute from an Asian country)." At that time, she already had returned to the Philippines. Many telephone calls to City Hall, the police, and the public health office poured in from residences in Nagano and also from those who had traveled to Nagano previously as people found out that the nightclub was in Matsumoto.

The Japanese government never did announce the name of the woman and nightclub officially. Nonetheless, many rumors spread. It caused some trouble, also, for people in that area. Trucks carrying vegetables and products from Nagano were refused entrance to the central market in Tokyo. A hotel in the northern part of Japan canceled the reservation of a tour group from Nagano. A travel agency in Matsumoto made reservations for tour groups from the area using the name of any other city or town except Matsumoto.

After this AIDS panic, 420 people received the blood test for HIV antibodies, and none of them were infected at that time.

15

National Considerations

C. Everett Koop and Michael Samuels

On February 5, 1986, President Ronald Reagan, in an address to the U.S. Department of Health and Human Services, directed the Surgeon General of the United States to prepare a major report to the American people on AIDS. In preparing this report, Surgeon General C. Everett Koop followed two parallel lines of inquiry. He consulted with the top clinical and research experts in the field, many of whom were in the Public Health Service (e.g., Dr. Anthony S. Fauci, director of the National Institute of Allergy and Infectious Diseases). At the same time he held private meetings with national organizations with specific interests in AIDS to listen to their concerns, share their insights, and build an informal consensus on how to inform the American people about AIDS.

The groups were: AIDS Action Council, National Coalition of Black Lesbians and Gays, National Minority AIDS Council, American Council of Life Insurance, Health Insurance Association of America, Washington Business Group on Health, National Association of Elementry School Principals, National Association of Secondary School Principals, National Association of State Boards of Education, National Educational Association, National Parent Teachers Association, American Dental Association, American Hospital Association, American Medical Association, American Nurses Association, American Osteopathic Association, American Red Cross, National Hemophilia Foundation, American Federation of Teachers, Association of State and Territorial Health Officials, National Association of County Health Officials, U.S. Conference of Local Health Officers, Southern Baptist Convention, National Council of Churches, Synagogue Council of America, U.S. Catholic Conference, and Service Employees International Union.

Every group contacted agreed to meet with the Surgeon General, and the final report contains insights and contributions from every group. After completion of the draft report, the Surgeon General had it officially cleared in record time. It was approved unanimously by the following individuals or groups in this sequence.

Assistant Secretary for Health—Dr. Robert E. Windom
Secretary of Health and Human Services—Dr. Otis R. Bowen
White House Working Group on Health—Dr. William L. Roper, Chairman
Domestic Policy Council—Attorney General Edwin Meese, Chairman
President Ronald Reagan

On October 22, 1986, Dr. Koop released the Surgeon General's Report on AIDS to the American people. The report described AIDs in laymen's terms and indicated that it was not communicated through casual contact. He identified intimate sexual contact and the sharing of intravenous needles as the principal means of spreading the disease. Citing the fact that there was no vaccine to prevent AIDS and no drug to cure it, our only weapon is education and information to change human behavior and contain the spread of the disease.

Dr. Koop clearly labeled the disease as a concern to everyone—hetero- and homosexual, male and female. He expressed concern about the disproportionate numbers of blacks and Hispanics with AIDS. He pointed out the plight of children born with AIDS.

The most controversial part of the Surgeon General's report has been, "Education about AIDS should start in elementary school and at home so children can grow up knowing the behavior to avoid to protect themselves from exposure to the AIDS virus: The fact that AIDS is a fatal disease gives the debate on sex education a new dimension that calls for resolution."

The release of the Surgeon General's Report on AIDS on October 22, 1986, was a historic day in the history of the fight against AIDS. The nation's physician called on all Americans to learn about AIDS, discuss it in frank terms, educate ourselves and our children about it, and adopt the preventive behavior necessary to contain the spread of the AIDS virus. His report set off a national, state, and local debate on all aspects of AIDS. This debate, fanned by media attention, appears to have raised the knowledge base of the American people. Only time will tell the full impact of the report.

Not content with just preparing and releasing the Surgeon General's Report on AIDS, Dr. Koop took the message directly to the American people via public appearances, radio, television, and the print media. This effort was temporarily halted by back surgery, but began anew in January 1987.

One of the best examples of this effort was Dr. Koop's speech before a joint session of the California Legislature on March 5, 1987. This activity shows the concern on the part of California Legislature about AIDS and their willingness to take action. Rarely does the Legislature extend an invitation for an individual to address a joint session. When the history of AIDS is written, the pioneering efforts of Californians in many areas will be highlighted.

The press release that accompanied the Surgeon General's Report on AIDS and the address to the joint session of the California State Legislature follow in their entirety, with the intent that the reader capture the flavor of the beginning of the Surgeon General's campaign as well as a later snapshot of his activities in interaction with the forces that shape our public opinion and policy.

STATEMENT BY C. EVERETT KOOP, MD, SURGEON GENERAL, U.S. PUBLIC HEALTH SERVICE, WEDNESDAY, OCTOBER 22, 1986, WASHINGTON, D.C.

Ladies and Gentlemen:

Last February, President Reagan asked me to prepare a report to the American people on AIDS. The report is now completed.

In preparing this document, I consulted with the best medical and scientific experts this country can offer inside and outside the Public Health Service. I met with the leaders of organizations concerned with health, education, and other aspects of our society to gain their views of the problems associated with

AIDS. A list of those organizations is in your press kit. The resulting report contains information that I consider vital to the future health of this nation.

Controversial and sensitive issues are inherent in the subject of AIDS, and these issues are addressed in my report. Value judgments are absent. This is an objective health and medical report, which I would like every adult and adolescent to read. The impact of AIDS on our society is and will continue to be devastating. This epidemic has already claimed the lives of almost 15,000 Americans, and that figure is expected to increase 12-fold by the end of 1991—only five years from now.

Our best scientists are conducting intensive research into drug therapy and vaccine development for AIDS, but as yet we have no cure. Clearly this disease, which strikes men and women, children and adults, people of all races, must be stopped. It is estimated that one and a half million people are now infected with the AIDS virus. These people—the majority of whom are well and have no symptoms of disease—can spread the virus to others.

But new infections can be prevented if we, as individuals, take the responsibility of protecting ourselves and others from exposure to the AIDS virus. AIDS is not spread by casual, nonsexual contact. It is spread by high risk sexual and drug-related behaviors—behaviors that we can choose to avoid. Every person can reduce the risk of exposure to the AIDS virus through preventive measures that are simple, straightforward, and effective. However, if people are to follow these recommended measures—to act responsibly to protect themselves and others—they must be informed about them. That is an obvious statement, but not a simple one. Educating people about AIDS has never been easy.

From the start, this disease has evoked highly emotional and often irrational responses. Much of the reaction could be attributed to fear of the many unknowns surrounding a new and very deadly disease. This was compounded by personal feelings regarding the groups of people primarily affected—homosexual men and intravenous drug abusers. Rumors and misinformation spread rampantly and became as difficult to combat as the disease itself. It is time to put self-defeating attitudes aside and recognize that we are fighting a disease—not people. We must control the spread of AIDS, and at the same time offer the best we can to care for those who are sick.

We have made some strides in dispelling rumors and educating the public, but until every adult and adolescent is informed and knowledgeable about this disease, our job of educating will not be done. Unfortunately, some people are difficult to reach through traditional education methods, so our efforts must be redoubled. Others erroneously dismiss AIDS as a topic they need not be concerned about. They must be convinced otherwise.

Concerted education efforts must be directed to blacks and Hispanics. While blacks represent only 12 percent of the U.S. population, 25 percent of all people with AIDS are black. Another 12 percent of AIDS patients are Hispanic, while this group comprises only 6 percent of the population. Eighty percent of children with AIDS—8 out of 10—are black or Hispanic. For optimum effectiveness in reaching minority populations, educational programs must be designed specifically for these target groups.

Many people—especially our youth—are not receiving information that is vital to their future health and well-being because of our reticence in dealing with the subjects of sex, sexual practices, and homosexuality. This silence must end. We can no longer afford to sidestep frank, open discussions about sexual practices—homosexual and heterosexual. Education about AIDS should start at an early age so that children can grow up knowing the behaviors to avoid to protect themselves from exposure to the AIDS virus.

One place to begin this education is in our schools. Every school day, more than 47 million students attend 90,000 elementary and secondary schools in this nation. Our schools could provide AIDS education to 90–95 percent of our young people. As parents, educators, and community leaders we must assume our responsibility to educate our young. The need is critical and the price of neglect is high. AIDS education must start at the lowest grade possible as part of any health and hygiene program. There is now no doubt that we need sex education in schools and that it include information on sexual practices that may put our children at risk for AIDS. Teenagers often think themselves immortal, and these young people may be putting themselves at great risk as they begin to explore their own sexuality and perhaps experiment with drugs. The threat of AIDS should be sufficient to permit a sex education curriculum with a heavy emphasis on prevention of AIDS and other sexually transmitted diseases.

School education on AIDS must be reinforced at home. The role of parents as teachers—both in word and in deed—cannot be overestimated. Parents exert perhaps the strongest influence on their youngsters' developing minds, attitudes, and behaviors. We warn our children early about the dangerous consequences of playing with matches or crossing the street before checking for traffic. We have no less a responsibility to guide them in avoiding behaviors that may expose them to AIDS. The sources of danger differ, but the possible consequences are much more deadly.

Before we can educate our children about AIDS, we must educate ourselves. The first thing we have to understand and acknowledge is that AIDS is no longer the concern of any one segment of society; it is the concern of us all. People who engage in high risk sexual behavior or who inject illicit drugs are risking infection with the AIDS virus and are endangering their lives and the lives of others, including their unborn children.

The Surgeon General's report describes high risk sexual practices between men and between men and women. I want to emphasize two points: First, the risk of infection increases with increased numbers of sexual partners—male or female. Couples who engage in freewheeling casual sex these days are playing a dangerous game. What it boils down to is—unless you know with *absolute certainty* that your sex partner is not infected with the AIDS virus—through sex or through drug use—you're taking a chance on becoming infected. Conversely, unless you are *absolutely certain* that you are not carrying the AIDS virus, you must consider the possibility that you can infect others.

Second, the best protection against infection right now—barring abstinence— is use of a condom. A condom should be used during sexual relations, from start to finish, with anyone who you know or suspect is infected.

I'd like to comment briefly on the issues of mandatory blood testing and of quarantine of infected individuals. Ideas and opinions on how best to control the spread of AIDS vary, and these two issues have generated heated controversy and continuing debate. No one will argue that the AIDS epidemic must be contained, and any public health measure that will effectively help to accomplish this goal should be adopted. Neither quarantine nor mandatory testing for the AIDS antibody will serve that purpose.

Quarantine has no role in the management of AIDS because AIDS is not spread by casual contact. Quarantine should be considered only as a last resort by local authorities, and on a case-by-case basis, in special situations in which someone infected with the AIDS virus knowingly and willingly continues to expose others to infection through sexual contact or sharing drug equipment.

Compulsory blood testing is unnecessary, unfeasible, and cost prohibitive. Furthermore, rather than aiding in prevention, testing could, in some instances, cause irreparable harm. A negative test result in someone who has been recently infected but not yet developed antibodies might give that person a false sense of security not only for him- or herself, but for that person's sexual partners as well. This could lessen the motivation to adhere to safe sex practices. Voluntary testing is available and useful for people who have engaged in high risk behaviors and want to learn if they are infected so that they can seek appropriate medical attention and act to protect others from infection.

You'll note that my report supports and reinforces recommendations by the Public Health Service on AIDS prevention and risk reduction. Although my involvement with AIDS is fairly recent, the Public Health Service has been deeply involved in the AIDS crisis from the start. In the past five years the PHS has made excellent progress in characterizing the disease, delineating the modes of transmission, and protecting our blood supply from contamination with the AIDS virus. Vigorous research into drug therapy and vaccine development continues, and, as you know, the drug azidothymidine—AZT—is being made available to thousands of people with AIDS who may benefit from this treatment.

Much remains to be done to stop this epidemic, and the Public Health Service will continue to work together with all elements of public and private sectors and use all our joint resources to the fullest to eradicate AIDS.

In closing, let me say that my report on AIDS is a document that people should read. It provides—in layman's terms—detailed information about AIDS, how the disease is transmitted, the relative risks of infection, and how to prevent infection. I'd like your help in letting the public know that this document is available and how they can get a copy of it. The address for requests is in your press packet. It also appears on this television public service announcement we are releasing today. I'd like to show it to you.

Thank you, and I'll take your questions now.

ADDRESS BY C. EVERETT KOOP, MD, SCD,* PRESENTED TO THE JOINT SESSION ON AIDS OF THE CALIFORNIA LEGISLATURE, SACRAMENTO, CALIFORNIA, MARCH 6, 1987

Mr. President, Mr. Speaker. . . to hosts, guests, friends, etc.)

It is an honor and a great privilege for me to address this joint session of the California Legislature. And while your invitation was addressed to me and I was pleased to accept it—I am here today—representing not just myself but

*Surgeon General of the U.S. Public Health Service and Deputy Assistant Secretary of Health, U.S. Department of Health and Human Services.

also the personnel of the U.S. Public Health Service. I want very much to share the honor of this moment with them, because so much of what I have to say is the product of their hard work.

Also, the relationship between local and state public health officers in California and my colleagues in P.H.S. is excellent. It *has* been over the years and I'm sure it will *continue* to be.

That's good for California. . .and it's good for the country.

This is an unusual event. . .an historic event. . .and I am moved by that consideration. Also, however, as I stand in this chamber, I am *most* mindful of the following. . .single. . .overwhelming and profoundly tragic fact:

That Californians were the *first* of our citizens, back in June of 1981, to be identified as being the victims of AIDS. . .they were among the first to die of the disease. . .and before the rest of our country knew about—or truly understood the nature of—this catastrophe, the people of California were already beginning to bury their dead.

I am deeply, deeply sorry that anyone—here or anywhere in the world—has had to die of this disease. And I am especially sorry that the people of this state have had to live with this grief the longest.

It hasn't been 6 years. . .yet, it seems like an eternity. . .since those first reports came in to our Centers for Disease Control in Atlanta. During that time. . .

We've seen the offending virus and we've named and renamed it. . .

We've developed a test to determine if the virus is present in someone's blood. . .

We've been able to galvanize a large, international army of biomedical researchers, among whom, I might add, are many men and women of genius who are working on the problem in laboratories right here in California. . .

And finally, over the past 6 years, we've developed a way of monitoring the spread of the disease so as to have some reasonable—although by no means perfect—basis upon which to plan the use of our resources tomorrow and for some years in the future.

That last point is a difficult one. . .especially for the elected representatives of a free people. But we know that the disease of AIDS—as it continues to spread throughout our population—will be drawing ever more heavily upon our social and political capital, as well as our medical and financial capital.

It's a difficult challenge for Americans. But we are a good people. Through 200 years of often stormy and tumultuous history, the people of the United States have clung to this society's fundamental values of personal freedom, mutual assistance, and national unity.

Those values have withstood every test, and they are being tested again. . .right now. . .by the infiltration of this lethal disease.

But I firmly believe that those values will once more be our guides for collective action and once more we shall survive a grave threat to our health and well-being.

And right here I must recognize the leadership already demonstrated by the Legislature of the State of California, by its Governor, George Deukmejian, and by the rank-and-file public health, medical, and nursing personnel throughout this state. Like the rest of us, you've only begun what appears to be a long and fearful journey. But you've made a very commendable start.

I'm thinking in particular of your early moves to establish mandatory reporting of the disease and a statewide registry of cases.

Within a week of the approval of the blood test for AIDS, California had its own emergency regulations in place to protect the blood supply. And your network of alternative test sites ought to be a model for every other state to follow.

And throughout this time, you've been very careful to build into the law a respect for confidentiality and an understanding of the overwhelming burden it can be for a person to learn that he or she has AIDS. . .and will soon die.

I've said it many times, that we are fighting a terrible disease. . .We are *not* fighting the people who have it, and by your actions, you have made the government of this state a strong ally in the campaign to make sure that Americans know and respect the difference.

I think California has done well in the way it has expended its social and political capital so far on the issue of AIDS.

But it's only been a few years. . .and this disease will be a burden to us for the rest of this century at least.

We need, therefore, to give some thought to the way we will care for the rising toll of AIDS victims. Among them will be those with high risk behavior—homosexual and bisexual men and IV drug abusers. But more and more heterosexual victims will be identified. Many of those will have been unknowingly infected by bisexual men or promiscuous partners.

One of the spin-offs from the high profile of Nancy Reagan's anti-drug campaign will be reducing the spread of AIDS. Anything that will stop drug abuse, stops the spread of the AIDS virus.

The number of babies born with AIDS will certainly rise. Some will die within the first year or two of life. We're seeing that occur already.

But other children will carry the virus and may not exhibit any symptoms of an AIDS-related illness until they are well into their school years.

Frankly, I don't think society has yet worked out how it wants to respond to the plight of these innocent young victims. Some have had to take the brunt of the anger and resentment directed at their parents. . .who've been better able to step out of the way.

Other children, abandoned by parents, have had to appeal through advocates for medical and social services that would have been routinely given children with any other disease.

We must generate a concern for these youngsters such as the First Lady has done with her campaign against drugs.

I do not believe that these examples will prove to be the rule, but the fact that they may have happened *at all* is reason enough for us all to feel some pain and contrition.

And the costs in dollars and cents is also going to mount. The federal contribution this year is $416 million. About $300 million of that is research. . .nearly $100 million is for public education and information. . .and about $10 million is for patient care.

As you well know, California by itself has spent nearly half the total dollars expended by all state governments on AIDS since 1983. . .some $56 million so far, apportioned among patient care, public information, and research.

Some of our experts estimate that, by 1991, the total national bill for the care of AIDS patients will be *$16 billion* a year. . .or nearly *twice* what we're spending *this* year to support *all* the programs of the entire U.S. Public Health Service.

How will we apportion those costs? What will be the Federal Government's share? What share is reasonable for the states to carry? And how much can we ask the individual and his or her family to pay?

Commercial insurors—both life and health—have raised questions about coverage for persons known to be carrying the AIDS virus. . .or who are members of one or another group practicing high risk behavior. While we can understand their concerns, from a strictly financial point of view, we need to ask ourselves how those concerns fit in with good public policy *in general*.

In other words, will our decisions regarding the way we pay to care for AIDS patients contaminate our entire social and political decision-making process *itself*? We must not allow that to happen. Such an effect on our public life would be in itself an "AIDS-related complex."

There is, of course, genuine alarm that the costs of AIDS could mushroom and bankrupt our health care economy. My advice is to take the issue seriously, but don't be frightened into taking action inconsistent with American values.

In addition, we must not let fear so paralyze us that we fail to do certain sensible and pragmatic things, such as developing alternatives to the high-cost terminal care that's given AIDS patients in our community and general hospitals.

In any case, the central question before us today. . .as it has been for over 200 years. . .is still this:

How can we live so that we may be *a humane and civilized people*?

I can't imagine this country ever becoming *financially* bankrupt. But our society—like every other society in human history—always runs the risk of becoming *morally and ethically* bankrupt.

And we must never let that happen.

Ordinarily, the Surgeon General of the United States doesn't worry about such things. He or she may be a moral and an ethical person—and certainly each of my predecessors was that kind of person and I hope I will be judged to have been one, also—but you know it's never been a requirement, as such, for holding this job.

But some things have appeared on my watch as your Surgeon General that have tested not only my understanding of medicine and health. . .but also my understanding of the nature of the American people.

Over the past 5 years I've had to wrestle with the ethical issues raised by "Baby Doe" and "Baby Fae". . .by little Katie Beckett. . .by our ability to transplant organs and prolong life for the terminally ill.

My latest challenge was given to me a year ago, in February 1986, when President Reagan asked me to gather together all the information on AIDS that was then available and put it into a plain-English report to the American people.

And that's what I did for the next 8 months. In the process, I met not only with doctors and nurses and public health people, I also met with representatives of concerned groups from across the spectrum of society. . .

Groups like the National Education Association and the National P.T.A. . . . .

The National Council of Churches and the Christian Life Commission of the Southern Baptist Convention. . .

The Synagogue Council of America and the National Conference of Catholic Bishops. . .

The National Coalition of Black Lesbians and Gays and the Washington Business Group on Health.

I talked with the representatives of 26 groups in all. Most of them knew quite a bit about the health threat posed by AIDS. But what they were deeply troubled about were the moral and ethical issues raised by this disease.

Yes, we all agreed that the only real weapon we had to fight with at this time—since we lacked a vaccine or an effective drug—was the weapon of education.

That's where we all agreed. Where we had some differences of opinion, was the *substance* and the *direction* of that education.

Everybody had said, Yes, we should teach about the dangers posed by the AIDS virus.

Most people said, Well, *maybe* we should teach about the methods by which AIDS is transmitted.

And quite a few people said that, of course, we might *possibly* teach young people something about their sexuality to begin with.

I listened to everybody and took very good notes.

You may recall that my entire report is not very long, and I only devoted 92 words to the topic of education. But those 92 words have captured most of the attention of the media, of parents, of educators, and of public officials at all levels of government.

The reason is clear enough: the issue goes to the heart of each person's own system of moral and ethical values. . .or lack thereof.

I introduced the subject in a straightforward way. I said in my report that. . .

"Education about AIDS should start in early elementary school and at home so that children can grow up knowing the behavior to avoid to protect themselves from exposure to the AIDS virus. The threat of AIDS can provide an opportunity for parents to instill in their children their own moral and ethical standards."

Some people were unduly alarmed by that phrase, "early elementary school." Would that include kindergarten? I'm afraid so.

I know of good, caring approaches to sex education that can be used—and in fact *are* used—in kindergarten and first grade.

However, I recognize that it's more difficult to do and, therefore, I would be willing today, some 4 months after publication, to make that single change in the report. . .That is, I would agree, albeit reluctantly, to take out the word "early" and just let the sentence read. . . "Education about AIDS should start in elementary school."

I concluded the report with exactly the same thought. I said. . .

"Education concerning AIDS must start at the lowest grade possible as part of any health and hygiene program. . . . There is now no doubt that we need sex education in schools and that it must include information on heterosexual and homosexual relationships. The threat of AIDS should be sufficient to permit a sex education curriculum with a heavy emphasis on prevention of AIDS and other sexually transmitted diseases."

And I would not change *any* of the words in that paragraph.

I am aware that the people of California, through their educational organizations, health organizations, and through their representatives in local and state government, have endorsed the need to begin teaching about AIDS no later than the 7th grade.

I think they're absolutely right and I applaud them for being clear-headed and public-minded on the issue.

I know, also, that many school districts in this state have adopted one or another curriculum elements that introduce human sexuality and reproductive health in a positive and caring way to children in elementary grades—generally speaking the 5th or 6th grades—and that should mean that local community standards, consistent with parental values, have been taken into account, which is as it should be.

And by the way, the School Health Task Force for Los Angeles County came to the same conclusion in January 1986, a good *10 months* before my own report was published. In *their* report, the Task Force members recommended the general adoption of a comprehensive school health education curriculum that routinely included sexuality right along with accident prevention, nutrition, and an understanding of the cardiovascular and gastrointestinal systems.

It's an eminently sensible recommendation, and it is an ethically positive recommendation as well. If we adults know something that could save the life of a child, then children have a right to that information. And we have the obligation to tell them.

If it makes us uncomfortable. . .if it is awkward to do. . .if it appears to conflict with other information that we might have, those are problems that *we* have to resolve in a way that enables us to *nevertheless* tell our children what they *need* to know and have a *right* to know.

I'm not saying it's easy. But it's far from impossible.

For example, I gave just these two precautions in my report. The *first* one is simple enough. It advises you to. . .

Find someone who is worthy of your respect and your love. . .give that person both. . .and stay faithful to him or her.

In other words, short of total abstinence, the best defense against AIDS is to *maintain a faithful, monogamous relationship* in which you have only one continuing sexual partner. . .and that person is as faithful as you are.

My *second* message is for people who don't yet have a faithful monogamous relationship for whatever reason. That message is. . .

Caution: It's important that you *know with absolute certainty* that neither you nor your partner is carrying the AIDS virus. If you're not absolutely certain, then you *must take precautions*, and the best one available—though far from perfect—is to use a condom from start to finish.

From my viewpoint, as a public health officer, I tell people that when they have sex with someone, they're also having sex with *everyone else* with whom *that* person has ever had sex. Naturally, if the "everyone else" is only you. . .you're very well protected from disease. . .and from a lot of other unpleasant surprises as well.

This all seems to be information that is clear enough and straightforward enough to tell children. There's nothing terribly esoteric about it. Yet, many adults—parents and teachers alike—are having trouble coming to terms with it all.

The more I've thought about this phenomenon, the more I've come to believe that the difficulty is not in the facts themselves concerning sexuality, human reproduction, and AIDS. The difficulty is in the *significance* of those facts relative to the totality of a *sensitive and affirmative* human relationship.

Such a relationship will include some fulfilling sexual activity, but it is not defined *only* *by* that activity. There's much more to a loving, caring, respectful, and tolerant human relationship than just "good sex." A relationship devoid of love and responsibility is like a piece of pie that's all crust and no filling. And young people ought to be advised of that.

Novelists call it "true love." Sociologists call it "marital fidelity." The Surgeon General calls it "monogamy." But whatever you call it, we all want that well-rounded, balanced, loving, and fully considerate relationship. . .a relationship that's enriched by sex, not overwhelmed by it or devoid of it either.

Such a relationship is an ideal. . .but "real life" isn't always like that. It's imperfect. . .it's give-and-take.

Without a compassionate understanding of the imperfect nature of many human relationships, a child's education will be. . .itself. . .very imperfect.

So if parents are to educate their children about human relationships—sexual and otherwise—they must first understand and accept the nature of their *own*. For many, that's hard to do.

Parents—and adults in general—are not very good about talking *to* *each* *other* about their sexuality. They feel frustrated, guilty, and even angry because they are unable to do the thing that they know—intellectually and emotionally— they *should* do.

But they can't.

And for me, that's the compelling reason why our schools, churches, synagogues, and other community institutions must do whatever possible to provide our children with the best available information. . .physical, sexual, emotional, and psychological. . .to help them negotiate their own way through the human condition.

You, as responsible legislators, are being called upon to contribute to that process, also, and I know that this legislature is indeed writing such a record in the indelible inks of compassion and duty.

I've delivered this message—and variations of it—many times in the past few months. But it doesn't get any easier.

It's essentially a grim message and I guess I'm something of a grim courier.

My only hope is that every American who hears or reads my message will believe it and do his or her part to stop the spread of AIDS. . .to protect and save the lives of people at risk, including and especially our unsuspecting young people. . .and that they will help return sexuality back to its rightful place in the spectrum of human experience: have it again be a *part* of the total complex of human, caring, interpersonal relations.

Such relations, in my book anyway, are known as "true love."

Which leads me to my final word. It's not mine really. It's the last sentence of *The Bridge of San Luis Rey*, the little novel written by the late Thornton Wilder, one of our greatest novelists and playwrights.

Wilder concluded that novel by observing. . .

"There is a land of the living and a land of the dead and the only bridge is love. . .the only survival, the only meaning."

Thank you.

16

The New Death among IV Drug Users

Don C. Des Jarlais, Cathy Casriel, and Samuel Friedman

INTRODUCTION

Intravenous (IV) drug users are the second largest group of persons to have developed AIDS in the United States and Europe. Of the 33,720 cases of AIDS in the United States, 5565 (17%) are among heterosexual IV drug users and 2550 (8%) are among male homosexual/bisexual IV drug users (reported through 6 April 1987).[1] In Europe, 600 (15%) of the 3898 cases have IV drug use as their primary risk factor, and 98 (3%) have IV drug use and male homosexual activity as risk behavior (reported through 31 Dec. 1987).[2] The metropolitan New York area has by far the greatest concentration of AIDS cases in which IV drug use is the primary risk factor, with 3248 cases in New York and 901 cases in New Jersey. These two states account for 75% of all U.S. cases in which IV drug use is the primary risk behavior.

There is great variation in HIV seroprevalence rates among IV drug users in different areas. High levels of seroprevalence—rates of 50% or greater—have been reported in the New York City area,[3,4] Edinburgh,[5] northern Italy,[6] and Spain.[7] Very low rates (4% or less) have been found in southern New Jersey,[8] London,[9] New Orleans,[10] and Glasgow.[11] At present there is no good explanation for this wide variation, although the date at which HIV was first introduced among IV drug users in a local area is undoubtedly one of the reasons.

Transmission of HIV among IV drug users occurs primarily through the sharing of drug injection equipment, with heterosexual transmission apparently playing a relatively minor role (see [12] for a review). The behavioral factors most frequently associated with HIV seropositivity are the frequency of drug injection[13-15] and the sharing of needles across friendship groups as in the use of "shooting galleries" (places where one can rent equipment which is then returned for other IV drug users to rent and use).[16-18] In cities where formally organized shooting galleries do not exist, the use of "house works" (injection equipment that a drug dealer keeps to lend to customers) may be the functional equivalent.

Once HIV is established among IV drug users in a local area, this group can become the dominant means of transmission to heterosexuals and perinatal transmission. In New York City, 87% of the heterosexual transmission cases have been from IV drug users to regular sexual partners who do not inject drugs, and 80% of the perinatal transmission cases have been in the children of IV drug users.[19]

The AIDS epidemic is having a very complex effect on IV drug users in Western societies. AIDS is leading to many changes in this subculture, some of which have been spontaneous and others of which have been in response to public health prevention efforts. The connection between IV drug users and heterosexual transmission of HIV is forcing many public health and political authorities to reassess previous attitudes regarding the nature and importance of illicit drug injection in society.

The theme of AIDS as a new way of dying for IV drug users will be used to integrate many (though clearly not all) of the effects of AIDS on the injection of illicit drugs. Consideration of death and IV drug use prior to the AIDS epidemic provides a good starting point for the analysis.

DEATH IN THE DRUG USE SUBCULTURE

Death was quite common in the IV drug use subculture prior to AIDS. The death rate for drug users in treatment was about 1.5% per year. Estimates of death rates among IV drug users out of treatment have ranged from 3.5% to 8% per year (see [20] for a review). The major factor accounting for the higher rate of out-of-treatment deaths was narcotic overdoses. In fact, prior to AIDS, an overdose was considered the prototype for the cause of death among active IV drug users.

Overdose deaths primarily come from taking a much stronger than usual dose of heroin, so that whatever tolerance has been developed is not sufficient to prevent a fatal respiratory depression. Heroin that can cause an overdose is thus also able to give a very good "high" (if the user exercises appropriate caution). This association between a strong dose of narcotic and overdose death has led many heroin dealers to name their personal "brands" with variations on the theme of overdosing-death. Black Death, Broken Hearted Killer, Death, Death Row, Death Wish, Killer, Killer 1, Kiss of Death, OD, OD (black star), Strangler, Suicide, and The Killer have all been used in the marketing of heroin in New York City.[21] Without being overly psychoanalytic, one may assume a fundamental ambivalence toward overdose deaths among IV drug users. While an overdose death clearly means facing the terrors of dying, as well as loss of the pleasures of using drugs, approaching this form of death also has a connotation of intense pleasure, and can be seen as a justifiable risk in the search for the peak of drug-induced euphoria.

AIDS VERSUS OVERDOSE DEATH

Death from AIDS is very different than death from an overdose. Table 1 presents some of these differences. The variation in the time duration between an overdose death and an AIDS death is fundamental. Death from a narcotic overdose will often occur within several minutes to an hour after taking the drug. During this time the person will usually be unconscious, so there is a very limited amount of time in which to realize/experience the overdose. In contrast, dying from AIDS is usually quite protracted. There may be many years from initial HIV infection to the development of clinical symptoms, days to years between the development of symptoms and the development of diagnosed AIDS, and then perhaps another year or more until death. Both an overdose or AIDS may lead to an IV drug user's death; it is, however, the relative lack of time between an overdose and death compared to the lengthy time between an AIDS

Table 1   Characteristics of overdose and AIDS deaths

Characteristics	Overdose death	AIDS death
Time duration	Immediate	Protracted
Physical characteristics	Euphoria	Pain, debilitation
Social reaction	Asocial	Isolation, strained relationships, potential intense guilt
Comparison to stressful life	Release	Worsening, leading to suicidal thoughts
Contingent on drug use	Stopping drug use eliminates risk	Often independent of continued drug use

diagnosis and death that leads to many of the differences in the psychology of the two forms of death.

The brief time span of an overdose is generally experienced as a narcotic euphoria (though there is some possibility that the IV drug user may become aware and alarmed about a potential overdose prior to losing consciousness). AIDS typically involves physical weakness and incapacitation, along with extended periods of pain associated with the opportunistic infections that arise as a result of the HIV-induced immunosuppression. The two types of dying may be considered almost complete physical opposites—sensations of intense pleasure versus extended debilitation and protracted pain.

An overdose death is basically asocial, although assistance to combat the overdose usually will be provided if others are present. Thus, to the extent that social relationships are involved in an overdose situation, they are likely to be supportive. The shortness of time between the taking of the overdose and loss of consciousness, however, does not provide much opportunity for social interaction; therefore, from the perspective of the person who has taken the overdose, the event as it occurs is primarily asocial.

The months from AIDS diagnosis to death permit many opportunities for social interaction between the IV drug user with AIDS and others. Despite the commitment and care of many of the health care providers, social interactions are likely to be extremely difficult for the IV drug user with AIDS. Friends who are also drug users may refuse to visit when the patient is in the hospital, out of (a mistaken) fear of casual contact transmission and a (generally correct) perception that current IV drug users are not welcome visitors in most hospitals. Family members may refuse to see the patient, again out of fear of casual contact transmission and also the emotional stress of an impending death. Friends and family may simultaneously feel guilt for not having done enough to prevent the drug dependency that led to AIDS and a "blame the victim" anger at the IV drug user for having brought the disease upon himself or herself.

If the IV drug user has a sexual partner who does not inject drugs, or has young children, there is the possibility of transmitting the virus to the partner and/or child. In this case the direction of any transmission is evident and there is the potential for extreme anger and guilt in all parties concerned. While an overdose death is essentially asocial, the interpersonal relationships after a diagnosis of AIDS are very complex and may cause as much distress and suffering as the physical symptoms of HIV infection.

These differences between overdose and AIDS deaths for IV drug users can be summarized as follows. An overdose death contains many elements of escape—it can be a quick and euphoric release from a troubled life. Death from AIDS, in contrast, is a prolonged experience in dying, combining physical debilitation, pain, and troubled interpersonal relationships. Many IV drug users, when comparing the two types of death, have expressed a preference for an overdose death, and have even suggested that they might deliberately take an overdose if they believed they had AIDS.

A word needs to be said at this point about the possible effects antiviral drugs such as AZT might have on the comparison between an overdose death and an AIDS death. Clearly, any antiviral drug that arrests the progression of HIV infection and prevents persons from dying from AIDS will change the psychology of HIV-infected individuals. The major difference between AIDS and overdoses, however, is in the time period prior to death. An antiviral drug with significant and unpleasant side effects, that requires frequent medical monitoring, and does not fully protect against transmission to others, and that must be taken frequently enough that others become aware of the person's condition, may actually heighten the differences between AIDS and an overdose. Thus much of the psychology of AIDS would still apply even if an antiviral drug that prevented death were readily available to IV drug users with HIV infection.

ACTUAL RESPONSES TO AIDS DIAGNOSES

Although the potentially traumatic effects of an AIDS diagnosis on the psychological functioning of IV drug users should not be underestimated, such a diagnosis very rarely leads to suicide or psychotic breaks. A more common reaction is the desire to regain health and to enter treatment immediately so that the period between diagnosis and death need not be spent trying to hustle drugs on the street. The stress of an AIDS diagnosis can be positive: it is clearly capable of eliciting great courage and strength among IV drug users and their families and friends. Some IV drug users have responded by joining AIDS prevention efforts aimed at current IV drug users.

RISK REDUCTION

Given that AIDS is a new form of death, one would expect IV drug users to have a significant interest in learning about AIDS and to show substantial behavior changes in order to avoid developing the disease. There is consistent evidence that IV drug users in New York City are relatively well informed about AIDS and that many have altered their behavior to reduce the risk of AIDS. In 1984, we conducted a survey of methadone maintenance patients in Manhattan.[22] Essentially all knew of AIDS, and over 90% knew that sharing drug injection equipment was a means of transmitting the virus. Thirty percent personally knew someone who had developed AIDS; 59% reported that they had changed their behavior to reduce their risk; 54% reported changes in their use of needles and syringes, with an increase in the use of sterile/cleaned equipment and a reduction in the number of persons with whom they would share injection equipment the most frequently mentioned changes.

Selwyn and colleagues[23] from Montefiore Medical Center in New York City conducted a similar study in 1985. It sampled IV drug users from a methadone maintenance program and from a prison detoxification service. The results were almost identical. Almost all subjects knew that AIDS was transmitted through the sharing of drug injection equipment, and over 60% had modified their use of injection equipment in order to protect themselves against AIDS. Again, increased use of sterile injection equipment and fewer numbers of people with whom one would share injection equipment were the two most common methods of risk reduction.

Validation of these self-reported changes in needle use behavior comes from our studies of the marketing of illicit sterile injection equipment in New York City. There has been a notable increase in the demand for and marketing of illicit sterile needles and syringes since 1984,[24,25] which supports the self-reports of greater use of such equipment in our own and the Montefiore studies.

These behavior changes among IV drug users in New York City occurred before the establishment of any large-scale prevention programs aimed at reducing AIDS within this group. This risk reduction should therefore be seen as a result of the general information about AIDS transmitted through the mass media and the oral communication networks of the IV drug use subculture rather than the result of any specific prevention campaigns.

Evidence that IV drug users alter their behavior to avoid AIDS is not limited to the New York area, where the large number of cases of AIDS among this group would serve as a signal of the need to reduce their risk. Ongoing research in Amsterdam and San Francisco shows that methods of risk reduction had begun in those cities *prior* to the development of many AIDS cases among IV drug users. Coutinho[26] reports increasing use of the "free needle exchange" program in Amsterdam in response to concern about AIDS in that city. Biernacki and Feldman[27] report that IV drug users in San Francisco were aware of AIDS by the end of 1985, and that a "significant minority" had changed their behavior to reduce the chances of developing AIDS.

REACTION OF DRUG ABUSE TREATMENT STAFF TO AIDS

AIDS as a new form of death has led to changes not only in the behavior of IV drug users themselves, but also in drug abuse treatment programs. In addition to the differences between an overdose death and an AIDS death summarized in Table 1, there is another that is particularly significant for drug abuse treatment programs. Stopping drug use eliminates the threat of an overdose death. Because of the long latency period between initial HIV infection and the development of clinical HIV disease, however, a person may stop drug use and still die from AIDS. This fact creates problems for drug abuse treatment staff in their attempts to motivate drug users to avoid IV drug use.

The reactions of drug treatment programs and staff in New York City have varied over time. Four stages have been observed in their responses to the AIDS epidemic (see [28] for a full presentation of these stages). These stages are similar to, but not identical with, the stages that Kübler-Ross[29] observed in medical patients who receive diagnoses of fatal conditions. They are also similar to the stages in response to stress that have been described by Selye.[30]

As within the Kübler-Ross schema, the typical first response among treatment staff to the AIDS crisis can be termed denial. Denial among drug abuse treatment staff consists of trying to continue treating IV drug users as if the epidemic were not affecting them. Initially this was done by simply not devoting any organizational resources (including staff time) to AIDS-related issues. Later, other methods, such as trying to screen out persons exposed to HIV from entry into the program, evolved.

It would be a fundamental mistake to see this denial as a simple failure to respond to a pressing issue. There are several psychological reasons for the reluctance of drug abuse treatment staff to address AIDS issues or to want to work with HIV-infected persons. The fear of casual contact transmission is one reason. While there is no evidence that HIV can be transmitted by casual contact, the reluctance of scientists to rule out absolutely any such possibility encourages the fear that it could happen. Drug abuse treatment often involves the collection of urine samples (in methadone programs) and the use of common eating facilities (in residential programs) both of which can serve as foci for fears of casual contact transmission.

Drug treatment staff generally have had very little training or expertise in working with infectious diseases, particularly incurable ones like AIDS. Previous experience with infectious diseases is likely to be confined to acute infections that are referred for medical treatment and are cured. They have had essentially no experience with counseling persons with long-term, fatal illnesses; they are neither professionally nor emotionally prepared for counseling persons who may die regardless of any behavior changes or medical interventions. Drug treatment staff are also not trained to counsel on sexual and/or perinatal risk reduction measures that are essential for effective AIDS prevention efforts among IV drug users.

Drug abuse counseling is already a task that is often emotionally frustrating. But there are certain rewards and feelings of accomplishment when, for instance, one sees reduction or elimination of drug use and improvement in the life situations of the clients. AIDS seems to ask drug abuse counselors to make a career change and become AIDS counselors. This new career involves hypothetical exposure to a deadly virus, confronting one's own sense of mortality, learning new counseling skills, and accepting the possibility that clients may die despite the best efforts of the client, the counselor, and medical personnel. Taking all these factors into account, denial can be considered a perfectly reasonable reaction to the AIDS epidemic; it should not be taken as an indication of lack of commitment on the part of drug abuse treatment staff.

It would be impossible to prevent all HIV-infected drug abusers from entering a specific treatment program. Ethical, legal, and technical reasons prohibit full exclusion. It then becomes a matter of time until someone in (or related to) the program develops an AIDS-related illness. This will provoke a second stage of response—panic. The fears of casual contact transmission become acute. Even for persons who do not have this fear, emotional difficulties in acknowledging their own mortality make for difficult interpersonal interactions with the AIDS client. During this stage, drug abuse treatment personnel have sometimes acted in ways that were actively harmful to the HIV-infected clients. They may have dismissed such people from the treatment program or, if allowed to stay, the persons with HIV infection may be required to attend at odd hours when they will not be seen by other clients in the program. AIDS need not occur in a person currently in treatment to provoke the panic stage among the staff. Panic has also arisen in response to HIV infection in the spouse of a current client, leading to the client being initially expelled from the program.

The third stage in the responses of drug abuse treatment staff to AIDS may best be termed coping. This stage includes full education about AIDS for all staff and active education/prevention efforts for all clients. Fears of transmission by casual contact, if not completely eliminated, are not permitted to interfere with the provision of drug abuse treatment services. Education includes acknowledging the fact that the great majority of persons in drug abuse treatment programs must be considered at risk for HIV infection either because they may continue to inject drugs if they are in outpatient programs or they may not successfully complete residential programs. Education efforts also include describing the dangers of heterosexual and perinatal transmission and explaining preventive measures which can be taken (such as the use of condoms, which may be distributed by the program). Effective liaisons are established to provide medical services to any persons who might develop HIV-related illnesses, while continuing their drug abuse treatment services.

The fourth stage, which has been observed among some drug abuse treatment personnel, may be termed burnout. Even after one has developed the necessary skills and prepared oneself emotionally, involvement with AIDS patients can be highly stressful. New cases of disease develop among previously infected persons. And as more IV drug users are infected, it becomes increasingly difficult to keep the remaining unexposed persons from being infected. Obviously the need for behavioral changes to prevent heterosexual and perinatal transmission also intensifies. Simply keeping current with new developments in the field can consume enormous amounts of time. The need for additional resources always seems to run ahead of the ability to develop new resources.

However, burnout need not be seen as inevitable among drug abuse treatment staff dealing with AIDS. Self-help groups composed of persons working in similar areas but in different organizations can be very useful for providing emotional support as well as practical problem-solving techniques. It must be realized, however, that when the coping stage is reached, all problems associated with adapting to the AIDS epidemic may not be resolved. The possibility of staff burnout still remains.

AIDS PREVENTION PROGRAMS FOR IV DRUG USERS

A wide variety of AIDS prevention programs for IV drug users have been established throughout the United States and Western Europe (see [31] for a review).

For the benefit of analysis, it is useful to categorize these AIDS prevention programs into two phases (an extended version of this analysis is presented in [32]). The first phase is general AIDS education. It focuses on informing people that AIDS is spread through the sharing of drug injection equipment and contains exhortations for IV drug users to stop injecting, or if they do continue, to stop sharing injection equipment. This information can be disseminated through the mass media, distribution of posters and pamphlets, and AIDS education sessions conducted in drug abuse treatment programs. It is then typically further spread through the oral communication networks of the IV drug use subculture.[33] This basic AIDS education does appear to motivate substantial numbers of IV drug users to alter their behavior, with increased utilization of available sterile injection equipment and a reduction in the number of persons with whom they share equipment being the most common changes. Such responses to AIDS information, however, are best described as risk reduction and not risk elimination. There is certainly no evidence that the amount of risk reduction that has occurred thus far has been sufficient to stop the spread of HIV among IV drug users in any geographic area.

The second phase of AIDS prevention among IV drug users is providing face-to-face education in conjunction with additional means to change their behavior. Face-to-face education about AIDS offers several potential advantages over general (mass media, pamphlets, posters) forms of education. Problems with language and the use of technical terms can be addressed because the participants have the opportunity to ask questions if there is something they do not understand. Of perhaps greater importance is the opportunity for nonverbal "emotional" communication in the face-to-face setting. The educator can assess the audience's emotional response to the content of the message and, if need be, modulate his or her presentation so that the seriousness of the AIDS threat can be conveyed without raising anxiety to the point where psychological denial of the problem becomes the dominant response. The AIDS educator can also convey nonjudgmental sincerity, explaining that AIDS really does require behavior changes and is not simply another scare tactic to try to get drug users to give up drugs. Ex-addicts can be used effectively as AIDS educators. They are positive role models—they have been successful in reducing their risk for developing AIDS—and have a greater ability to communicate with drug users who can identify with them.

The face-to-face situation allows the health educator to probe for the aspects of AIDS that are of greatest concern to the individuals in the program. It may be the threat of infecting the drug user's children, the pain and debilitation of AIDS, or the difficulty of hustling drugs when ill. Preliminary data from an ex-addict health educator/outreach program in New York indicate that the ex-addicts have been adopting this strategy of tailoring the prevention message to the concerns of the individual recipient, and that this leads to greater interest in seeking additional counseling and greater expressed intentions of behavior change.[34]

Once IV drug users have been motivated to modify their behavior to avoid AIDS, the means for those changes must be provided. That public officials have shown increased willingness to provide these services is an indication of the effect the AIDS epidemic is having on attitudes toward IV drug use. Supplying IV drug users with sterile drug injection equipment is one way to help IV drug users change behavior that puts them at risk for AIDS. Sterile needles and syringes can be purchased legally in most Western European countries and in the great majority of the states in the United States. Prescriptions for the sale of needles and syringes are required in Sweden and in many of the states here that have large concentrations of IV drug users. The lack of a prescription requirement, however, does not necessarily mean that sterile injection equipment is actually available to IV drug users. Pharmacists in many areas have typically refused to sell needles and syringes to persons suspected of injecting drugs, and there are also laws against the possession of "narcotics paraphernalia" in many jurisdictions. The laws requiring prescriptions have been changed in Switzerland[35] and France[36] specifically as measures to reduce AIDS among IV drug users.

"Needle exchange" systems, in which IV drug users can exchange used injection equipment for new sterile equipment are a way of increasing the means for risk reduction among IV drug users with the advantage of providing for safe disposal of many of the used needles and syringes. Needle exchange systems for the prevention of AIDS have been established in Holland, the United Kingdom, and Australia. (The needle exchanges in Holland were actually established as hepatitis control measures prior to the AIDS epidemic, but have been greatly expanded because of AIDS.)

Needle exchange systems (or changing laws that restrict the legal availability of sterile injection equipment) have not yet been instituted in the United States. They have been considered and rejected in New Jersey and California, and, as of April 1987, an exchange system is under consideration in New York. The American alternative to making sterile injection equipment legally available is teaching IV drug users how to sterilize used injection equipment. Bleach, alcohol, and boiling in water can all be used to sterilize injection equipment. There are programs in San Francisco, New York, New Jersey, Chicago, Baltimore, and Washington, D.C. that instruct IV drug users in sterilization procedures. Most of these programs use trained ex-addicts as the instructors. (The instructors also provide general AIDS instruction, emphasizing that stopping drug injection altogether is a better way to reduce the risk of AIDS.)

Provision of additional drug abuse treatment is another method of increasing the means for AIDS-related behavior change among IV drug users. To the extent that treatment leads to the cessation of IV drug use, the risk of exposure to HIV through the sharing of injection equipment has been eliminated. Even if treatment does not lead to complete elimination of further drug injection, it might still be successful in terms of AIDS prevention. Following "safe injection" procedures appears to be most difficult when a person is using drugs at the level of physical addiction (where sudden cessation of drugs will be followed by withdrawal symptoms). Withdrawal symptoms are sufficiently unpleasant that almost all IV drug users report that if they are in withdrawal and do have drugs to inject, they will use whatever injection equipment is readily available.[37] Thus, if treatment leads to levels of drug use less than those associated with physical addiction, the likelihood of risk-reduction behavior is greatly increased. More treatment programs for drug abuse have been created in New York, New Jersey, San Francisco, and Sweden as an AIDS prevention measure. The National Institute on Drug Abuse in the United States and several European countries, including the United Kingdom and the Federal Republic of Germany, are planning to expand treatment facilities.

As noted earlier, there is consistent evidence that phase one—basic AIDS education—leads to risk reducing behaviors among IV drug users. Measuring the effectiveness of the phase two prevention programs is clearly a much more difficult task, as the effects of these programs must be separated from the ongoing behavioral changes associated with basic information about AIDS and the effect that ever-increasing numbers of HIV-infected persons has on IV drug users. While it is too early to determine the efficacy of the phase two AIDS prevention programs, there are a number of aspects that are worth noting. The programs appear to be well accepted by IV drug users. Reports of the face-to-face education programs indicate that current IV drug users show considerable interest in learning more about AIDS and that the educators have relatively little difficulty in establishing rapport.[38-40]

Many IV drug users are extremely responsive to the face-to-face education programs. As previously mentioned, many of these programs provide education on how to sterilize drug injection equipment (or, as in Europe, actually provide free sterile equipment). Prior to the establishment of these programs, the objection was made that providing means for "AIDS safe injection" would "encourage drug abuse." Contrary to this expectation, the available data show that the programs have either no effect on the levels of drug injection or actually influence many IV drug users to seek treatment to reduce their levels. There is no evidence that the needle exchanges in Amsterdam[41] and in Liverpool[42] have led to any increases in illicit drug injection in these cities. In Amsterdam, the number of IV drug users entering treatment has increased during the period the needle exchange programs (data is not yet available on entry into treatment for other cities with needle exchanges). Early reports on the face-to-face education programs also indicate that many current IV drug users respond to these programs by seeking treatment to reduce their levels of drug injection.[43-45] Thus, while the data still must be considered preliminary, it appears that AIDS prevention programs that include methods of "AIDS safe injection" do not "encourage drug abuse," and may in fact serve to motivate drug users to enter drug abuse treatment programs.

It is clear that AIDS is provoking behavior changes among IV drug users as no other health threat has ever done before. The AIDS prevention programs, however, have generally presented AIDS as a fatal threat to IV drug users and have not usually focused on the differences between AIDS and other threats to the lives of drug users. More research needs to be done to determine what specific aspects of AIDS are most likely to lead to sustained risk reduction and how to individualize the prevention messages to reach different IV drug users. The face-to-face education programs do present a good mechanism for both obtaining data on the responses of current IV drug users to various aspects of AIDS and for presenting individualized prevention messages.

THE NEW DEATH AND NEW IV DRUG USERS

One particularly important aspect of AIDS as a new form of death is how it affects recruitment into IV drug use. There is a relatively high turnover among IV drug users. Within a "stable population" of IV drug users, an estimated 10–20% leave active IV drug use annually,[46] through death, successful treatment, or simply their own efforts to stop injecting drugs. These people are then replaced by new IV drug users. Because of this high turnover, control of HIV within the IV drug use population will require either that the number of new drug injectors is reduced or that new injectors adopt "AIDS safe injection" practices as they are initiated into IV drug use.

How concerns about AIDS are incorporated into IV drug recruitment is particularly interesting, since initial IV drug use almost invariably involves sharing injection equipment,[47] and "fear arousal" techniques have traditionally been ineffective in preventing youth from drug experimentation.[48] (The failure of the possibility of death to prevent drug use applies to legal drugs such as nicotine and alcohol as well as to illicit drugs.)

A research project in New York City is examining new recruitment into IV drug use through a longitudinal study of persons who are heavy users (but not injectors) of heroin and cocaine.[49] The central experimental component of this project is a training group that prepares heroin and cocaine "sniffers" (persons using the drugs intranasally) to manage situations that might otherwise trigger their initiation into drug injection. The training is based on drug prevention efforts developed from social learning theory. Experimental and control subjects are monitored over time to evaluate the training group's success in preventing drug injection and exposure to HIV.

Data from the first 40 heroin sniffers recruited for the study revealed complex but generally positive attitudes toward heroin use. Twenty-five of the subjects had no prior drug treatment history. While few actively opposed treatment, many felt they could control their use and therefore did not need treatment. Ten were trying to stop using heroin; the rest planned to continue using it.

Although subjects were knowledgeable about AIDS and needle transmission, fear of AIDS was rarely the primary reason for remaining a sniffer. Rather, subjects were averse to needles, considering injection a more advanced stage of addiction. Sniffing was seen as less dangerous, less addicting, and easier.

Subjects had rejected encouragement by IV drug users to inject for the "rush." Yet over half thought they might indeed inject "to get a better high." Eleven said they might inject because of peer pressure and ten to avoid withdrawal. A small but disturbing number (eight) thought they might inject if clean needles were available. Other reasons cited for injecting were: to appease curiosity, to conquer a phobia, and to minimize drug-induced damage to one's nose. Thus it would appear that AIDS has not yet become a dominant reason for avoiding drug injection, even in New York City, where over 3000 cases of AIDS have occurred among IV drug users.

The first group randomly selected to participate in the training showed a very positive response. Out of ten people contacted by telephone, eight came to the first session and seven of these made a commitment to return. There was a 98% attendance record over the course of the training, and the group collectively decided to extend the number of meetings from four to six to cover additional AIDS/drug use issues. While AIDS was not initially considered a major reason for not injecting drugs, the subjects were quite responsive to the intervention designed to reduce their risk of developing AIDS.

A major concern about the connection between IV drug use and AIDS has not yet emerged in the young people who are at high risk to begin injecting drugs and who live in the city with the largest number of IV drug-related AIDS cases. There does, however, appear to be an underlying receptivity to AIDS/IV drug use prevention efforts. Much more research is needed to determine the best methods for utilizing that receptivity.

"NON–AIDS" DEATHS AMONG INTRAVENOUS DRUG USERS

AIDS-related illnesses and AIDS deaths are already having a profound impact on IV drug users, drug abuse treatment programs, and medical care facilities in the New York City area, Spain, and Italy. Given this impact, it is almost ironic to note that there is probably a major underestimation of the amount of HIV-related mortality among IV drug users.

There has been a dramatic increase in deaths among IV drug users in New York City since HIV was first introduced into this group in the middle to late 1970s. The death rate among the group has increased from 257 in 1978[50] to approximately 2000 in 1986.[51] Half of these deaths can be attributed to diagnosed AIDS or ARC.[52] The others have been caused by various factors, including epidemic increases in tuberculosis, non-pneumocystis pneumonia, and endocarditis. Research is currently underway to examine the relationship between these greater numbers of death and HIV infection. At present, the best estimate is that HIV-related deaths among IV drug users are at least 50% greater than the official AIDS/ARC counts.

CONCLUSION

IV drug users are a critical group in efforts to control HIV infection in the United States and Europe. They form the second largest group of persons who have developed AIDS, and they are the major sources of heterosexual and perinatal transmission. The threat of AIDS has already led to much more risk reduction behavior among IV drug users than would have been expected, considering their behavior with respect to other health threats. When AIDS is thought of as a new way of dying much of the data on IV drug user behavior changes and the reactions of drug abuse treatment staff to the AIDS epidemic can be comprehended. Further exploration is needed to discover how best to incorporate the unique aspects of AIDS into prevention programs—particularly prevention programs for persons who are not yet injecting drugs—and what the full range of effects of HIV infection will have on the health of IV drug users.

REFERENCES

1. Centers for Disease Control. AIDS Surveillance. Personal communication, 1987.
2. Brunet J. B. WHO AIDS European Coordinating Center. Personal communication, 1987.
3. Marmor, M.; Des Jarlais, D. C.; Cohen, H.; Friedman, S. R.; Beatrice, S. T.; Dubin, N.; El-Sadr W.; Mildvan, D.; Yancovitz, S.; Mathur, U.; Holtzman, R. Risk factors for infection with human immunodeficiency virus among intravenous drug users in New York City. *AIDS: An International Bimonthly Journal.* Forthcoming.
4. Weiss, S. H.; Ginzburg, H. M.; Goedert, J. J.; et al. Risk for HTLV-III exposure and AIDS among parenteral drug abusers in New Jersey. Paper presented at the International Conference on the Acquired Immunodeficiency Syndrome (AIDS), Atlanta, 14–17 April 1985.
5. Robertson, J. R.; Bucknall, A. B. V.; Welsby, P. D., et al. Epidemic of AIDS related virus (HTLV-III/LAV) infection among intravenous drug users. *British Medical Journal* 292:527–529 (1986).
6. Angarano, G.; Pastore, G.; Monno, L., et al. Rapid spread of HTLV-III infection among drug addicts in Italy. *Lancet* ii:8467:1302 (1985).
7. Camprubi, J. SIDA: Prevalencia de la infeccion por la IVH en los ADVP: Situacion actual y posibilidades de la actuacion. *Comunidad y Drogas* 2:9–22 (1986).
8. Weiss, S. H., et al. Risk for HTLV-III exposure and AIDS among parenteral drug abusers in New Jersey.
9. Jesson, W., et al. Prevalence of anti-HTL-III in UK risk groups. *Lancet* i:155 (1986).
10. Ginzburg, H. NIDA. Personal communication, 1986.
11. Follett, E. A. C.; McIntyre, A.; O'Donnell, B. HTLV-III antibody in drug abusers in the west of Scotland: The Edinburgh connection. *Lancet* i:8478:446–447 (1986).

12. Des Jarlais, D. C.; Friedman, S. R.; Marmor, M.; Cohen, H.; Mildvan, D.; Yancovitz, S.; Mathur, U.; El-Sadr, W.; Spira, T. J.; Garber, J.; Beatrice, S. T.; Abdul-Quader, A. S.; Sotheran, J. L. Development of AIDS, HIV seroconversion, and co-factors for T4 cell loss in a cohort of intravenous drug users. *AIDS: A Bimonthly Journal*. Forthcoming.

13. Follett, E. A. C., et al. HTLV-III antibody in drug abusers in the west of Scotland.

14. Weiss, S. H., et al. Risk for HTLV-III exposure and AIDS among parenteral drug abusers in New Jersey.

15. Schoenbaum, E. E.; Selwyn, P. A.; Klein, R. S.; et al. Prevalence of and risk factors associated with HTLV-III/LAV antibodies among intravenous drug abusers in methadone programs in New York City. Paper presented at the International Conference on AIDS, Paris, 23–25 June 1986.

16. Marmor, M., et al. Risk factors for infection with human immunodeficiency virus among intravenous drug users in New York City.

17. Selwyn, P. A.; Cox, C. P.; Feiner, C., et al. Knowledge about AIDS and high-risk behavior among intravenous drug users in New York City. Paper presented at the International Conference on AIDS, Paris, 23–25 June 1986.

18. Chaisson, R. E., Moss, A. R.; Onishi, R.; Osmond, D.; Carlson, J. R. Human immuno-deficiency virus infection in heterosexual intravenous drug users in San Francisco. *American Journal of Public Health* 77:169–172 (1987).

19. New York City Department of Health. Personal communication, 1987.

20. Des Jarlais, D. C. Research design, drug use, and deaths: Cross study comparisons. In *Social and Medical Aspects of Drug Abuse*, edited by G. Serban, New York: Spectrum, 1984.

21. Goldstein, P. J.; Lipson, L.; Preble, E.; Sobel, I.; Miller, T.; Abbott, W.; Paige, W.; Soto, F. The marketing of street heroin in New York City. *Journal of Drug Issues* 14:553–566 (1984).

22. Friedman, S. R.; Des Jarlais, D. C.; Sotheran, J. L., et al. AIDS and self-organization among intravenous drug users. *International Journal of the Addictions*. Forthcoming.

23. Selwyn, P. A.; Cox, C. P.; Feiner, C.; Lipschutz, C.; Cohen, R. Knowledge about AIDS and high-risk behavior among intravenous drug abusers in New York City. Paper presented at the Annual Meeting of the American Public Health Association, Washington, D.C., 18 November 1985.

24. Des Jarlais, D. C.; Friedman, S. R.; Hopkins, W. Risk reduction for the Acquired Im-munodeficiency Syndrome among intravenous drug users. *Annals of Internal Medicine* 103:755–759 (1985).

25. Des Jarlais, D. C., and Hopkins, W. Free needles for intravenous drug users at risk for AIDS: Current developments in New York City. *New England Journal of Medicine* 313:23 (1985).

26. Coutinho, R. A. Preliminary results of AIDS studies among IVDA in Amsterdam. Paper presented at Workshop on Epidemiological Surveys on AIDS: Epidemiology of HIV Infections in Europe Spread among Intravenous Drug Users and the Heterosexual Population, Berlin, 12–14 November 1986.

27. Biernacki, P., and Feldman, H. Ethnographic observations of IV drug use practices that put users at risk for AIDS. Paper presented at the XV International Institute on the Prevention and Treatment of Drug Dependence, Amsterdam/Noordwijkerhout, the Netherlands, 6–11 April 1986.

28. Des Jarlais, D. C. Stages in the response of the drug abuse treatment system to the AIDS epidemic in New York City. *Journal of Drug Issues*. Forthcoming.

29. Kübler-Ross, E. *Living with Death and Dying*. New York: Simon and Schuster, 1981.

30. Selye, H. *The Stress of Life*. New York: MacMillan, 1978.

31. Friedman, S. R.; Des Jarlais, D. C.; Goldsmith, D. S. An overview of current AIDS prevention efforts aimed at intravenous drug users. *Journal of Drug Issues*. Forthcoming.

32. Des Jarlais, D. C., and Friedman S. R. AIDS prevention among intravenous drug users: Phases one and two. Forthcoming.

33. Des Jarlais, D. C.; Friedman, S. R.; Strug, D. AIDS among intravenous drug users: A socio-cultural perspective. In *The Social Dimensions of AIDS: Methods and Theory*, edited by D. A. Feldman, and T. A. Johnson. New York: Praeger, 1986.

34. Mauge, C. Personal communication, 1987.

35. Ancelle, R. Personal communication, 1986.

36. Brunet, J. B. WHO AIDS European Coordinating Center.

37. Des Jarlais, D. C., et al. AIDS among intravenous drug users: A socio-cultural perspective.

38. Kleinman, P. H. Personal communication, 1987.

39. Feldman, D. A. Personal communication, 1987.

40. Jackson, J. New Jersey Department of Health. Personal communication, 1987.

41. Buning, E. Amsterdam's drug policy and the prevention of AIDS. Paper presented at the Conference on AIDS in the Drug Abuse Community and Heterosexual Transmission, Newark, N.J., 31 March–1 April 1986.

42. Parry, A. Needle swop in Mesey. *Druglink, The Journal on Drug Misuse in Britain* 2(1):7 (1987).

43. Kleinman, P. H. Personal communication.

44. Feldman, D. A. Personal communication.

45. Jackson, J. Personal communication.

46. Frank, B.; Schmeidler, J.; Johnson, B.; Lipton, D. S. Seeking truth in heroin indicators: The case of New York City. *Drug and Alcohol Dependence* 3:345–358 (1978).

47. Des Jarlais, D. C., et al. AIDS among intravenous drug users: A socio-cultural perspective.

48. Schaps, E.; DiBartolo, R.; Churgin, S. *Primary Prevention Research: A Review of 127 Program Evaluations*. Walnut Creek, CA: Pyramid Project, Pacific Institute for Research and Evaluation, 1978.

49. Des Jarlais, D. C., Friedman, S. R.; Casriel, C.; Kott, A. AIDS and preventing initiation into intravenous (IV) drug use. Unpublished manuscript.

50. Des Jarlais, D. C., et al. Risk reduction for the Acquired Immunodeficiency Syndrome among intravenous drug users.

51. New York City Department of Health. Personal communication.

52. Stoneburner, R.; Guigli, P.; Kristal, A. Increasing mortality in intravenous drug users in New York City and its relationship to the AIDS epidemic: is there an unrecognized spectrum of HTLV-III/LAV-related disease? Paper presented at the International Conference on AIDS, Paris, 23–25 June 1986.

17
Hemophilia- and Transfusion-Associated AIDS

Terence Chorba and Bruce Evatt

INTRODUCTION

In 1981, the first cases of acquired immune deficiency syndrome (AIDS) in the United States were identified in male homosexuals[1] and intravenous drug abusers.[2] Because of the high incidence of hepatitis B generally observed in persons in both of these groups, hepatitis B was suggested as a model of transmission for an infectious etiologic agent. In 1982, the development of AIDS in persons who had received blood products added support to that model.[3] By the end of 1987, over 50,000 U.S. patients with AIDS were reported to the Centers for Disease Control (CDC).[4] In 1789 of these (506 persons with hemophilia and 1283 persons who were transfused with blood or blood products for other reasons), the principal risk factor for developing AIDS was transfusion with blood or blood products. Most of these persons underwent transfusions (1) before March 1983, when the U.S. Public Health Service guidelines regarding transfusions and donor-deferral were first implemented, or (2) before March 1985, when human immunodeficiency virus (HIV) antibody test kits were licensed for blood donation screening, or (3), in the case of persons with hemophilia, before the availability of heat-treated factor concentrates.

INFECTIOUS COMPLICATIONS OF TRANSFUSIONS

In 1943, Beeson first suggested an infectious etiology for cases of jaundice observed in patients within 4 months of transfusion with blood or plasma.[5] The list of infectious agents transmitted by blood now includes many bacterial and parasitic agents (Table 1) and numerous viruses. The transmission of different infectious agents by transfusion of blood products depends on the ability of laboratories to screen for infection, the biology of the infective organisms, the methods of blood component storage, and the application of inactivating procedures for infective agents. Both cellular and noncellular blood products have been associated with the transmission of several known viral agents, including cytomegalovirus (CMV), human parvovirus B19, hepatitis B virus, delta agent, and the virus(es) of non-A, non-B (NANB) hepatitis.[6-8] Another predominantly intracellular virus, Epstein-Barr virus (EBV), has been transmitted by fresh blood, platelets, and leukocyte transfusions but has not been observed in association with transfusion of fresh-frozen plasma or factor VIII or factor IX concentrates.[6] Consequently, most U.S. blood banks screen for hepatitis B surface antigen (HBsAg) and syphilis in addition to antibody assays for HIV and,

Table 1 Infectious agents transmitted by transfusion

Viruses	Treponemes
Cytomegalovirus	Syphilis
Delta agent	Parasites
Epstein-Barr virus	Babesiosis
Hepatitis A	Filariasis
Hepatitis B	Malaria
Hepatitis non-A, non-B	Toxoplasmosis
Human parvovirus B19	Trypanosomiasis
Human immunodeficiency virus	Bacteria
Human T-lymphotropic virus type I	Multiple organisms
Human T-lymphotropic virus type II (?)	

in the case of special pediatric units, CMV. In the United States, screening procedures taken to reduce the risk of transmitting infectious agents have limited significant transfusion-associated infections, and only hepatitis viruses and CMV still caused much concern for U.S. physicians before the retroviruses were identified.

The appearance and identification of the retroviruses have raised new concerns regarding the safety of the various blood products.[9] Cellular and noncellular blood products appear to carry divergent risks of infection with different retroviruses. HIV, the causative agent of AIDS, has been transmitted by transfusion of blood and of noncellular blood components, e.g., non-heat-treated factor concentrates, and by the exclusive use of cryoprecipitate.[10] Although human T-cell lymphotropic virus type I (HTLV-I) has been reported to be transmitted by transfusion of whole or cellular blood components, it may be much more difficult to transmit with cell-free blood products[11] transmission by transfusion with factor concentrates does not appear to occur.[12] The American Red Cross is currently conducting studies of blood samples from randomly selected donors in geographically divergent regions of the United States to determine if there is evidence of infection with HTLV-I in the U.S. blood donor population.[13] There is also now serologic evidence that blood-borne exposure may result in infection with HTLV-II, another retrovirus, for which no mode of transmission has definitively been described.[14] In 1986 a second retroviral strain (HIV-2) with biological properties similar to the prototype strain of HIV (HIV-I) was isolated from AIDS patients in West Africa. CDC and the Food and Drug Administration (FDA) initiated surveillance for HIV-2 in the United States in January 1987. In December 1987 the first reported case of AIDS caused by HIV-2 was diagnosed in a West African woman living in New Jersey.[15] As of September 1988 two other cases of HIV-2 had been identified in West African women residing in the United States (CDC, Dr. Scott Holmberg, personal communication). CDC and FDA surveillance for additional cases of HIV-2 infection in persons residing in the United States continues.

HIV INFECTION AND CELLULAR BLOOD PRODUCTS

In 1982, the first case of AIDS associated with a cellular blood product transfusion was reported.[16,17] The patient was a 20-month-old child who developed severe cellular immune deficiency and multiple opportunistic infections after receiving several blood component transfusions for hemolytic disease of the newborn (erythroblastosis fetalis). The occurrence of *Pneumocystis carinii* pneumonia in three adult transfusion recipients in mid-1982 strengthened the hypothesis that a potentially transfusable agent caused AIDS.[17] Investigations of other blood transfusion-related cases demonstrated a consistent pattern. For AIDS cases associated with cellular blood product transfusion, the male-to-female ratio approached 1:1, and the geographic distribution of cases resembled that of cases in the original two risk groups and was consistent with the source of the blood donations. All of the first 18 transfusion-associated AIDS cases without hemophilia occurred in persons who had received more than one type of blood product including packed cells, fresh-frozen plasma, whole blood, or platelet concentrates. Six of the first seven patients who developed transfusion-associated AIDS had at least one blood product donor from a group at increased risk for AIDS, and all seven were exposed to a donor subsequently found to have a decreased T-helper/T-suppressor lymphocyte ratio. Consequently, in March 1983, the Public Health Service recommended that members of groups at increased risk for AIDS or persons with symptoms suggestive of AIDS refrain from donating blood or plasma.

HTLV-I has limited antigenic cross-reactivity and genetic homology with HIV. In 1984, Jaffe et al. reported a higher prevalence of antibodies to the membrane antigens (MA) of cells infected with HTLV-I in serum of donors of blood to transfusion-associated AIDS patients than among a control group of blood donors.[18] These antibodies appear to have been directed against HIV-encoded glycoproteins that cross-react with HTLV-I antigens.[19] When HIV-antibody assays were developed, similar work was important in supporting the hypothesis that HIV causes AIDS and is potentially transmissible from an infected blood donor to a susceptible recipient.[20,21] Isolation of HIV from blood donor-recipient pairs confirmed that the etiologic agent was a retrovirus.

HIV has been isolated from at least one peripheral blood specimen in 67–95% of persons with specific antibodies to HIV.[22] Because HIV infection has been demonstrated in asymptomatic persons, presence of HIV antibodies is considered presumptive evidence of current infection and a potential carrier state. This hypothesis has received recent support from the work of Ou et al., who, by means of a selective DNA amplification technique called polymerase chain reaction (PCR), found HIV sequences in 64% of DNA specimens isolated from peripheral blood mononuclear cells of seropositive virus-culture negative men.[23] Surrogate laboratory tests have been evaluated to distinguish HIV-infected blood donors from noninfected blood donors, including T-helper/T-suppressor cell ratios, antibody to hepatitis B core antigen, alanine aminotransferase, and immune complexes, but the present assays for HIV antibodies are more sensitive and more specific.[24] The development of inexpensive, commercially available enzyme-linked immunosorbent assay (ELISA) kits for detecting the presence of antibodies to HIV has limited the risk of HIV transmission by blood transfusion. The Western blot assay for HIV has also proved effective in detecting the presence of antibodies to HIV but has not been easily adaptable for mass screening.[25] The more sensitive PCR technique may eventually be used to complement or replace viral isolation and antibody assays as a routine method for determining HIV infection.[23]

In January 1985, the CDC recommended that all blood used for transfusion or for the manufacture of blood products be screened for HIV. In March 1985, the Secretary of the Department of Health and Human Services (HHS) announced the licensure by the FDA of the ELISA test as an HIV screening test for use in blood and plasma centers. FDA has reported data from a survey of more than 2.5 million units of blood collected and tested for HIV antibodies by 155 centers from April to November 1985 using the licensed ELISA tests.[26] Of this total, 8443 units (0.34%) were repeatedly reactive for HIV antibodies. CDC and the Atlanta region of the American Red Cross also surveyed 67,190 blood donors of whom 171 (0.23%) were repeatedly reactive for HIV antibodies by ELISA.[27] Specimens from 150 of these repeatedly reactive units were tested at CDC; 45 (30%) demonstrated strong reactivity by ELISA; 38 (84%) of these 45 were also positive by Western blot; 40 of the 45 had lymphocyte cultures for HIV completed, and of those 40, 22 (55%) had positive cultures for HIV. One of 111 donors whose EIA tests were repeatedly reactive but subsequently negative on Western blot assay had a positive HIV culture. Of the 150 ELISA-positives, 40 (27%) were HIV-positive by Western blot or culture. If one conservatively assumes that these were the only true positives in this study, no more than 131 (0.19%) of the 67,190 units were falsely positive, which indicates a minimum calculated test specificity of 99.81%. There are now data indicating that most blood samples that are HIV antibody-positive by ELISA but negative by Western blot are false positives.[28] It is thought that the "false" reactivity may be directed against antigenic determinants of the H9 lymphoid cell line used to grow HIV for the ELISA.[29-32] Such cross-reactivity may be eliminated by recent technology.

The HIV ELISA appears to be quite sensitive. In persons attending a sexually transmitted diseases clinic in San Francisco, none of 70 high-risk men with negative HIV antibody tests had a positive HIV culture, whereas 43 (60%) of 72 with repeatedly positive tests had a positive HIV culture. Of these 72 antibody-positive individuals, all but two were highly reactive for HIV by ELISA, and 97% of those tested had a positive Western blot test for HIV.[33] Other trials of test performance in symptomatic HIV-infected persons conducted before licensure obtained a sensitivity of 95%,[34] but this may actually underestimate the true sensitivity, as persons with AIDS may lose detectable HIV antibodies.[35]

In March 1985, screening procedures were introduced by blood and plasma collection centers in the United States to decrease the transmission of HIV through transfusions. Potential donors are now informed that if they have a risk factor for HIV infection, they should not donate, and blood or plasma accepted from donors is screened for antibodies to HIV. Donor deferral recommendations also now include any man who has had sex with another man since 1977, including those who may have only had a single contact, and men or women who have engaged in prostitution since 1977 and persons who have been their heterosexual partners within 6 months. These categories were added because many individuals with confirmed positive HIV antibody tests had engaged in prostitution, were males who had sexual relations with another male, or were sexual contacts of homosexual males, bisexual males, or prostitutes.[36-38]

In 1985, 0.04% of U.S. blood donations were positive for HIV by Western blot assay.[37] Although the number of HIV-infected donors was probably lower in earlier years, if 0.04% of blood component units donated in the year prior to screening had been infected with HIV, then about 7200 of 18 × 10⁶ blood component units transfused in 1984 were potential vehicles for HIV transmission.[39] It is estimated that about 12,000 persons now living in the United States acquired a transfusion-associated HIV infection between 1978 and 1984.[40]

The risk of HIV transmission by blood transfusion in the United States was low, even before screening, and has been greatly reduced with the application of the ELISA test in the routine screening of donated blood and plasma and with the use of donor deferral criteria by blood banks. In the United States, blood banks try to obtain confirmation of ELISA reactive tests by using Western blot prior to notifying donors, and plasmapheresis facilities usually notify donors when a repeatedly reactive ELISA test result is obtained. At least 16 European nations have also developed HIV screening programs for donated blood and plasma.[32] However, a few new cases of transfusion-associated AIDS will continue to appear for several reasons: (1) A "window phase" of weeks to months exists between exposure to HIV and the subsequent detectability of antibodies by EIA. Some persons infected with HIV by transfusions before the availability of EIA methods may develop clinical symptoms and later progress to AIDS. Using mathematical modeling, the mean incubation period for transfusion-associated AIDS has been estimated to be 4.5 years, with a 90% confidence interval ranging from 2.6 to 14.2 years.[41] (2) The technology and biology of seroconversion may limit the sensitivity of detection methods. HIV transmission has been reported in a few cases by transfusion of infected units of blood negative for HIV antibodies by ELISA.[40,42] One of these donors appears to have had a recent infection through a single homosexual contact 3 months before blood donation, which demonstrates the importance of donor deferral strategies in excluding blood from high-risk and potentially recently infected donors who lack detectable HIV antibodies.[43] Current estimates are that 3–4% of infected potential donors will not have developed antibodies to HIV, because they are still in the "window phase."[38] Because antibody to the major core protein (p25) of HIV tends to appear before antibody to the envelope glycoprotein (p41), ELISA tests to the core protein may have an advantage over those to the envelope glycoprotein in terms of sensitivity. (3) As the virus disseminates into heterosexual populations, donor deferral programs will be hampered by lack of knowledge among donors who may not know that they have been exposed to the virus.

Clearly, means of virus inactivation and more sophisticated virus testing will be desirable. Improvements in the design and use of HIV antibody and antigen detection assays are inevitable.

HIV INFECTION AND CELL–FREE PRODUCTS

By the end of 1982, there was considerable evidence to indicate that transfused non-heat-treated factor VIII preparations could transmit HIV. AIDS cases had occurred in persons with hemophilia with no known risk factor other than transfusion with non-heat-treated factor VIII preparation. Hemophilia-associated AIDS cases initially occurred among persons who were heavy users of the factor VIII concentrate, and immune abnormalities were found to be associated with high usage of factor concentrate.[44] Unlike other transfusion-associated cases, the national distribution of hemophilia-associated AIDS cases was not related to the distribution of cases in other risk groups.

By September 1988, 740 cases of hemophilia-associated AIDS had been reported to the CDC. Of these, 649 (88%) had hemophilia A (factor VIII deficiency), 63 (8%) had hemophilia B (factor IX deficiency), 17 (3%) had Von Willebrand's disease, 11 (1.5%) had an acquired inhibitor of factor VIII or another factor deficiency as their primary coagulation disorder. The majority of the patients with hemophilia A had severe functional factor VIII deficiency (<1% factor activity). The number of reported cases of AIDS in persons with hemophilia represents an attack rate of about 5 per 100 of the 12,000–17,000 persons with hemophilia in the United States, with an incidence rate of about 1800 cases per 100,000 persons with hemophilia per year in 1987. AIDS now exceeds hemorrhage as the leading cause of mortality in the United States for persons with hemophilia.

As with AIDS patients whose risk factor was cellular blood product transfusion, in the laboratory a high prevalence of HTLV-MA antibodies was initially found in the sera of hemophilia patients treated with non-heat-treated factor concentrates.[45] When HIV antibody assays became available, seropositivity was demonstrated in the majority of asymptomatic persons with hemophilia,[46] and a temporal relationship was demonstrated between seroconversion among hemophilia patients and expansion of infection with HIV in the general population.[47] The first HIV exposure in persons with hemophilia in the United States appears to have been in 1979, soon after the first retrospectively identified U.S. AIDS cases developed. Most U.S. hemophilia A patients developed antibodies to HIV by 1983.[48–51] Similar seroconversion has been observed in hemophilia patients in the United Kingdom[52] and the Federal Republic of Germany.[53] In 1985, 92% of persons with hemophilia A and 52% of those with hemophilia B in a U.S. cohort had antibodies to HIV.[54] Data available from France for 1986 indicate seropositivity in 51% of persons with hemophilia A and 47% in persons with hemophilia B, which may reflect the fact that since 1980, most patients with hemophilia in France have been treated with domestic concentrate preparations.[55]

Previous exposure to allogeneic proteins and other infectious agents, HIV inoculum size, and differences in inoculum strain have all been proposed to explain differences in seroconversion intervals observed for hemophilia patients relative to other risk groups.[56,57] The kinetics of the development of serologic markers in the early stages of HIV infection that have been worked out in exposed hemophiliacs include detectable antigenemia as early as 2 weeks after exposure, followed within a month by development of antibodies to the viral envelope and then to the core protein.[58] One study suggests that most seroconversions in hemophilia patients would be detectable by or before 26 weeks.[59] The prognosis for seropositive persons with mild or no symptoms remains unknown, although in one study of 78 seropositive homosexual men followed over 4 years, 23 (29%) developed appreciable immunologic abnormalities, and nine (12%) were diagnosed with AIDS.[60] As for seropositive persons with symptoms, a recent CDC study of 75 seropositive homosexual men with lymphadenopathy demonstrated a 5-year cumulative AIDS incidence rate of 29%.[61] Although HIV has not been isolated from factor concentrate preparations, there is little doubt that factor concentrate provided the principal exposure to HIV among most patients with hemophilia. Unfortunately, HIV antibodies do not consistently convey significant neutralizing activity in serum, even when antibodies to viral membrane antigens are present in high titer.[62]

Most patients who receive multiple transfusions, such as persons with hemophilia, thalassemia, or sickle cell disease, have abnormalities of cellular immunity similar to those of AIDS patients. Commonly they have an alteration in the numbers and proportion of T-lymphocyte subsets with a decrease in the T-helper/T-suppressor cell ratio, decreased in vitro lymphocyte responses to antigens and mitogens, and increased levels of circulating immunoglobulin.[63,64] Because these patients are repeatedly exposed by their therapy to a variety of viral infections, including hepatitis B and NANB hepatitis, it is possible that infection with these viruses may account for some of the observed immunologic abnormalities. It has also been proposed that the antigenic load of transfused proteins may also be contributory to a dysregulation of the immune system.[64]

HIV Inactivation Studies

The development of AIDS in persons in the absence of known risk factors or exposures other than the use of non-heat-treated factor VIII concentrates implicated such preparations as potential vehicles of HIV transmission. Any given lot of commercially prepared factor VIII concentrate may contain plasma from between 2500 and 25,000 blood or plasma donors;[65] if not heat-treated, the concentrate could present the patient with a greater chance of exposure to an infectious agent than would cryoprecipitate, which is a clotting factor-containing product obtained from one or only a few persons. However, HIV is very heat labile, and when added to lyophilized antihemophilic factor and the mixture is heated to 60°C, 90% of HIV is inactivated in about 30 min.[66] Heat treatment of factor concentrates in lyophilized form for 30 h at 60°C inactivates HIV without significantly altering the plasma recovery or plasma half-life.[67,68] There are some variations in heat treatment procedures used by different manufacturers: one manufacturer applies heat to lyophilized concentrate suspended in the organic solvent n-heptane; another heats the concentrate earlier in the moistened state (commonly referred to as "wet" heating).[68]

Several studies have documented a lack of HIV seroconversion in hemophilia patents treated with U.S. heat-treated factor VIII concentrates, indicating that proper heat treatment should reduce the potential risk of HIV transmission.[69-71] However, concern has been raised that in some circumstances, heat treatment may fail to inactivate HIV. There have been reports of prolonged HIV seroconversion in several hemophilia patients treated strictly with heat-treated intermediate- and/or high-purity factor VIII concentrate from a single manufacturer.[72-73] At least 18 reports of HIV seroconversion have met CDC's operational criteria for probable association with heat-treated factor concentrates.[74] Ten of the 18 cases meeting the CDC criteria occurred before initiation of donor screening. The other eight patients had received donor-screened factor concentrates that were heat treated in lyophilized form at 60°C for 30 h ("dry" heating). All eight of these had received nonscreened products at some time, but the timing of the seroconversion implicated the donor-screened, heat-treated product. However, estimates for the present annual incidence rate of HIV seroconversion associated with donor-screened, virus-inactivated, clotting-factor products are less than 1 per 1000.[74] In a 2 1/2 yr study of 1489 European patients who received approximately 75 million units of American- or European-manufactured, virus-inactivated, donor-tested factor concentrates, none have seroconverted.[74]

No HIV seroconversion has yet been reported among hemophilia patients who have used or are using only donor-screened, heat-treated products, but the transition to donor-screened, heat-treated factor therapy has been recent, and longitudinal studies are under way to substantiate the additional margin of safety provided by HIV screening of plasma used in the manufacture of factor concentrates.[56]

Monoclonal antibody technology is currently being used to produce a factor VIII concentrate that is 1000–3000 times purer than most factor VIII preparations have been, by precipitating out monoclonal antibody/factor VIII/von Willebrand factor complexes. This procedure alone, before heat treatment, results in marked reduction of virus quantities. The resultant product is currently being given to hemophilia patients on an experimental basis.[75] A similar, highly purified factor IX preparation is also being developed.

A major shortcoming of heat treatment methods used in preparing factor concentrates has been failure to eliminate NANB hepatitis viruses. NANB hepatitis and chronic liver disease are serious problems for persons treated with factor concentrates.[76–79] Investigators are exploring alternative ways of virus inactivation aimed specifically at NANB hepatitis that may also help further reduce any possibility of HIV surviving the inactivation process. Ultraviolet light and beta propriolactone (BPL) together will inactivate virus.[68] BPL-treated factor IX prothrombin-complex concentrates are commercially available in Europe. Since BPL causes extensive protein denaturation, reduced yields of clotting factor have somewhat discouraged interest in this method.[80] Other investigators have shown the ability of tri-N-butyl phosphate (TNBP) plus detergents to inactivate viruses having lipid-containing envelopes; the added agents are removed from the processed proteins using chromatographic methods. This method appears to be useful for HIV, hepatitis B virus, and one strain of NANB hepatitis virus.[68] Another process in which factor VIII concentrate is heated in the presence of glycine and sucrose in solution at 60°C for 10 h before final lyophilization has also yielded a promising, clinically effective concentrate; no evidence of hepatitis or serologic evidence of infection with hepatitis B, hepatitis A, CMV, EBV, or HIV was found in 26 seronegative hemophilia patients who were treated only with this concentrate preparation and followed over a period of 12 months.[81]

Immune Globulin Preparations

Since April 1985, all donor units used in making immune globulin products have been screened for antibodies to HIV, and all repeatedly reactive units have been discarded. Immune globulin preparations—e.g., immune globulin (IG), hepatitis B immune globulin (HBIG), intravenous immune globulin (IVIG), and Rho (D) immunoglobulin (RhoGAM)—have not been implicated in transmission of HIV or other infectious agents when produced by plasma fractionation methods approved for use in the United States.[82] Several studies have evaluated recipients of HBIG and IG, including recipients of lots subsequently found to be positive for HIV antibodies.[82,83] Transient low levels of passively acquired HIV antibodies have been detected after receiving immune globulin preparations that were strongly positive for HIV antibodies,[84] but long-term seroconversion to HIV antibody positivity and/or development of signs or symptoms suggestive of HIV infection in persons receiving IG, HBIG, and IVIG has not been observed.[85] HIV seropositivity has been observed in one HBIG recipient of 183 recipients of IG and/or HBIG who were enrolled in long-term CDC follow-up studies of persons with needle-stick exposures since August 1983. No preexposure serum was available for this individual, and seroconversion may have occurred before the needle-stick exposure and prophylaxis.[82] Current epidemiologic and laboratory evidence indicates that these preparations carry no discernible risk of transmitting HIV, even if manufactured before 1985, when preparations were derived from plasma of donors who were not screened for HIV. The current indications for the clinical use of immune globulin preparations should not be altered because of concerns for HIV exposure.

It has been estimated that plasma of HIV-infected persons contains less than 100 in vitro infectious units (IVIU)/ml.[82] In one study, the geometric mean titer in plasma from 43 HIV-infected persons was 0.02 IVIU/ml.[86] The standard fractionation processes[87,88] used in producing immune globulins result in HIV removal of more than 1×10^{15} IVIU/ml and thus appear to provide a considerable margin of safety with respect to removal of infectious HIV.[82]

Hepatitis B Vaccine

There has been concern that the hepatitis B vaccine might transmit HIV, because the plasma-derived vaccine is manufactured from pooled plasma of persons who are chronic carriers of hepatitis B and may be in high-risk groups for AIDS. This preparation is a suspension of inactivated HBsAg particles purified from the plasma. Inactivation is a threefold process using 8 M urea, pepsin at pH 2, and 1:4000 formalin. Studies have demonstrated inactivation of human retroviruses and representatives of all other known virus classes by the inactivation steps routinely used in the vaccine manufacturing process,[89,90] and epidemiologic data have corroborated the lack of transmission of HIV or any other known human pathogen by the vaccine.[89] A nonplasma-derived yeast-recombinant hepatitis B vaccine was recently licensed by the FDA and is now available.[91] It appears to be as effective as the plasma-derived vaccine in preventing hepatitis B infection and the chronic carrier state, and its method of manufacture obviates concerns about HIV transmission.

NEW CONSIDERATIONS FOR TRANSFUSION

The use of blood and blood products in the United States has declined significantly since 1982, in large part reflecting more judicious use of transfusion therapy by physicians. Health care providers are now much more aware of the importance of using substitutes for blood where feasible, such as crystalloid solutions, synthetic colloids, or albumin, if circulatory volume expansion is indicated.

There is uniform agreement that autologous blood transfusion is the safest form of cellular blood transfusion therapy,[92] provided the recommendations of the AMA Council on Scientific Affairs[93] and the American Association of Blood Banks standards[94] are observed; this practice has been endorsed by the American Medical Association and the American Red Cross. The American Blood Resources Association recommends that blood banks and blood centers "make this option available to all qualified healthy people with a scheduled elective operation, simplify the donation process to the extent possible, and inform physicians and patients about the advantages and mechanics of this approach."

Autologous transfusion can be achieved either (1) through predonation, that is, donation of the required amount of blood by the patient before surgery, or

(2) through intraoperative salvage. In addition to completely eliminating the risk of HIV transmission, it averts the risks of transfusion reactions and alloimmunization. Autologous transfusion of blood donated prior to surgery can be achieved with liquid products, and storage can be extended up to 42 days with additive solutions. With a 3-week lead time, most patients given oral iron therapy can predeposit two or three units of blood.[92]

More problematic is the freezing of blood for persons with no foreseen need for transfusion. With increasing demand due to fear of AIDS or HIV infection, it is feared that this practice will reduce the number of blood donors available to the general community,[95] even though FDA regulations permit frozen storage for only 3 years. Whereas at least 1000 U.S. hospitals and almost all of the 200 regional blood centers in the United States now offer autologous predonation and transfusion services,[92] blood-banking organizations do not endorse the practice of donor designation—i.e., where a potential recipient designates specific donors other than himself. The contention is that this practice would complicate blood storage procedures, reduce the pool of donated blood, and create the appearance of a double standard of quality in blood sources.[96]

Heat-treated material from HIV-screened donors remains the recommended therapy for clotting factor replacement at present. Future methods of viral inactivation will eliminate the present concerns with HIV infection and NANB hepatitis.

RECOMBINANT FACTOR CONCENTRATES

The gene for factor VIII has been isolated and cloned.[97–99] It is 186,000 nucleotides long. The coding information for circulating factor VIII is spread among 26 separate coding blocks (exons). DNA clones encoding the complete 2351-amino acid sequence for human factor VIII have been isolated.[97] The extreme length of the gene and the necessity for extensive posttranslational modification discouraged the use of recombinant bacteria in manufacturing this protein. Initial attempts to produce the protein in vitro have necessitated using cultured mammalian cells, and the resulting recombinant factor VIII has many immunological characteristics of serum-derived factor VIII. It also has full activity in that it corrects the defect caused by the missing protein in hemophiliac plasma. In hemophiliac dogs, the recombinant product circulates with a half-life similar to that of native factor VIII. Clinical trials of this recombinant product began in March 1987.[100] The gene in factor IX has also been cloned, and several groups are trying to develop a bioengineered factor IX product.[85,101]

RISKS OF HIV TRANSMISSION

Heterosexual transmission of AIDS in the United States has primarily been from men to their female partners.[32] Possible risk to hemophilia patients' family members was first considered following the development of AIDS in the wife of a hemophilia patient who subsequently developed AIDS[102] and in a child of an HIV antibody-positive hemophilia patient.[103] In two studies, three (10%) of 30 sexual partners of hemophilia patients in 1984 had antibodies to HIV, acquired presumably through exposure by intimate contact.[104,105] As of September 1988, 25 female sexual partners of male hemophiliacs, one male sexual partner of a woman with coagulopathy, and six children born to women who were sexual partners of hemophilic males had developed AIDS. This growing secondary epidemic has a similar epidemic curve to that of the primary epidemic that was first recognized four years earlier.[106]

The risk of transmission to family members (other than those who are sexual contacts or exposures that occur in utero) appears to be small, as demonstrated by the absence of antibodies to HIV in family members of hemophilia patients other than sexual partners, children born to hemophilia patients after the start of the epidemic, or persons who had HIV infection acquired outside the household. Several studies of family members of HIV-infected patients have found no HIV transmission to adults who were not sexual contacts of the infected patients or to older children who were not subject to perinatal transmission.[105,107-109] There is still no evidence of transmission by arthropods[110] or by close contact[109] other than intimate sexual or blood exposures.

Because HIV-infected persons are at risk for developing AIDS or related conditions themselves and may transmit HIV to others, the U.S. Public Health Service has recommended that physicians should consider offering HIV antibody testing to some patients who received transfusions between 1978 and late spring of 1985, based on the likelihood of infection in a recipient and the likelihood of potential HIV transmission to others, especially if the patient is sexually active.[39] In addition, some blood collection agencies in the United States have begun notifying hospitals that have received units of blood from donors who were later found to be positive for HIV, for the purposes of identifying and counseling some recipients who may have been exposed.

Although public awareness of the potential modes of HIV transmission has continued to increase, the importance of education and counseling remains paramount. In a multicenter study conducted in 1985 by the CDC and the National Hemophilia Foundation, adult patients with hemophilia recognized the risks of HIV infection for themselves and their sex partners less than they recognized the risk for persons in other risk groups.[111] The Mental Health Committee of the National Hemophilia Foundation (NHF) has issued specific recommendations for counseling hemophiliacs and their sexual partners regarding intimacy and sexual behavior.[112] The use of condoms and the avoidance of rectal intercourse are recommended for hemophiliacs and their sexual partners. For uninfected individuals likely to have continued sexual exposure to HIV, the use of condoms is recommended based on data that indicate that condoms are effective barriers to viruses, including HIV,[113] and on data that suggest that sexual partners of persons infected with HIV may be protected by the use of condoms.[107]

RECOMMENDATIONS FOR PREVENTION

As of September 1988 the recommendations of the Public Service for reducing potential risk of transmitting HIV by transfusion, transplantation, other parenteral exposure, or artificial insemination[36,74,114-119] include:

1. Blood and/or plasma donation by persons in high-risk groups for AIDS should be deferred. Persons at increased risk also include sexual partners of persons at high risk, prostitutes and their sexual contacts, and persons with positive tests. These persons should not donate body organs, other tissues, or semen regardless of the result of antibody testing.

2. All donated blood and plasma, and blood or serum from donors of organs, tissues, or semen intended for human use, should be appropriately screened for HIV antibodies.

3. Blood or plasma that is reactive for HIV should not be transfused or used for manufacture into injectable products capable of transmitting infectious agents.

4. Devices that have punctured the skin should be safely discarded or sterilized by autoclave before reuse, and whenever possible, disposable needles and equipment should be used.

5. Desmopressin (DDAVP®) should be used whenever possible by patients with mild or moderate hemophilia A. When feasible, an alternative to concentrates may be cryoprecipitate prepared from one well-screened and repeatedly tested donor or from a small number of such donors.

6. Clotting factor concentrates that are heated in aqueous solution (pasteurized), treated with solvent/detergent, purified with monoclonal antibody, heated in suspension in organic media, or dry heated at high temperatures for long periods are preferred. These products are at substantially reduced risk of transmitting HIV.

7. For patients with severe factor IX deficiency, NHF continues to recommend the use of virus-inactivated factor IX concentrate. For patients with mild or moderate factor IX deficiency, when feasible, an alternative would be fresh, frozen plasma prepared from one well-screened and repeatedly tested donor or from a small number of such donors.

Other interventions for the prevention of HIV infection and AIDS include the avoidance of unprotected sexual contact and of needle sharing with HIV infected persons.

In summary, until a cure is found or a vaccine becomes available, the principal modes of preventing spread of HIV must be behavioral restraint, appropriate use of barrier methods, and proper transfusion practices.

REFERENCES

1. Centers for Disease Control. Kaposi's sarcoma and *Pneumocystis* pneumonia among homosexual men—New York City and California. MMWR 1981;30:305–308.

2. Wormser GP, Krupp LB, Hanrahan JP, et al. Acquired immunodeficiency syndrome in male prisoners. New insights into an emergency syndrome. Ann Intern Med 1983;98:297–303.

3. Centers for Disease Control. *Pneumocystis carinii* pneumonia among persons with hemophilia A. MMWR 1982;31:365–367.

4. Centers for Disease Control. Acquired immunodeficiency syndrome (AIDS) weekly surveillance report—United States, September 5, 1988, p. 1.

5. Beeson PB. Jaundice occurring one to four months after transfusion of blood or plasma: Report of seven cases. JAMA 1943;121:1332–1334.

6. Soulier JP. Diseases transmitted by blood transfusion. Vox Sang 1984;47:1–6.

7. Enck RE, Betts RF, Brown MR, et al. Viral serology (hepatitis B virus, cytomegalovirus, Epstein-Barr virus) and abnormal liver function tests in transfused patients with hereditary hemorrhagic diseases. Transfusion 1979;19:32.

8. Mortimer PP, Luban NLC, Kelleher JF, et al. Transmission of serum parvovirus-like virus by clotting factor concentrates. Lancet 1983;ii:482–484.

9. Sandler SG. HTLV-I and -II: New risks for recipients of blood transfusions? JAMA 1986;256:2245–2246.

10. Centers for Disease Control. Changing patterns of acquired immunodeficiency syndrome in hemophilia patients—United States. MMWR 1985;34:241–243.

11. Okochi K, Sato H, Hinuma Y. A retrospective study on transmission of adult T cell leukemia virus by blood transfusion: Seroconversion in recipients. Vox Sang 1984;46:245–253.

12. Chorba TL, Jason JM, Ramsey RB, et al. HTLV-I antibody status in hemophilia patients treated with factor concentrates prepared from U.S. plasma sources and in hemophilia patients with AIDS. Thromb Haemostas 1985;53:180–182.

13. American Red Cross. The Red Cross studies HTLV-I among blood donors. Blood Services Bull 1986;19:23.

14. Robert-Guroff M, Weiss SH, Giron JA, et al. Prevalence of antibodies to HTLV-I, -II, and -III in intravenous drug abusers from an AIDS endemic region. JAMA 1986;255:3133–3137.

15. Centers for Disease Control. AIDS due to HIV-2 infection—New Jersey. MMWR 1988; 37:33–35.

16. Ammann AJ, Cowan MJ, Wara DW, et al. Acquired immunodeficiency in an infant: Possible transmission by means of blood products. Lancet 1983;i:956–958.

17. Curran JW, Lawrence DN, Jaffe HW, et al. Acquired imunodeficiency syndrome (AIDS) associated with transfusions. N Engl J Med 1984;310:69–75.

18. Jaffe HW, Francis DP, McLane MF, et al. Transfusion-associated AIDS: Serologic evidence of human T-cell leukemia virus infection of donors. Science 1984;223:1309–1312.

19. Groopman JE, Salahuddin SZ, Sarngadharan MG, et al. Virologic studies in a case of transfusion-associated AIDS. N Engl J Med 1984;311:1419–1422.

20. Feorino PM, Kalyanaraman VS, Haverkos HW, et al. Lymphadenopathy associated virus infection of a blood donor-recipient pair with acquired immunodeficiency syndrome. Science 1984;225:69–72.

21. Jaffe HW, Sarngadharan MG, DeVico AL, et al. Infection with HTLV-III/LAV and transfusion-associated acquired immunodeficiency syndrome. JAMA 1985;254:770–773.

22. Feorino PM, Jaffe HW, Palmer E, et al. Transfusion-associated acquired immunodeficiency syndrome: Evidence for persistent infection in blood donors. N Engl J Med 1985;312:1293–1296.

23. Ou C–Y, Kwok S, Mitchell SW, et al. DNA amplification for direct detection of HIV-1 in DNA of peripheral blood mononuclear cells. Science 1988;239:295–297.

24. McDougal JS, Jaffe HW, Cabradilla CD, et al. Screening tests for blood donors presumed to have transmitted the acquired immunodeficiency syndrome. Blood 1985;65:772–775.

25. Carlson JR, Bryant ML, Hinrichs SH, et al. AIDS serology testing in low- and high-risk groups. JAMA 1985;253:3405–3408.

26. Kuritsky JN, Rastogi SC, Faich GA, et al. Results of nationwide screening of blood and plasma for antibodies to human T-lymphotropic III virus, type III. Transfusion 1986;26:205–207.

27. Ward JW, Grindon AJ, Feorino PM, et al. Laboratory and epidemiologic evaluation of an enzyme immunoassay for antibodies to HTLV-III. JAMA 1986;256:357–361.

28. Fang CT, Darr F, Kleinman S. Relative specificity of enzyme-linked immunosorbent assays for antibodies to human T-cell lymphotropic virus, type III, and their relationship to Western blotting. Transfusion 1986;26:208–209.

29. Hunter JB, Menitove JE. HLA antibodies detected by ELISA HTLV-III antibody kits. Lancet 1985;ii:397.

30. Sayers MH, Beatty PG, Hansen JA. HLA antibodies as a cause of false-positive reactions in screening enzyme imunoassays for antibodies to human T-lymphotropic virus type III. Transfusion 1986;26:113.

31. Peterman TA, Lang GR, Mikos NJ, et al. HTLV-III/LAV infection in hemodialysis centers. JAMA 1986;255:2324–2326.

32. Peterman TA. Transfusion-associated acquired immunodeficiency syndrome. World J Surg 1987;11:36–40.

33. Food and Drug Administration. Progress on AIDS. FDA Drug Bull 1985;15:27–32.

34. Marwick C. Use of AIDS antibody test may provide more answers. JAMA 1985;253:1694–1699.

35. Sarngadharan MG, Popovic M, Bruch L, et al. Antibodies reactive with human T-lymphotropic retroviruses (HTLV-III) in the serum of patients with AIDS. Science 1984;224:506–508.

36. Centers for Disease Control. Testing donors of organs, tissues, and semen for antibody to human T-lymphotropic virus type III/lymphadenopathy-associated virus. MMWR 1985;34:294.

37. Schorr JB, Berkowitz A, Cumming PD, et al. Prevalance of HTLV-III antibody in American blood donors. N Engl J Med 1985;313:384–385.

38. Anon. FDA revises donor screening guidelines; recommends confidential unit exclusion. Council of Community Blood Centers Newsletter, October 31, 1986.

39. Centers for Disease Control. Human immunodeficiency virus infection in transfusion recipients and their family members. MMWR 1987;36:137–140.

40. Peterman TA, Lui KJ, Lawrence DN, Allen JR. Estimating the risks of transfusion-associated acquired immune deficiency syndrome and human immunodeficiency virus infection. Transfusion 1987;27:371–374.

41. Lui KJ, Lawrence DN, Morgan WM, et al. A model-based approach for estimating the mean incubation period of transfusion-associated acquired immunodeficiency syndrome. Proc Natl Acad Sci USA 1986;83:3051–3055.

42. Zuch T. Greetings—with comments on lessons learned this past year from HIV antibody testing and from counseling blood donors. (Editorial.) Transfusion 1986;26:493.

43. Centers for Disease Control. Transfusion-associated human T-lymphotropic virus type III/lymphadenopathy-associated virus infection from a seronegative donor—Colorado. MMWR 1986;35:389–391.

44. Tsoukas C, Gervais F, Fuks A, et al. Immunologic dysfunction in patients with classic hemophilia receiving lyophilized factor VIII concentrates and cryoprecipitate. Can Med Assoc J 1983;129:713–717.

45. Evatt BL, Stein SF, Francis, DP, et al. Antibodies to human T cell leukemia virus-associated membrane antigens in haemophiliacs: Evidence for infection before 1980. Lancet 1983;i:698–701.

46. Ramsey RB, Palmer EL, McDougal JS, et al. Antibody to lymphadenopathy-associated virus in haemophiliacs with and without AIDS. Lancet 1984;i:397–398.

47. Evatt BL, Gomperts ED, McDougal JS, et al. Coincidental appearance of LAV/HTLV-III antibodies in hemophliacs and the onset of the AIDS epidemic. N Engl J Med 1985;312:483–486.

48. Knutsen AP, Bouhasin JD, Lawrence DN, et al. Time relationship of immune changes to HTLV-III/LAV seroconversion in patients with hemophilia. Ann Allergy 1986;57:376–384.

49. Eyster ME, Goedert JJ, Sarngadharan MG, et al. Development and early natural history of HTLV-III antibodies in persons with hemophilia. JAMA 1985;253:2219–2223.

50. Evatt BL, Gomperts ED, McDougal JS, Ramsey RB. Coincidental appearance of LAV/HTLV-III antibodies in hemophiliacs and the onset of the AIDS epidemic. N Engl J Med 1985;321:483–486.

51. Lederman MM, Ratnoff OD, Evatt BL, McDougal JS. Acquisition of antibody to lymphadenopathy-associated virus in patients with classic hemophilia (factor VIII deficiency). Ann Intern Med 1985;102:753–757.

52. Machin SJ, McVerry BA, Cheingson-Popov R, Tedder RS. Seroconversion for HTLV-III since 1980 in British haemophiliacs. Lancet 1985;ii:336.

53. Gurtler LG, Wernicke D, Eberle J, et al. Increase in prevalence of anti-HTLV-III in haemophiliacs. Lancet 1984;ii:1275–1276.

54. Jason J, Holman RC, Kennedy MS, et al. Longitudinal assessment of hemophiliacs exposed to HTLV-III/LAV. In: Program and Abstracts of the 26th Interscience Conference on Antimicrobial Agents and Chemotherapy, New Orleans, Louisiana, Abstract 97, 1986.

55. Allain J-P. Prevalence of HTLV-III/LAV antibodies in patients with hemophilia and in their sexual partners in France. N Engl J Med 1986;315:517.

56. Centers for Disease Control. Survey of non-U.S. hemophilia treatment centers for HIV seroconversions following therapy with heat-treated factor concentrates. MMWR 1987;36:121–124.

57. Ho DD, Sarngadharan MG, Resnick L, et al. Primary human T-lymphotropic virus type III infection. Ann Intern Med 1985;103:880–883.

58. Allain J-P, Laurian Y, Paul DA, et al. Serological markers in early stages of human immunodeficiency virus infection in haemophiliacs. Lancet 1986;ii:1233–1236.

59. Ludlam CA, Tucker J, Steel CM, et al. Human T-lymphotropic virus type III (HTLV-III) infection in seronegative haemophiliacs after transfusion of factor VIII. Lancet 1985;ii:233–236.

60. Taylor JMG, Schwartz K, Detels R. The time from infection with human immunodeficiency virus (HIV) to the onset of AIDS. J Infect Dis 1986;154:694–697.

61. Kaplan JE, Spira TJ, Fishbein DB, et al. Lymphadenopathy syndrome in homosexual men. JAMA 1987;257:335–337.

62. Weiss RA, Clapham PR, Cheingsong-Popov R, et al. Neutralization of human T-lymphotropic virus type III by sera of AIDS and AIDS-risk patients. Nature 1985;316:69–72.

63. Gascon P, Zoumbos NC, Young NS. Immunologic abnormalities in patients receiving multiple blood transfusions. Ann Intern Med 1984;100:173–177.

64. Jason J, Hilgartner MW, Holman RC, et al. Immune status of blood product recipients. JAMA 1985;253:1140–1145.

65. Levine P. AIDS in individuals with hemophilia. Ann Intern Med 1985;103:723–726.

66. McDougal JS, Martin LS, Cort SP, et al. Thermal inactivation of the AIDS virus, HTLV-III/LAV, with special reference to antihemophilic factor. J Clin Invest 1985;76:875–877.

67. Heldebrant CM, Gomperts ED, Kasper CK, et al. Evaluation of two viral inactivation methods for the preparation of safer factor VIII and factor IX concentrates. Transfusion 1985;25:510–515.

68. Gomperts ED. Procedures for the inactivation of virus in clotting factor concentrates. Am J Hematol 1986;23:295–305.

69. Rouzioux C, Chamaret S, Montagnier L, et al. Absence of antibodies to AIDS virus in haemophiliacs treated with heat-treated factor VIII concentrates. Lancet 1985;ii:271–272.

70. Mosseler J, Schimpf K, Auerswald G, et al. Inability of pasteurized factor VIII preparations to induce antibodies to HTLV-III after long-term treatment. Lancet 1985;i:1111.

71. Felding P, Nilsson IM, Hansson BG, et al. Absence of antibodies to LAV/HTLV-III in haemophiliacs treated with heat-treated factor VIII concentrate of American origin. Lancet 1985;ii:832–833.

72. Van den berg W, ten Cate JW, Breederveld C, et al. Seroconversion to HTLV-III in haemophiliac given heat-treated factor VIII concentrate. Lancet 1986;i:803–804.

73. White GC, Matthews TJ, Weinhold KJ, et al. HTLV-III seroconversion associated with heat-treated factor VIII concentrate. Lancet 1986;i:611–612.

74. Centers for Disease Control. Safety of therapeutic products used for hemophilia patients. MMWR 1988;37:441–444, 449–450.

75. Terry WD. New methods for purifying factor VIII. National Hemophilia Foundation Newsnotes, September 1986, p. 14.

76. Colombo M, Mannucci PM, Carnelli V, et al. Transmission of non-A, non-B hepatitis by heat-treated factor VIII concentrate. Lancet 1985;ii:1–4.

77. Mannucci PM, Capitaneo A, DelNinno E, et al. Asymptomatic liver disease in haemophiliacs. J Clin Pathol 1975;28:620.

78. Aledort LM, Levine PH, Hilgartner M, et al. A study of liver biopsies and liver disease among haemophiliacs. Blood 1985;66:367–372.

79. Hay CRM, Preston FE, Triger DR, Underwood JCE. Progressive liver disease in haemophilia: An understated problem? Lancet 1985;i:1495–1498.

80. Prince AM, Horowitz B, Brotman B. Sterilisation of hepatitis and HTLV-3 viruses by exposure to tri (n-butyl) phosphate and sodium cholate. Lancet 1986;i:706–710.

81. Schimpf K, Mannucci PM, Kreutz W, et al. Absence of hepatitis after treatment with a pasteurized factor VIII concentrate in patients with hemophilia and no previous transfusions. N Engl J Med 1987;316:918–922.

82. Centers for Disease Control. Safety of therapeutic immune globulin preparations with respect to transmission of human T-lymphotropic virus type III/lymphadenopathy-associated virus infection. MMWR 1986;35:231–233.

83. Tedder RS. Uttley A, Cheingsong-Popov R. Safety of immunoglobulin preparation containing anti-HTLV-III. Lancet 1985;i:815.

84. Piszkiewicz D. HTLV-III antibodies after immune globulin. JAMA 1987;257:316.

85. Jaye M, De la Salle H, Schamber F, et al. Isolation of a human anti-haemophilic factor IX cDNA using a unique 52-base synthetic oligonucleotide probe deduced from the amino acid sequence of bovine factor IX. Nucleic Acids Res 1983;11:2325–2335.

86. Wells MA, Wittek A, Marcus-Sekura C, et al. Chemical and physical inactivation of human T lymphotropic virus, type III (HTLV-III). Transfusion 1986;26:110–130.

87. Cohn EJ, Strong LE, Hughes WL Jr, et al. Preparation and properties of serum and plasma proteins. IV. A system for the separation into fractions of protein and lipoprotein components of biological tissues and fluids. J Am Chem Soc 1946;68:459–475.

88. Oncley JL, Melin M, Richert DA, et al. The separation of the antibodies isagglutinins, prothrombin, plasmonogen and beta-lipoprotein into subfractions of human plasma. J Am Chem Soc 1949;71:541–550.

89. Centers for Disease Control. Hepatitis B vaccine: Evidence confirming lack of AIDS transmission. MMWR 1984;33:685–687.

90. Gerety RJ. U.S. licensed hepatitis B vaccine; regulatory perspective. In: Overby LR et al. (eds). Viral Hepatitis: Second International Max von Pettenkoffer Symposium. New York: Marcel Dekker, 1983.

91. Stevens CE, Taylor PE, Tong MJ, et al. Yeast-recombinant hepatitis B vaccine. Efficacy with hepatitis B immune globulin in prevention of perinatal hepatitis B virus transmission. JAMA 1987;257:2612–2616.

92. Surgenor DMN. The patient's blood is the safest blood. N Engl J Med 1987;316:542–544.
93. Council on Scientific Affairs. Autologous blood transfusions. JAMA 1986;256:2378–2380.
94. Oberman HA (ed.) Standards for Blood Banks and Transfusion Services, 11th ed. Washington, D.C.: American Association of Blood Banks, 1986.
95. Greenwalt TJ. Autologous and aged blood donors. JAMA 1987;257:1220–1221.
96. Matthews GW, Neslund VS. The initial impact of AIDS on public health law in the United States—1986. JAMA 1987;257:344–352.
97. Wood WI, Capon, DJ, Simonsen CC, et al. Expression of active human factor VIII from recombinant DNA clones. Nature 1984;312:330–336.
98. Vehar GA, Keyt B, Eton D, et al. Structure of human factor VIII. Nature 1984;312:337–342.
99. Toole JJ, Knopf JL, Wozney JM, et al. Molecular cloning of a cDNA encoding human antihaemophilic factor. Nature 1984;312:342–347.
100. Roberts HR, Macik BG. Factor VIII and XI concentrates: Clinical efficacy as related to purity. In: Verstracte M et al. (eds). Thrombosis and Haemostasis 1987. Leuven: Leuven University Press, 1987, pp. 563–581.
101. Kurachi K, Davie EW. Isolation and characterization of a cDNA coding for human factor IX. Proc Natl Acad Sci USA 1982;79:6461–6464.
102. Pitchenik AE, Shafron RD, Glasser RM, Spira TJ. The acquired immunodeficiency syndrome in the wife of a hemophiliac. Ann Intern Med 1984;100:62–65.
103. Ragni MV, Urbach AH, Kiernan S, et al. Acquired immunodeficiency syndrome in the child of a haemophiliac. Lancet 1985;i:133–135.
104. Melbye M, Ingerslev J, Biggar RJ, et al. Anal intercourse as a possible factor in heterosexual transmisson of HTLV-III to spouses of hemophiliacs. N Engl J Med 1985;312:857.
105. Lawrence DL, Jason JM, Bouhasin JD, et al. HTLV-III/LAV antibody status of spouses and household contacts assisting in home infusion of hemophilia patients. Blood 1985;66:703–705.
106. Lawrence DN, Jason JM, Holman RC, et al. Sex practice correlates of human immunodeficiency virus transmission and AIDS incidence in heterosexual partners and offspring of U.S. hemophilic men. Am J Hematol 1989; in press.
107. Fischl MA, Dickinson GM, Scott GB, et al. Evaluation of heterosexual partners, children, and household contacts of adults with AIDS. JAMA 1987;257:640–644.
108. Friedland GH, Saltzman BR, Rogers MF, et al. Lack of transmission of HTLV-III/LAV infection to household contacts of patients with AIDS or AIDS-related complex with oral candidiasis. N Engl J Med 1986;314:344–349.
109. Centers for Disease Control. Antibodies to a retrovirus etiologically associated with acquired immunodeficiency syndrome (AIDS) in populations with increased incidences of the syndrome. MMWR 1984;33:377–379.
110. Curran JW, Morgan WM, Hardy AM, et al. The epidemiology of AIDS: Current status and future prospects. Science 1985;229:1352–1357.
111. Hargraves M, Jason JM, Chorba T, et al. Patient knowledge assessment study, Abstract 719. Proceedings of the International Conference on AIDS, Paris, June 1986.
112. National Hemophilia Foundation, Hemophilia Information Exchange. Hemophilia and acquired immune deficiency syndrome (AIDS): Intimacy and sexual behavior. Med Bull 1985;27.
113. Conant M, Hardy D, Sernatinger J, et al. Condoms prevent transmission of AIDS-associated retrovirus. JAMA 1986;255:1706.
114. Centers for Disease Control. Semen banking, organ and tissue transplantation, and HIV antibody testing. MMWR 1988;37:57–58, 63.
115. Centers for Disease Control. Education and foster care of children infected with HTLV-III/LAV. MMWR 1985;34:517–521.
116. Centers for Disease Control. Acquired immune deficiency syndrome (AIDS): Precautions for clinical and laboratory staffs. MMWR 1982;31:577–580.
117. Centers for Disease Control. Acquired immunodeficiency syndrome (AIDS): Precautions for health-care workers and allied professionals. MMWR 1983;32:450–452.
118. Centers for Disease Control. Recommendations for prevention of HIV transmission in health-care settings. MMWR 1987;36(25):35–185.
119. Centers for Disease Control. Update: Universal precautions for prevention of transmission of human immunodeficiency virus, hepatitis B virus, and other blood-borne pathogens in health-care settings. MMWR 1988;37:377–382, 387–388.

18

Pediatric AIDS

Moses Grossman

The enormous worldwide attention and publicity that have attended the AIDS epidemic have essentially bypassed the problem presented by infants and children. There are good reasons for this. The number of cases of AIDS reported in both children and adolescents in the United States as of March 1, 1988, is less than 2% of a total number of some 54,000 cases. The number of children infected with human immunodeficiency virus (HIV) not yet meeting the diagnostic criteria for AIDS is much larger. Recent surveys in Massachusetts and New York suggest that as many as one-half to two percent of newly delivered mothers have HIV antibody. Much of the political and legislative focus has been on the homosexual and bisexual transmission of the disease, which does not include children. The number of adults and children infected by blood and blood products has been relatively small and will not grow, because of the success in screening and protecting blood and blood products from contamination by HIV. The principal pool of infected children has come from infants born to infected women, most of them intravenous drug users; these cases have been concentrated in a very few communities—New York, Newark, Miami, and Los Angeles.[1,2] The country at large has so far had no need to face this difficult problem.

This has not been the case in Central Africa, however. There the disease has affected many men and women in almost equal numbers, and a large number of children have become infected by vertical transmission.[3] It has now become clear that heterosexual transmission is not an exclusively African phenomenon, and the expectation is that the United States may also see an increase in heterosexual transmission and thus an increasing number of affected children.

EPIDEMIOLOGY

There are four ways in which children can acquire infection with the HIV virus: through vertical transmission from the mother, through infection carried by blood, blood products, or transplanted organs; through child abuse; and, for adolescents, through sexual intercourse—homosexual or heterosexual with an infected partner. By far the most important route of transmission is the perinatal one. Some 75–80% of the 865 cases reported to date are due to perinatal transmission from infected mothers. This infection is transmitted during pregnancy, labor, and delivery from mothers infected with the virus, who themselves may or may not have symptoms.[4] The risk of infection to a baby born to an HIV-infected mother has not been firmly established. If a mother is HIV-positive and has had one baby with AIDS or has the disease herself, the risk of infection of the newborn appears to be 30–60%. In the case of an asymptomatic pregnant woman with an HIV infection, the risk is somewhat lower but has not been quantified. What determines whether the infant will or will not be infected is not known.

Early statistics from the Centers for Disease Control showed that 18% of children reported to have AIDS acquired this infection from blood or blood products. Many were hemophiliacs receiving factor VIII or IX concentrates, some had open heart surgery, and some had transfusions in the newborn nursery. This percentage will go down significantly, since essentially no new infections have been occurring as a result of the screening of all blood donors.

There is no published information on HIV infections as a result of child abuse. An unconfirmed report suggests that three children have been infected by this route. A prospective study is currently in progress.[5] As for adolescents getting infected as a result of sexual intercourse, clinically the issues are no different from those in adult infection. Legally and socially, the issues are quite different, because the adolescents are minors in the eyes of the law. It is important to emphasize that not a single youngster has been found to be infected as a result of *casual* contact. Several well-controlled studies involving well over 100 children have confirmed that children living in households with family members who have the disease have not acquired the infection over 2 or 3 years of exposure.[6-9]

CLINICAL CONSIDERATIONS

The large majority of reported cases of children who acquire HIV infection from their mothers have appeared normal at birth. A few infants have been reported by Marion et al.[10] from New York who appear to have unusual dysmorphic features—growth failure, microcephaly, hypertelorism, prominent forehead, flat nasal bridge that might represent an embryopathy due to this infection. However, the majority of infants appear normal, have a normal weight gain, and are asymptomatic for the first 8 or 9 months of their life. During this asymptomatic period the infant is truly "in limbo" as far as the diagnosis is concerned. The HIV antibody test is positive, but during this period it is not clear whether these are solely maternal antibodies or the infant is making antibodies as well. After a year of life, maternal antibodies disappear, and antibody positivity at that point is tantamount to indication of infection. The recovery of HIV virus from the infant is diagnostic of an infection, but viral cultures can only be done in a relatively few research laboratories at the present time. A test for HIV-IgM antibodies would be enormously helpful diagnostically. Such a test is not available at present; it is possible that this test or a test for the presence of the virus not requiring culture techniques (antigen detection or DNA probe) will become available soon. That would certainly help to clarify the infant's status and help with issues of placement, foster care, and adoption.

At the present time (April 1988), an infant of an infected mother can be considered to be free of infection if by the age of 15 months the infant does not manifest any clinical signs or symptoms of HIV and is negative for HIV antibodies.

Infected infants begin to be symptomatic somewhere between 8 and 15 months of age. Initial signs and symptoms are failure to thrive, chronic diarrhea, and developmental delays. Lymphadenopathy, hepatomegaly, and splenomegaly develop. Unlike adult patients, these children are peculiarly susceptible to common bacterial infections such as otitis media and pneumonia. Two findings peculiar to children are parotid swellings and lymphocytic infiltrative pneumonitis.[2] As the disease progresses, opportunistic infections that are the hallmark of this disease appear. These include *Pneumocystis carinii* pneumonia; infection with *Mycobacteria*, principally of the avium intracellulare group; candidiasis; toxoplasmosis; and many others. The brain is infected with HIV, resulting in many neurologic manifestations.[11] A common laboratory finding is hypergammaglobinemia. Lymphopenia, an almost constant hallmark of the adult disease, is uncommon in children. The reversal of the ratio of T-suppressor cells (T4) to T-helper cells (T8) is not as reliable a diagnostic sign in children as it is in adults.[12,13]

The spectrum of infection ranges from asymptomatic individuals through ARC (AIDS-related complex) and AIDS, the most serious form of the infection. The CDC definition of pediatric AIDS has recently been expanded and[14,15] is currently not as restrictive as it was 2 or 3 years ago, when very significant numbers of symptomatic children failed to meet the diagnostic criteria. At the present time there is no standard definition of ARC in children. These are symptomatic children with HIV infections who fail to qualify for the strict definition of AIDS.

The prognosis in children has been as dismal as it has in adults. The majority live less than 3 years and die with opportunistic infections. Infants with vertically transmitted disease who become symptomatic in the first year of life usually live less than a year after symptoms appear. Hemophiliacs who have acquired their infection from blood products seem to have a very long period of being asymptomatic. But even among the infants who are the products of infected mothers, a few have survived longer, as long as 8 years. Their clinical course is often complicated by very serious social circumstances including serious illness and often loss of the mother from the same disease.

There is no specific treatment for the infection at the present time. Attention to nutrition and prompt treatment of both the common and opportunistic infection are important. The administration of prophylactic trimethoprim/sulfamethoxazole to prevent *Pneumocystis* infection should be attempted. The adverse reaction rate is not as high as it is in adult patients. Some advocate monthly prophylactic intravenous gamma globulin in an attempt to prevent the occurrence of common infections, an approach that makes sense but that has not yet been demonstrated to be effective. Specific anti-HIV viral drugs, azidothymidine (AZT) in particular, are just beginning to be tested in children.

PERINATAL ISSUES

Management of perinatal HIV infections has to begin with education of women in the high-risk group. At the present time it is a fairly clearly defined group— intravenous drug users, sexual contacts of infected men or men in a high-risk category, and recipients of blood or blood products between the years 1979 and 1985. As heterosexual transmission of HIV infection spreads, such educational efforts will have to involve an ever enlarging group. The first steps are (1) to have the potential mothers-to-be consider whether they might want to get tested before they contemplate pregnancy and (2) to provide information about the effect of HIV infection on the infant. Women in the high-risk group who become pregnant should be strongly counseled to be tested for HIV infection during the first trimester; those who are positive may wish to consider the interruption of pregnancy because of the deleterious effect of the pregnancy on the immunologic status of the mother herself as well as the serious import for the infant.[4]

We recommend repeating the antibody test during the third trimester for those women who were negative earlier. This second test will identify women whose antibodies to HIV develop later in pregnancy. We feel that it is very important to inform the delivery room personnel when delivery by an infected woman is imminent. While HIV infection is not spread by *casual* contact, the massive presence of bodily fluids and placenta, all of them containing virus, requires that infection control precautions be taken to protect delivery room personnel.[16-18] It is equally as important to inform the pediatrician if the mother is antibody-positive. The baby is not infectious once the first bath has been given. The only precautions necessary in the nursery are in the handling of blood and body fluids. However, more important for the infant, if the infant is at risk of having been vertically infected, would be more vigorous treatment of minor infections. One would also wish to consider the use of live virus vaccines. It is advisable to give the infant the killed (Salk) polio vaccine, mostly because of the concern for probable immunocompromised adults in the household. Measles, mumps, and rubella (MMR) live attenuated vaccine is recommended for infected infants whether symptomatic or not.[19,20]

A special problem arises if the baby requires shelter or foster care, a situation that arises commonly in this group because of maternal medical and social problems. In that setting one would urge voluntary disclosure on the part of the mother of the antibody status to a single responsible person with assurance of maximum confidentiality. If the mother is unwilling to do so, court-mandated testing of the baby might be considered. This is a serious decision that requires consideration of the likelihood of the baby's being vertically infected, the risk of negatively labeling the baby, and the benefit of the medical caretaker and the foster parent being able to provide better, more enlightened medical care for the infant.

The adoption of babies from this high-risk category presents similar problems. Considering the grave nature and cost of the disease and the high mortality, it is only right that the adoptive parents should understand all of the facts, including the infant's antibody status. Detailed guidelines for these considerations have been published.[17,21]

Foster care placement of infants positive for HIV antibodies has been a very difficult issue in several communities. Despite convincing evidence that the infection is not transmitted by casual contact, foster parents have been reluctant to accept these infants in their homes. Some communities have been successful in appealing to better-educated foster parents, in some cases with a background of health care education, to accept these infants. Other communities have had to resort to some form of institutional care for these infants, an alternative that is less likely to meet their developmental and emotional needs than an individual foster home.

DAY CARE

The guidelines of the Centers for Disease Control[21] suggest that children with HIV infections be allowed to lead as normal a life as possible and that the advantage of receiving an education in the regular classroom outweighs the risk of being in school and being exposed to infections. We need not consider the risk to others, because the evidence that HIV infection is not transmitted by casual contact is really quite strong.[6,7,9] The CDC guidelines do mention that for preschool children or neurologically disabled children who cannot control their body secretions, a more restrictive setting might be advisable.

Perhaps of even greater importance is the fact that children attending day care centers have a greatly increased incidence of infections of all types. Shielding these HIV-infected children from excessive exposure to common infection might have quite an important bearing on how or if their HIV infection progresses to the clinical phase. For all these reasons we feel that as a general practice, children with HIV infections should not be in regular day care settings until they are 3 years old. If child care is needed, individual arrangements for one-to-one or one-to-two child care should be made. After the age of 3 years, each child's medical situation should be reviewed, and optimal placement in day care should be recommended.[21] For the majority of these children, regular day care placement will probably be suitable.

PREVENTION

Although research on developing various treatment modalities and the development of a vaccine is important, the only realistic approach to the problem of AIDS at this time is prevention. In the case of pediatric AIDS, this means the prevention of infection of women of childbearing age and the avoidance of pregnancy in women known to be infected, as well as the consideration of interruption of pregnancy when it is diagnosed in HIV-infected individuals. To this end the stress on education is of paramount importance. The education of women in high-risk categories as well as general education of young people about HIV infection and its consequences must be pursued with great vigor. No group is more important than early teenagers. This is the time of life when sexual experimentation is prevalent, the use of contraceptive devices including condoms is mostly neglected, and the "magical" thinking of the teenager suggests that she or he is immune from consequences. We hope that educational efforts with this group will be more successful in preventing the birth of children with AIDS than they have been in preventing teenage pregnancies.

REFERENCES

1. Rogers MF: AIDS in children: A review of the clinical, epidemiologic and public health aspects. Pediatr Infect Dis J 4:230, 1986.
2. Rubinstein A. Pediatric AIDS. Curr Prob Pediatr 16:365–409, 1986.
3. AIDS in Africa (editorial). Lancet ii:192, 1987.
4. Scott GB et al. Mothers of infants with the acquired immunodeficiency syndrome. JAMA 253:363, 1985.
5. Dattel B, Coulter K. Personal communication.
6. Friedland GH, Saltzman BR, Rogers MF, et al. Lack of transmission of HTLV-III/LAV infection of household contacts of patients with AIDS or AIDS related complex with oral candidiasis. N Engl J Med 314:344–349, 1986.
7. Kaplan JE, Oleske JM, Getchell JP, et al. Evidence against transmission of human T-lymphotropic virus/lymphadenopathy-associated virus (HTLV-III/LAV) in families of children with the acquired immunodeficiency syndrome. Pediatr Infect Dis 4:468–471, 1985.

8. Mann JM, Quinn TC, Francis H, et al: Prevalence of HTLV-III/LAV in household contacts of patients with confirmed AIDS and controls in Kinshasa, Zaire. JAMA 256:721–724, 1986.

9. Sands MA. Transmission of AIDS: The case against casual contagion. N Engl J Med 314:380–382, 1986.

10. Marion RW, Wiznia AA, Hutcheon RG, et al. Human T-cell lymphotropic virus type III (HTLV-III) embryopathy: A new dysmorphic syndrome associated with intrauterine HTLV-III infection. Am J Dis Child 140:638–640, 1986.

11. Epstein LG, Sharer LR, Oleske JM, et al. Neurologic manifestations of human immunodeficiency virus infection in children. Pediatrics 78:678, 1986.

12. Shannon KM, Ammann AJ: Acquired immune deficiency syndrome in childhood. J. Pediatr 106:332–342, 1985.

13. Ammann, AJ. The acquired immunodeficiency syndrome in infants and children. Ann Intern Med 103:734–737, 1985.

14. Classification system of human immunodeficiency virus (HIV) infection in children under 13 years of age. MMWR 36:225, 1987.

15. Centers for Disease Control: Revision of the CDC surveillance case definition for acquired immunodeficiency syndrome. MMWR 36:25, 1987.

16. Centers for Disease Control: Recommendations for assisting in the prevention of perinatal transmission of human T-lymphotrophic virus type III/lymphadenopathy-associated virus and acquired immunodeficiency syndrome. MMWR 34:721–732, 1985.

17. City and County of San Francisco Department of Public Health Perinatal and Pediatric AIDS Advisory Committee: Guidelines for control of perinatally transmitted human T-lymphotrophic virus-type III/lymphadenopathy-associated virus infection and care of infected mothers, infants, and children. San Francisco Epidemiol Bull 2(1):1S–16S, 1986.

18. Grossman M. HIV infections in children. Public health and public policy issues. Pediatr Infect Dis 6:113, 1987.

19. Immunization Practices Advisory Committee: Immunization of children infected with human immunodeficiency virus. MMWR 37:181, 1988.

20. Halsey NA, and Henderson DA. HIV infection and immunization against other agents. N Engl J Med 316:383, 1987.

21. Centers for Disease Control: Education and foster care of children infected with human T-lymphotropic virus type III/lymphadenopathy-associated virus. MMWR 34:517–521, 1985.

22. Committee on Infectious Diseases, American Academy of Pediatrics. Health guidelines for the attendance in day care and foster care settings of children infected with HIV. Pediatrics 79:466, 1987.

19

Contact Tracing

Dean F. Echenberg

The strategies used to deal with the AIDS epidemic must evolve as our knowledge of the epidemic evolves. We must continually evaluate what we are doing and how we are going to do it. The interventions will be very different depending upon the local situation.

The goal of an AIDS prevention program is to prevent transmission of human immunodeficiency virus (HIV) infections. A broad range of intervention programs will be needed to attain this goal. Programs must be appropriate to the particular circumstances of each community in which they are implemented. Although no single strategy will be successful everywhere, education must be the cornerstone of each effort. Devising the appropriate education program is critical. This education must be focused on targeted groups or individuals, on those who are either infected or at risk of becoming infected.

One factor which will determine how this education is to be applied in any population depends upon the prevalence of the disease in that population. When many are infected, obviously mass education directed to the entire affected population is one of the most important methods. When there are very few infected, additional attempts must be made to locate these individuals and then educate them individually. In San Francisco two strategies have been developed to deal with both a high and low prevalence situation.

The AIDS epidemic has spread with great rapidity in certain areas. The first cases of what came to be diagnosed as AIDS were reported in Los Angeles in June 1981.[1] One month later similar cases that had presented in the previous 30 months were reported from New York and San Francisco.[2] All of these cases had appeared in young homosexual or bisexual men who lived in urban settings. Many of them used drugs and were affected by various infectious agents. Reviews of case reports and hospital records of the previous 10 years in New York and San Francisco revealed almost no cases during that period in men in similar age groups.

In the absence of a reliable test for AIDS, the Centers for Disease Control (CDC) established a working case definition. The definition incorporated two major features: It was a disease at least moderately predictive of a defect in cell-mediated immunity, and it occurred in a person with no known cause for diminished resistance to that disease. Although CDC did not include the full spectrum of disease subsequently known to be caused by the virus, the initial definition provided a useful classification for establishing an intensive surveillance system.

A look at the epidemiology of AIDS in San Francisco reveals how different control strategies evolved. A cohort of homosexual men in San Francisco recruited from the municipal sexually transmitted disease (STD) clinic has been followed since 1978.[3,4] These men were voluntary participants in a hepatitis B study. In 1984 it was learned that many of these men were infected with the AIDS virus. They were subsequently asked to consent to participate in an AIDS study and to agree to an examination of their blood serum saved from 1979 and 1980.

One of the most tragic aspects in this overall tragedy is that by the time the first publication on AIDS appeared in the medical literature in July of 1981, 30–40% of the men in this cohort were already infected.[5] It took another year before the sexual mode of transmission was more clearly understood, at which time 40–50% of the cohort was infected.

The strategies that evolved in San Francisco in that high prevalence situation were obviously very different than those that would be used where the prevalence is much lower. In addition there is now a blood test to detect seropositivity.

PREVENTION

The goal of an AIDS prevention program is to prevent transmission of and infection with the AIDS virus. Accurate knowledge of the nature and extent of the virus must be the cornerstone for stopping both the AIDS epidemic and hysteria. Other related goals are to reduce morbidity and premature mortality in those who are already infected. The prevalence of infection and disease in each geographical area or group should determine, in part, where the emphasis should be placed in any prevention or education campaign.

In order to effectively prevent transmission one of two basic approaches is used. First, an assumption can be made that everyone in a geographical area or group is infectious through certain actions. Education about prevention of transmission should be aimed at everyone in these areas or groups. This approach is particularly suited if the prevalence is high.

In the initial stages of the epidemic in San Francisco, a strategy was evolved that said, in effect, all people in the classic high risk group should consider themselves infectious through sexual contact. This included not only homosexual and bisexual men, but also included hemophiliacs and intravenous (IV) drug users.

Education targeted to broad population and identity groups has been relatively effective. Mass education has had a great impact in decreasing the frequency of unsafe sexual activities that can transmit the virus.[6] For example, an average of 382 cases of rectal gonorrhea were seen each month during 1982 at the sexually transmitted disease clinic in San Francisco. By the end of 1986 the monthly case totals had decreased to less than 30 per month.[7]

A second generation approach to prevention education program strategy is to target education to individuals who have a high likelihood of being infected. (This will obviously increase the effectiveness of the intervention as well.) This is a classic approach that has been used in the control of a variety of infectious diseases. The smallpox eradication campaign, for instance, uses case-finding techniques and sexually transmitted disease programs utilize a contact-tracing strategy. However, for smallpox and most sexually transmitted diseases, interventions are available in the form of either vaccination of contacts or treatment of infected individuals. With AIDS there is no vaccine, nor is there available treatment in the classic sense. Therefore, individuals who are infected with the AIDS virus must be educated and properly counseled as to their risk of transmitting the disease to others in the community. This education will be most effective if it focused on those individuals known to be infected.

Individual education is especially important in areas where disease prevalence is low, because care providers in the general community might not yet be aware of the salient issues of AIDS prevention. In contrast, when disease prevalence is high, the death rates are also high, and mass education programs can rapidly raise the level of awareness and of concern that probably results in behavioral changes. Where the prevalence is low such changes cannot be expected to occur when mass education programs are applied.

In San Francisco, when it became apparent that cases could also occur in individuals outside of the classically defined "high risk" groups (those in low prevalence groups such as the general heterosexual population), it was realized that other strategies were needed. An estimated 50% of all homosexual men in San Francisco are infected with HIV.[8] In the general heterosexual population, the prevalence of HIV infection is currently less than a fraction of one percent. For heterosexuals, the progression of the epidemic may prove more insidious than for homosexuals and bisexuals, because heterosexuals won't suspect or know that they are infected.

The incubation period for AIDS is thought at this point to be as long as seven years, and possibly even longer.[9] An infected individual can unknowingly carry the virus and infect others for the entire incubation period. The immediacy of the epidemic among heterosexuals is very different than it has been among homosexual and bisexual men. Many individuals in the homosexual and bisexual community have become ill and died as a consequence of HIV infection. This widespread morbidity and mortality has not yet occurred in the heterosexual population. Therefore, mass education campaigns designed for the heterosexual population are not likely to result in the dramatic decrease in unsafe sexual activity observed in the homosexual and bisexual community.

Attempts must be made to locate heterosexuals who have been unknowingly exposed. These individuals should be offered risk reduction education and serological testing. San Francisco has established a model for heterosexual contact-tracing.[10] Without contact notification, rivulets of undetected AIDS virus infections will extend unchecked into the general heterosexual population, leading to problems of much greater magnitude in the future.

A tracing program for heterosexual contacts of HIV-infected persons has been in place in San Francisco since late 1985.[11] This program is part of an active surveillance program to locate all cases of AIDS in San Francisco. All individuals who have been diagnosed with AIDS are interviewed and asked to provide the names of their heterosexual partners so they can be contacted and informed of their exposure to HIV infection and its possible consequences. The program employs sensitive, trained investigators with experience in STD control. The investigators get a very high degree of cooperation. The identity of the initial case is never revealed to the contacts. The program is completely voluntary: any individuals who choose to inform their sex partners themselves have that option, or, if in some cases they'd rather not participate directly, that is their prerogative (although such an occurrence has been rare).

In San Francisco, these same tracing techniques have been used for over 6000 cases of syphilis and gonorrhea. Although there is no treatment for AIDS as there is for syphilis and gonorrhea, intervention is still possible. People who would not otherwise realize that they might have been infected can be so informed. A major assumption underlying the program is that an individual would not want to infect others unknowingly. Several women who were infected but unaware that they had been exposed to the AIDS virus were located with this program. To date, most of the individuals named as heterosexual partners are women of childbearing age. A contact-tracing program is especially important in preventing perinatal transmission of HIV as well as further transmission through sexual or parenteral means.

Twenty-seven heterosexual contacts have been investigated since the beginning of this program.[12] Seven of these were HIV antibody positive. Almost all of these were women of childbearing age. It is interesting that about half of the women had concerns about being infected even prior to their being contacted by our investigators. They thought they were at risk because of their sexual activities and were greatly relieved when the blood tests proved to be negative. Those who actually were positive did not know they were infected.

It is extremely important for anyone who is contemplating this type of program to understand the necessity for maintaining confidentiality. There must be very strong legal protections to safeguard this information from all subpoenas. In addition, there is a need for a precise, technical approach based on knowledge of HIV transmission along with very sensitive, well-trained investigators.

In addition to contact-tracing of the heterosexual partners of people with AIDS we have begun a similar program of contact-tracing of individuals who have become infected after receiving contaminated blood and for mothers of pediatric AIDS cases. In addition, all HIV-infected persons are encouraged to refer their partners for education, counseling, and testing.

In conjunction with individual contact-tracing and partner referral programs, other components are essential to HIV prevention.

1. *Community education.* In both low and high prevalence situations education on risk reduction must be developed for the entire community. It is important to stress both how the disease is transmitted and who is at risk, as well as how the disease is not transmitted and who is not at risk.

2. *Health provider education.* Education for health care providers about the prevention of AIDS transmission is extremely important. In high and low prevalence areas all health care providers must know who is at risk and who is not. In addition to knowing how to counsel individuals, they must understand when it is appropriate to suggest a test for the HIV antibody. When they find an individual who is infected in a low prevalence situation, the providers must understand the importance of stressing that the patient inform his or her sexual contacts. This is especially important in areas where HIV infection is not reportable and public health officials are not involved in contact-tracing programs.

3. *Risk group education.* Just as any clinical intervention involves a dialogue with the individual patient, a public health intervention involves a dialogue with the affected community. The most effective way to establish this dialogue and develop educational strategies for a community is to involve members of

that community. This is especially true in the AIDS epidemic, a tragedy which has been compounded in that it has struck communities that have been historically suppressed. In many places in the United States where AIDS spread rapidly and entire segments of the community were infected, programs were established in the community, in collaboration with local public health departments, to disseminate information rapidly and effectively.

One of the most important aspects of any prevention program is the establishment of strong constraints against the misuse of the information obtained by public health officials. If there is not effective governing legislation that prevents inappropriate disclosure of confidential information, disease control programs based on ascertaining the prevalence of infection in the community are doomed to fail. Without strong protections of individual rights, infected individuals will have cause to stay away from health providers and control programs. This may result in increased spread of the virus within the community.

INAPPROPRIATE INTERVENTION

Precise information must be gathered in order to plan appropriate intervention techniques. Inappropriate interventions can also hasten the spread of the disease. Unlike tuberculosis, AIDS is spread by consensual acts. Except in the case of perinatal transmission it takes two willing individuals to transmit the disease. AIDS cannot be spread by casual contact. If there are good community education programs, an individual will not unknowingly be infected with the AIDS virus— he or she will be aware that he or she is taking a risk. Education programs should ensure that discrimination does not occur with AIDS-infected individuals. It is important that public health officials remain firm in the face of demands for restrictive actions to stem the epidemic; such actions are inappropriate. Actions must be based on scientific information and sound principles of public health.

REFERENCES

1. Gottleib, M. S.; Schanker, H. M.; Fan, P. T., et al. Pneumocystis pneumonia. *Los Angeles, Morbid Mortal Weekly Report*, 30:250–252 (1981).

2. Friedman-Kien, A.; Laubenstein, L.; Marmor, M., et al. Kaposi's sarcoma and pneumocystis pneumonia among heterosexual men. *New York City* and *California, Morbid Mortal Weekly Report* 30:305–308 (1981).

3. Jaffe, H. W.; Feorino, P. M.; Darrow, W. W., et al. Persistent infection with HTLV-III/ LAV in apparently healthy homosexual men. *Annals of Internal Medicine* 102:627–628 (1985).

4. Jaffe, H. W.; Darrow, W. W.; Echenberg, D. F., et al. AIDS, AIDS-related conditions, and infection with HTLV-III in a cohort of homosexual men: A 6-year follow-up study. *Annals of Internal Medicine* 103:210–214 (1985).

5. Echenberg, D. F.; Rutherford, G. W.; O'Malley, P., et al. UPDATE—acquired immunodeficiency syndrome in the San Francisco cohort study 1978–1985. *Morbid Mortal Weekly Report* 35 (1985).

6. McKusick, L.; Wiley, J. A.; Coates, T. J., et al. Reported changes in the sexual behavior of men at risk for AIDS, San Francisco 1982–1984: The AIDS behavioral research project. *Public Health Report* 100:622–628 (1985).

7. *San Francisco Epidemiologic Bulletin*, Rectal gonorrhea in San Francisco, Oct. 1984–Sept. 1986. Vol. 2, No. 12 (December, 1986).

8. Winkelstein, W.; Lyman, D.; Padian, N., et al. Sexual practices and risk of infection by the human immunodeficiency virus. The San Francisco men's health study. *The Journal of the American Medical Association* 257:321–325 (1987).

9. Jaffe, H. W., et al. AIDS, AIDS-related conditions, and infection with HTLV-III.

10. Echenberg, D. F. A new strategy to prevent the spread of AIDS among heterosexuals. *The Journal of the American Medical Association* 254:2129–2130 (1985).

11. Echenberg, D. F. Education and contact notification for AIDS prevention. *New York State Journal of Medicine* 87:296–298 (1987).

12. Ibid.

V

PSYCHOLOGICAL ASPECTS

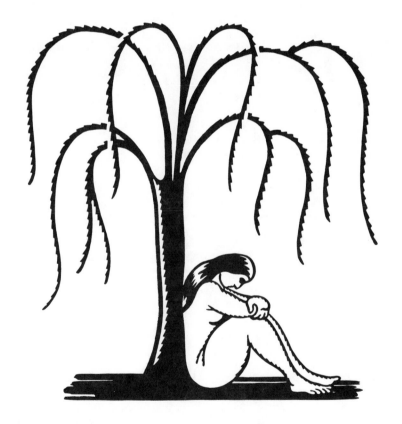

Psychological Aspects
Bereaved, a solitary figure sits under a bare willow tree.

20

The Treatment of People with AIDS: Psychosocial Considerations

Zelda Foster

INTRODUCTION

The impact of AIDS in our society is a continuing personal and social tragedy that is still unfolding. Never before in the history of a disease have so many physical and social forces collided with such a catastrophic outcome. The threatening personal and social context of this disease creates multiple dynamics that determine who becomes infected, how the disease is spread, the extent of its influence on the larger population, and societal responses. Thus, psychosocial considerations are of major consequence, playing a pivotal role in the treatment of persons with AIDS, the effects on their families and social networks, as well as on the health care providers who themselves are affected participants. The psychosocial considerations are complex but readily identifiable and can help determine meaningful psychosocial treatment approaches. The challenge for health care providers and relevant health and social organizations is to generate the strength, direction, and determination required to respond to these encompassing needs and demands.

Psychosocial considerations for individuals who have a diagnosis of AIDS or ARC, for their loved ones, and for those who have the responsibility for providing social and health care are extremely profound. Much has been written describing themes that pervade the experiences of each risk group and these provide meaningful generalizations about psychosocial issues and treatment implications.[1-3] The anguish, the physical and emotional devastation, and the frequent collapse of economic and social supports of people with AIDS are prevailing themes. There are also, however, examples of remarkable efforts to cope with these agonizing changes and threats to survival. These include using the experience of having AIDS or being closely associated with people who have AIDS in a positive manner by advancing new programs and trying to change the public's attitudes.[4]

The current and anticipated impact of the AIDS crisis on individuals, families and loved ones, social networks, the general community, and the health care system is almost immeasurable due to a number of key factors characterizing this disease. People who develop AIDS at this time in medical history have a debilitating, often fatal illness. Most of these people are relatively young and are members of stigmatized populations—homosexuals and intravenous drug users. AIDS was contracted in the great majority of cases either by sexual transmission or by the sharing of infected needles. At risk therefore are sexual partners as well as babies who may be infected perinatally. The lack of full knowledge about the etiology, incubation, transmission, possible changes in the virus itself, and treatment makes AIDS a mysterious and extremely threatening disease.

This chapter will focus on both the problem-specific and the more universal psychosocial issues and psychosocial treatment considerations for members of population groups who are facing a possible diagnosis of AIDS. The risk groups considered are homosexuals, IV drug users, families and their children diagnosed with AIDS, and people who received contaminated blood products. Although these groups may have a number of overlapping members, there are major differences that warrant addressing each respective group's distinct concerns separately.

Two important phenomena must be considered in any discussion of the psychosocial impact of AIDS: one is the very real concern about the ever-increasing spread of AIDS and the second is the stigmatizing and stereotyping of people with AIDS.

There are forecasts in the mass media and the professional literature of anticipated growth in the number of people who will develop AIDS to epidemic proportions.[5] There also will be simultaneous shifts in the population groups at risk for contracting and spreading this disease.[6,7] The resultant psychosocial considerations have monumental implications for individuals, families, friends, and for all of our social institutions. The projections of the sheer numbers and the populations at risk highlight a critical and dramatic need for a massive and comprehensive public health campaign that must deal with community education, prevention, and global and specific changes in our health care delivery system. The potential for ill-considered and inadequate social health policy development threatens the quality of our lives and the communities in which we live. Continuing negative public reaction to AIDS can have serious consequences by discouraging people to come forward for testing, educational, and preventive help. Repressive and retaliatory public policy toward those with AIDS or in high risk groups is a possible future negative outcome.

The second phenomenon is the negative impact of stereotyping and stigmatizing persons with AIDS. Stereotypes and deep-seated prejudices about homosexuals and IV drug users have allowed the general population to be detached and unempathic. These stereotypes are extremely destructive. The wish on the part of the "unaffected" population is for protection and separation from groups whose behavior and practices will ultimately "ravage innocent people." It is easier, for example, to view the IV drug user as a heroin addict who was infected by using dirty needles in an anonymous shooting gallery, rather than as a possible past drug user who is part of a family, a parent to young children. Similarly, the homosexual can be seen as a person involved in promiscuous, compulsive sexual activity in bathhouses rather than as a creative, useful member of society. Certain ethnic and racial groups also have strong indictments against homosexual practices. For example, there are prohibitions in some segments of black and Hispanic cultures against homosexuality.

Other strong social prejudices are prevalent in perceptions of the "AIDS threat." IV drug abuse is closely associated with black and Hispanic populations; therefore, already existing negative feelings toward these populations may be further heightened. It is crucial that individuals in each risk group not be stereotyped. The Gay Men's Health Crisis, AIDS Institute, AIDS task forces, social agencies, and self-help networks are working hard to eradicate, or to at least modify, stereotypes, deal with discrimination, and provide necessary services to all affected groups.[8]

There is neither a monolithic population at risk nor a monolithic disease. Who gets it, how it develops and progresses, and the response to biopsychosocial treatment must be looked at in each individual set of conditions.

The following discussion should not have as its outcome a universalizing of "truths" but is presented instead as a guide and focal point for a deepened grasp of the meaning of the behaviors, needs, and helping conditions relevant to the community of people personally and professionally touched by AIDS.

COMMON CONCERNS

People with AIDS experience common concerns and face a multitude of obstacles that can severely damage their coping capacities. The diagnosis of AIDS immediately threatens long-term survival and predicts a remaining quality of life jeopardized by severe debilitation, extreme susceptibility to infections, hospitalizations, disfigurement (in the case of Kaposi's sarcoma), and multiple and staggering personal losses. These losses are intensified by feelings of rejection and self-blame. The anticipated decline and fear of loss of life evident in patients with incurable cancer is not nearly as overwhelming as the stigmatization faced by AIDS patients who are associated with being part of a group whose promiscuous behavior or drug abusing practices has brought this disease upon themselves and who may in turn transmit it to the general public. There is also increasing clinical evidence of AIDS patients who are exhibiting signs of dementia as a result of direct effects of the virus on the central nervous system.[9] The staggering management and care problems of this patient group create additional burdens on social support and health care delivery systems. This situation of limited resources for an infected and stigmatized population facing debility and death and causing transmission to others is the general climate surrounding the lives of persons with AIDS. Members of each risk group have distinct and specific characteristics that influence their care and treatment. These will be discussed below.

IV DRUG USERS WITH AIDS

Intravenous (IV) drug users are a major risk group with far-reaching implications for effective and productive psychosocial treatment. Personality as well as behavioral and social patterns severely obstruct how help is sought and accepted in this group.[10] Most health and social agencies have not yet embraced this population in outreach efforts and have not forged relationships in ways which are sufficiently responsive. Public health issues emerge as a particularly serious aspect of treatment. Most IV drug users are seropositive (at least 62%) and 30% are women who are largely of childbearing age.[11] Additionally, a portion of these reportedly are prostitutes. The transmission of AIDS through the use of infected needles and heterosexual sexual activity increases the probability that members of this population will develop AIDS and also infect others.

Women who are IV drug users, prostitutes, or who are associated with men who are IV drug users, are not only at risk themselves but also risk giving birth to babies infected with AIDS. The increasing number of babies born with AIDS to infected mothers is a cause for alarm. The mother may be asymptomatic (not manifest signs of AIDS or ARC) but may be a carrier and, possibly, susceptible to future illness.

IV drug users, whether male or female, are clearly carriers of the virus and are often ill and at extreme risk. A population of probable disease carriers presents agonizing dilemmas in terms of social policy (for example, mandatory testing). It also presents enormously difficult ethical and treatment issues since the IV drug user may refuse to consider using safe practices to protect partners and children yet to be born. Health care treatment teams need to emphasize this responsibility to partners; they must also know how to offer help to partners who have developed AIDS or become seropositive.

This population of drug users—who are likely to be carriers and who may be facing serious debilitation and death—are characterized by alienation, antisocial behavior, poor economic situations, inadequate social supports, severed personal bonds, and chaotic and sometimes criminal lifestyles. Consequently, there are substantive questions regarding how to effectively engage and offer this population treatment. Difficulties in trust, in forming relationships, in expressing feelings, and in recognizing anxiety would be a barrier to productive treatment under most circumstances.[12] In these situations, heightened anxiety and immobility makes patterns of avoidance and denial less achievable but desperately sought by patients as they try to cope with intolerable feelings of pain and anxiety. The likelihood of ongoing opportunistic infections and a rapid physical decline further compromises the time available and the capacity to work on problem resolution.[13] Increased demanding and manipulative behavior, and the creation of chaos and crisis are often present in these treatment situations. Many health care workers are not accustomed to such behaviors and may react in ways which increase the potential for negative interaction.

Effective psychosocial treatment strategies require addressing both the internal and external influences on patients as well as how the reactions of the health care providers influence the success or failure of treatment. The central issue in each individual situation is how a person can be sustained, nurtured, and offered medical and psychosocial treatment while facing the extreme likelihood of severe incapacity and death. Of critical importance is the strengthening of social supports including a place to live, home care, financial management and income from entitlement programs, care management services, a consistent treatment team with follow-up responsibilities, and an alternative to hospitalization programs (hospices, residential drug programs, half-way houses, supportive housing, hospital-based home care). It is advised to involve the IV drug user in a drug treatment program whether the person is drug-free, on methadone maintenance, or a current user. The person who is drug-free may be at great risk to return to drugs and may be considered for methadone at this crisis point or for a referral to a drug-free program.[14] Whichever specific program is chosen is perhaps less important than connecting the person with AIDS to programs that offer clear, consistent, and firm structures while providing supportive help. However, some drug treatment programs will need special consultation to learn more about dealing with the physical decline and the emotional issues for both staff and patient that are stirred up by this overwhelming disease.[15]

Infectious disease staffs and primary health care staffs also need consultation from the drug treatment programs to better grasp how to engage and manage patients with these personality/behavioral characteristics. This points to the value of a strong investment in "sharing" patients, in interdisciplinary teams in collaboration rather than functioning as fragmented or competitive providers. There is a convergence of unique and usually separated factors and of health care providers who are usually not closely related to one another in practice. New teams may be designed which encompass skill in responding to death and dying concerns, drug use/behavior, infectious disease, and primary care. Coordination and communication is an essential dimension in offering care. These new resources and partnerships will take work, investment, and a lack of territoriality to establish and nurture. While a most intensive and concerted thrust is needed for educational and preventive services, there will be a growing population of seriously ill and dying people.

There is much to learn from hospice and death and dying conceptual frameworks. How people face their remaining days and death, how families might be reconciled, and what settings offer the best opportunities for care are known. Relevant for treatment of the former or current drug user is the professional obligation to conceptually spell out effective treatment interventions for this population. Approaching the emotional life of drug users is not easy. How does one and should one deepen relationships, open up anxious and conflicting feelings, search for opportunities for reconciliation with family, and explore for meaning and purpose in the face of death? The past or present drug user with AIDS who is viewed as having a fatal disease will present a dilemma for staff. The wish to be nurturing and all-giving might be best tempered and balanced by limits and holding to guidelines. The patient's struggle with trust and involvement may test the limits of the program. There are many questions. The patient may need anxiety reduction drugs but will this induce a flight back into drug dependency? When is methadone a treatment of choice? How do you involve the patient in considering safe sexual practices, birth control, and possibly abortion? How might these patients become more active in political advocacy for increased services and also in establishing more self-help networks? Do Vietnam Era veterans with AIDS have additional needs and other networks to draw on? How does one deal with low frustration tolerance, need for immediate gratification, and manipulative behavior while attempting to maintain the patient in treatment? What help do family members and patients need as they feel regret and bitterness for a troubled past, a difficult present, and a sorrowful future? Discussions with health care providers report a wide spectrum of experiences. These must be evaluated, considered theoretically, and incorporated into treatment concepts and approaches that can be disseminated among the interdisciplinary professionals working in this area.

HOMOSEXUALS WITH AIDS

This disease has had devastating impact on a community of people tied together by lifestyle and social networks. Drawn by the anonymity, opportunities, and acceptance permitted in a number of major U.S. cities, many gay people have gathered together and established their own separate communities within them. This has led to the simultaneous consequence of significant numbers of members of these communities either having died of AIDS, being ill with AIDs or ARC, being seropositive for the AIDS virus, or being at future risk. Bereavement overload and heightened anxiety are evident. There has been a monumental effort made for collective action to stem the transmission of the disease by practicing "safe sex" and to develop services for people with AIDS regardless of risk group. Services developed by the Gay Men's Health Crisis in New York City and many other networks and task forces cover a wide range of needs, including companion help, support groups, and legal action to deal with discriminatory acts.[16]

Irrational fear and reaction to homosexuality existed prior to the occurrence of AIDS and was then intensified when AIDS, initially thought to affect only homosexuals, appeared. The existence of AIDS accentuated and deepened the rage toward and fear of homosexuals. Societal blame, attacks, and terror create an environment which holds danger for homosexuals with AIDS in the form of abandonment, social ostracism, isolation, and damaging discriminatory behavior. Homosexuals themselves are experiencing self-blame, fear, loss of social networks, and changed lifestyle patterns.[17] They are confronted daily by the death of loved ones and other members of their community. Self-hatred, guilt, and loss of self-esteem are concomitant reactions to these societal judgments. Self-help organizations and groups act as counterforces to the internalization of perjorative and condemnatory reactions. Further complexity is created for some by the secret of their homosexuality hidden from families and/or irreconcilable differences in life patterns causing estrangement and conflict between family members and partners. Families, even when reconciled to the knowledge, may live far away. Other families are confronted with their son's (brother's) homosexuality and dying at the same time.

Many situations have been reported where the parents have been summoned to a major city to learn that their son is dying and they must then simultaneously cope with the diagnosis of AIDS, the secret homosexual lifestyle, and a kinship circle of loved ones (partner, friends) who are alien to the parents. For the patient, the parent, and the partner, there are disturbing and powerful feelings which need resolution. Sometimes it's possible for parents to provide care, for parents to join with partners, or for current partners to assume major responsibility. Current partners may have varied abilities to assume responsibility. For other patients there is no one available and they are alone and isolated except for the limited help of support networks and health care systems.[17,18] For these, housing, financial management, and supportive housing services are required.

Other situations have been reported where bisexual men involved in current marriages or other heterosexual relationships have developed AIDS. This is an especially traumatic event when the partner did not know of the past or present homosexual practice and now is at risk herself. If she remains emotionally and physically involved in the continuing relationship, there are many decisions which need to be made and there is much with which to cope. Some women have contracted AIDS as a result of sexual relationships with bisexual men. For them, there is the reality of the disease as well as the feelings of betrayal, rage, and shame.

Treatment considerations must be encompassing, reaching inner feelings while offering practical and comprehensive help with the management of the illness and current existence.[19] All related networks must be included and encouraged to work cooperatively on behalf of the patients who are torn further apart by conflict and guilt. This requires a high level of skill and sophistication on the part of the health care providers responsible for psychosocial treatment. For many patients, there is a struggle to cope with multiple losses, fear of dying, exposure of homosexuality, self-recrimination, family conflicts, and changing relationships with loved ones.[20] These are issues which can be meaningfully helped with counseling. Psychosocial treatment must begin at the point of the diagnosis and continue throughout the course of the diseases and in bereavement help to the survivors.

How people face terminal illness and what are effective helping interventions are well documented.[21] The nature of AIDS and its social context influence the number, intensity, and complexity of the issues. The feelings of self-blame, rage, lowered self-esteem, loss of status, sense of expendability, alienation, discriminatory acts, knowledge of one's infectiousness, and the existence of two separate kin networks (family and partners/friends) change the scope and dimensions of the dynamics involved. Unresolved conflicts around homosexuality, one's role in causing the disease because of lifestyle, and the impact of exposure of homosexuality to employers/family and others are areas with which counseling can be effective, helping provide a greater sense of peace and acceptance. Treatment considerations must encompass and integrate these additional dynamics while relating to the struggle to cope with decline and dying. Intensive therapy is indicated to encourage sharing of feelings, decision-making, working through of denial, and processing of critical life events. Each physical and emotional phase during the course of the illness will require specific address. Patients evidencing signs of dementia will benefit from early assessment, clear guidance, and therapy. Liaison psychiatry must have an ongoing role in treating these neuropsychiatric manifestations. Psychiatric consultation will also be valuable in offering diagnostic help and treatment regimens including prescribing psychotrophic medication. Hypnosis, positive imaging, relaxation techniques, diet, rest, holistic medicine, and spiritual help are all possibilities worthy of being offered at relevant times to appropriate patients. Needed services and connections to peer support groups can be sought with the patient's participation in both establishing treatment directions and in problem-solving efforts. It is vital for patients to find new ways to socialize, deal with sexuality, and maintain relationships.

This disease strikes relatively young people who have in the main been financially independent, vocationally productive, and contributors to their environments. Losses in every sphere, unrelenting psychosocial stressors, and confrontations with one's severe debility and mortality create struggles for treatment staff as well, as they attempt to cope with their own feelings of distress, grief, and vulnerability.

THE IMPACT OF AIDS ON FAMILIES AND THEIR CHILDREN

The ratio of people with AIDS who are or were IV drug users is increasing as compared with the homosexual population. A significant portion are women IV drug users with some accounts claiming a 30% ratio of women among IV drug users.[22] Other women with AIDS, ARC, or seropositivity have been infected by heterosexual contact, most often by men who are IV drug users. The risk to themselves, to the babies born to them, and to their current and future male partners presents at this juncture a major public health concern.

The psychosocial implications are anguishing. Most mothers and their families are poor and black or Hispanic. They often live in inadequate housing, have had poor access to health care, and rely on marginal and stressed social supports. Entitlement programs are fragmented and are unable to provide a comprehensive scope of services. Each mother who has a baby with AIDS is herself at risk. Either she has AIDS, ARC, or at the very least, is seropositive. The mother will need to consider issues relating to her own sexuality, fertility, and infectiousness. Cultural factors are relevant to feelings and decision making in these areas. These mothers may be experiencing their own illness either full-blown or in beginning signs. There certainly is an ever-present fear of developing the illness which results in living day to day with uncertainty and fear.

There are hundreds of cases of infants left in hospitals when the mothers because of illness, death, or lifestyle patterns (addicts, prostitutes) cannot care for their children. These children are virtually abandoned and receive care from either hospital staffs or the foster care system. Children who do go home live with mothers and in families beset with overwhelming problems in everyday management. In some families a number of the family members are ill, there is poverty, and multiple sociocultural barriers exist to going outside to obtain needed resources, for example, hospital, clinics, schools. There is a reliance on social service and home care agencies which do not resolve the terrible living conditions or traumatic family relationships. There are examples of extended families, neighbors, and helpful social agencies but the totality of the problems encountered in the care of a sick, often dying, child living in poor, inadequate conditions and frequently with other ill family members speaks to the scope of counseling and practical help which must be made more totally and readily available.

The illness of the child is directly related to the mother's transmission of the disease. This dynamic is added to the horror of coping with the illness and anticipated death of one's child. The care and management of the child is complex as problems in physical and psychological growth emerge, as dependency on educational, health, and social agencies increases, and as the family unit tries to function against what seem to be unsurmountable attacks on it.

There are examples of health care agencies behaving responsively, of entitlement programs devising specific and earmarked services, and of the young mother's parents, partner, and neighbors rallying. Yet, for many this help is insufficient or not available. The social and emotional cost to these mothers is infinite. If there is an involved father or a current partner, this relationship has a most significant role in treatment and planning.

Psychosocial treatment has focused on the provision of services including public assistance, home care, and support groups. To be fully effective, each situation must be assessed so that help is directed to the entire network of concerned members including grandparents, siblings, and extended family. The impact of current drug use, the capacity to provide care, and how the mother and child are coping can be assessed while practical services are being made available. Feelings of unbearable grief, self-blame, helplessness, and rage may be expressed. At the same time, the mother may be able to provide some care and to give love to her child, and in this giving of love, some hope and restoration may be possible. Bereavement help is vital to the mother and other family members to encourage a more successful working through of grief in its acute and long-term forms. The pain and grief attached to the loss of a child always remains and although never fully resolved, can be made less damaging to functioning and present relationships.[23]

In situations where the mother cannot cope, where the mother is ill or has died, or where the child is abandoned, another set of problems emerges. Boarder babies in hospitals, difficulties in finding foster homes, and children not thriving and in obvious great peril, are the victims and social consequences of this disease. The development of safe and caring environments where children can thrive as best as is possible is one of the greatest challenges facing the social welfare system and the humanity of our social organizations.

AIDS AND CONTAMINATED BLOOD PRODUCTS

People who become seropositive or develop ARC or AIDS due to receipt of contaminated blood products consider themselves unaware and innocent victims of an evil and cruel fate. They also, in the role of carrier, pose a great threat to partners, spouses, and infants born to infected mothers. They may be developing or have developed a disease to which great stigma is attached and which threatens current existence and survival. Their loved ones also may be in jeopardy. Dealing with a blow of this nature and facing the course of an illness so devastating and incomprehensible without rage and despair is not possible. The skill of solid and well-developed psychosocial treatment services is key with this population as well as with the previously described ones.

Although the reported number of hemophilia-related AIDS cases is not presently increasing, the high degree of seroprevalence is cause for concern.[24] It is no doubt a population at risk for developing AIDS, as possible carriers may be jeopardizing those with whom they are in sexual contact. Educational assistance and therapeutically directed counseling is essential to reach those affected to help deepen coping and problem-solving abilities and to enlist available resources to enable the most positive emotional adaptive outcome possible.

FURTHER TREATMENT IMPLICATIONS

The pressure to offer effective psychosocial treatment to increasing numbers of people in need is mounting. Extreme stress is being placed on health providers as they become part of the lives of this young, stigmatized, and often dying population. The likelihood of health care providers feeling overwhelmed, guilty, and helpless suggests the value of instituting planned and ongoing staff support services. Hospice experience has shown that recognizing the needs of staff has important application to staff effectiveness. The work and treatment environments for most professional caregivers is either in acute hospitals or home care agencies. Both environments have unique sets of stressors and large numbers of health care staffs who are not prepared for the extent of death and dying issues confronting patients and themselves.

The form of supportive help for staff can take many shapes. Opportunities to increase self-awareness and knowledge, share reactions and disturbing feelings, seek mutual help from peers, obtain ongoing supervision and consultation, and have respite periods away from the work are possible ways for recognizing needs and helping staff to better cope. The role of hospice also must be evaluated as a resource which can be expanded but which will require an investment in careful training, resource development, and a program balance between cancer patients who are the usual candidates for hospice,[25] and persons with AIDS (who also have an especially limited life span). Hospice philosophy values the role of the caregiver and promotes caregiver support through groups, volunteers, and respite services. Caregivers of patients with AIDS face difficult symptoms and concerns regarding infectiousness and encounter stress on every level.

The focus on practical and psychotherapeutic help needs to be balanced so that community resources are developed which meet the wide range of services needed to maintain an ill population while recognizing that enhancing coping abilities go beyond the provision of concrete services. Help to multiple networks of involved relatives, lovers, and friends, recognizing the value of and providing support group and bereavement services are important aspects of a treatment program.

There is an imperative to provide preventive and educational services, especially as one considers the vast numbers of people who are seropositive and therefore contagious. At the same time, persons with AIDS will continue to require extensive, intensive helping services. Advocacy work in changing health care delivery systems and in responding to discriminatory acts becomes an important part of the professional role.

Coordination is necessary to promote the development of inpatient and outpatient comprehensive interdisciplinary teams and also for the integration between hospital and community services. Hospitals which are designated AIDS centers may be able to accomplish this more easily but sound planning, program development, and communication to assure more effective service delivery remain as challenges.

Well-organized interdisciplinary teams can lend strength to its members and to those treated. Multidisciplinary physician specialists, nurses, and social workers have core roles in providing treatment, ongoing care management, and psychosocial coordination.[26] Chaplains, dieticians, psychologists, and other health professionals must join in offering their expertise. Drug programs, task forces, self-help groups, social agencies, and AIDS service/research/educational institutes all have key roles to play.

Health care providers will have a major voice in how AIDS as the major biopsychosocial problem of these times is treated. They will bear witness to suffering beyond comprehension and will participate in shaping how care is offered. To be effective, health care providers need to speak with a voice which is unified, well organized, and powerful in its leadership. AIDS is one disease which requires response on individual, institutional, and societal levels. All in health care will be called upon to find a commitment to service never before asked. AIDS will test the systems in which we live and work and, ultimately, each individual's values and capacities.

REFERENCES

1. Furstenbert, A., and Olson, M. Social work and AIDS. In *Social Work in Health Care*. New York: The Haworth Press, Inc., 1984:45–61.

2. Christ, G., and Wiener, L. Psychosocial Issues in AIDS, In *AIDS: Etiology, Diagnosis, Treatment, Prevention*. Philadelphia: Lippincott Co., 1985:275–297.

3. Lehman, V., and Russell, N. Psychological and Social Issues of AIDS and Strategies for Survival. In *Understanding AIDS: A Comprehensive Guide*. New Brunswick, NJ: Rutgers University Press.

4. Health Letter 5. Gay Mens Health Crisis Inc., May 1985.

5. World Drive on an AIDS Pandemic. *The New York Times*, November 23, 1986.

6. The AIDS Epidemic, Future Shock. *Newsweek*, November 24, 1986.

7. Heterosexuality and AIDS: The Concern Keeps Growing. *The New York Times*, October 28, 1986.

8. Persons with AIDS Coalition. *Newsline*, December 1986.

9. Perry, S., and Jacobsen, P. Neuropsychiatric Manifestations of AIDS-Spectrum Disorders. *Hospital and Community Psychiatry*, (February 1986):135–141.

10. Angel, S. From Action to Reflection, New Depth in Psychotherapy with Drug Addicts. *Clinical Social Work Journal*:151.

11. Drucker, E. AIDS and Addiction in New York City. *American Journal of Drug and Alcohol Abuse* 12(1 and 2) (1986):165–181.

12. Cohen, M., and Weisman, H. A. Biopsychosocial Approach to AIDS. *Psychosomatics* 27(4) (April 1986).

13. Maayan, S., et al. Acquired Immunodeficiency Syndrome (AIDS) in an Economically Disadvantaged Population. *Archives Internal Medicine* 145 (September 1985):1607–1612.

14. Personal communications with Melodye Schoonmaker, Chief of Counseling, U.S. Navy Family Service Center, Roosevelt Rd., Puerto Rico (Formerly AIDS Coordinator, VAMC, Bronx, NY); and Rose Jacobs, Supervisory Social Worker, VAMC, Bronx, N.Y.

15. Editorial. AIDS and the Substance Abuse Treatment Clinician. *Journal of Substance Abuse* 2 (1985).

16. Violence vs. Homosexuals, Rising Groups Seeking Wider Protection. *The New York Times*, November 23, 1986.

17. Nochols, S., et al. *Acquired Immune Deficiency Syndrome*. Washington, DC: American Psychiatric Press, Inc, 1984.

18. Merin, S.; Charles, K.; Malyan, A. The Psychological Impact of AIDS on Gay Men. *American Psychologist* 39 (November 1984):1288–1293.

19. World Drive on an AIDS Pandemic. *The New York Times*.

20. Health Letter/5.

21. Furstenbert, A., et al. Social Work and AIDS.

22. Drucker, E. AIDS and Addiction in New York City.

23. Arnold, J., and Buschman, P. *A Child Dies: A Portrait of Family Grief*. Rockville, MD: Aspen Systems Corp., 1983.

24. Surveillance Maintained on Hemophilia-Associated AIDS. *Oncology Times*, January 15, 1987.

25. National Hospice Organization Policy Statement—AIDS.

26. Psychosocial Treatment of Patients with Acquired Immune Deficiency Syndrome (AIDS). VA Clinical Affairs Letter IL 11-86-15. September 1986.

21

In Need of Comfort: AIDS Patients on Psychiatric Units

Judith Bograd Gordon and Sheila Dollard Pavlis

Who art thou, that thou art afraid of man who shall die,
And the son of man that shall be made as grass
And has forgotten the Lord, thy maker . . .
He that is beat down shall speedily be loosed;
And he shall not go dying into the pit,
Neither shall his bread fail . . .
How shall I comfort thee?
(Isaiah, Chapter 51: 12, 14)[1]

As we begin to address the plight of people grappling with AIDS on psychiatric inpatient units, it is appropriate to remember that fear of the ill and dying is as old as humankind. In earlier eras the afflicted, as Isaiah reminds us, turned to a Lord who comforted as well as punished and who forgave as well as damned. But, although the prophet urged that the dying not be deprived of bread, human beings have not always heeded such injunctions. Individuals with AIDS, like others throughout history who have suffered from diseases that are feared, have the burden of dying among the living who mask their own fears of mortality by blaming the victim and isolating those who care for and about them. Today AIDS patients are being attacked in the name of public health and religion by those who have forgotten to ask the question: How shall I comfort thee?

The purpose of this paper is to look at the complex interplay of biography, social organization, and history that takes place on psychiatric inpatient units as members of this society encounter AIDS and death. The personal troubles of both patients and staff reflect the psychosocial issues that shape the interactions on the unit itself. For, as Jung observed, "In insanity, we do not discover anything new or unknown. We are looking at the foundations of our own being, the matrix of those vital problems on which we are all engaged.[2]

We gratefully acknowledge the thoughtful comments and suggestions of the following colleagues who graciously reviewed drafts of this chapter: Drs. Boris Astrachan, Department of Psychiatry, Yale School of Medicine; Alvin Novick, Department of Biology, Yale University; Ellis Perlswig, Yale Child Study Center, Yale School of Medicine; Rabbi James Ponet, Yale University Hillel, and Dean Ralf Carriuolo, School of Special Studies and Continuing Education, University of New Haven.

THE SOCIOCULTURAL MATRIX

To be human is to be influenced by culture and society, since no human being lives alone. Sociologists interested in what has been called interpretative sociology point to the dialectic that occurs between the institutional structures that confront the individual and the consciousness of individuals.[3] Clearly, the meanings given to AIDS are complicated sociocultural constructions which shape an individual's experience of this disease.[4]

Culture is, as anthropologists point out, a system of shared understandings and symbols that groups use to provide frameworks for making sense of lives and deaths.[5] Different religions, for example, offer believers different systems of understandings in regard to gender roles, family structure, sexual behavior, and social policy.[6] Given the complexity of our culture and the conflicting schemes of interpretation used by various groups within the United States, it is no wonder that some persons dealing with AIDS-related problems, with and without neuropsychiatric diseases, find their way into inpatient psychiatric units. Some of the tasks of the unit, therefore, are shaped by the complex ways in which the members of society give meaning to the syndrome, the "victims," and their treatment.

AIDS, as others in this volume point out, is terrifying in itself. Indeed, the growing numbers of the "worried well" give testimony to the fearfulness that has been created by the emergence of this disease which as yet has no cure, no effective pharmacological treatment for the symptoms, and no prevention. AIDS often strikes young adults. It devastates not only their lives, but the lives of those who love them. Even if some of these people have engaged in life styles that other members of this society may condemn, their suffering is so horrible that the most reasonable of observers engage in compassionate efforts to help.

In an era when medical science has been able to eliminate some devastating diseases and to control or cure others including sexually transmitted diseases such as syphilis, the emergence of AIDS reveals again the limitations of our medical knowledge. If human beings were entirely rational creatures, the discovery of AIDS should have immediately precipitated significantly increased funding for scientific efforts to mitigate the ravages of this disease, particularly given its similarities to other devastating incurable diseases such as Alzheimer's. It did not.

As Freud pessimistically argued, civilized human beings are not always rational.[7] Many Americans, for example, have preferred to deny that anyone can die except the old.[8] The death of young people with AIDS sharply confronts us with the cost of such denial. Like the young who suffer from progressive neurological disorders, AIDS patients in the United States also encounter a society that has propagated the myth that only the old need chronic care. And the inadequacy of the long-term care for the elderly with chronic conditions is well documented.[9]

As the staff of psychiatric inpatient units know, AIDS patients are not unique in their painful discovery that their lives are being further complicated by a health care system primarily designed to provide acute care. Our society has yet to develop adequate health care systems for chronic illness, either physical or mental.

Current cutbacks in health and human services threaten the development of such a system even for the "deserving frail elderly."[10] The majority of the first cohort of AIDS patients consisted of members of stigmatized groups such as homosexuals and intravenous drug abusers. Not everyone agrees that these people are deserving of care, especially if such care requires government funding. Even those who initially come from nonstigmatized groups face added suffering. Children with AIDS have been cruelly rejected by schools and neighbors; some die abandoned on pediatric wards. Adults who contract AIDS via blood transfusions or intercourse with an unsuspected affected partner find that AIDS is an additional handicap they face as they encounter the same hardships confronted by people of all ages who need long-term care.

This additional burden of suffering has been created because the publicity surrounding the discovery of this syndrome has precipitated a kind of social hysteria which resembles the medieval reaction to the Bubonic Plague. As others in this book report, the terrified and self-righteous among us punish the ill and, increasingly, those suspected of being ill by the loss of employment, housing, social support, and health insurance, compounding the effect of AIDS itself.

Given the stress of both the disease and the social reactions to it, some people dealing with AIDS pass through psychiatric treatment settings in their transitions from physical health to illness or life to death. American culture, after all, has medicalized much of human suffering. And these patients are indeed sick, not only in body, but sometimes in mind or spirit. Surely, psychiatric inpatient units can be viewed as appropriate places for some to come to terms with the meaning of their disease, the reactions of others in the social world, and their own destiny.

But not everyone agrees with such a conclusion. The stigma attached to madness has also attached to the setting where madness is treated, and vice versa. Mental-health personnel are not always viewed as allies by members of the "high-risk groups" AIDS has first affected. Some advocates for homosexuals, the minority poor, and women have pointed to "oppressive" features of psychiatric treatment which they claim is often delivered by people who are consciously or unconsciously racist, sexist, homophobic, or class biased.[11,12] Streetwise people such as addicts may weigh the benefits of being labeled "crazy" in a time of tight resources.[13] Although some drug addicts desperately demand inpatient psychiatric treatment, others reject efforts by mental-health professionals or courts to engage them in therapy.[14] Middle-class patients may realistically fear the adverse effect of a psychiatric hospitalization on their employment, compounding the problems they already face. Physicians have frequently viewed psychiatric hospitalization as inappropriate for dying patients. Negative stereotyping of inpatient psychiatric units has not made them easy places to which someone may turn. Which AIDS patients, then, make use of such units?

THE FIRST COHORT—THE ARRIVAL OF AIDS PATIENTS ON PSYCHIATRIC INPATIENT UNITS

At present there is no systematic way of knowing the precise number of AIDS-related cases treated in psychiatric inpatient services, since most state reporting procedures identify the hospital but are not unit-specific. Some do not believe such statistics should be readily available, given issues of confidentiality, the repercussions of a double stigma for the patient, or fear of adverse publicity for the unit. The published literature suggests that the number of cases on any

particular unit is relatively small. However, the cumulative total is steadily growing as AIDS and HIV infection rates rise; the numbers are projected by the
Surgeon General to continue to increase.[15]

The pathways to a psychiatric unit are varied. A psychiatric unit can be a
known place through which patients have passed before, suffering from a psychiatric condition that preceded their contracting AIDS. Others, although never
before hospitalized, have encountered mental-health systems since childhood or
adolescence in outpatient clinics or in drug treatment units. It is a part of such
lives to be repeatedly under psychiatric care. For some who had no need of
psychiatric treatment before, a psychiatric hospitalization is yet another humil-
iating and terrifying experience that grows out of the complication of contracting
the AIDS virus.

The first cohort of AIDS-related psychiatric referrals includes a wide spectrum
of people ranging from the "worried well" to those who have a full-blown case
of AIDS. Some have ARC. Still others have HIV serum positivity. Some are
admitted for drug detoxification after diagnosis; others because of a prior psychiatric diagnosis complicating their response to AIDS. If not screened out as
medically inappropriate, neurologically impaired patients present as well for
diagnostic evaluation. For those who have been diagnosed as having AIDS for
a considerable length of time prior to admission, signs of organicity, changes in
coping ability, increased life stresses, new losses, sudden development of severe
depression, or suicidal tendencies are grounds for admission. However, many
cases of HIV-associated organicity remain unreferred.

Patients who present immediately after diagnosis are usually agitated or extremely anxious. They may be in a state of shock or overwhelmed, devastated,
or despairing. Occasionally, they show symptoms of acute psychotic thinking
and are delusional, paranoid, manic, or suicidal. Some have precisely the same
response after being diagnosed with ARC, being found to be HIV-positive or
prior to testing for the virus.

Patients with previous psychiatric diagnoses may be physically well but need
admission because their terrified response to the possibility of contracting AIDS
has exacerbated their psychiatric conditions. Some of these people fear adverse
consequences from their experimentation with drugs or sex. Others find that
their attempts to make money at prostitution or to find intimacy have brought
them into contact with individuals who are in high-risk groups or ill.

In theory, anyone should be admitted if an inpatient psychiatric unit is the
least restrictive setting in which assessment and treatment can occur. But, in
fact, we know that not everyone who needs mental-health services will choose
to use them. Nor are services necessarily accessible for all who need or want
them.[16]

We need to know much more about the socioeconomic, organizational, and
geographical variables that influenced the composition of the first group of
patients treated on psychiatric units. Are the small numbers of AIDs patients
on particular units simply a reflection of the newness of the disease? After all,
until recently, AIDS patients were a novelty and not routine. Or, as Cecci
suggests, are the numbers small because psychiatric-unit chiefs have been unwilling to accept AIDS patients?[17] Since physicians do not routinely refer patients
with medical conditions such as AIDS for inpatient psychiatric care, how do
they determine whom they do refer? Are there special characteristics about

those drug addicts, homosexuals, or prostitutes who voluntarily turn to such units for help? And what about those who are involuntarily admitted? Most published reports simply specify membership in the high-risk groups and give little information about other variables that have led to admission.

Much of the early literature focused on those situations in which patients were admitted on the basis of events over which the treatment staff had little control.[18] Some patients' entry into a psychiatric treatment setting, for instance, was forced by a compassionate hospital administrator who insisted that AIDS patients were entitled to treatment. Even units that wish to cannot always exclude AIDS patients. Units cannot always screen out potential AIDS cases. Some found themselves dealing with AIDS inadvertently after it was discovered that patients suffered from AIDS or ARC after being admitted for other reasons. Patients themselves as well may find that a problem they believed to be purely psychological had this unanticipated or denied cause.

All things considered, it is impossible to claim that AIDS patients in psychiatric units are necessarily representative of the AIDS population as a whole. But, regardless of the specific characteristics of the sample, as staff have been faced with the specter of growing numbers of AIDS patients, attention has been turned to the issues and concerns the staff have about treatment of the person with AIDS.

STAFF CONCERNS

The staff of the psychiatric unit, too, need comfort. As members of the society at large, they are not immune from the general fears of AIDS. But, unlike the staff of nursing homes or general hospitals where victims of equally terrifying diseases of unknown etiology are treated, the staff of psychiatric units did not expect to grapple with dying patients and their diseases. Traditionally, good mental hospitals were places where life was renewed. As Stanton and Schwartz put it, it is common for patients to enter psychiatric units "disturbed, confused or terrified to such an extent that ordinary support and reassurance have failed . . . in bringing them relief . . . for many, hospitalization means a new beginning rather than an end."[19] When working well, psychiatric inpatient units have been places where people regained hope in themselves and renewed courage to live their lives in spite of the stigma that is frequently attached to the place where this effort occurs.

Even if the ideals of treatment are not always the reality, psychiatric units, at the very least, try to offer rapid relief from symptoms. Patients are offered medication and brief therapy. Social skills may be taught, health education provided, and social support networks mobilized in the hope that follow-up will be available on an outpatient basis. It is not that the staff of such units are unaccustomed to confronting those who, in despair, long for death. But their task has been to save lives and prevent death. Staff do not always view the dying as appropriate patients.

Physically ill patients have also posed problems. They require a different kind of nursing care and attention to new issues. AIDS patients are no exception. However, these patients focused attention on infection control procedures which, in the past, may not have been as salient for the staff.

Ironically, unlike patients with physical problems, such as an infected stump,

chronic obstructive pulmonary disease, or diabetes, which may require complicated and time-consuming nursing management, AIDS patients frequently need
only minimal and specific protocols which do not greatly intrude on the work
of the staff.[20] However, because of the fear of contagion, these procedures are
often fraught with great symbolism in a health care system that too often ar-
bitrarily separates mental and physical illness. Other patients who have HIV
spectrum disorders, of course, may challenge medical and nursing staff with
complex and sometimes puzzling symptoms pertaining to secondary opportunistic infections and diseases, which demand careful analysis and appropriate
treatment.[21] As well, the task of determining accurate diagnoses of both psychiatric and medical conditions can prove particularly difficult because presenting
symptomatology can sometimes signal either psychological or physiological conditions, the differential sorting is not always clear-cut, and the treatment choices
can differ significantly.

The inpatient psychiatric staff currently have other burdens as well. The rapid
escalation of hospital inpatient costs has turned attention to the use of prospective
payment systems to contain hospital costs. For instance, the Social Security
Amendments of 1983 introduced diagnosis-related groups to establish hospital
charges for Medicare patients. Although psychiatry was exempted, it is clear
that fiscal policies may be developed that can radically revise, generally down-
ward, the capacity of psychiatric inpatient units to care for the poor or severely
ill.[22]

In addition, public thinking about disability and outpatient psychiatric care
has been influenced by those who demand more stringent disability determinations and cost containment.[23,24] Paradoxically, funding for outpatient social
services dwindles while the demands for such services grow, as inpatient units
accommodate to the call for cost containment by shortening the length of stay.
Psychiatric inpatient staff may therefore be faced with new constraints on their
ability to care for AIDS patients if a prospective payment system is developed
that further limits the time such patients can spend on the unit.

The projected cost of treating AIDS further complicates the picture. One
suggestion has been to turn from acute-care settings to home care, long-term
care settings, and hospices.[25] The anticipated growth in the number of people
with organic brain problems resulting from the HIV virus raises new problems.[26]
Although it may be a good idea, in theory, to treat people in the community,
there is in fact a shortage of appropriate alternative settings that meet the needs
of those AIDS or ARC patients who can benefit from inpatient psychiatric
assessment or treatment.

If this social context is ignored, psychiatric staff can be as stereotyped as their
patients. For example, some advocates assume that gay men on such units
encounter homophobia when they are not discharged to optimal community
settings. But, added to the current problems of finding housing for the mentally
ill and poor are the problems created by the fear of AIDS in the community.

Like others, the anxieties of the staff reflect the gaps in what is known about
AIDS and its possible danger to themselves, even if they are not members of
the high-risk groups. After all, increasing numbers of people who were once
considered low-risk are flocking to have HIV antibody tests to determine whether
they have been exposed. For some this brings relief; for others, fear. Moreover,

the majority of the staff are aware of the test's limitations. A small percentage of the staff may react to the deviant status of the patient in less than helpful ways.[27] When all is said and done, patients and staff alike must struggle to do the best they can in a society that has yet to find solutions to the difficult social and ethical problems AIDS raises. What, then, in the social organization of the psychiatric unit makes it a place where AIDS patients can be helped?

SOCIAL ORGANIZATION AND CULTURE OF PSYCHIATRIC INPATIENT UNITS

With all its problems and pressures, the therapeutic milieu approach rests on the belief that human beings can form communities that facilitate social integration and mutual support.[28] Few brief treatment units, even those dominated by a biomedical model, are organized around an approach in which patients are expected to deal individually with their problems alone with a doctor, apart from a "community." A milieu, recognized or not, always exists. The staff in units that adhere to the therapeutic community approach frequently view the unit as a microcosm of the exterior world in which patients react "as if" it were that external reality, reflecting the troubles and issues that brought patients there and to which they will return. In psychiatric units, the rich and the poor; old and young; men and women; heterosexuals and homosexuals; blacks, Hispanics, and Anglos; Jews, Christians, Moslems, and atheists; ethnic minorities; and dominant-group members can find themselves mingling, linked by the fact they encounter each other in search of comfort, symptom relief, and health.

The staff, as part of its own practice, continually observes itself and its reactions to patients, including those with AIDS-related conditions. In theory, the unit is designed to counter prejudices, reaffirm an individual's worth, and reassert a belief in a common humanity while also confronting the problems posed in the world "outside." This orientation can be of great benefit in the treatment of patients who have AIDS. The restoration, in Lifton's words, of the broken connections[29] between self and others is especially needed by those people grappling with AIDS whose quality of life may increasingly depend on their abilities to utilize existing social resources.

However, the social organization of psychiatric units is shaped by other factors besides treatment ideologies. For instance, units located in for-profit general hospitals are different from public hospitals and community mental health centers that are mandated to accept anyone in a catchment area, regardless of their ability to pay. Voluntary acute-stay wards affiliated with universities and teaching hospitals are different from units in hospitals to which people are committed against their will. Some units are directed by young physicians whose lives may be quite similar to those of young AIDS patients from similar socioeconomic backgrounds. Others are directed by older, foreign physicians whose own lives and families may bear little resemblance to the social worlds of the patients they treat. Some units have more sophisticated or better academically prepared staff or a mixture that includes individuals from many different backgrounds. Staff education about AIDS will need to take account of these differences. On some units, AIDS patients provide an opportunity for research and career advancement. On others, such activity is viewed as intrusive or irrelevant.

The roles of the professional specialties on such units can also vary. In some places, a team approach resembles a football team in which the physician is the quarterback and calls the signals. In others, the milieu is the responsibility of the nursing staff. In still others, nurses primarily monitor medical care. The work of relating the unit and patient to the "outside" is customarily delegated to a psychiatric social worker rather than to clinical sociologists or medical anthropologists. Rehabilitation or vocational counselors may or may not be part of the core treatment team. Psychotherapy may be emphasized or minimal. Psychoanalytic psychodynamic formulations may be important or viewed as unnecessary. Psychological tests may or may not be administered. Physicians on some units work with patients only while social workers work with the family.

In short, psychiatric units are not all the same. Each has its own unique culture, its own strengths and weaknesses. The treatment of all patients, including those who must deal with AIDS, is shaped by the complex interplay of treatment philosophy, organization, available resources, politics, specialties, and personalities that influence the actions of both patients and staff.

Within all these diverse settings, however, staff struggle to communicate with each other and patients. As always, the forms of talk are complicated.[30] Both formal and informal communication lines exist. There are general and unspoken norms governing to whom one talks and under what circumstances, what should be talked about, what should be done about what is said, and what is not said at all.

Patients and staff alike develop ways of doing things that are both shared and secret. According to Belitsky and Lieberman,[31] the details of a patients' history and condition are confidential on a short-term psychiatric unit, and it is up to the patient to decide how much should be shared with others. Patients are usually encouraged to do so as part of their treatment. However, longer term settings, such as those designed for intensive treatment of adolescents/young adults, may view disclosure of such information as an expectation, given the prolonged interdependancy and intimacy of the group on the unit, the age group involved, and the ever-present issues of impulsiveness and sexuality. Other units that subscribe to a private model in which a private psychiatrist conducts individual psychotherapy with patients and the treatment setting is seen simply as a place to monitor symptoms and adjust medications may strongly discourage sharing of such personal information, even among unit staff. Moreover, as Yalom has noted, the opportunity to help others is one of the curative features of both inpatient and outpatient group therapy.[32] AIDS patients are, after all, not alone in grappling with the powerlessness, loneliness, and fear of a biological condition that alters life plans and hopes. As biological explanations of mental disease become more accepted, others, such as people diagnosed schizophrenic, can share a recognition of some of the aspects of the AIDS patients' social plight. But do patients have a right to know if the afflicted person chooses not to confide in them? And, conversely, does the afflicted person have the right to remain silent if he or she does not believe the response of the others will be helpful?[33]

The presence of AIDS patients forces attention on the taken-for-granted understandings of appropriate talk within the worlds of staff, patients, and community. Each unit must find ways of framing these patients in order to incorporate them into the units ongoing work and to formulate treatment plans.

FRAMING AIDS PATIENTS

According to Goffman,[34] during an interaction, actors (to use the sociological term) cognitively "frame" a situation by enclosing it within a series of definitions of what exists and what should transpire. Goffman theorized that this was analogous to a picture frame which places a border around the subject matter thereby containing it. Framing takes place at multiple levels and can be an ongoing process by which people make sense of what is transpiring and develop expectations of what should occur[35].

The initial framing of AIDS patients also framed the staff. Staff were immediately targeted as being in need of education. The first task was to frame the disease in such a manner that the staff could handle their own fears and work out proper procedures. Programs were launched to give accurate information and education to the staff about the changing knowledge about the virus and syndrome as it pertained to the activities of the unit. The medical aspects of psychiatric treatment were reinforced by directing staff attention to the task of properly assessing patients, particularly those from high-risk groups, to ascertain whether they suffered from AIDS, ARC, or the fear of an AIDS syndrome that had yet to manifest itself. Infection control officers were called on to quickly develop means of protecting others, including staff, while maximizing the patient's ability to participate in unit activities. Issues of confidentiality were debated within the context of the development of such protocols, some of which were more stringent than others. By use of such interactions, treatment staff were reinforced in their primary roles as health care providers. However, both clinical and nonclinical staff sometimes remain quite skeptical of the medical team members' efforts to reassure them by framing AIDS in this way.

A second frame grew out of the categories developed by the Centers for Disease Control (CDC). Following the categorization of patients developed for epidemiological purposes, patients were framed by membership in the high-risk groups, and educational programs were targeted on the basis of such categories. The gay community, in particular, was most influential in developing strategies to address the presumed homophobia of the staff and in initiating a search for ways to mitigate this assumed prejudice or fear. Much of the published literature at hand primarily discusses the homosexual AIDS patients without much reference to socioeconomic class or life style. Early efforts were devoted to empathically framing homosexual patients by calling attention to the cruel repercussions of AIDS in their lives. As attention to IV drug users increased, so did an awareness for more targeted approaches to this subpopulation. But, increasingly, articles are appearing that note that social types constructed from the CDC categories may oversimplify the task of understanding a person in the everyday world whose encounter with AIDS is one life event among others.[36]

Given the vast literature on the influence of socioeconomic status, ethnicity, gender, color, and diagnosis on disease and psychiatric treatment, it has been perplexing to find that so much of the initial literature intended to influence the meanings that staff give to AIDS patients glossed over such variables.

By the time the book in which this paper is published goes to press, it will have been over two years since the article was written. In the natural history of the AIDS epidemic this is a very long time, indeed. Given the rapidity of new information about AIDS, an article can become dated before it is read. For instance, when we initiated our literature review, the only article identified in a 1986 Med-Line search and published in a social work journal stated that "for purposes of presentation" the dilemmas of a gay male patient can be used to represent "most of the issues" involved in the treatment of all patients with AIDS.[37] We now note an impressive increase in the literature.[38]

People confronting mortal illness do share a common situation. But there is a growing recognition of the fact that the everyday problems of a poor black unwed mother dying from AIDS are different than those of a white professional man whose wealthy lover is steadfastly standing by to help and care. People in real life belong to multiple groups, play many roles, and occupy more than one status. The responses of staff, family, friends, and community shape the social world in which persons with AIDS find themselves and the options that are available to them.

It is also noteworthy that, in reflecting on what we had originally written, we were struck by the constancy of many of the issues. Given the delay in publication, this paper is already a historical document that reflects the social, moral, ethical, legal, and professional concerns at one point in time. It also serves as a more enduring expression of the fundamental questions regarding HIV germaine to psychiatric settings.

For some purposes, it may have been necessary to gloss over such complexities by discussing AIDS patients in the broad categories epidemiologists were using. But if we want to influence the meanings that shape the practical work of a psychiatric inpatient staff, it is these very complexities that matter. And so, the search must continue for additional frames to augment staff thinking and to enhance treatment.

One such frame is provided by what sociologists have called the theory of social action, which directs attention to the analysis of social relationships. As actors, staff and patient encounter each other while engaged in a complex human endeavor. Although dealing with AIDS is a commonality, each actor comes to the unit with different life experiences. While sharing time and space, the lives of patient and staff intersect. Their effect on each other exposes the complexity of the shared enterprise which is psychiatric treatment. We can illustrate this best while protecting confidentiality of both patients and staff by turning to case vignettes we have created to provide glimpses of interaction on such units.

GLIMPSES OF LIVES: SOCIAL INTERACTIONS ON INPATIENT PSYCHIATRIC UNITS

The components of the theory of social action are actors, a situation of action, and the orientation of actors to that situation.[39] All three matter. Patients with AIDS, like those with other diagnoses, bring their own individual traits to the unit. The social structure of the unit is in place, as is its relationship to the society outside its walls. But human beings have the unique capacity to give meanings to their situations. It is through these definitions of the situation "that human lives are shaped and transformed,"[40] as the following vignettes illustrate.

1. A white Protestant graduate student became depressed after it was discovered that he had AIDS. He was referred by the university health service.

His stay on the unit was marked by the fact that the university was located far from his family and he had to choose between being cared for by his lover or his parents. It was impossible for his lover, without great personal sacrifice, to move where his parents lived. This dilemma, which equals that of Solomon's, tormented both him and the treatment staff. Some of the staff favored his remaining with his lover; others thought he belonged with his family. The social worker did not view the lover as equivalent to a spouse and spent a great deal of time in efforts to convince the young man to go back to his parents' home. Eventually he did so. When he died, his major department held a memorial service which members of the unit staff attended. His death was mourned by the unit as well as by his parents, lover, relatives, teachers, classmates, and friends.

2. A 32-year-old Hispanic man on disability diagnosed schizoaffective arrived on the unit contemplating suicide after finding out his blood test for HIV was positive. The unit staff was dismayed. The patient had first been treated at 18. He had returned over and over again as he worked out his sexual orientation. At one point, he fled from the small town in which he lived to a major metropolitan center where he experimented with homosexuality by going to bathhouses. At another, in fury with his family, who attacked him for not working, he spent a brief period of time employed as a gay prostitute. With the help of a caring young therapist, he made peace with his homosexuality and entered into a constructive loving relationship for the first time in his adult life. The relationship was jeopardized by the findings of the blood test. Faced with the need to tell his lover and to deal with the ambiguity of the implications of the test, he became suicidal, as he had been in the past. He voluntarily returned to the inpatient unit in order to come to terms with his fear of AIDS in the company of those staff members who had watched him grow up and who could comfort him in this horrifying, unanticipated consequence of the work done together during past hospitalizations. He openly discussed his fear with the members of the therapeutic community, and some other patients benefited from supporting him. When he was discharged, his relationship with his lover remained unresolved, and the staff anticipated further hospitalizations.

3. A single black mother came to the unit from a community hospital. Her life had never been easy. She grew up in a series of foster homes, and it was suspected that she had been sexually abused in the last one. She bolted from it into the arms of a drug-using pimp and became a mother at age 14. From 14 on, the only social support she received came from drug addicts, as she supported herself and child through prostitution. She herself became an IV drug user. At varying points in time, she voluntarily entered drug treatment programs only to fail. She was expelled from one such program because she missed group sessions claiming she was "too tired to come." AIDS had not yet become an issue in this center, and the group leader, an ex-addict, did not realize that this fatigue was an early symptom of AIDS. As information about AIDS spread through the shooting gallery, she came to the emergency room and was subsequently diagnosed with ARC and admitted to the hospital. There she encountered a volunteer from a community project who was willing to help her place her child in the home of a friend in the same school district. But, the hospital social worker did not agree with the placement. She nullified it with the help of Protective Services, placing the child in a foster home far from the school he attended.

The foster parents were not known by the mother. The social worker made it clear that the volunteer had overstepped his boundaries and that discharge planning must remain in the hands of the paid professional staff. The patient became suicidally depressed, made an abortive attempt to cut her wrists, and was transferred to psychiatry.

She was tormented by her failure to protect her child and by her ties to her pimp and drug-using friends. In addition, she confronted the fast-moving progression of her disease and its effect on her child's future. The social worker on this unit recognized the magnitude of problems this woman posed, not the least of which was housing. Unlike her colleague, she was delighted that a community AIDS project existed and recontacted the volunteer the patient had liked. At discharge, she was linked into a network of competent and caring people who became her allies. Ironically, she lacked such social resources before contracting AIDS. Although her life remained difficult, her child's future seemed less bleak as the volunteer helped her reestablish contact and reopened the child's placement. Although this patient was both a prostitute and an IV drug user, she viewed herself as a loving mother. Her therapist's recognition of that role helped her regain the courage to live with her disease, caring for her child as well as she could.

4. A young homosexual Polish-American man who had become psychotically depressed upon diagnosis used the hospitalization to come to terms with his anticipated death, as he had been found to have full-blown and rapidly progressing AIDS. Because the staff did not know how to resolve the conflicting demands of his right to confidentiality and the other patients' right to know, they utilized an infection control procedure which isolated him from the community. He himself abided by these restrictions, some of which were unnecessary, and voluntarily obeyed all precautionary measures. He did not talk about his disease with other patients. A few, however, let it be known that they were aware of his condition and made themselves available to him as caring others. The majority did not appear to be affected by his presence. At first, he thought he would become involved in efforts to shape public opinion about AIDS and decided to make a videotape telling the story of his life. But his parents were horrified. Not only did they resent having to deal with the fact that their son was gay and now ill with a contagious, socially unacceptable disease, but he was also in a psychiatric ward. They insisted that he have no further contact with the treatment team and urged early discharge. He abided by their wishes and canceled the taping. The unit staff learned of his death by reading the obituary. His primary therapist mourned in private, unknown to the family, friends, or community project volunteers.

5. A 25-year-old white single mother of a 2-year-old daughter was admitted for depression and withdrawal from IV drugs. On the 4th hospital day, she confided in her clinician that she felt "guilty" because she had not told the staff her child had diagnosed ARC and she had a number of ARC symptoms herself.

She was placed on precautions, was provided education and took advantage of the opportunity to discuss her experiences with the community. She then revealed that prior to admission she had an abscessed tooth. After telling the dental clinic staff about her illness, she had been "stalled" in one clinic and rejected from another. She was then given a list of dentists who accepted AIDS patients, but none would take Medicaid. In desperation, she finally set up an appointment at another hospital clinic near a relative's home without stating she had ARC. Her experiences of rejection had led her to believe honesty was not the best policy. She desperately wanted to be detoxified to care for her child.

6. A 26-year-old white separated woman who was a prostitute was to be admitted to the unit. She had become a public figure because of her refusal to stop her work after her disease was diagnosed. She had a turbulent treatment career, deliberately scratching and spitting at the medical staff who cared for her. To the relief of all, she died before she was admitted to the psychiatric unit. Of the cases reviewed, she received the least sympathy, as her fury at both her death and life alienated her from staff. Unlike the gay men whose deaths were mourned, her death was welcomed, as staff did not want to have to deal with an angry "sociopathic borderline" who physically attacked them in hopes they, too, would contract the disease.

7. A 41-year-old physician was called out of a team meeting by an urgent phone call from his daughter. She had mentioned at work during a coffee break that her father worked with AIDS cases, and her supervisor had stormed into her employer's office to demand she be terminated from her summer job. She wanted her father to call immediately and reassure the employer that she could not "give them AIDS."

8. A psychiatric technician accompanied a patient who had HIV serum positivity to the ER for a medical consultation. The young physician encountered problems with the syringe while drawing blood. He became increasingly upset, finally snapping at the technician, "This patient better not have AIDS or the virus, or I'll sue you all." He stormed from the room, leaving the patient with the syringe stuck in his arm as the blood streamed out. The technician, quite shaken, dashed out to find a nurse. The patient rose to the occassion and reassured the technician on the way back, "Things like this just happen; it wasn't your fault."

9. A 33-year-old black homosexual professional man became psychotically depressed after learning he had ARC. He lived alone and currently had no close sustaining relationships other than with his family, who did not know he was gay. He was particularly worried about his mother's reaction, as she was a devoutly religious Christian. To his surprise, she arrived in the company of her minister, who had come to pray with her and her son. The minister assured the patient that the entire congregation was concerned about his welfare and were praying for his recovery. He urged the patient to return to church and to put himself in "the Lord's hands." The patient was greatly relieved by the visit. Although his therapist was concerned by what he saw as increased "religiosity," he helped the patient to formulate discharge plans that included his return to active participation in church prayer meetings, study, and community service projects.

Daily, as these examples reveal, the social world unfolds as people grappling with AIDS interact with each other. The situation in which these interactions take place is indeed difficult. Why, then, do some choose to turn from suffering human beings while others display such compassion and courage?

The need to understand how we choose among contending alternatives is important to both social science and psychiatric treatment. As Schutz, among others, has argued, it is by studying the meanings given to social action that we can understand and shape social processes.[41] It is through these processes that the social environment becomes transformed into a field of possibilities in which human choices are made. Given all that remains to be learned, we can only conclude that attention to the experiences of patients and staff struggling with AIDS on psychiatric inpatient units enables us to reflect on the relationships between self and society that affect our choices.

CONCLUDING REFLECTIONS

The experiences of people encounterng AIDs demonstrate both the glories and the agonies of social interaction. Psychiatric inpatients units provide one setting in which we can observe people giving meaning to themselves and their social worlds. There is much we can learn from such observations.

As we have seen, psychiatric units are not paradises. The conflicts, prejudices, and contradictions of the everyday social world are mirrored on the unit. That social world is constantly changing as knowledge and politics influence the meanings given to AIDS. We must take account of the complex interplay of history, social organization, and biography. To study, understand, and evaluate the experiences of people coping with AIDS on psychiatric units, we must look at the ways lives are embedded in the fluctuating social matrix that shapes the responses to AIDS itself.

We note that the term "high-risk group" is being replaced in the literature by "high-risk behavior," calling attention to individual variations in behavior. This change in terminology will mean that the experiences of one cohort of patients may vary from those of the next due to the rapidly changing ways in which persons with AIDS are framed and treated. Therefore, the social processes by which knowledge is formulated, distributed, and used have great bearing upon the struggles and acts of both staff and patients on inpatient units. Such changes and their impact must be studied continually.

Furthermore, patients vary in regard to the stage of the disease at which they present. Responses of staff, patient, families, friends, and lovers vary, too. We cannot discuss AIDS patients on psychiatric units without acknowledging the heterogeneity of those involved. We must continually locate those interacting on these units in both time and space.

Despite this complexity some people struggling with AIDS can learn the social skills necessary to give and receive comfort. Those who can empathically take account of others' feelings fare better both within and outside the hospital. Whether patients are gay, drug users, or prostitutes is less significant than whether they alienate the people on whom they must depend. Given this, we should celebrate the accomplishments of AIDS patients faced with an untimely and terrible death who emerge from despair and use what is offered them during the hospitalization creatively to reconstitute meaningful lives, no matter how brief.

We can also appreciate the accomplishments of other patients on the unit, who by accident of fate find themselves sharing time and place with an "AIDS victim." In the face of a disease that is so feared, those hospitalized psychiatric patients who reach out and empathically reaffirm the worth of another human being who must deal with AIDS are impressive indeed. We only wish that all on the "outside" who think of themselves as normal, sane, healthy, and God-fearing could respond as well.

We recognize the courage of those members of the inpatient psychiatric staff who in the face of their own death anxieties find ways to overcome their fears, offering as much as their science, their professions, their humanity, and their social worlds make possible. They help people struggling with AIDS to summon the strength to live and, when necessary, to die.

Observers can affirm the accomplishments of those families, friends, and lovers who loyally stand by and use the unit to find the support necessary to continue to help while grieving. And we celebrate the existence of community projects staffed by "brave, generous, and caring people"—the volunteers who work so diligently and at such great cost to themselves to provide the follow-up care that makes it possible for some discharged patients both to live and to die with dignity.[42]

It is these very strengths that expose the impoverishment of a society that too often turns away from human need. It is ironic that it may only be through a psychiatric hospitalization precipitated by AIDS that some members of this society experience the full richness of a complex yet caring community. Why should social support and human connectedness be dependent on the emergence of a dread disease? Do not all people need to know that they will not lack hospital or home care if they become ill and cannot work? Do not all families need to be assured they will be housed adequately, even if they or the head of the family becomes ill? Why must any human being die in misery alone? Why should any of us mourn the loss of the life of someone we love apart from a community made up of comforting others who acknowledge our grief? We all need a compassionate society.

At best, psychiatric inpatient units provide a model of a community that reawakens a vision of what a society can be. For members of a truly therapeutic community, the age, sex, sexual preference, color, religion, alcohol or drug abuse history, occupation, ethnicity, or marital status of a human being does not negate an empathic response to human suffering. Such communities can indeed be microcosms of the world outside of the hospital that permit us to examine the tasks of understanding the human condition and shaping social relationships that can accept adversity while going beyond it.

One unanticipated consequence of paying attention to AIDS patients has been the reemphasis of the connections between biology and society. Since this paper's completion, an initiative undertaken by the American Psychiatric Association in the summer of 1987 explicitly advocates use of a biopsychosocial model to frame AIDS. As Novick recently noted,[43] the psychiatric treatment of persons with AIDS exposes the awful problems physicians face when working with people struggling with an incurable and stigmatized disease. The biomedical treatment of any illness, including AIDS, provides hope for cure, at best, or prolongation of life with the disease. But each individual human life, regardless of its duration, is lived with others. And so we return to the connections between personal troubles and social issues with which we began.

Human beings cannot will away the horror of diseases like AIDS or eliminate the tragedy of death. But we do have the power to reach out to each other at times of grief and let others know as they die or watch loved ones die that they are not alone and that the community will not abandon them. The encounters of people struggling with AIDS on psychiatric inpatient units remind us of the fragility of human existence and the power of social bonds. It is a complicated task to give meaning to such encounters and to adequately frame both patients and staff. And yet recognition of this complexity is essential. Our own reflections have led us to reemphasize the linkages between individuals and the social world. After all, it is on understanding and shaping this connectedness that the quality of all our lives and deaths depends.

REFERENCES

1. Isaiah (117). *The Holy Scriptures According to the Masorctic Text* (LXI, 12, 14) Philadelphia: Jewish Publication Society, 1952.
2. Lutruff, D., Everest, H. (1985). The myths in mental illness. *J. Transpersonal Psychol.* 17(2):123–125.
3. Kasper, A. (1986). *Consciousness re-evaluated: Interpretive theory and feminist scholarship. Sociol. Inquiry* 56(1):30–49.
4. Bayer, R. Fox, D., Willis, D. (1986). AIDS: The public context of an epidemic. *Millbank Q.* (Suppl. 1).
5. Kaufman, S. A. (1986). *The Ageless Self: Sources of Meaning in Late Life*, p. 14–16. Madison: University of Wisconsin Press.
6. Hsu, F. (1985). The self in cross-cultural perspective. In A. Marsella, G. DeVos, F. Hsu (eds.) *Culture and Self: Asian and Western Perspectives*, pp. 24–55. New York and London: Tavistock Publications.
7. Freud, S. (1962). *Civilization and Its Discontents.* New York: W.W. Norton (first American ed.).
8. Riley, M.W., Riley, J.W. Jr. (1986). Longevity and social structure: The potential of added years. In A. Pifer, L. Bronte (eds.) *Our Aging Society*, pp. 57–78. New York: W.W. Norton.
9. Harrington, C. et al. (1985). *Long Term Care of the Elderly: Public Policy Issues.* Newbury Park, California: Sage Publications.
10. Callahan, D. (1986). Health care in the aging society: A moral dilemma. In A. Pifer, L. Bronte (eds.) *Our Aging Society*, pp. 319–340). New York: W.W. Norton.
11. Bayer, R. (1981). *Homosexuality and American Psychiatry: The Politics of Diagnosis.* New York: Basic Books.
12. Lerner, M. (1987). Public interest psychotherapy. *Utne Reader* 1(20):39–45.
13. Estroff, S.E. (1981). *Making It Crazy: An Ethnography of Psychiatric Clients in an American Community.* Berkeley: University of California Press.
14. Peyret, M. (1985). Coerced voluntarism: The micropolitics of drug treatment. *Urban Life* 13(4):343–365.
15. Koop, C.E. (1987). *Surgeon General's Report on Acquired Immune Deficiency Syndrome.* Washington: U.S. Department of Health and Human Services, pp. 1–36.
16. Greenlee, J., Musse, L. (1986). Help-seeking and the use of psychiatric Services. Paper presented at the Meeting of the Society for the Study of Social Problems, New York.
17. Cecchi, R.L. (1986). Health care advocacy for AIDS patients. *Qual. Rev. Bull. J. Qual. Assurance* 12(8):297–303.
18. Polan, H.J., Hellerstein, A., Jess, M.D. (1985). Impact of AIDS-related cases on an in-patient therapeutic milieu. *Hosp. Community Psychiatry* 36(2):173–176.
19. Stanton, A., Schwartz, M. (1954). *The Mental Hospital*, p. 3. New York: Basic Books.
20. Pavlis, S. (1986). Blood/body fluid precautions, CMHC. (Available from S. Pavlis, 34 Park Street, New Haven, CT 06510.)
21. Flaskerud, J.H. (1987, December). Neuropsychiatric complications, *J. Psychosocial Nursing* 25(12): pages.
22. English, T., Scharfstein, S., Scherl D., Astrachan, B., Muszynski, I. (1986). Diagnosis-related groups and general hospital psychiatry: the APA study. *Am. J. Psychiatry* 143(2):131–139.
23. Stone, D. (1984) *The Disabled Society.* Philadelphia: Temple University Press.
24. Sharfstein, S. (1986). Commentary on "Prospective payment for out-patient mental health services evaluation of diagnosis related groups by Wood and Beardmore." *Community Ment. Health J.* 22(4):292–293.

25. Harding, A. (1986). Planning for the health care needs of patients with AIDS. (Editorial.) *J. Am. Med. Soc.* 56(22):3140.

26. Wolcott, D. (1986). Neuropsychiatric syndrome in AIDS and AIDS-related illnesses. In L. McKsusick (ed) *What To Do About AIDS,* pp. 32–45. Berkeley: University of California Press.

27. Douglas, C.J., Kalman, C.M. Kalman, T.P. (1983). Homophobia among physicians and nurses: an empirical study. *Hosp. Community Psychiatry* 36(12):1309–1311.

28. Alice, J., Griffith, E.H. (1986). The psychiatric unit as a dynamic model for change. *J. Nat. Med. Assoc.* 78(1):33–38.

29. Lifton, R. (1979). *The Broken Connection.* New York: Simon and Schuster.

30. Goffman, E. (1981). *Forms of Talk,* Philadelphia: University of Pennsylvania Press.

31. Belitsky, R., Lieberman, P. (1985). The psychiatric patient with AIDS: New issues and challenges for the in-patient unit. *Yale Psychiatr. Q.* 8(3):4–17.

32. Yalom, I. (1983). *In-Patient Group Psychotherapy.* New York: Basic Books.

33. Novick, A. (1986). AIDS virus infection: Issues of confidentiality and counseling. *AMS News* 52(12):610–612.

34. Goffman, E. (1974). *Frame Analysis.* New York: Harper and Row.

35. Turner, J. (1986). The mechanics of social interaction. *Sociol. Theory* 4(1):901.

36. Perry, S., Markavitz, J. (1986) Psychiatric interventions for AIDS-spectrum disorders. *Hosp. Community Psychiatry* 37:1001–1006.

37. Furstenberg, A. L., Olson, M. (1984). Social work and AIDS. *Social Work in Health Care* 9(4).

38. Koshland, D., Ed. (1988). The AIDS Issue, *Science* 239:541, 573–622.

39. Parsons, T., Shils, E. (eds.) (1951). *Toward a General Theory of Action.* New York: Harper Torch Books.

40. Schutz, A. (1962). *The Collected Papers, I. The Problem of Social Reality.* M. Matanson (ed. and tr.). The Hague: Martinus IV Hoff.

41. Schutz, A. (1967). *The Phenomenology of the Social World.* G. Walsh, F. Lehnert (tr.). Evanston, Il: Northwestern University Press, pp. 57–69.

42. Perlswig, E. (1986). *AIDS Project New Haven Newsl.* 15:2.

43. Novick, A. (1988). The ethics of AIDS: The doctor-patient relationship under stress. Unpublished paper presented at Yale University, Department of Psychiatry Continuing Education Program, April 28, 1988, New Haven, Connecticut.

22

The Stress of AIDS Care Giving: A Preliminary Overview of the Issues

Leonard I. Pearlin, Shirley J. Semple, and Heather Turner

In this chapter we shall describe some of the stressful problems experienced by care givers to AIDS patients. In the effort to understand AIDS and its consequences, research to date has been directed almost entirely toward those who actually host the malady. However understandable this attention is, it has left out of consideration other crucial actors in the AIDS drama—namely, the care givers. There are several reasons why it is important to examine the conditions that affect the well-being of those who provide care. One concerns the enormous economic costs of hospital and institutional care. To the extent that care giving extends the time the patient can remain outside these settings, incalculable economic benefits accrue to community and society. Moreover, we can see that many of the needs of AIDs patients are better met in the care systems of the community than in the labyrinths of the hospital care system. However, such care is typically given with considerable stress and emotional and physical cost to the care givers. If we seek to maximize and prolong care giving, as we should, it behooves us to understand what these stresses are and how care givers, through the use of supports and coping strategies, manage to constrain their magnitude and intensity. The purpose of this chapter is to contribute to such understanding.

It should be recognized at the outset that care givers comprise a rather diverse group whose members stand in very different relationships to the recipient of the care. One distinction that needs to be drawn is between informal and formal care givers. In the case of homosexual patients and care givers, the informal care givers are usually lovers of the patient or are drawn from the ranks of friends, neighbors, or family. They give care because of their attachment to and love for the person or as an expression of the commitment they feel to the community of homosexuals. By contrast, formal care givers, although they often are drawn to the role by compassion and an urgent sense of mission, approach the recipient as trained workers contractually engaged to do a job. That they stand in a formal relationship to the recipient does not mean that they are impervious to emotional pain. However, although formal care givers may also be exposed to stress and its consequences, it is the well-being of the informal care givers that is most at risk, for it is this group that has the greatest emotional stake in the fate of the victim. For this reason, our focus in this chapter is primarily with informal care givers, principally intimate friends and lovers of homosexual AIDS patients.

Although this focus is easily justified by the vulnerability of informal care givers to stress, the formal and informal exist hand in hand in the dynamics of caring for patients. Thus, the problems encountered by informal care givers and their efforts to manage and cope with these problems cannot be viewed as being separate from the system of formal supports that is available. The nature and range of informal care-giving activities and the psychological and physical toll they exact are, to a substantial measure, conditioned by the availability of formal supports. How the informal care giver performs his role, what he must attend to, and what he can ignore are largely governed by the formal resources and services that are available. The tight interweaving between the informal and formal systems of care will be made clearer in a later section where we describe some of the formal services and resources that are available in San Francisco.

Before discussing the stresses and coping behavior of AIDS care givers, a few caveats are in order regarding the limits of our observations. To some extent, our interest in the stresses experienced by AIDS care givers is an extension of our established program of research into the stresses experienced by general populations and, more recently, of our study of care giving to people suffering from chronic diseases—Alzheimer's disease in particular. Much of the theoretical orientation that has guided earlier stress research can be applied to AIDS care givers. However, although certain features of the stress process impinge on everyone alike, the stress experienced by AIDS care givers is sufficiently unique that what has been learned elsewhere cannot fully describe this group. Indeed, although AIDS and care giving are certainly present in heterosexual populations, care giving in the homosexual community has its own special problems that do not apply to others. Since we wished to learn about these problems, we conducted our inquiry by intensively interviewing several people who represent the ranks of both formal and informal care givers in the homosexual community. Although a great deal has been learned from these interviews, we want to emphasize that we are only at the beginning of our inquiry. To capture the complexities and nuances of AIDS care-giver stress, a much more systematic study is required.

It also needs to be underscored that what we have learned of care-giving stress in San Francisco is not necessarily generalizable to other urban areas. Most importantly, San Francisco probably differs from other cities by the density of its community organizations providing formal support to AIDS patients. These community resources, in turn, help to shape the form and nature of informal care giving. Therefore, at both the formal and informal levels, it is doubtful that what is found in San Francisco is duplicated in other locales. The generalizability of our observations, then, is limited by the considerable variation between locales with regard to their systems of formal care giving and the effects of these on informal care giving.

Generalizability is also limited by variation in the commitments of informal care givers and the situational contexts of their care giving. For example, some care givers are fully involved in virtually every aspect of care throughout the entire course of the illness, from diagnosis to death. They participate in medical care decisions, in the running of the household, in feeding the patient and providing him nursing care, in managing finances and legal matters, in serving as the liaison between the patient and the patient's family, friends, and social network, and in seeing to the arrangements following death. The inclusiveness and durability of such commitment depend not only on love and intense motivation but also on access to critical resources. Obviously, even when armed with intense devotion, some care givers must eventually yield many of the tasks to the formal care system. Some care givers withdraw at a time when the patient cannot participate in his own care, when he becomes incontinent, or when he needs more continuous medical care. Others may have to yield the care-giver role earlier, simply because the housing arrangements, the financial resources, or the care giver's occupation do not permit the prolonged and intense use of time and energy for care giving. Finally, there are still other potential care givers who almost immediately separate themselves following the diagnosis of AIDS, either out of fear of contagion or because there was not initially a strong attachment to the patient. This chapter cannot capture these important differences in the commitments of care givers and the conditions that influence the duration of care giving.

Here we shall limit ourselves to considering care-giving stress from the perspective of the fully committed care giver who continues in the role over all or most of the course of the illness. We do this not out of any sense that this will describe most care givers; frankly, we do not know at this time how care givers are distributed along continua of commitment and duration. We believe that by looking at the most difficult and stressful care-giver situations we shall be in a better position to understand the types of challenges and emotional tolls that, to greater or lesser degrees, are experienced by most care givers.

Because of the limited scope of our interviews, the geographical location of the inquiry, the fact that it is directed only at the homosexual community, and the complex variation in the situational contexts of care giving, the reader should be alert to the fact that what we observe may lack generalizability. It is our hope, nonetheless, that even this preliminary undertaking will succeed in focusing on a particularly crucial and vulnerable group and in providing a useful conceptual framework for understanding their experiences.

SOURCES OF STRESS IN AIDS CARE GIVING

What is stressful about giving care to a friend or lover who has AIDS? In answering this query, it is useful to distinguish three types of problems that the care giver may encounter. Each alone is capable of arousing symptoms of stress and in combination, they will almost certainly lead to depression, anxiety, physical illness, or all three. The problems that can result in the care giver's having such symptoms are: first, those that are directly anchored in the demands of caregiving; second, those that stem from certain intrapsychic processes, especially processes of identification with the patient; and, finally, problems that are created in other important areas of life, such as job and finances, which we refer to as attendant life strains. We shall take up each of these in turn and, following this, consider how care givers use social supports and personal coping strategies to deal with such problems.

The Care-Giver Role

Looking at the care-giver role itself, it can be described simply: it is increasingly demanding as the AIDS progresses, it pushes against the limits of energy, it is relentless, it is emotionally depleting, and, eventually, it is defeating. Depending on the stage of the illness, of course, the care giver may be called on to act as friend and confidant, lover, housekeeper, nurse, and paramedic. Moreover, he may be required to act as a liaison with the patient's family, the doctors and clinics in which the patient is involved, the compensatory systems (e.g., Social Security, medical insurance) on which the patient depends, and the social networks of which one or both might be a part. In short, the notion of role overload finds quintessential expression in AIDS care giving.

Given the variety of hats that the care giver must wear and the variety of individuals and institutions with which he must contend, the potential for conflict is great. Some of this conflict is internal, resulting from the necessity to act in one relationship to the patient while wanting to act in another. For example, it is not a simple matter to have a relationship involving the reciprocities of a friendship that is periodically interrupted by the necessity to enforce a medication regimen. But whatever intrapsychic conflicts are aroused by the multiple components of the care-giver role, these are likely to be overshadowed by the conflicts that arise between the care giver and the patient. The patient may come to resent the care giver in direct proportion to the loss of autonomy and control he experiences. It is our impression that resentment and conflict of this sort are particularly likely to occur in the earlier stages of the disease, declining as health itself declines and the patient must acknowledge his dependency on others. The relationship between the informal care giver and the patient is one that goes through radical restructuring, a process likely to produce sharp antagonisms, however transitory they might be.

Relationships with friends also become spheres of conflict. One would ordinarily think that friendships would be nurtured during the long course of care giving, since friends—whether the care giver's, the patient's, or those jointly held—are potential sources of support and assistance. However, it also happens that friendships are sometimes abandoned by the care giver, because the usable support he receives does not balance his expenditure of time and energy. The care giver can come to feel that his friends are unable or unwilling to provide the kind of help that is most needed, that they do not fully appreciate the burdens he bears or the seriousness of the patient's illness, and that they disrupt the routines of the household. The care giver may also be placed in the position of having to give reassurance and support to erstwhile supporters, a role reversal that is resented and that acts as a force to withdraw from such friendships. The care giver simply may not have the reserves that would allow him to continue with supporters who do not support.

The contacts of the care giver with the family of the patient may also be problematic. Care givers on occasion do encounter disdain. The regrets and recriminations that the family might harbor regarding the patient's homosexuality or life style can be directed toward the care giver. He may be totally ignored by the family, treated as an insignificant person, or be the object of overt hostility. The care giver, who is likely to see himself as someone sacrificing his present life for the patient, is understandably left with a sense of outrage when he encounters the contempt of relatives from whom the patient himself might feel psychologically distant. The antagonisms between the care giver and the patient's family may be even more acute in instances where the family first learns of the patient's homosexuality at the time they learn of his AIDS. However, as in virtually every aspect of care-giver stress, there is a good deal of variation in the relationships of care givers and relatives, with some families providing support to the care giver and demonstrating compassion and acceptance. Under adverse circumstances, however, the management of family contacts represents one of the difficult and stressful tasks of the care giver.

An overview of the care-giver role, then, reveals it as one involving a large number of tasks, each of them possessing such urgency that the care giver may be hard put to maintain order and managerial control over the role. Instead, he experiences a situation of overload, where his scarce time and energies are not equal to the urgent demands he must satisfy. The magnitude of the overload, moreover, increases with the course of the disease process. In addition, the care giver is thrown into relationships with formal systems, friends, and family that are often adversarial and conflictive. It is a patently stressful role, one calling for intense motivation, heroic effort, the sensitivity of a diplomat, and a very thick skin.

Intrapsychic Processes and Identification

The observer is necessarily struck by an aspect of AIDS care giving that sets it apart from care giving for people with other diseases, such as cardiovascular disease or Alzheimer's. In the homosexual community, the AIDS care giver has often been exposed to the same risk factors for the malady as those encountered by the patient. He may have been the lover of the patient or might have followed a similar life style and patterns of sexual practice. Under these circumstances, it is understandable that when the giver of care looks at the recipient of care, he may see himself as he fears he will become in the future. This element of identification makes AIDS care giving unique. Furthermore, we believe that such identification adds many degrees of stressfulness to what is already an intensely stressful role.

What are the added burdens associated with identification? One, certainly, is the stark confrontation with one's own vulnerability to disease and death. There is a general mantle of death that solemnly hangs over the gay community, resulting in its own depressive effects. When death is brought home, literally, to the care giver, depression and anxiety are virtually inescapable. It is not only the loss of a loved one that is painfully difficult; that loss, additionally, can represent a terrifying marker of the care giver's own future. Being embedded in the same life style as the victim and, hence, being exposed to the same ruthless system of probabilities heightens identification with the victim to a degree where the care giver is uncertain whether he is witnessing the decline of a lover or friend or his own inexorable movement toward death. There are instances where an individual might have been a principal or secondary care giver to more than one victim. In such cases, where an individual repeatedly sees friends or lovers become ill and die, the processes of identification with the victims and the consequent sense of threat to one's own life probably become even greater.

It needs to be underscored here that care givers may see an even more difficult future for themselves than they witness in the illness and decline of the patient. As they contemplate their own possible futures as victims of AIDS, they foresee a situation in which there will be no one left to give them the same care that they now provide to another. This view of the future is generated not only by the loss of a person who may be closer to them than any other but also to an awareness of the wide swath cut by the advance of AIDS in the homosexual community. As the incidence of AIDS increases, the number of people needing care also increases. Moreover, as the number of people needing care increases, the number of people able to provide it decreases. The burgeoning incidence of AIDS, coupled with the attenuation of informal networks, leaves the care giver in a profound state of anticipatory isolation. Today's care giver may see himself as tomorrow's patient, but without the benefit of care from a loved person.

It is probably typical, then, that because the care giver has shared the same risks as the patient, he is likely to see the patient's plight as the scenario for his own fateful future. Indeed, he may foresee a future that is more bleak and lacking in care than the current situation of the patient. It is no contradiction that even as the care giver's view of his future is shaped by his identification with the patient, he is also keenly aware of the salient difference that separates them. Specifically, he sees himself as different from the patient by virtue of the crucial fact that, unlike the patient, he does not have AIDS. Although he might have taken the same risks as the patient, he has somehow escaped, at least for the present. Indeed, the victim's suffering may magnify the care giver's feeling of being specially anointed. The disparity between the patient's pain and the care giver's health, fragile as it may be, can lead the care giver to rejoice— consciously or not—that it is not he who has AIDS. It is not unlike combat, where at the very time that the soldier feels remorse over his buddy's mortal wounds, he is also delighted that it is not he who is lying on the ground. AIDS can be likened to the capricious bullet that as it seeks out one, spares the other. Although we can only speculate, it would seem that the care giver is vulnerable to a burden of guilt over his own relative good health. He who is spared does not necessarily escape the anguish of survivorship, an anguish made all the more severe by the close identification of the care giver with the patient.

Both the similarities and the differences the care giver sees between himself and the patient are potentially serious sources of stress. The inherent duality in the role relations can shackle the care giver to feelings of terror over his future, on the one hand, and to guilt over his present advantage in health, on the other. These emotional polarities, especially when joined with other ambivalences in the care giver–patient relationship, understandably lead to outbursts of anger and hostility, as well as expressions of deeply felt compassion and love. Although we are able at this time only to chart in a provisional way the problems and stressors that arise out of processes of identification and disidentification, it seems clear that care givers are beset by a host of psychological cross-pressures.

Attendant Life Strains

One is usually not only a care giver but other things as well. He may be a worker, a breadwinner, a participant in a social network, a son or brother, a person with interests pursued in leisure time, and so on. Normally, time and energies are distributed among our multiple roles such that the demands and enticements of each role can be satisfied. Where there is conflict between multiple roles, people are often able to fine-tune their activities to reconcile incompatible demands. AIDS care givers depart from these norms in two respects. First, care giving can be imperialistic—intruding on other roles and gradually diminishing their scope. Second, there is little the care giver can do about this as long as he continues to give care to someone whose needs can only increase with time. Thus, care giving inexorably affects other roles, creating additional problems and stressors for the care giver.

We refer to these additional stressors as attendant life strains, a term that conveys the fact that for the care giver, problems in one pivotal role are likely to cause problems in other roles. The care giver is left to carry not only the enormous burden of care giving itself and the psychological dilemmas that go with it, but also the added weight of job problems, economic problems, the attenuation of important relationships, and the abandonment of interests. Moreover, as problems in these roles mount, each becomes an independent source of stress, incrementally adding to anxiety and depression.

The conflicts entailed in being a care giver and a jobholder provide clear examples of how the burdens of the former create attendant dislocations and problems in other roles. From our earlier description of the many dimensions of the care-giver role, it is obvious that even its minimal demands can easily consume the attentions, energies, and time of the individual. As these demands grow, they can only be satisfied at the expense of other activities and commitments, such as those involved in one's occupation. Care givers report a loss of concentration on the job; they begin to lack the stamina and strength required by the work; they engage in more absenteeism; and they evaluate their own work performance as being below par. The lowered quality of work, in turn, can induce a sense of inadequacy, diminished self-esteem, and threatened job security.

Since AIDS care givers are relatively young, they lack both the economic resources and control over their work lives that older and more established workers might enjoy. Unless they have unusually understanding employers and supervisors (as some do), they are able to exercise little choice and flexibility in how much or when they work. Thus, they are probably obliged to work while engaged in care giving, usually at the expense of the quality of job performance. The demands on the person as a care giver, therefore, stand a very good chance of being incompatible with those of the occupational role. To the extent that he satisfies one role, he risks failure at the other. The result is an ongoing dilemma, leaving him with a sense of inadequacy wherever he places his efforts. The sense of failure, fueled by this relentless dilemma, must eventually push the care giver toward a state of helplessness and powerlessness—states that open the floodgates to depression.

There are many examples that document the emergence of attendant strains in other areas of the care giver's life. They all converge on the same general point: the care-giving role becomes a powerful focal point around which other roles come to be organized. The results are constellations of interrelated stressors, each capable of adversely affecting the care giver's well-being. The speed and extent of this diffusion of problems through the life space of the care giver depend, of course, on the dependency of the patient and the commitment of the care giver to the role. Where the AIDS is at its advanced stages and where one is fully committed to the role, virtually no corner of the care giver's life will remain unaffected.

In sum, there is unfortunately no scarcity of ways in which stress can arise in the lives of care givers. Most that we have been able to identify stem directly from the inordinate demands of the care-giver role itself. Others arise from the processes of psychological identification that are set in motion—especially when the care givers have engaged in sexual practices and life styles similar to those followed by the AIDS sufferers. Still others result from the generation of attendant life strains. The picture we paint is dark. However, for committed care givers who are able to maintain the role to the end, it is an accurate picture. It was our intent to portray the experiences of people at the extreme end of the care-giving gradient, for this portrait is likely to capture at least some of the experiences of those whose care giving is less inclusive or for shorter periods of time. Yet, even at the extreme, people manage to sustain a functional level of integration, despite the ordeals of the care-giver role. How do they do it? Partly as a result of their use of social support and partly through their own coping efforts, to which we now turn.

THE MEDIATORS OF CARE–GIVER STRESS

Social support, both formal and informal, and coping are referred to as mediators of the stress process. This label calls attention to people's capacity to regulate the impact of the stressors to which they are exposed. Thus, two individuals who face similar hardships may exhibit very different stress responses; one may become deeply distressed while the other fares better. Such differences may be explained in part by differences in their access to and use of social and economic resources and by their coping repertoires. Clearly, if we are to understand how people are able to maintain their roles as care givers, we must understand the conditions that materially and emotionally sustain them in the face of these arduous circumstances.

With regard to formally organized, community-based support, we can assert unequivocally that this is a necessary condition for the functioning of informal support and care giving. That is, without the formal system, other systems would be insufficient to keep patients out of hospital settings to the extent that they are now able to do. To catalog the formal resources available in San Francisco is far beyond the purpose and scope of this chapter. A partial view of their diversity and range can be conveyed by a brief description of programs under the aegis of Shanti, an organization that receives part of its funding from the city. Under the umbrella of this single organization are the following: an emotional support program staffed by a pool of about 400 volunteers who have undergone an intensive training regimen; a practical support program with up to 125 volunteers providing material assistance such as shopping and light housekeeping; a residence program that accommodates about 50 patients in 10 houses, two of them functioning as hospices providing 24-h care; a counseling service, entailing both a hotline that receives up to 450 calls a day and face-to-face contact with patients at San Francisco General Hospital; and, finally, client support groups that primarily are aimed at patients but also operate for family, friends, and lovers. Although this is only a modest sample of formal resources, we do not wish to create the impression either that there are sufficient resources to meet the needs of all patients and their care givers or that all patients and care givers take equal advantage of what is available. What we want to emphasize is that there is a network of organizations that make a substantial difference in the lives of many patients and that ease some of the burdens and stresses of care givers. The constellations of community resources represent crucially important stress mediators at an organizational level.

Let us now consider the care giver's informal supports. These may come from his own friends, from the patient's friends, or from the patient's family. As we have seen, the availability of friends and relatives does not automatically assure that they will be appropriately supportive or that the support they give will compensate what the care giver must reciprocate in time and energy. The care giver may indeed become alienated from his network should it fail his expectations and needs, and it is also possible that some people in the network become "burned out" by the care givers' endless appetite for help and assistance. Despite the forces that attenuate the system of informal support, it remains a very powerful mediating force in the stress process. Care givers do draw on this network for day-to-day logistical help, and it is used, too, to provide the care giver the opportunity for occasional respite. Moreover, it is a source of emotional sustenance. The sheer solidarity of purpose and concern can be uplifting and helpful to the care giver in reinforcing and validating his commitments. In addition, within the network, care givers may find sexual partners with whom they can safely satisfy their needs for intimacy and expressiveness. Informal support, then, may periodically lift some of the burden from the shoulders of the principal care giver. More importantly, it can emotionally sustain the care giver through expressions of esteem and affection.

As crucial as the systems of formal and informal support are, the survival of the care giver may eventually come to rest on his own coping abilities. Three general functions of coping can be recognized: it can function to *change or manage the situation* that is giving rise to the threatening life problems; it can serve to *change the perceived meaning* of the situation such that its threat is reduced; and it can *provide relief from the symptoms* of stress.

It is in relation to the first function, changing the situation, that the limitations of coping are most apparent. Many of the stressful situations in which people are located are simply not amenable to change through individual effort. Care givers face two situations, one involving their own health and the other the health of the patient. Coping that functions to prevent or minimize damage to the care giver's health may be more effective than that aimed at protecting that of the patient. For example, the care giver might alter his life style, enhance his physical health, or engage in sexual practices that entail less risk. These kinds of actions represent highly efficacious ways of coping with situations that can adversely affect the care giver. However, the demands of taking care of the AIDs patient largely defy coping. Present knowledge indicates that once AIDS is contracted, individual coping efforts—on the part of either the patient or the care giver—will not alter the malady or its course. Care givers can and do organize their activities in ways that enable them to be more efficient and to conserve precious time and energy. These managerial coping techniques are important for both care giver and patient, but they do not alter the forward movement of the disease process or the intensification of care giving that occurs over time.

Consequently, there is a heavy reliance on coping techniques having the second function, the management and change of the meaning of the situation, in ways that reduce its threatening qualities. There are a number of perceptual and cognitive devices used to reduce the threatening meaning of the situation. For example, during the early phases of the illness, care givers and patients alike might adopt a very "positive" view of things. This view may be fed by the belief that positiveness cures or retards disease whereas negativism speeds its course. In effect, it enables people to cling to the very important notion that they can control their own fate. To support a positive outlook, it is usually necessary to engage in some denial of encroaching signs that belie the outlook. For example, in one household the patient and care giver terminated the services of hospice personnel because they felt that their presence promoted an air of pessimism. However, denial and the optimism it permits must eventually yield to mounting evidence that the situation is worsening.

Instead of trying to maintain a rosy view of the patient's future, the care giver might attempt to block out the future from consciousness. If he follows the trajectory of events into the future, he may find little reason to continue the struggles of care giving. He could easily be so discouraged that he gives up the fight. Consequently, the care giver is likely to become largely oriented to the present, essentially adopting the "one day at a time" coping strategy. The care giver does not contemplate next month or next week but instead devotes himself totally to what needs to be done here and now. The very multiple demands of care giving that can so stress the care giver may also aid his temporary salvation. He is able to allow himself to become so totally preoccupied with what immediately confronts him that he is able to screen out the bleaker and more frightening future.

The ideologies and value systems of the care giver may also be involved and bent in a way that controls the meaning of the situation, to make it less threatening and more acceptable. The care giver might come to appraise his activities not only as an act of compassion toward an individual but also as one that is consistent with larger moral precepts. For example, the care giver may view the patient as family or as a comrade in a group to which he has complete allegiance. When one is bound by such important ties, there are few limits to the sacrifices that one makes. Care giving is not a choice; instead, it is a calling. The very hardships and deprivations one suffers stand as testimony to the nobility of one's moral commitments. Far from being degraded by the hardships, the care giver may be elevated by the pride he feels in unswervingly responding to the call and in fulfilling his duty. The care giver may be bloodied, but he can stand unbowed.

It should be noted that some self-interest might be mixed with the genuine altruism and spirit of community that underlie the care giver's motives. Care givers may see their commitments as an expenditure of currency that might be recalled in the future. Being a care giver legitimizes the expectation that should the need arise in the future, one will also be the recipient of informal care. Correspondingly, if one shirks one's duty now, one abrogates future claims. It is a "do unto others . . ." appraisal of the situation.

As we emphasized above, close identification with the victim can leave the care giver very frightened of his own vulnerability to AIDS. It is not surprising that to weaken such identification and its threats, care givers find ways to differentiate themselves from the patient. One way is to evaluate the patient as having been more susceptible to AIDS because he dwelled on the malady and was particularly fearful of becoming its victim. He might also call attention to the importance of diet and nutrition, evaluating the patient's eating habits as less healthy than his own. Additionally, he may come to believe that the patient's immunological system is simply less resistant to the virus than his own. This is a belief that is especially supported in instances where there is a chance that the care giver was the source of the patient's AIDS. Such instances invite the care giver to speculate that the absence of active symptoms reflects his own biological capacity to resist AIDS. Whatever the specific difference the care giver focuses on, it serves a clear purpose: to perceptually exempt the care giver from the same probabilities of AIDS as the patient confronted. These exemption techniques essentially represent important coping strategies that enable the care giver to avoid being immobilized by fears that would otherwise result from close psychological identification with the victim.

The general point to be understood is that there is a host of beliefs, values, understandings, and appraisals that the care giver typically calls upon. All of these function either to ease the ominous meaning of the patient's illness or to fend off the fears that the care giver has about his own future well-being. The use of these devices is dynamic, with some being drawn into prominent use at one stage of the disease process and later abandoned as the course of the illness advances to another stage. We know from other research that coping with the meaning of the situation can be very effective. Nevertheless, this coping function is not likely to completely spare the individual over the long run. Unavoidably, the care giver is likely to experience a substantial measure of stress in spite of the efficacy of this kind of coping.

This brings us to the third coping function, coping that manages or controls the symptoms of stress. There is an almost limitless array of behaviors that enable the individual to avoid being overwhelmed by stress. Essentially, these behaviors all function to keep the symptoms of stress, such as tension and despair, within manageable bounds. Almost any behavior that helps the individual remove himself temporarily from the intrusive awareness of the threat can serve this function. The care giver may immerse himself in television at every opportunity; he may meditate, jog, consume alcohol, or smoke marijuana; or he might seek relief in sexual activity. Similarly, one's occupation might be used as a haven to which the care giver flees. As we pointed out, the quality of his work might suffer because of the demands of care giving, but some care givers still look forward to work as the one place to which they can legitimately retreat. This kind of coping obviously does not change the situation, nor is it likely to change the meaning of the situation. However, to the extent that it succeeds in releasing from consciousness the relentless presence of stress, it helps the care giver to nurture and remobilize his inner resources.

This brief overview of coping functions and their mechanisms describes some of the practices and strategies care givers use to deal with the problems and hardships encountered in their roles. Although eventually patients die, death does not necessarily free the care giver of stress. It usually serves only to substitute some problems for others. In place of the endless care-giving activities are feelings of loss, grief, and continuing, perhaps intensified, fears for one's own future. We know very little of the lives of care givers after approximately a year following the patient's death. From fragmentary indications, former care givers do reassemble the pieces of their lives and go forward. It is not easy and is probably never fully accomplished. It is our guess that even if former care givers escape AIDS, they will constitute a growing group of people whose mental and physical health are at serious risk as a result of the prolonged and intense stresses they have experienced.

23

The Hidden Grievers

Patrice Murphy and Kathleen Perry

The "hidden grievers"—an intriguing title!

Who are they? This article will explore the concept of hidden grievers in the AIDS epidemic from the prospective of the St. Vincent's Hospital and Medical Center Supportive Care Program in New York City. The Supportive Care Program recognizes the lovers/partners and family members of those dying from AIDS as the "hidden grievers." This recognition has occurred through the experiences of staff working with persons with AIDS and their significant others in their grieving process.

The largest percentage of the population afflicted thus far with AIDS are homosexual men and intravenous drug abusers. Whereas persons in either category are cared for and followed by St. Vincent's, the homosexual population comprises a larger proportion of the AIDS population probably owing to the location of the medical center in Greenwich Village, a largely gay community. The experiences drawn upon, then, are mainly related to homosexual AIDS patients and their loved ones.

Certainly over the years there has been no lack of censure in the press and media, by churches and the clergy, by politicians, and by professionals in all walks of life for the gay community. The reasons for this censure are as varied as those expressing them. How, then, can we expect those lovers/partners who may have had lengthy, monogamous, satisfying, life-enriching relationships with their loved one to be other than hidden in a society that, first of all, is extremely uncomfortable in the face of death and grief, and second, fails to recognize what is frequently a spousal relationship deserving of acknowledgment.

Parents, siblings, aunts and uncles, wives and children are also hidden grievers, because their child's or brother's or husband's death is a secret. Or the cause of death and its circumstances are kept a secret because of their uneasiness with their loved one's sexual orientation or the history of substance abuse that made them vulnerable to the AIDS virus. Family members are afraid of society's censure; they are embarrassed or ashamed or feel guilty or angry, and they shed their tears, swallow their sobs, and try to be "normal" although their hearts are heavy and their spirits are burdened. They are indeed "hidden grievers."

These are the grieving loved ones to whom the bereavement component of the Supportive Care Program has sought to offer support, comfort, counseling, and education. Recognizing the importance of expressing sorrow and confronting one's sense of loss, of verbalizing feelings of guilt and anger, and learning to relinquish the emotional ties to the deceased despite the attending pain and sorrow are essential to the healing process.[1] Bereavement counselors realize the importance of being present emotionally as well as physically, of assisting the griever to express and identify feelings, of listening nonjudgmentally and with permissiveness and acceptance, and of allowing their genuine concern and caring to show.[2]

But before we discuss in greater detail the problem of these grieving persons, two other groups of hidden grievers must be identified. They also grieve—their sorrow unidentified or poorly identified, recognized, or acknowledged. Sometimes it is forgotten that the patients—all dying patients, but in particular those with AIDS—are grieving. If grief is defined as "an emotional reaction to the perception of loss,"[3] then the person with AIDS meets the criterion, for his or her perceived losses are many, and there has been little education or preparation for them. AIDS generally strikes the young, usually between 20 and 40 years of age. The illness with its multisystem manifestations and devastation almost always causes loss of energy, physical attractiveness, control, and independence.

AIDS almost always alters the person's body drastically, resulting in a body no longer seen as friend but rather as enemy. The sense of selfhood contracts over and over again.

Persons with AIDS may have already felt the withdrawal of parents, relatives, and friends because of their sexual orientation and/or drug-abusing life style. They may have deprived themselves of possible relationships with their parents and other family members to protect themselves from what is perceived as an unwelcome reality. Now another process of loss is beginning in relation to the world of events, persons, and relationships.

Persons with AIDS have roles, and many have lost or relinquished their roles as son, brother, grandchild, husband, father. If in addition this illness means that the patient is an actor who cannot act, an artist who cannot paint, a physician who cannot heal, the person is further diminished by the loss of still another role. If an individual cannot do the things that he or she identifies with the fact of his being, he or she may no longer feel whole.

Each of us has a perceived future for himself, one's talents and energies and loved ones. There is hope in this element of being, and tremendous suffering attends the loss of hope. In many ways the grief processes of the AIDS sufferer parallel those of the bereaved, and the patient who cannot be cured of his or her illness struggles with the same tasks as a mourner following a death. It is imperative that care givers anticipate, recognize, and acknowledge this grief and be aware of its manifestations so that the dying/grieving may be assisted in dealing with the dying process and facing death "retaining his/her dignity and self respect, relinquishing the unattainable, respecting him/her self for what one has been and helping him/her move away from life as it known to death with its unknowns in peace and acceptance."[4]

There is yet another group of "hidden grievers" who are expected to face death and life—perhaps a number of times in each day and night—and still retain their equanimity and professional decorum despite the cost to their personal feelings and thoughts. They are the nurses, physicians, and other care providers who have lived and died a little with each dying patient for whom they have cared. In the song "No Man Is an Island," the words "each man's grief is my own" ring true to those who truly care. Although the world will go on expecting the caring professional to be a "super" man or woman, it is important that we recognize and acknowledge the losses—the deaths—of our patients and reach out to one another with an empathy, caring, and thoughtfulness that is supportive, consoling, and meaningful. There need not be hidden grievers among care givers if we care a little more for one another.

Although this article focuses on our use of support groups for those grieving the loss of a person with AIDS, there are a small number of individuals for whom a group is not appropriate or desirable. On an individual basis, with the person seeking assistance, we arrive at the best option, whether that may be a referral for individual counseling with a focus on bereavement, the assignment of a bereavement volunteer from our program to the individual, and/or regular phone contact for a 13-month period by our bereavement follow-up team. For those family members whose loved one died in New York City but who live out of town, attempts are made to connect them with a bereavement program in their home town. It is our feeling that most people welcome this outreach and support. Support groups serve a very special purpose for persons struggling with the problems and stresses of life. At St. Vincent's the Supportive Care Program's bereavement component has reached out in a variety of ways to the loved ones of those who have died from AIDS, the bereavement support group being one major and effective way. The purpose of the bereavement group is to provide a safe and supportive place where people who are grieving may come together and share their experience and feelings. There is a special need to provide this kind of support to those whose loved ones have died of AIDS, because, as has been stated previously, these individuals frequently lack the usual support and sympathy extended to bereaved persons.

BEREAVEMENT GROUPS

We have met the need of our community by organizing and leading bereavement groups for men who have lost a lover to AIDS as well as for families who have lost a son, daughter, brother, sister, or husband or wife to AIDS. Over 25 such groups have been developed since late 1983.

The groups have an average of seven or eight members, meeting for 90 min once a week for 8 weeks. The meetings are held in our offices adjacent to St. Vincent's Hospital in Greenwich Village, New York City. Originally, we received most of our referrals from the Gay Men's Health Crisis (GMHC). Although the GMHC still refers many people, we now also get referrals from members of previous bereavement groups who recommend the group to their newly bereaved friends. Of course, our own Supportive Care Program generates a number of referrals.

We begin the group process by having a prospective group member come in for a brief interview. In this way we begin our relationship with the person hearing the person's "story" and briefly assessing his situation. This interview is also a time for the group member to ask any questions about what to expect in the group. Usually, we give the person an overview of the group and issues usually discussed and speak of the helpfulness to the individual of being involved in a group.

The first group meeting is the only meeting of the eight in which we as coleaders have an "agenda." At this meeting, we speak of the purpose of the group, our roles as coleaders, the importance of confidentiality, and our availability as resource people during the 8 weeks to answer questions about AIDS or the grieving process. At this meeting, we ask all persons present to introduce themselves and to tell their story; to take a few minutes to tell the group about the person they loved, how long they were together, some details about his or her illness and death; and to share with the others how they have been doing since the death. This is usually a very emotional time, and we recognize how difficult it is for each person present to listen to all the others' grief when they themselves are barely able to manage their own feelings. But we feel it is an important activity, necessary for the group's bonding and cohesiveness. We also ask people to share their expectations of the group experience.

Following each group meeting, the coleaders spend time together talking about the evening's meeting, sharing concerns, supporting one another, and reflecting on the overall direction and nature of the group. We believe this is essential to being effective leaders of a grievers' group. During the next 7 weeks we open and close the meetings, prevent any one person from dominating the group, draw into group interaction any quiet or reluctant member, and give feedback and support as appropriate. We observe the group process. We assume an educational role, describing the process of grieving, the normalcy of thoughts and feelings, and, on request, share a bibliography we have developed. We have a number of handouts: *How to Grieve, Coping with the Holidays, Tasks of Mourning*, as well as various articles written by bereaved persons who have attended our groups. We answer questions about AIDS and the various opportunistic infections, medical procedures, and medications, and occasionally about the experimental therapies available (both medical and holistic). We make every effort to be supportive, to make clear the purpose of the group as a self-help support group, and to be facilitators in the group.

The issues that come up in the group over the 8 weeks are ones that arise in any bereavement group. But there are two very striking and distinct differences: the stigma attached to the AIDS diagnosis and the youth of the victims and their lovers. These men have little or inadequate support from family, friends, and work environment—supports that would normally be available to a person whose loved one has died. They do not have the usual supports, because people do not fully recognize or acknowledge gay relationships and because people are reacting to stigma and fear of the disease. Many family members deny how important the deceased was to the bereaved lover. "Even my own brother, who had visited us many times in our apartment over the 10 years we were together, said he had no idea of our emotional commitment to one another," reported one group member. That people are unable to recognize the loss for what it is (in the case of a gay man—loss of a spouse) speaks to society's inability to deal with and accept homosexual relationships.

Family members often withhold information about the AIDS diagnosis and therefore obtain the customary support that any father or mother, husband or wife, brother or sister would receive at the time of a death. But then they live with anger and guilt, compounded by the fear that they will be "discovered." Fear of people's finding out the true diagnosis, especially for wives whose husbands have died of AIDS, has prompted many to protect themselves and their children with a web of secrecy unknown in their previous life. Harboring "their secret," being unable to talk about what is really on their minds, hampers resolution of the grief and compounds the agony. Those individuals who are courageous and allow the diagnosis to be known suffer rejections and judgments similar to what the lovers experience. "My husband's family never mentions his name, as if he never existed, and he's only been dead 5 months," cried one widowed woman whose husband of 23 years was bisexual. "His live style, once realized by them, and the fact that he had AIDS, was so unacceptable that they denied all he meant to them as son or brother and all that they meant to him."

Friends of gay men frequently have no idea how to befriend the bereaved. Given that they are young people who have had little or no experience with losing a loved one, it is understandable. They feel their role as a friend of the bereaved is to distract them from their grief. The bereaved find they have to tell their friends "what helps." Group members share with one another the various ways that they have coped with well-intentioned but uninformed friends who want to be supportive but end up espousing cliches or platitudes that are inappropriate. The general population seems to fell that a person should "get on with his or her life" within a few months of the death and anything to the contrary is viewed as dwelling on the loss or as unfounded, lingering depression. We assist group members to be more realistic about how long it takes to "feel like yourself again." Having a framework of recovery is helpful. It prevents the bereaved from expecting too much of themselves too quickly and helps them to understand the process.

Another issue that comes up in every group is the fear of having or getting AIDS. The gay men are in the high-risk group by virtue of their sexuality. The fact that their lover died of AIDS puts them at even higher risk. Newly bereaved gay men frequently speak of a preoccupation with their health. The slightest bruise is quickly construed to be a Kaposi's sarcoma lesion, and the merest sniffle to be *Pneumoncystis carinii* pneumonia. Physical symptoms of stress seen in all bereaved persons (insomnia, diarrhea, gastrointestinal upset, headaches, fatigue) are quickly interpreted as symptoms of AIDS. Although we point this out, we are careful not to be too reassuring, as realistically, it is impossible to know the reasons for their discomfort. Learning that physical symptoms occur with all losses of significance does seem to keep some of the anxiety in check. We encourage all to be under a physician's care, but the anxiety of becoming ill and having no one to care for them as they lovingly cared for their lover is overwhelming. For some there is a period in which they wish they would die—to end the pain of grief and as an attempt to join their loved one. Sharing their thoughts and feelings and learning that others in the group feel similarly is cathartic and reassuring.

Dealing with your own mortality when you are 20–35 years old is not age-appropriate, but it is sobering and maturing. All seem to confront death and become stronger, less fearful than before their loved one died. Many group members share their philosophical and religious thoughts, talk about their coping strategies, and draw on their past experience of coping with being homosexual as a way of successfully coping with their current crisis.

GUILT AND GRIEF

The issues that arise in the group that are not unlike those of other bereaved persons still have some uniqueness and often much poignancy. Feelings of guilt are often verbalized particularly in relation to not being present at the time of the person's death. Most often lovers have spent every available minute at their loved one's bedside—all time except that spent at work or getting a few hours' sleep. Not infrequently, the patient dies at a moment when the lover is not present and the unanswered questions—"Was he in pain?" "Did he call out or reach for me?"—cause much pain and guilt, frequently expressed as "If only I stayed instead of going home," "I promised him I'd be with him." "I never said the final, 'I love you.'"

Bereaved persons, often quite young, and grieving a major loss for the first time, find it almost impossible to comprehend that grief is a time-consuming process with a beginning, middle, and end or resolution. Surrounded as we are with "instant" everything, young people find it difficult to wait and to view grief as work—particularly because it is painful. This attitude emerges as a shortcoming of an "instant" society, and must be presented for what it is over and over again. Aware as we are of the death- and grief-denying society surrounding us, these attitudes should not surprise us. Over and over again, we may need to reiterate that grief work is very individual, that grievers are not in competition to see who can finish fastest, and that the length and intensity of grief are strongly influenced by many factors unique to each individual relationship.

Guilt is manifested throughout the grief process. One of the times that it is strongly experienced by the bereaved is when they begin to feel a little less sad, when the tears have only come once instead of three or four times in a day, when they see humor in a situation or even actually laugh out loud. Then suddenly they are remorseful—"How could I have?"—and see their laughter as a symptom of forgetting or being disloyal to the loved one instead of what it really is—a step toward recovery.

Guilt may occur again further along, when the bereaved person may meet a new person, be attracted to him or her, and accept an invitation to dinner or a movie. Frequently when this happens there are inner silent recriminations about disloyalty, and "How could I?" reflections. It is extremely important, then, that the healthiness of this openness to connecting in some new way with another be emphasized as well as its significance as another milestone in the grief process. Reassurance at this time is also imperative—reassurance that the deceased person will always have a special place in the bereaved's thoughts and heart and reassurance also that, although the grieving person will never be the same again, he or she will have grown significantly in many inner ways and be more mature, sensitive, and compassionate.

Another recurrent theme is the physical changes that occur as a result of disease progression. AIDS is a devastating disease; wasting effects and sometimes gross neurological changes transform the person with AIDS—formerly young, attractive, and healthy into an unrecognizable vision of themselves—like victims of concentration camps. The bereaved lovers and family members have a difficult time remembering their loved ones like this. The images persist, and for a while the bereaved may suffer flashbacks of the ill person, weak and frail and unable to perform the simplest tasks for himself. "I can only remember him sick, suffering the indignities of incredible weakness and fatigue: unable to open the Thermos of cool water at his bedside, unable to feed himself or hold a napkin. My strong, handsome son dying such a death as this at his young age. I can't get the horror of it out of my mind." Gradually this image changes for the bereaved, but while it continues, it is reassuring to know that it is a common problem. It is an image with which many bereaved have to deal, but it is more pronounced and common with AIDS patients. Those whose loved one has been deceased for a longer period of time frequently share how the image of the sick person gradually gives way to a well image of the person prior to the illness.

There are many day-to-day issues that are difficult to face in the period of bereavement including disposing of possessions and celebrating holidays. Disposing of the deceased's possessions and belongings is always a stressful task. With the gay men whose lovers have died, the task can be complicated by relatives and family members who do not recognize the lover as a "spouse" or significant other. Sometimes the family has never accepted the gay relationship. The lover has to deal with the anger and frustration of coping with an estranged family who may have come in and taken all the lover's belongings. Not infrequently these family members have been out of touch for long periods of time and were quite unsupportive during the deceased one's illness. These same relatives often go ahead with funeral plans which may be very different from what the deceased had wished, and to compound the injury, do not invite or prohibit the bereaved lover from attending. Being left with only memories, these group members express profound sadness at their inability to perform the rites of holding on and letting go of their loved ones' clothes, books, photographs, records, and personal belongings.

Dealing with holidays, birthdays, and anniversaries seems impossible for most newly bereaved persons to even imagine, but it is even more difficult for men in a gay relationship, because they have created their own holiday celebrations over the years and find themselves at a terrible loss when it comes to facing these dates and times alone. If they are newly bereaved, they are still so sad and depressed at their loss that they cannot image being in a mood of joy and happiness. For others, looking back at past celebrations may be too painful and the future too uncertain and unknown. For all, it is a trying time which must be recognized and acknowledged. Similar fears arise at vacation times; some have never traveled alone or taken a vacation without their lover. Facing this time without their partner can be upsetting and frightening. As group leaders we try to make suggestions, some general guidelines to help the bereaved through these times.

Group members on the whole have shown a willingness to talk and share their thoughts, feelings, and experiences in a very open and revealing way. They are eager to explore and confront themselves (and one another) with a desire and fervor we do not usually see in our bereavement work.

Many bereaved persons find they are questioning their religious or spiritual beliefs at the time of the patient's death and afterward. Some express being "angry with God" having "an inability to pray" or "an aversion to church." Certainly this crisis time does allow for rethinking and reformulating one's beliefs. Group members try to respond to one another's questions and to direct their anger in constructive ways. These interactions provide support during the bleakest moments for those who feel "abandoned" by God and church. Others have the exact opposite experience with a feeling of renewed belief and a growing strength in their faith. The amount of support and help a person receives from his religious community certainly seems to enhance the opportunities for a person to have a positive spiritual experience in this time of crisis.

Over the past 3 years, we have felt privileged to know the people who have been in our bereavement groups. Hospice workers will quickly recognize that feeling of being witness to heroes—courageous people who have cared for with great love and then grieved their loved one with great pain. Because of the youth of these bereaved and the obstacles to dealing with a disease that has so much stigma attached to it in a society that is frequently not supportive and comforting but rather judgmental and punitive, these groups testify to the enormous value of self-help groups. We have heard story after story of love and devotion, of lives that have been ripped apart by loss but then slowly reconstructed—recovery and growth the bereaved could never have suspected possible.

The growth and strength we witness in the course of conducting these groups give us the motivation and courage to begin yet another group. Our lives have been greatly enriched, and we have indeed been privileged to do this work.

REFERENCES

1. Rando, T. A. Concepts of death, dying, grief and loss: Participants manual. In *Hospice Education Program for Nurses*. Washington DC: U.S. Government Printing Office, 1981, module III, p. 129.
2. *Ibid.*, pp. 156–157.
3. *Ibid.*, p. 135.
4. *Ibid.*, p. 143.

VI
SOCIOCULTURAL AND ETHICAL ASPECTS

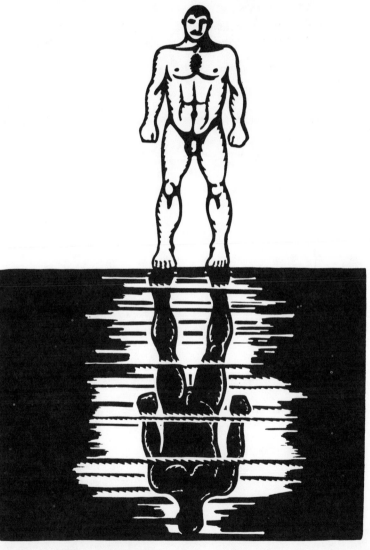

Sociocultural and Ethical Aspects
This white figure reflecting back his black brother is a metaphor for an anguished community absorbed in self-reflection and reassessment.

24

Epidemic Control Measures for AIDS:

A Psychosocial and Historical Discussion of Policy Alternatives

David G. Ostrow, Michael Eller, and Jill G. Joseph

INTRODUCTION

The epidemic of acquired immune deficiency syndrome (AIDS) is an unprecedented occurrence in recent medical history. The increasing incidence of the typically fatal syndrome, its transmissibility through sexual and blood contact, and the continuing lack of either an effective vaccine or cure have created a broad series of challenges.[1] In spite of the relatively rapid isolation of the etiologic agent, human immunodeficiency virus (HIV; formerly referred to as HTLV-III/LAV), and the development of antibody detection assays,[2,3] many of these challenges are predominantly psychosocial in nature. Some are well recognized; for example, increasing attention is being paid to the extent and determinants of behavioral changes required to reduce HIV infection[4,5] and to the complex social and psychological needs of those diagnosed with AIDS or who are HIV-seropositive.[6,7] Another set of issues, largely unrecognized in the medical and social science literature, deals with the relationship of those at risk for AIDS to the broader social and political environment. As the majority of AIDS cases have occurred in stigmatized groups—homosexually active men, intravenous drug users, and immigrants—it is not surprising that there have been attributions of blame and countercharges of discrimination. There has been little scientific discussion of this phenomenon, its origins, and its possible consequences.

This paper examines ways in which the attitudes and activities of the majority, heterosexual culture may impede or facilitate the adaptation of homosexual/bisexual men to the crisis of AIDS. Although specific to this particular risk group, comments offered here may be more broadly applicable to others at risk. These impressions are based on a systematic review of qualitative data collected across a period of 2½ years in a cohort of approximately 1000 homosexual or bisexual men at risk for AIDS. This discussion will be prefaced by a more general historical description of social responses to epidemic disease and will be followed by comments on the potential for responsible and positive choices by all of us confronting the problem of AIDS.

This work was supported by research funding from the National Institute of Mental Health (2 RO1 MH3936-O2A1) and the University of Michigan.

The authors thank the men in the Coping and Change Study whose participation makes this research possible.

HISTORICAL CONTEXT

Epidemics and their psychosocial consequences are not new. Furthermore, there is a predictable series of events that can occur as epidemics threaten the sense of control and mastery implicit in most forms of social organization. By examining historical parallels it may be possible to understand our current situation better, thus minimizing the fear and discrimination that subvert the formulation of effective public health policy. In the discussion that follows, special attention is paid to the ways in which "epidemic control" measures (such as quarantine) may arise more from a need to blame or control than from an accurate epidemiologic assessment of risk.

The potential threat produced by epidemic disease can be profound, particularly when the existing social order appears impotent to provide the protection it implicitly promises. Such implicit promises may arise from the theological bases of a feudal system or from the assumed biomedical-technological hegemony of our own society. The extreme social reaction to epidemic disease in such a context will only be exacerbated by the well-described phenomenon of misestimating health risks.[8,9] Research evidence suggests that we optimistically underestimate risk that arises from our own behavior,[10,11] while the opposite is true of external threat. External risk is frequently misperceived as more threatening and serious than is factually accurate. Therefore, when the epidemic is seen to originate from infected "others" (some stigmatized and easily identifiable subgroup), the sense of risk or threat is likely to be further increased, thus intensifying the need for more stringent "control" measures. Three historical antecedents illustrating these points are discussed below.*

THE PLAGUE IN MEDIEVAL EUROPE

Beginning in the 14th century, pandemics of plague afflicted Europe, recurring at regular intervals until well into the 17th century. Although estimates of the proportion of the population dying vary, it is apparent that these epidemics were devastating. There were profound effects on the religious, political, economic, and social order which have been well documented but will not further concern us here. For example, local dramatic decreases in the supply of labor had the potential to shift economic organization toward the concept of wage rather than servitude. Of greater interest for our purpose were the complex and largely abortive attempts to control dissemination of the disease. Attempts to quarantine affected villages have been carefully described, as has the frequent neglect of those stricken. While these measures likely increased the suffering of those taken ill, there is no evidence that they slowed or halted the spread of plague in Europe. Such efforts were based on an understandable but inaccurate assessment of the mode of transmission of plague. Except for the pneumonic form of the disease, transmission was from fleas carried by the commonly occurring brown rat. Thus, the isolation of individuals or communities was largely ineffectual. Similarly, the reaction of some physicians was both exaggerated and unnecessary. For example, physicians, in parts of France wore full-length leather cloaks and wide-

---

*Material for the historical section below was taken from a limited number of major sources. Rather than our repetitively citing each, the interested reader is referred to references 12–17.

brimmed hats and used pointers to avoid close contact with plague victims. Quite by coincidence, the only value of such practices may have been to avoid close contact with fleas.

By the 15th century, yet more distressing social phenomena were apparent. As the epidemic toll continued erratically but largely unabated, more extreme measures were used to preserve the prevalent theistic world view. Bands of devout pilgrims appeared in large numbers, moving through the major population centers of Europe, stripped to the waist and publically whipping themselves. These flagellants, perceiving plague as punishment for previously unrecognized sin, sought relief in their mortifications. By voluntarily submitting to self-imposed pain and suffering, they believed that the wrathful God punishing them could be propitiated. Simultaneously, they turned on the vulnerable and stigmatized Jewish population. Although fundamentally inconsistent with the concept of plague as divine retribution, flagellant groups simultaneously held Jews to be responsible for transmission of the disease. Flamed by an inability to control the epidemic even through penance, rumors of well-poisoning and other malicious activities by Jews spread rapidly. Flagellants therefore felt further justified in systematically seeking out and murdering large Jewish populations. For example, in Brussels, following a procession by flagellants, the entire Jewish population was massacred. Indeed, within a decade there were virtually no Jews left in either Germany or what later became Belgium.

In spite of desperate "control measures," largely based on a misunderstanding of disease transmission or a theology of retribution, epidemics of the plague continued at irregular intervals. Ultimately, by the late 17th century they abated, for reasons that remain largely unexplained.

CHOLERA

In August of 1817, an epidemic was documented in the British possession of India, in a district approximately 70 miles from Calcutta. Whether previously endemic in the Indian subcontinent or not, it is certainly true that the modern history of cholera begins with this episode. Carried both overland and by sea, the disease soon penetrated Russia and the Austro-Hungarian Empire. The rapid dissemination of this new and lethal affliction again prompted the search for those who could be blamed for its occurrence. In central Europe rumors spread that the rich were deliberately infecting peasants or poisoning their water supply. More commonly, however, it was the poor themselves who were seen as the source of disease. Writing in 1832, an English physician described the reasons he believed his locality was susceptible to an epidemic of cholera. "Our population may be described as vicious, immoral, and miserable; a full half being liable to the vice of all others the most destructive to religion and morals—I mean drunkenness."[15] He went on to suggest that not only drunkenness but Catholic emancipation in 1829 might further explain why cholera was inevitable. The dual notions of moral and physical filth placing a group at risk were also expressed in the United States, where it was reported regarding cholera, "Drunkards and filthy, wicked people of all descriptions, are swept away in heat, as if the Holy God could no longer bear their wickedness, just as we sweep away a mass of filth when it has become so corrupt that we cannot bear it."[17]

In addition to general notions regarding classes of people who were responsible for or susceptible to the epidemic, there was a consistent attempt to identify specific individuals who brought the disease to a previously unaffected location. Three shoemakers were reportedly responsible for the introduction of cholera to Scotland. Similarly, a woman known to be a public drunkard was blamed for bringing the disease to the Isle of Bute off the coast of Scotland. A young woman who traveled to the home of her mother although desperately ill with cholera, was dragged from her bed for fear she would bring cholera and sent in a cart to a foundry, where she died. (Her mother was subsequently forced out of her home, which was burned with all its contents.)

In the United States a general pattern of response to the threat of cholera emerged. First, attempts were made to prevent transmission of the disease, usually including institution of a quarantine. Although medical opinion of the time held that no disease was contagious and that therefore such measures were unnecessary, popular opinion generally supported their adoption. Second, there was an attempt to clean towns of the accumulated waste and garbage typically littering the streets. Often the garbage was deposited in local rivers or simply left outside city limits to rot. Finally, medical facilities and personnel were generally made available for the poor who became ill.

Although there was a general agreement that such facilities were necessary, there was often a similar agreement that they should be available in someone else's neighborhood. Measures as innocuous as petitions and as lethal as arson were used to dissuade the establishment of cholera hospitals. These attitudes arose not only from a fear of disease but from the prevalent attitude well described in the words of one observer who reported, "The visitor finds few others in those receptacles than the inpenitent sot and debauchee."[17] Finally, because personal habits were believed to be an important cause of cholera, it became the duty of public officials to protect the community from perceived human excesses. Connecticut physicians demanded that the Board of Health have "the power to change the habits of the sensual, the vicious, the intemperate."[17] In addition, in most communities affected by cholera, the sale of certain foods was forbidden, including unripe fruits, cucumbers, and corn in New York. These, as well as alcohol, were held to increase the likelihood of cholera.

SYPHILIS

With the discovery of the *S. pallida* in 1905, the Wasserman test in 1906, and arsphenamine (Salvarsan or "606") in 1909, the way was paved in the United States for public health control programs aimed at controlling syphilis. Persons with syphilis were frequently viewed as unclean and deserving of their affliction, because they had chosen illicit sexual behaviors despite the threat of disease. Although men with syphilis were rarely quarantined, women accused of "solicitation" were forced to undergo Wasserman testing and, if positive, were detained and treated until considered noncontagious. The use of preventive measures such as condoms and urethral disinfectants were opposed by moralists, who believed they promoted promiscuity. It was only during wartime, with increasing morbidity in soldiers due to syphilis and gonorrhea, that the military began to promote prophylactic measures widely. Nonetheless, prevention was also linked to chastity, and American soldiers were urged to "discipline" their sexual urges. This was illustrated in an extreme form by the government order issued in July 1917 that made contraction of venereal disease by soldiers a punishable offense.

Between 1935 and 1938, 26 states passed laws requiring premarital syphilis testing and prohibiting seropositive persons from marrying. Despite evidence against nonsexual transmission of syphilis, ordinances requiring food handlers and domestics to be tested were commonplace. Quarantine of prostitutes, although substantially abandoned earlier, was reimposed, and employment restrictions were effectively ended only with the availability of penicillin in the late 1930s. Nonetheless, ordinances from the 1920s and 1930s regulating control of sexually transmitted diseases (STDs) remain and are often referred to as the basis for AIDS control measures. Recently, bills have been introduced in many state legislatures that would mandate premarital HIV serotesting and prohibit seropositive individuals from marrying.[18] Similarly, state and federal proposals for mandatory reporting on HIV seropostivity and contact tracing of partners of seropositive individuals are based on the methods used in the 1930s and 1940s for syphilis controls.

Such measures as mandatory reporting of syphilis cases and contact tracing to control venereal disease had been avoided by those who were able to use private physicians. Such physicians were less likely to report patients by name to public health authorities, resulting in underreporting of STD statistics. With the development of effective treatment for syphilis, the emphasis switched from reporting and contact tracing to ensuring effective treatment of persons suspected of exposure. In the 1970s and 1980s, there was a significant increase in the proportion of syphilis reported due to homosexual transmission and in attempts to apply contact tracing and prophylactic treatment to this population. However, the anonymous nature of many homosexual contacts, as well as the reluctance of gay men to have their names or those of their partners reported to public health authorities, rendered such measures generally ineffective as they sought care from private practitioners willing to protect their identity.[19] This was only untrue where local health authorities worked cooperatively with the homosexual subculture and gay community to establish trust in their ability to provide both confidentiality and needed medical treatment.

It is apparent that many of the current proposals for "controlling" the AIDS epidemic recapitulate earlier, unsuccessful experiences. Adequate control of transmission must inevitably take account of both the characteristics of the pathogen and the social context within which it is appearing. Failure to appreciate the vector for transmission of plague led to inappropriate control measures which increased human suffering while still failing to halt the spread of the epidemic. This failure, in turn, fueled the need to identify a group that could be blamed and punished. The emerging consensus about HIV transmission must influence the development of public policy and provide the impetus for further scientific investigations. This virus is comparatively difficult to transmit and is not usually spread by contact other than that which involves sharing blood or sexual activity.

Early attempts to control cholera are also instructive. Illness and contagion reinforced existing, moralistic sterotypes regarding the poor, the alcoholic, or the immigrant. The emerging concern for the indigent ill competed sharply with the desire to protect one's own neighborhood from the perceived threat of epidemic illness. Once again, basic facts about transmission were unavailable, and in this vacuum, preexisting world views became the basis for social and political responses to the epidemic. Currently, unnecessary attempts to exclude children with AIDS from schools and to prevent the establishment of hospices have been documented; these demonstrate that knowledge of transmission may not be well assimilated and/or heeded and that the current panic can lead to actions that even do violence to pervasive norms of compassion for the young and the dying. The homosexual male is without doubt at great risk for "scapegoating" in this milieu, and such social responses make attempts to control the epidemic only more difficult. Attempts to develop effective public health policy must take into account these extreme and often morally derived reactions. It is essential for scientists and health care providers to join the policy debate; our failure to recognize the social reactions to this epidemic, to take such reactions seriously, and to counter inappropriate policies will have consequences as adverse as ignorance of basic biomedical data.

Finally, the history of syphilis should sharpen awareness of the need to think clearly about the presumed effectiveness of proposed policies. When test reporting and contact tracing are mandated, those with the means to do so avoid the public sector and the services provided there.[19] The likelihood that sexual contacts will be accurately reported declines in an atmosphere of repression and is less likely yet when no definitive prevention or cure is available. For example, there is already excellent anecdotal evidence that use of alternative test sites decreases dramatically when mandatory reporting and contact tracing are instituted or even rumored.

Control measures based on other transmission models may be ineffective and even damaging. They can distract from the real and expensive work of education in high-risk groups and can alienate those in need of such educational programs. All proposed measures short of quarantine, but including contact tracing, mandatory testing, or even tattooing the seropositive, postpone but do not obviate the need for effective educational efforts. By whatever means one learns that either a proposed partner or oneself is seropositive, the issue remains one of education; it is necessary to understand what this information means and to regulate relevant behaviors. Thus, the need for effective education reasserts itself after a potentially expensive and distracting delay. Furthermore, this attempt to locate those needing education can neither mandate honest reporting nor ensure the success of the educational effort itself. It is especially important to recognize that no evidence is available demonstrating that knowledge of one's serologic test results decreases the likelihood of risk-related behavior. This remains an issue urgently requiring investigation. What is known is that *all* those at risk ought to avoid behaviors linked to HIV transmission.

These brief historical discussions highlight the ways in which periods of epidemic are psychological, social, and political events as well as biomedical phenomena. Inappropriate and ineffectual attempts to control an epidemic are often derived from the sense of disease as deserved punishment as well as extreme and exaggerated fear of personal harm. This produces a social climate in which certain vulnerable groups, ranging from Jews to prostitutes to homosexuals, become targets for scapegoating. In addition, attending appropriately to the needs of those who are already ill becomes difficult in the moralized environment that perceives illness as punishment. Many of these themes have reemerged during the AIDS epidemic. In the next section of the paper we discuss ways in which such social reactions, although unnecessary and inappropriate, impinge upon the ability of at-risk gay men to adapt to the current crisis.

ADAPTATION AND FEAR

Data were obtained from a cohort of 950 Chicago homosexual and bisexual men participating in both a biomedical and a psychosocial study of AIDS risk. On a semiannual basis, participants are seen for an extensive medical-epide-miological-virological evaluation and are given a psychosocial questionnaire to complete approximately 2 weeks following this evaluation. The delay between the clinic visit and completion of the questionnaire was established to obtain a more accurate assessment of psychosocial functioning. (Pretesting suggested biomedical evaluations often heightened concerns about AIDS and could transiently increase psychological distress.) The structured questionnaire examines behavioral, social, and psychological responses to the threat of AIDS. It also documents perceived needs for, and impact of, community support programs, personality, and interpersonal dynamics on coping and change. At the time of enrollment, April 1984 to March 1985, the cohort was 92% white and had a mean age of 36 years and an average of 16.4 years of education.

In addition to the structured closed-form questions, an open-ended question asks: "Is there anything else you would like to tell us about yourself or about AIDS?" Approximately 250 men in each of the first four waves of the study responded to this question, and all responses have been reviewed and characterized by the authors. In addition, participants are given the opportunity to express any concerns of distress to the on-site research associate. Participants with significant distress or who request help are evaluated, and appropriate intervention or referral is provided. Both written comments at the conclusion of the questionnaire and notes of discussions with participants provide the basis for comments offered in this report.

We have previously characterized the phenomenology of AIDS as including extreme threat, uncertainty, and stigmatization.[20] Major stressors experienced by persons at high risk of AIDS include fears of transmitting and developing a fatal illness, loss of friends or partners with associated grief, and the stress of radical life style changes, as well as concerns regarding the effectiveness of such changes. Motivation for effective behavioral risk reduction necessitates perceiving one's vulnerability, yet such perceptions are often distressing. Participants struggle to maintain a positive adaptation balanced to include both appropriately altered behaviors and the maintenance of psychological health and social networks.

Furthermore, although there were few reported incidents of frank discrimination or ill treatment, there were consistently increased fears of anticipated discrimination, antigay violence, and employment or health care difficulties because of AIDS. For example, in mid-1985, 39% of the cohort reported fears of police harassment, 41% cited concerns about workplace hostilities, and 56% were worried that heterosexuals generally perceived gay men as diseased. Over one-third of the participants (38%) reported worries that their families were uncomfortable because they were gay. These specific concerns were paralleled by reports of general AIDS-related worries. The cohort described these concerns as often intruding on their thinking (47.3%), as interfering with their ability to relax (20.2%), or as making them feel uncomfortable with other gay men (22%). Between one-quarter and one-half of all participants reported feeling tense (26.6%), angry (31.6%), or worried (46.1%) because of AIDS.[21]

When open-ended responses were analyzed for all four waves, it was apparent that many participants attempt to discern some positive effect of this devastating epidemic. In the words of one participant, "AIDS has become a modern-day plague that has affected all of us in some way . . . . The only thing positive about AIDS (is that) people are becoming more aware of the disease and wanting to learn and educate others. It has brought more caring and concern among the gay community." Similarly, many develop an altruistic attitude, reporting volunteer activities in the community or among those already affected with AIDS. One participant typically commented, "I am trying to do whatever I can to make someone's life a little more happy, to be there for others."

Reasonably enough, considerable sadness and anger are also expressed by participants. This was perhaps best explained by the participant who wrote, "Living with AIDS is living with a time bomb. You can only hope it doesn't explode inside you." Another stated, "I have always believed that love created life and that love sustains and nurtures life. Now I see a dilemma, where love destroys life." Occasional participants have developed clinically significant depression, often related to the death of friends or lovers due to AIDS or a sense of mortal threat to their own lives. In perhaps its most ironic form, the psychological distress is experienced as an internalized, self-directed homophobia. One participant wrote, "The thought of getting AIDS sets off my guilt at being homosexual. In a way, I guess I almost do view it as "God's punishment," since I was taught that being gay is bad."

In gay men the complex process of adaptation to the AIDS crisis is constantly being disrupted by negative events in the broader social environment. One participant wrote, "To be gay and have to read day after day about AIDS only adds stress and fear to an already difficult life." Another commented, "After Rock Hudson died, rumors circulated at work that I have AIDS. One co-worker even addressed me with, 'Hi, Rock.' " As proposals were discussed in the media regarding mandatory HIV antibody testing, one participant responded, "I am very scared that the availability of the test could open up a crisis where forced testing for jobs, insurance, housing, etc. would be required." Another participant suggested during the same time period, "Lately, with talk of quarantine, I have a fear of concentration camps. It's scary and anger-provoking; I want both to run and to fight." Another reported, "These fears of discrimination definitely take their toll on one's emotional well-being." There were dramatic increases during late 1985 in such comments expressing fear or anger over society's responses to AIDS. This increase in hostile or fearful responses corresponded to increased media coverage in Chicago of proposals for mandatory AIDS testing, reporting, and quarantine during that same period.

We believe that such information reported by our participants highlights a progressively evolving set of social stressors and their negative psychological consequences. We chose to call this phenomenon "fear of holocaust" to differentiate it from previously reported sources of AIDS-related stress in gay men.

It seems likely that our participants are responding to a wide-ranging set of legislative, corporate, and social responses which are currently occurring or being publicly debated. Such actions or proposals can clearly create a social milieu that adds significantly to the already identified chronic stress experienced by gay men.

This social milieu might be expected to lead to increased psychological distress in our participants through at least two mechanisms. By directly adding to the burden of fear experienced by persons at high risk of AIDS, "fear of holocaust" would significantly increase the intensity and extent of AIDS-related chronic stress. In addition, this new form of stress frequently indicates rejection of the person at risk from the "general society;" therefore, the person perceiving himself the object of these proposals can feel more isolated and vulnerable, with less access to medical and psychological care. Unless effective interventions are found for both society's ill-informed anxiety and our subjects' sense of social isolation, increasingly extreme psychological responses can be expected. Whether or not actual physical quarantine or other repressive responses to AIDS do occur in the United States, the perception of their plausibility by an increasing proportion of the general public and by at-risk populations significantly intensifies the negative psychosocial consequences of the AIDS epidemic.

Although quarantine generally did not contain the transmission of those diseases discussed earlier, it nonetheless offered an illusory sense of protection from perceived external threat. It is, however, consistent and well-validated epidemiologic data regarding HIV transmission that should inform the formulation of public health policy. In particular, as we have already emphasized, only blood exchange and certain sexual behaviors (whether homosexual or heterosexual) can serve as effective routes of HIV transmission. Thus, individuals can effectively eliminate their risk of AIDS by regulating their own behavior rather than that of others. Unfortunately, misguided and unnecessary policies continue to be discussed. Inevitably, these have a negative impact on those men attempting to adapt to this crisis. One respondent expressed this clearly but dramatically when he wrote, "I remember the Jews who were shot in World War II. They wore a yellow star. I also remember the gays who were shot in World War II. They wore a pink triangle. Last week in the (Chicago) *Tribune* they talked about quarantine for gays. That is the third article that I have seen in 2 weeks. Next, we will all have to wear pink triangles as in WW II and be shot." There can be little doubt that, however inappropriate such policies as quarantine, their discussion can increase the distress of gay men.

FUTURE PROSPECTS: RESPONSIBILITY AND CHOICE

Clearly, the solution to the AIDS epidemic is currently behavioral. Given that HIV can insert into human DNA, probably for a lifetime, such behavioral changes will need to be extremely long-range. Therefore, it is in the interest of all that we encourage and facilitate such behavioral changes. There is already good evidence that gay men are reducing the sexual behaviors that transmit HIV.[22,23] The salient question is how both those who are at risk and those who are not can work together to produce a society in which a positive adaptation to the AIDS crisis is possible. It is this issue that will be discussed in this final section of the paper.

In many ways the current AIDS crisis recapitulates past experiences of epidemic disease. Currently defined risk groups are seen as diseased, dirty, and morally destitute;[24] collectively, they are perceived as a source of dangerous threat not only to health but to the existing social order. Such stereotypes, rather than available and accurate epidemiologic information, provide the basis for the extreme and unnecessary "epidemic control measures" being proposed. Paradoxically, such suggestions not only are unnecessary but may well impede control of this epidemic. The fragile coalition between the majority (and often medical) culture and the currently defined at-risk populations is disrupted by such proposals. Furthermore, they create an added burden of distrust, anxiety, and anger which is potentially disruptive to the establishment of safer life styles. At their worst, they have the potential for alienating gay men from those services and the care providers whose help may be so essential to them. For example, an individual who believes that HIV antibody testing is personally valuable may be likely to avoid such testing if the potential legal and financial consequences seem extreme and outweigh any personal gain. Put succinctly, insofar as we behave punitively, we will drive this epidemic "underground," and insofar as it is "underground," it will be more difficult to control.

What then might be a role for those who themselves are not members of at-risk groups? We would argue that all of us are confronted with the possibility of making responsible choices that may alter the course of this epidemic. For at-risk gay men, these choices have been well discussed, focusing on the alteration of sexual behavior. For too long, however, our society has seen its task as control of the "other"—the homosexual, the intravenous drug user, the immigrant. This external focus might more appropriately be replaced by a careful examination of our own attitudes and behaviors. In this way it may be possible to identify potential changes that could positively influence the course of this tragic epidemic. By mastering our own sense of impotence and futility, it may be less necessary to support or even give credence to the politically extreme and epidemiologically naive proposals for control of AIDS. Our own experience in working with groups as diverse as school administrators, prison guards, health care providers, and major employers suggests that this is indeed the case. Mastery of basic biomedical and epidemiologic information is within the grasp of everyone and can provide the foundation for a more appropriate and less anxious approach to the issues surrounding AIDS. Unions, employers, and workplace supervisors need to have not only access to such information, but the appropriate policies required to reinforce acceptable behavior. Already, hospitals have found that the combination of information, supportive counseling, and clear behavioral guidelines has done much to mitigate workplace anxiety and discrimination.

In addition to knowledge and behavior, it may also be possible that those in the majority culture are able to change equally important attitudes. There has been considerable censure of gay men for their sexual behavior, which has been perceived as "promiscuous" or "fast-track." Less attention has been paid to the ways in which the dominant society may contribute to certain components of such homosexual behavior. There has been a suggestion in cross-cultural research that homophobic attitudes in a society are correlated with increased numbers of homosexual partners and decreases in long-term, stable coupling.[25] Although it is obvious that the determinants of both heterosexual and homosexual behavior are complex, this issue may provide an important opportunity for dealing with one aspect of the AIDS epidemic. In a society that condemns the open, social, and sensual bonds between gay couples, it may be more likely that men turn to closeted, clandestine, and brief sexual encounters. For example, it is ironic that those who condemn sexual activity outside of traditional marriage may be even more distressed by the prospect of sanctioning gay marriages. Change is possible. In general, staffs of hospitals, particularly intensive care units and specialized AIDS treatment facilities, have come to accept and support gay relationships. The value of such acceptance is readily observed in these circumstances and needs to be extended. Perhaps instead of focusing on the "other" and the imperative for change elsewhere, it is time that we each examine our own attitudes and priorities. This lesson, too, has been learned however relucently and late, in other epidemics. It is exactly such lessons that may facilitate rather than impede control of the AIDS epidemic.

REFERENCES

1. Curran JW: The epidemiology and prevention of AIDS. Ann Intern Med 103:657–662 (1985).

2. Barre-Sinoussi F et al: Isolation of a T-lymphotropic retrovirus from a patient at risk of acquired immunodeficiency syndrome (AIDS). Science 222:861–871 (1985).

3. Popovic M, Sardgadharan M, Read E, Gallo R: Detection, isolation and continuous production of cytopathic retroviruses (HTLV-III) from patients with AIDS and pre-AIDS. Science 224:497–500 (1984).

4. Emmons CA, Joseph JG, Kessler RC, Wortman CB, Montgomery SB, Ostrow DG: Psychosocial predictors of reported behavior change in homosexual men at risk for AIDS. Health Educ Q 13:331–345 (1986).

5. Martin JL: AIDS risk reduction recommendations and sexual behavior patterns among gay men: A multifactorial categorical approach to assessing change. Health Educ Q 13:347–358 (1986).

6. Deuchan N: AIDS in New York City with particular reference to the psycho-social aspects. Br J Psychol 145:612–619 (1984).

7. Nichols SE: Psychosocial reactions of persons with the acquired immunodeficiency syndrome. Ann Intern Med 103:765–667 (1985).

8. Kirscht J, Haefner D, Kegels S, Rosenstock I: A national study of health beliefs. J Health Hum Behav 7:248–254 (1966).

9. Harris D, Guten S: Health protective behavior: An exploratory study. J Health Soc Behav 20:17–29 (1979).

10. Weinstein N: Why it won't happen to me: Perception of risk factors and susceptibility. Health Psychol 3:431–457 (1984).

11. Kasper RG: Perceptions of risk and their effects on decision-making. In "Societal Risk Assessment: How Safe Is Safe Enough?" RC Schwing, WA Albers (eds). New York: Plenum (1980).

12. Brandt AM: "No Magic Bullet: A Social History of Venereal Disease in the United States Since 1880." New York: Oxford University Press (1985).

13. Cipolla CM: "Cristofano and the Plague: A Study in the History of Public Health in the Age of Galileo." Berkeley: University of California Press (1973).

14. Delaporte F: "Disease and Civilization: The Cholera in Paris, 1832." Cambridge, MA: MIT press (English translation: 1986).

15. Longmate N: "King Cholera: The Biography of a Disease." London: Honish Hamilton (1966).

16. Nohl J: "The Black Death: A Chronicle of the Plague." New York: Harper and Row (English translation: 1969).

17. Rosenberg CE: "The Cholera Years: The United States in 1832, 1849, and 1866." Chicago: University of Chicago Press (1962).

18. Gostin L, Curran WJ: Legal control measures for AIDS: Reporting requirements, surveillance, quarantine, and regulation of public meeting places. Am J Public Health 77:214–218 (1987).

19. Darrow WW: Social and psychologic aspects of the sexually transmitted diseases: A different view. Cutis 27:307–311 (1981).

20. Joseph JG, Ostrow DG: The crisis of AIDS: Implications for health care providers. In "Biobehavioral Control of AIDS." DG Ostrow (ed). New York: Irvington (in press).

21. Ostrow DG, Eller M, Joseph JG: Fears of a new holocaust: Emerging AIDS-related psychosocial issues. Paper presented at the Second International Conference on AIDS, Paris (June 1986).

22. McKusick L, Horstman W, Coates TJ: AIDS and sexual behavior reported by gay men in San Francisco. Am J Public Health 75:493–496 (1986).

23. Martin JL: Sexual behavior patterns, behavior change, and occurrence of antibody to LAV/HTLV-III among New York City gay men. Paper presented at the Second International Conference on AIDS, Paris (June 1986).

24. Hastings GB, Leather DS, Scott AC: AIDS publicity: Some experiences from Scotland. Br Med J 294:48–49 (1987).

25. Ross MW: Predictors of partner numbers in homosexual men: Psychosocial factors in four societies. Sex Transm Dis 11:119–122 (1984).

25

AIDS: Seventh-Rank Absolute*

Robert Fulton and Greg Owen

INTRODUCTION

Images of what threatens to be a major human catastrophe were presented to the American public in 1986 in the form of a 2-h PBS "Frontline" documentary entitled, "AIDS." It featured a *cinéma verité* presentation of the life of an afflicted black male homosexual prostitute—Fabian Bridges. The program offered the viewer a microcosm of the world within which Fabian found himself: a medical establishment confronted with a new, lethal disease for which there is no known cure or vaccine; a public health service threatened with being overwhelmed by AIDS patients; legislators pulled in different ways by their constituents to respond to the epidemic; and an embattled homosexual community aware that its members currently represent more than two-thirds of all AIDS patients. Following the film, a panel of medical experts, a legislator, a public health official, and representatives of several gay-rights organizations were asked to comment on the scenes of Fabian moving about the city of Houston making contacts with men and engaging in sexual acts. The general confusion and unpreparedness of civic authorities to deal with the disease or the civil rights issues it raised were highlighted by the inability of public officials to prevent Fabian's behavior or remove him from the street. While the program recognized that the AIDS virus was indifferent to race, sex, income, or age and that others (IV drug users and transfused individuals) were also afflicted with the disease, the film footage and the discussion focused primarily on the male homosexual. Some panel members expressed deep concern that the film depicting Fabian's life would merely serve to exacerbate homophobia across the country and intensify the hysteria that has surfaced in reaction to this still largely unknown disease. They objected to what they perceived to be a distorted vision of the behaviors of persons with AIDS and felt the film did not reflect actions typical of gay men in the community.

The authorities' treatment of Fabian following his arrest for simple theft reflects these several concerns. He was kept in solitary confinement; the materials he handled (paper, pen, cutlery, etc.) were destroyed; he was not physically touched by any of the police or court officers; and to make certain that he did not constitute a threat to the local community of Houston, the charges against him were dropped, and the police department purchased one-way airfare

---

*In the game of chess, when a player places a rook on an opponent's seventh rank, thereby severely limiting the mobility of the opponent's king and threatening checkmate, the positioning of the rook is called the seventh-rank absolute. Similarly it could be said that AIDS has positioned itself on humankind's seventh rank, for it not only severely limits our options as to what we can do, it also possesses the potential for checkmate.

for him to Cleveland, where he had relatives. To ensure Fabian's departure, the presiding judge personally contributed $20 toward the fare.

BACKGROUND

In 1981 the initial report of *Pneumocystis carinii* pneumonia (PCP) among five male homosexuals in Los Angeles marked the recognition of what has come to be known as AIDS. In 1984 a human retrovirus, HTLV-III/LAV (human T-cell lymphotropic virus type III/lymphadenopathy-associated virus), now called HIV (human immune deficiency virus), was determined to be the etiologic agent of AIDS, and in 1985 serologic tests for antibodies to the virus were developed and made available.[1]

Over this relatively short period of time, AIDS cases have been reported in all 50 states, the District of Columbia, and four territories. As of January 1, 1988, 48,139 residents of the United States were on record as being ill with the disease. It is estimated that there are upwards of 2 million people in the United States infected with HIV and that 20–30% of them are expected to develop AIDS within 5 years. By the end of 1991 it is projected that the cumulative cases of AIDS in the United States meeting the Centers for Disease Control (CDC) surveillance definition will total more than 270,000 cases and that more than 145,000 individuals will require medical attention for AIDS. It is expected that of this number, 54,000 will die. The CDC cautions, however, that the empirical model upon which these estimates are based may underestimate the morbidity and mortality attributable to AIDS by as much as 20%.[2]

In the last half decade, AIDS has reached pandemic proportions. More than 129 countries report the presence of the disease, with some European countries such as Belgium and France reporting a threefold increase in the incidence of the disease yearly.[3] It is estimated that upwards of 1 million Europeans and more than 5 million Africans are infected with the virus.

SOCIAL RESPONSE

When the mode of transmission was initially identified with the particular sexual practices and reported promiscuity of homosexuals, many persons viewed the disease as a consequence of immoral and self-destructive behaviors by a socially disreputable group. The same was true with respect to the intravenous drug user. Religious attitudes toward homosexuality and the social and legal disapproval of drugs also helped to define the AIDS epidemic in its early stages as a disease that was essentially self-inflicted. The historical condemnation of homosexuality and its designation as a felony in over 25 states in the United States also permitted many persons to disregard the illness and its consequences.

The interpretation of illness as a punishment for immoral behavior and the impulse to blame the victim have a very long history in Western culture. Susan Sontag, in her book *Illness as Metaphor*, describes illness as the "night side of life."[4] She reminds us that throughout history, disease has frequently been taken as metaphor, that it has often been represented as supernatural punishment or demonic possession. Death among the Greeks, for instance, was often seen as a consequence of personal fault or as a result of an ancestor's wrongdoing. With the advent of Christianity, the association of disease with divine judgment became even more specific, and illness came to be seen as appropriate and just punishment. This is most vividly illustrated in the general response to the Bubonic Plague of the 14th century. Reactions took two separate directions. First, the plague was treated as an act of God—as a judgment upon sinners, in the way Sodom and Gomorrah were reported to have been destroyed as a result of God's displeasure. In response to such a belief, groups of flagellants appeared in different parts of Europe and beat themselves and others bloody in acts of propitiation and atonement. Anti-Semitism also flared, and Jews were attacked and killed because of the belief that they were responsible for spreading the pestilence. On the other hand, there were those who reacted to the plague passively. The death and misery associated with the plague were seen as the quintessence of order and control. The view taken was that while illness was indeed a punishment God inflicted on whom He willed, He granted clemency to the faithful.[5]

In *Shoah*, a recent documentary on the Nazi holocaust, one hears repeated these ancient ideas that have reverberated through history. In the film, the annihilation of the Jews is justified by some of those interviewed as a consequence of Divine judgment: they were killed as a result of their moral corruption and their adamantine refusal to accept Jesus as the Messiah.

So, too, the idea of God's justice is heard in the United States today in relation to the AIDS epidemic. Throughout the country, particularly among fundamentalist Christians, the disease called AIDS is presented as God's scourge levied against homosexuals, drug users, and prostitutes. Various references to the Old Testament are made to support this view:

> If a man also lie with mankind, as he lieth with a woman, both of them have committed an abomination: they shall surely be put to death; their blood shall be upon them.
>
> *—Leviticus 20:13*[6]

> Neither shalt thou bring an abomination into thine house, lest thou be a cursed thing like it, but thou shalt utterly detest it, and thou shalt utterly abhor it; for it is a cursed thing.
>
> *—Deuteronomy 7:26*[7]

Theological judgment with respect to AIDS is also related to the traditional prohibitions against fornication and abortion. From the point of view of some religious communities, abortion clinics, family planning, and sex education programs are essentially all of a piece. They are viewed as a falling away from God's ordinances concerning the sanctity of marriage and procreation. In contrast, the view is held that responsibility for, and guidance in, the moral and ethical education of children belongs solely to the parents and not to the government or other agencies. Even educational programs that attempt to check the spread of AIDS are seen not only as an assault on parental rights with respect to the moral education of a child but also as introducing libertarian views and inducements for immoral behavior.

American society today is challenged to strike a balance or make a choice between the community's responsibility to prevent the spread of illness through various educational and public health measures and the rights of parents to decide how and in what form their children will receive sex education. Despite the Surgeon General's recent national television appearance recommending that children from the earliest grades be informed about the risks associated with sexual intercourse and that they be fully instructed to ensure the maximum safety for themselves and their sexual partners, many religious groups in the country not only are failing to respond to the issue of AIDS but also are attempting to terminate such sex education programs as do exist.[8]

Although it is clear that AIDS is a sexually transmitted disease, sex education alone is not sufficient to change the customs and mores associated with sexual behavior or the extent to which various precautions will or will not be observed. Research has shown, for example, that otherwise sexually knowledgeable young women will avoid birth control measures in order not be perceived as promiscuous by their sexual partners.[9] Moreover, for some men and women, engaging in sex without birth control is a way of both expressing and calling forth commitment.

The struggle to direct the minds and the sexual behavior of the young is fraught with other difficulties as well. Of significance is the fear among some blacks that sex education programs and family planning information may constitute a conspiracy on the part of the white community to perpetrate genocide against them. The first author encountered this largely unspoken concern when as a guest speaker at Dr. Martin Luther King's Alma Mater, Morehouse College in Atlanta, some years ago, he had occasion to address a group of preseminary students on the topic of death and dying. He was challenged by several students who questioned him sharply about the white community's efforts to restrict black population growth. In any program dealing with sex education in the schools, this issue must be addressed if black support for AIDS education is to be successful.

Although we have observed that the black community fears that family planning organizations have hidden agendas, it must also be recognized that this fear is present in a somewhat different form among white groups. There is a concern that blacks, Hispanics, Asians, and Roman Catholics have greater birth rates than white Protestants, and that promotion of birth control can only aggravate a situation in which particular white groups see their numbers overwhelmed by growing minority populations.

Containment of the epidemic, however, is not the only challenge that AIDS presents to American society. The role of professional care givers is also brought into question. Because of the relative newness of the disease, few health care professionals have had prior training or experience in treating AIDS patients. Information and technologies concerning the disease increase at a rapid rate. Professional care givers are often hard pressed to keep current. Moreover, the psychological, neuropsychiatric, and broader psychosocial aspects of AIDS are still emerging. In the face of the fact that over 70% of AIDS patients develop psychiatric or neuropsychiatric signs and symptoms, lack of appropriate therapies often diminishes the professional care givers' sense of efficacy. As a consequence, many are expressing growing unease about the AIDS epidemic.[10] In turn, this has led in some instances to a refusal to accept acutely ill AIDS patients, a reluctance to carry out invasive procedures and autopsies, or a refusal to admit a seropositive person for medical treatment.[11]

Studies are also beginning to show that care givers are becoming less tolerant of AIDS patients, particularly homosexuals. In one study, three-quarters of the respondents felt that special units for AIDS patients would provide better care then those available in ordinary hospitals, but only 11% said they would be willing to work in such units.[12]

FEAR OF AIDS

The general public, too, displays increased fear and anxiety in the face of the specter of AIDS. Almost daily the news media report incidents or issues involving the disease. The frequency of these reports is in response to the public's growing awareness and concern. These concerns include the risk that children afflicted with AIDS pose to their schoolmates, the advertisement of condoms on television, the distribution of free needles to drug addicts, and the legal and civil propriety of identifying persons seropositive for the virus in official records. Still other reports and news stories tell of persons with AIDs who have lost their jobs, their homes, their medical insurance, or the support of their families and friends.

Individuals from all groups and classes of people seem to fear the disease. Dr. Elisabeth Kubler-Ross, the noted psychiatrist who is recognized worldwide for her work among the dying, was forced to end a presentation early when her largely sympathetic and middle-class audience in Virginia demonstratively opposed her suggestion that the community establish a hospital for the care of abandoned children afflicted with AIDS.[13]

It is ironic that AIDS has appeared at a time in history when American youth, who are more sexually aware and liberated than their forebears, are to a great extent insulated from the immediate experience of death. The present cohort of young men and women often referred to as the "baby boom generation" have, for the most part, experienced death at a distance. Life expectancy for these persons is beyond 70 years. This generation has received the maximum benefits of an urbanized and technologically advanced existence, as modern health care institutions have protected them from general exposure to illness and disease. For them death has been invisible and abstract. In fact, this is the first generation in history in which there has been only a 5% chance that an immediate family member would die before a member of the "baby boom generation" reached adulthood.[14] Although death today can be said to be generally an experience of the aged, the advent of AIDS threatens to effect a profound change in the mortality rates of the young.

In contrast to Sontag's thesis that illness has historically been viewed as supernatural punishment, this age group would explain the AIDS epidemic as a result of failure to practice proper hygenic measures with respect to both sex and drug use. As in so many other aspects of our culture, the "baby boom generation" thinks of illness as something that can be controlled by the individual or prevented, if not cured, by medical science. Such an attitude, however, fails to recognize the extent to which our collective well-being is often dependent on the goodwill of strangers. Surgical patients, for example, must rely on the generosity of those who regularly volunteer their blood and, as sociologist Richard

Titmuss has pointed out in his prescient monograph, *The Gift Relationship*, they have traditionally been assured the greatest margin of safety when the blood they received was donated rather than purchased.[15]

Recently, however, the American Medical Association has come out in favor of a system of private blood banking, the storing of the patient's own previously donated blood, so that persons anticipating the need for surgery may eliminate the risk of receiving contaminated blood from an anonymous donor. Although this may be useful in some cases, where a limited amount of blood will be needed and where the scheduling of the operation can be both planned and controlled, it poses serious limitations in other circumstances. Some of these limitations are: the shelf life of whole blood is only 6–8 weeks; an individual is limited in the amount of blood that can be safely withdrawn over a 12-month period; the blood must be stored within reasonable proximity of the patient in the event of need; at least 1½ h is required for blood to be thawed; and, finally, the cost of such a program may be prohibitive for many.

Over and above these considerations, however, the AMA's recommendation evokes a specter of a new mind-set for the American people: a world of the future in which one donates only to oneself or to immediate family members, who in turn must show evidence of being AIDS-free in order to reciprocate. The proposal offers the prospect of a new definition of community—one characterized not by civic responsibility and neighborliness, but by a dramatic shift toward self-preservation and "lifeboat" ethics and measured in terms of blood purity.

Titmuss's study of blood donation reminds us of the importance of the voluntary act, especially the gift of blood. Such donations, he argues, serve not only to bind a society together but to identify it. When we recall the blood philosophy and policies of the Nazi regime, as well as the American public's own attitudes toward race and blood (i.e., until 1942 the American Red Cross identified and kept separate white and black blood), the prospect of such a program threatens to assault the sense of community and militate against the tradition of altruism and volunteerism.

Community is, at best, a fragile thing. Research shows both its strength and its weaknesses, its substance and its volatility. Extensive studies have shown that communities will respond quickly, vigorously, and sympathetically to victims of accidents and to victims of natural disasters such as floods, hurricanes, or earthquakes.[16]

On the one hand, people who are sick or injured are not blamed for their illnesses, particularly if they act in ways that indicate their desire to get well. Rather, they are described as victims or suffering from diseases over which they have no control. On the other hand, persons who contract a disease such as AIDS or who are perceived to have brought their illness on themselves by their living habits are generally held responsible for contracting the disease, not only by the public but also by health care personnel. This opprobrium is in sharp contrast to the concern manifested for athletes who incur injuries in the course of "play." This comparison clarifies for us that it is the taboo sexual behavior or intravenous drug use that are anathema and not merely the involvement in the development of the disease or injury. Were it simply the latter, individuals who develop lung cancer following years of smoking would be treated with the same degree of disrespect. The negative evaluations of AIDS patients not only result in ostracism, but as research has indicated, also threaten their abandonment by care givers.[17]

The challenge of care, given the psychosocial and neurological sequelae of the disease, presents a configuration of problems and tasks that care givers have difficulty confronting. In addition to the fears and apprehensions care givers may harbor, the patients themselves can display a spectrum of problems ranging from irritability and noncompliant behavior to anger and depression. Furthermore, the patient may also manifest such neurological symptoms as aphasia, seizures, blindness, and dementia, which create further problems in patient–care giver relationships.

At a recent meeting of the American Academy of Arts and Sciences, Paul Volberding, director of the AIDS program at San Francisco Hospital, cautioned his audience that the health care system is San Francisco is showing severe signs of stress.[18] While the rest of the nation has come to look upon San Francisco as a model for coping with the AIDS crisis, Volberding is concerned that the burnout of health care workers, the ever increasing number of AIDS cases, the competing needs of other patients and the lack of coordinated long-range planning may overwhelm the San Francisco health care system. Part of the problem he identifies is the sheer burden of caring for this group of patients, given increasing numbers of patients and limited resources, and the emotional stress on care givers of watching so many young persons die. Though he notes that the most pressing current problem is one of chronic care, the situation will inevitably worsen, he predicts, as the number of AIDS patients increases, making both the acute and the chronic care systems "hopelessly inadequate." In the face of these and other considerations, the moral and ethical cement that has traditionally bound care givers to patients threatens to crumble.

HISTORICAL PERSPECTIVE

History records the challenges that plagues and pestilences have presented to humankind. In his study *Plagues and People*, William McNeill cites the many instances of death dealing epidemics among human populations.[19] Importantly, he notes that one advantage the West had over the East in the face of deadly epidemics was the role of caring for the sick, which among Christians was a recognized religious duty. As he observes, elementary nursing care, even when all normal services broke down, greatly reduced mortality. The simple provision of food and water by the care givers allowed many persons to survive who would otherwise have died of starvation. Moreover, the effect of a prolonged epidemic more often than not strengthened the church when other social institutions were discredited for not providing needed services. McNeill further observes that the teachings of the Christian gospel made life meaningful, even in the immediate face of death: not only could survivors find spiritual consolation in the vision of heavenly reunion with their dead relatives or friends, but God's hand was also seen in the work of the life-risking care givers.[20]

The United States, too, has had its share of plagues and epidemics, one of the most notable of which was the outbreak of yellow fever in Philadelphia in 1793. During the course of that long summer and fall, thousands of citizens of the city perished. William Powell, in his currently relevant book, *Bring Out Your Dead*, written in 1965, vividly describes the scene that Philadelphia presented at that time: the dying were abandoned; the dead were left unburied; orphaned children and the elderly wandered the streets in search of food and shelter. Nearly all who could, fled the city, including the President, leaving the victims of the fever to their fate. Among those who remained, however, were Dr. Benjamin Rush, a cosigner of the Declaration of Independence; the mayor; a handful of medical colleagues and their assistants; and an appreciable number of clergy. With the help of a small but redoubtable group of ordinary laborers and craftsmen, they undertook the enormous tasks of maintaining law and order and providing medical care, food, and shelter to the sick and helpless as well as gathering up and burying the dead.[21] From reading Dr. Rush's diary and voluminous correspondence written during the time of the epidemic, Powell was able to report that what kept Dr. Rush and the others at their posts, even though many of them were made ill by the fever and others died, was their overriding sense of professional obligation, as well as a conviction inspired by the precepts of the New Testament.[22] Unlike the Old Testament, with its stern and unforgiving ordinances currently being invoked to validate a punitive or passive reaction to the AIDS epidemic, the New Testament calls forth a different view of illness and a different vision of the sick:

> Blessed are the merciful, for they shall obtain mercy.
>
> *Matthew 5:9*[23]

> Jesus went about all Galilee, teaching in their synagogues, and preaching the gospel of the kingdom, and healing all manner of sickness and all manner of disease among the people. And his fame went throughout all Syria; and they brought unto him all sick people that were taken with diverse disease and torments, and those who were possessed with demons and those who were epileptics, and those who had the palsy; and he healed them.
>
> *Matthew 4:23–24*[24]

But even this vision, shared by Christians for centuries, which distinguished sickness from sin and which along with a sense of professional commitment permitted Dr. Rush and his fellow Philadelphians to risk their lives in the care of victims of yellow fever, may not be sufficient to persuade contemporary care givers to stay at their posts. The "baby boom generation," well educated, highly secular, and self-oriented, has learned to blame AIDS on groups whom the society defines as deviant and on the fringes of the community—homosexuals and drug users. There is a very strong likelihood, therefore, that today's young health care giver may turn away from those perceived as undeserving of care despite the fact that a 1981 Gallup Poll of the religious beliefs and practices of 14 countries shows that the United States leads the world not only in church membership but also in voluntary service.[25]

The situation is made problematical by the fact that professional care givers perform their duties by reason of the ethics and standards of their professions, beyond whatever religious or moral commitments they may embrace. Moreover, as more is understood about the transmission of the disease, personal health risk to the care giver and subsequent fear of contracting the disease are reduced. Other considerations, however, conflict with the traditional code for professional conduct. In addition to holding homosexuals and IV drug users responsible for the problem of AIDS, care givers are beginning to see them as self-seeking, imprudent, and acting without regard for the condition or well being of others. Concern for the health of one's family members, as well as the anxiety felt by family members and friends for the AIDS care giver, threatens to diminish the care giver's commitment to the task of serving persons with AIDS. Finally, moderate and enlightened Christian care givers who subscribe to the ethic of grace and compassion are again challenged in their distinction between the "sickness and the sin" by the New Testament theology proclaimed by Paul in Romans 1:27:

> And likewise also the men, leaving the natural use of the woman, burned in their lust one toward another, men with men working unseemliness, and receiving in themselves that recompense of their error which was due.[26]

Given such a perception, acts of altruism can become strained and may cease to be offered.

A singular challenge in this regard is the problem of AIDS among incarcerated populations, where homosexual behavior is extensive, and the fact that a substantial number of prison inmates fall within identified high-risk groups for AIDS as well. As with society at large, AIDS within a prison is more than a simple health problem. Decisions concerning prevention, education, identification, and treatment, as well as legal and ethical issues related to medical care and its costs, are but some of the problems that confront the correctional administrator.[27]

As of October 1, 1987, there have been 1964 confirmed cases of AIDS reported in 70 federal and state prison systems.[28] A recent *New York Times* article reports that in New York State, AIDS is now the leading cause of death among all prisoners.[29] The threat of AIDS has raised a multiplicity of problems that would have been unimaginable just a few years ago. For example, some defendants report being deprived of their civil rights because court officers refuse to go near them or even take them into court, while other defendants are released or the charges against them dismissed, because they are dying of AIDS. In fact, judges and parole boards are beginning to question whether persons with AIDS should even be prosecuted and whether dying inmates should not be released.

At Riker's Island correctional facility in New York State in 1986, it is estimated that of the 50,000 inmates who were sentenced or were pending indictment, between 11,000 and 12,000 were infected with the AIDS virus. Nevertheless, despite the call by correctional officers for the screening of all prisoners for AIDS, state and city policies prohibit such testing. The result is that infected inmates with no confirmed diagnosis are housed with the general prison population. The significance of this policy becomes clear when examined in light of the National Institute of Justice Report on AIDS in correctional facilities which estimated that prior to the advent of AIDS, 30% of all inmates engaged in homosexual activity and 10–20% of the overall prison population are subject to rape or other involuntary sexual acts.[30] Unless these behaviors are modified, the prospect of AIDS continuing to spread among prison populations is great, and with it is an increase in fear among prison staff and administrators.

General concern, moreover, is heightened by the fact that blacks and Hispanics, who make up 39% of all persons identified with AIDS in the United

322   R. FULTON AND G. OWEN

States, are also overrepresented in prison populations. This awareness has sparked
some minority leaders to demand greater resources to educate minority communities.

ROLE OF SOCIAL SCIENCE

In the face of this burgeoning pandemic for which there is currently no vaccine
for prevention or medication for cure, the question before us is what can social
science contribute to the understanding and mitigation of the wide range of
social and psychological as well as clinical problems associated with AIDS.

If education is one of our major lines of defense against this lethal disease,
it is our challenge as professionals and as citizens to determine what the major
social issues are and to bring to them the knowledge requisite to increased
understanding and, hopefully, resolution.

Sociologists have already begun to address the challenge of AIDS, both as
educators and as researchers. An organization known as the Sociologists AIDS
Network (SAN) has been formed and an agenda drawn up that includes the
development of a bibliography on the social dimensions of AIDS, the publication
of a newsletter, and the compilation of a directory of sociologists working in
the area.[31]

Karolynn Siegel directs sociological research on AIDS at Memorial Sloan-
Kettering Cancer Center in New York and is studying the sexual behavior of
gay men. Siegel and others have also made a content analysis of AIDS brochures
published around the country. It is their judgment that many brochures fail to
inform successfully or to motivate for change. In order to effect a change in
behavior, they conclude, anxiety levels must be high enough to promote change
but not so high that they trigger denial.[32]

Albert Chabot, a medical sociologist whose area of specialty is the sociology
of death, has established a program called "Wellness" that provides training for
volunteers who offer personal attention to individuals with AIDS. The program
also provides them with information about relevant medical and social resources
in the Detroit community.[33]

Jill Joseph, an epidemiologist, with her colleagues at the University of Michigan School of Public Health, is studying 1000 sexually active gay men from the
Chicago area. The study is designed to determine to what extent gay men are
changing or modifying their attitudes and behaviors in response to the perceived
risk of AIDS. Preliminary findings indicate that about 80% of the subjects have
changed their behavior in some way to reduce the risk of contracting AIDS.[34]

Levi Kamel, a former director of AIDS services in California, designs AIDS
education programs. He works in small towns where gay populations are largely
invisible. By drawing on his skills in qualitative research methods, he is able to
estimate the size of the gay community and its level of consciousness about the
epidemic.[35] Such ethnographic research makes it possible to design and estimate
the costs associated with proposed educational programs.

Samuel Friedman, of Narcotic and Drug Research, Inc., is conducting research on the potential for organizing education and self-help programs among
IV users. There are several strong inhibitors to self-organization among IV drug
users. On the one hand, the illegality of the activity makes organization dan-

gerous; on the other hand, time, money, and attention to their addiction leave few resources for other activities.[36]

Medical and sociological research teams have made significant progress since 1981. Over this brief period to time, the etiologic agent of AIDS has been identified, serologic tests to check the blood supply have been developed, and recommendations for the prevention of AIDS have been published. Sociological understanding came first, however. It was the early research of William Darrow, a research sociologist at the Centers for Disease Control, and others that enabled the development of sociograms of sexual contracts which linked AIDS patients in different cities. By questioning these homosexual men, specific behaviors and sexual practices were uncovered, which allowed for greater understanding of the manner in which AIDS was transmitted. This information was critical and continues to be of the utmost importance for AIDS education and prevention programs.[37]

Social scientists actively involved in AIDS education and research programs have expressed concern, however, that neither public policy nor behavioral scientists are responding as is demanded by this social problem.[38] The World Health Organization recently went on record to state that AIDS is the greatest catastrophe of the 20th century.[39] In the face of this lethal disease and the absence of an effective cure, our only recourse to limit the spread of the disease is effective educational programs directed at prevention of the transmission of the virus. Even if these programs are successful, others will be needed that focus on the mitigation of the many social and psychological problems that follow in the wake of the diagnosis of AIDS. Given our current knowledge, it will be a test of our professional skills and our human capacity to respond to this challenge that will determine whether or not AIDS will put our society in "check" and thereby change it irretrievably.

REFERENCES

1. *Public Health Reports*, July–August 1986, Vol. 101, No. 4. Washington, D.C.: U.S. Government Printing Office, 341–342.

2. *Ibid.*, 342. (See also *American Journal of Public Health*, April 1988, Vol. 78, No. 4, 10.)

3. Serrill, Michael. "In the Grip of the Scourge." *Time*, February 16, 1987, 58–59.

4. Sontag, Susan. *Illness as Metaphor*. New York: Farrar, Straus and Giroux, 1977, 3.

5. *Ibid.*

6. *Holy Bible*, Authorized King James Version, New Scofield Reference Edition. New York: Oxford University Press, 1967, 153.

7. *Ibid.*, 227.

8. *Minneapolis Star and Tribune*, November 28, 1986.

9. Thorton, Arland, and Marlene Studor. "Adolescent Religiosity and Contraceptive Usage." *Journal of Marriage and the Family*, February 1987, 117–128.

10. Mckusick, Leon. *What to Do About AIDS: Physicians and Mental Health Professionals Discuss the Issues*. Berkeley: University of California Press, 1986.

11. "Odyssey of AIDS Victims Ends in Death." *American Medical News*, November 4, 1983, 3. (See also T. C. Gayle and D. G. Ostrow, "Psychosocial and Ethical Issues of AIDS Health Care Programs." *Quality Review Bulletin*, 1986, Vol. 12, No. 8, 284–289, 292–294.

12. Douglas, C. J., and T. Kalam. "Homophobia Among Physicians and Nurses: An Empirical Study." *Hospital and Community Psychiatry* 36:1309–1311 (1985).

13. Engel. Wayne. "AIDS: Dealing with the Hysteria." *Virginia Medical* 113:222 (April 1986).

14. Fulton, Robert, and Greg Owen. "Death and Society." *Omega*, 1987, Vol. 18, No. 4, 375–395.

15. Titmuss, Richard. *The Gift Relationship*. New York: Vintage Books, 1971, 22.

16. Pijawka, K. David, Beverly Cuthbertson, and Richard S. Olson. "Towards an Understanding of Human Adaptation to Extreme Events: Emerging Themes in Natural and Technological Disaster Research." *Omega*, 1988 (in press).

17. Gayle. T. C., and D. G. Ostrow, *op. cit.*

18. Deborah Barnes. "AIDS Stresses Health Care in San Francisco." *Science* 235:964 (1987).

19. McNeill. William H. *Plagues and Peoples*. Garden City, NY: Anchor Press, 1976.

20. *Ibid.*, 108.

21. Powell, J. H. *Bring Out Your Dead*. New York: Times Books, 1965.

22. *Ibid.*, *passim*.

23. *Holy Bible*, *op. cit.*, 998.

24. *Ibid.*, 997.

25. Analytica, Oxford. *America in Perspective*. Boston: Houghton Mifflin, 1986, 121–124.

26. *Holy Bible*, *op. cit.*, 1211.

27. National Institute of Justice, *AIDS in Correctional Facilities: Issues and Options*. Washington, D.C.; Department of Justice, U.S. Government Printing Office, 1986, 10–13.

28. National Institute of Justice, *AIDS in Correctional Facilities: Issues and Options*, 3rd Ed., prepublication copy. Washington, D.C.; Department of Justice, U.S. Government Printing Office, 1988.

29. *New York Times*, March 5, 1987.

30. National Institution of Justice, *op. cit.*, 1986, 15.

31. Berg, Ellen. "Sociological Perspectives on AIDS." *Footnotes* 14(9):8, 1986.

32. *Ibid.*

33. *Ibid.*

34. *ISR Newsletter*, Autumn 1986, 3.

35. Berg, *op. cit.*, 8.

36. *Ibid.*, 9.

37. *Ibid.*, 8.

38. *Ibid.*

39. *New York Times*, November 21, 1986, p.8.

26

AIDS: A Jewish View

Terry R. Bard

Despite initial thoughts and some irresponsible media coverage, AIDS is neither a "gay disease" nor a disease limited to members of other high-risk groups. The mode of HIV transmission seems clear,[1-3] and anyone, regardless of race, gender, or sexual preference, is susceptible to the contagion during intimate sexual relationships, the sharing of needles, or other means of transferring infected blood. Nonetheless, today's attitudes are clouded because the public has been influenced by the *initial* press which stigmatized persons with AIDS.[4-6] These news reports and releases still establish the idealized framework within which most people consider the disease. Consequently, the following discussion will focus on Jewish attitudes toward health and disease and homosexuality as the backdrop against which current attitudes toward AIDS may be understood.

Like other ethnic, cultural, and religious groups, the Jewish community eludes simple and singular description; it is inherently pluralistic.[7] Although many Jews appear to subscribe to similar central concepts and shared myths[8] such as the centrality of Torah, a corporate history, and a common culture, the Jewish polity is better understood by its variety. The American Jew is shaped by cultural legacies from idiosyncratic Ashkenazic, Sephardic, and Oriental histories as much as he or she has been molded by social and cultural changes in the American landscape.[9-11] Shared foundations in Jewish history as well as Jewish legal and legendary literature help to create an apparent corporate (or group) Jewish mindset. Nonetheless, such foundations are not the basis for the dominant thinking mode or social style of most of America's Jews. Consequently, attempts to grasp, formulate, and understand the variety of specifically Jewish responses to all life experiences and especially to catastrophic experiences such as AIDS are met with initial frustration.

Further complicating such attempts, illnesses like AIDS unearth fundamental human concerns that touch the most protected and defended dimensions of the psyche.[12] Such disparate observers of human behavior as Sigmund Freud (*Totem and Tabu* and *The Future of an Illusion*) and Woody Allen ("Love and Death" and "Annie Hall") have suggested that basic fears of being homosexual, becoming impotent, and dying underlie much of life's thoughts. Many of our daily activities are metaphoric attempts to deny or mask these basic fears and deny the reality of death.

This broad ethnic, cultural diversity and the personal human response are necessary background against which any attempt to understand, to explain, and to assist Jews in their responses to AIDS should be made. Since a detailed analysis of these components would require a major treatise, this paper will focus on the intersect between Jewish cultural diversity and psychic frailty. Further, it will pose problems and solutions for Jewish responses to AIDS.

Whereas Jewish biblical and talmudic (halakhic-legal) literature contains a variety of values, one value, the *preservation of life*, appears paramount. Life is good,[13] meant to be perpetuated,[14] and meant to be maximized. Even though death is inevitable, and some theoretical excursions into the possibility of life after death have been focal in some postbiblical Judaisms, all Jewish systems of belief and practice are life-affirming. Biblical accounts describe death from polar extremes as a natural event[15] and as the sign of absolute punishment for blasphemy, bloodshed, or incest. Job represents a watershed between naturalistic and casuistic thinking. His "friends" and "comforters" implore Job to curse God and die. Job refuses charges of any culpability. A standoff between Job and God/Satan ensues as the biblical author poses the ancient human question— Why do the innocent suffer?

Like death, illness can be considered either a natural event or the consequence of wrongdoing. The many biblical concerns about leprosy are one example[16] expressing the extremes of such polar thinking. Either way, that which is considered inexplicable is potential grist for the human fantasy mill. Most people think casuistically—viz., cause and effect. When no apparent cause exists, the human mind is quick to fill the gap. Cultural reinforcement of shared bewilderment creates a milieu mind-set[17] for mythic and superstitious thinking. Demons begin to lurk in the distant abyss, behind every tree, and in dark places. They are poised, ready to do their nasty deeds, wreaking havoc in an otherwise orderly world.[18]

To compound matters, early rabbinic thinkers were both inheritors of biblical thought and savvy observers of humankind. Recognizing that people are capable of good and evil, they concluded, in almost gnostic fashion, that the human psyche is composed of two major inclinations, the "inclination toward good" (*yezer ha-tov*) and the "inclination toward evil" (*yezer ha-ra*). People's activities and thoughts can be categorized within these two classifications. Whatever the etiology of such activities—demons, deity, or determinism—the act itself could be placed into categories. Freud's *id* and *super ego* are interesting correlates to such thinking. It is noteworthy that both the rabbis and Freud allied the sexual drive with the negative component. If sexuality is a component of the *yezer ha-ra* and the *libido* an acting-out of the *id*, homosexuality clearly finds its place on the evil side of the human psychic equation. It is an easy next step that such a view become culturally enshrined by future generations. Such enshrinement is especially likely to occur, if psychoanalytic insight has any veracity, when homosexuality is regarded as a latent repressed human fear at least as intense as the fear of death. Thus the individual Jew in his or her cultural surroundings throughout the millenia has been able to deny and repress any overt acknowledgment of and giving any legitimacy to homosexuality. It is difficult to assess whether this resistance constitutes pathological homophobia or simply workable denial. Either way, the result has been a Jewish cultural and religious attitude that has denied homosexuality a legitimate place in Jewish life.

Biblical condemnations of homosexuality and inappropriate sexual practice (i.e., coitus interruptus) include references to Onan's crime[19] and Levitical prohibitions of same-sex cohabitation.[20] Historical responses have differentiated between the homosexual person and the homosexual act. The homosexual person is regarded as sick and capable of "cure" or "rehabilitation," but the act itself is condemned.[21-24]

Much of the literature about the gay population and their families frequently notes a sense of parental failure; recent articles suggest problematic fathering. For the Jewish family, this sense of failure is heightened. Jews for centuries have prided themselves on family coherence; it is one of the functional myths of Jewish society. The gay person is outcast to this family system; it jeopardizes the corporate myth.

The existence of AIDS challenges every dimension of contemporary society. AIDS poses specific threats to many Jews and the Jewish community at every level—cultural, social, religious, and psychic. Despite the increasing incidence of AIDS, communal denial has characterized the institutional Jewish reaction and thwarted formal Jewish responses to AIDS until recently. In fact, had AIDS proved to be limited to the gay, IV drug abusing, or non-Jewish population, it is unlikely that any programmatic Jewish response would have developed. Likewise, it is not surprising that some of the early Jewish institutional responses arose out of the liberal movement. Jewish institutional responses to AIDS remain slow, except for some of the Jewish community-sponsored hospitals.

To date (Nov., 1986), the Union of American Hebrew Congregations (UAHC) and the Central Conference of American Rabbis are the only major international Jewish organizations to address the AIDS issue programmatically. In 1985, Rabbi Alexander Schindler, President of the UAHC, proposed the formation of a national Jewish task force on AIDS. Such a task force now convenes regularly to learn about the disease and to create a national educational program for the UAHC's constituency. Rabbis and clinical personnel including physicians, biochemical researchers, social workers, and laity meet to create national programming to address issues posed by AIDS. A packet of basic information and resources has been developed and sent to all member congregations and reform rabbis in the country. Regional meetings of congregations and rabbis have included formal programming on AIDS.

At this writing, the Northeast Council of the UAHC has been one of the most active in the Reform Jewish community. The Massachusetts Board of Rabbis, in the fall of 1985, sponsored an educational forum for its membership inclusive of Reform, Conservative, Reconstructionist and some Orthodox branches of Judaism; attendance was small. The next formal meeting was sponsored by the Boston Area Reform Rabbis. An educator joined by two members of the Boston gay Jewish community discussed attitudes toward gay men and women and provided information about the disease. During this session a sexual-attitude survey was completed by the rabbis present, one of whom was female.[25] This survey was a poor research tool; nonetheless, a quick tabulation of responses suggested that some degree of homophobia existed in approximately 33% of those surveyed. Shortly after this meeting, the social action coordinator of the UAHC initiated a programmatic Jewish response. Meetings ensued, and a lay pastoral care givers' program was developed.

In the fall of 1986, Reform Jewish congregations and their rabbis were invited to recruit volunteers for this visitation program. Of the 40 congregations solicited, seven individuals attended. Two evening training sessions took place under the direction of the Director of Pastoral Services of Beth Israel Hospital, Boston. Each lasted for 2½ h. The first session addressed myths and medical facts about

AIDS and attitudinal concerns within the Jewish community. The second session focused on the practical details of how interventions and interviews with patients with AIDS or their family members or significant others were to be conducted, how confidentiality would be preserved, and how referrals would be made. A follow-up workshop took place in the winter of 1987. At that meeting several new volunteers participated in an accelerated introductory program. Topics discussed included AIDS problems in the law and in the workplace as well as the latest medical research findings. Then a "debriefing" of participants' experiences during the previous 6 months took place. Currently the services of this group are underutilized, although information about the group was published in the Boston papers, the Anglo-Jewish press, the gay press, and through AIDS support groups. Additional training programs are contemplated in Hartford, CT, and Albany, NY.

Increasing evidence that the AIDS virus is indiscriminate and epidemiologists' warnings that the incidence of the virus is increasing geometrically in all populations make it less possible for individuals to deny susceptibility. The virus's quick mutability is equally scary. In this context, the veneer of denial within the Jewish community is beginning to peel away just as earlier denials of Jewish susceptibility to alcoholism, homosexuality, divorce, intermarriage, and child and wife abuse peeled away as these have become recognized as unfortunate realities of social integration into American society.[26]

Although the Jewish response to AIDS has been slow in developing, training and education will hasten an acknowledgment that AIDS is also a problem that occurs among Jews. When formal acknowledgment occurs, programmatic responses will likely arise across the spectrum of Jewish life.

REFERENCES

1. Groopman, J.E., et al.: HTLV-III in saliva of people with AIDS-related complex and healthy homosexual men at risk for AIDS. *Science* 1984;226:447–449.

2. Hirsch, M.S., et al.: Risk of nosocomial infection with human T-cell lymphotrophic virus III (HTLV-III). *N. Engl. J. Med.* 1985;312:1–4.

3. Friedland, G.H. et al.: Lack of transmission of HTLV- III/LAV infection to household contacts of patients with AIDS or AIDS-related complex with oral candidiasis. *N. Engl. J. Med.* 1986;314:344–349.

4. Morin, S.F., and Batchelor, W.F.: Responding to the psychosocial crisis of AIDS. *Public Health Rep.* 1984;99:4–9.

5. Brandt, E.N., Jr.: The concentric effects of the acquired immune deficiency syndrome. (Editorial.) *Public Health Rep.* 1984;99:1–2.

6. Fornstein, M: The psychosocial impact of the acquired immune deficiency syndrome. *Semin. Oncol.* 1984;11:77–82.

7. Sklare, M. *Understanding American Jewity*, Transaction Books, New York, 1982.

8. The term "myth" as used in this paper does not mean fable or fantasy tale. Myth means a central organizing principle that may or may not be based in an event but has become focal over time. The myth itself thus becomes a conceptual artifact of a civilization.

9. Sklare, *op. cit.*

10. Dawidowiscz, L. *On Equal Terms—Jews in America 1881–1981*. Holt, Rinehart and Winston, New York, 1984.

11. Neusner, J. *American Judaism*. Prentice-Hall, Englewood Cliffs, New Jersey, 1972.

12. Morin and Batchelor, *op. cit.*

13. Deuteronomy: "I have set before you life and good, death and evil, therefore *choose life*" (italics added).

14. Genesis: The first biblical command, "Be fruitful and multiply."

15. See biblical accounts of the death of the patriarchs and matriarchs in Genesis as well as the references to Moses' death in the last chapter of Deuteronomy.

16. Preuss, J. *Biblical and Talmudic Medicine.* (Fred Rosner, ed.) Hebrew Publishing Company, New York, 1983.

17. Eliade, M. *Cosmos and History.* Harper Torch Books, New York, 1961.

18. Trachtenberg, J. *Jewish Magic and Superstition.* Jewish Publication Society, Philadelphia, 1970.

19. Genesis 38:6. Current understanding is that Onan's sin was not masturbation but coitus interruptus.

20. Leviticus 18.

21. Jakobovitz, I. *Jewish Medical Ethics.* Bloch Publishing, New York, 1959, 1975.

22. Feldman, D. *Health and Medicine in the Jewish Tradition.* Crossroads Publishing, New York, 1986.

23. Bleich, D. and Rosner, F. (eds.). *Jewish Bioethics.* Sanhedrin Press, New York, 1978.

24. Freehoff, S. *Current Reform Responsa,* 1969; *Contemporary Reform Responsa,* 1974; *Modern Reform Responsa,* 1971; *Reform Responsa and Recent Reform Responsa,* 1973. Hebrew Union College Press, Cincinnati.

25. McHugh, G. and McHugh, T.G., "A Sex Attitude Survey and Profile." Family Life Publications, 1976.

26. Although the frequency is unknown, such problems appear to have existed at earlier times but were most often repressed, denied, and sublimated.

27

Development of AIDS Awareness: A Personal History

Angie Lewis

"I heard about the strangest disease today. It's a rare skin cancer that usually happens in old men, but I understand they are beginning to find it in young gay men. A doctor from New York talked about it and the information was so new that he used hand-drawn slides!" I remember the conversation so well. I also remember the day. It was a beautiful Saturday afternoon in June 1981, and as a friend and I chatted, driving over the Golden Gate Bridge, we never thought that within five years this disease would attract the attention and concern of the entire world.

Later that summer, I attended two medical rounds on "Kaposi's Sarcoma in Gay Men" that were presented where I work, the Medical Center at the University of California, San Francisco. I was one of a very few women, and perhaps the only nurse, in the audience. As I sat and tried to listen to the clinical discussion, my thoughts were occupied with a deep concern for the men experiencing this condition. In particular, I thought about how difficult it would be to be gay and terminally ill. I am a lesbian, and I know what it is like to be closeted. I remembered the emotional turmoil I experienced during two hospitalizations, especially the one in the small hospital where I worked in Florida during the mid-sixties. At that time I was literally terrified that someone would guess I was "queer." I didn't want my lover to be around when I went to the operating room because I felt it would look unusual; I was so preoccupied with that concern that I didn't stop and realize that many people have a friend visit before they leave for the operating room. I was careful about how we addressed each other, even when talking on the phone, and holding hands was reserved for times when the door was closed and bed curtain drawn. I was deep in my secret closet and felt I could only trust or confide in others whom I knew were in the same situation.

A man with KS (as Kaposi's sarcoma was being termed) didn't have the choice of staying in the closet—not with those purple marks—he was out; he was a homosexual. What would it be like to be young (most patients were in their twenties or thirties), reaching that time in life which should be the most productive, and then to be diagnosed and openly identified? In a society obsessed with physical attractiveness, how would it feel to begin developing ugly purple spots? Already the prognosis was grim and the media were beginning to discuss a "gay plague". If you haven't come out to your family, or yours friends, or on the job, what must it be like to do so under these circumstances?

After the second lecture on KS, I introduced myself to the speaker, explaining that I was both a Nurse Educator in Nursing Education and Research and a lesbian who would be willing to visit patients and/or provide a perspective of and connection to the gay/lesbian community. In retrospect, that quite political act was very atypical of me. I certainly never considered myself an activist nor was I "connected" to the San Francisco gay community. But I had been a lesbian and a nurse for over 15 years and I knew firsthand the isolation that the health care system could impose on people who didn't "fit."

I was invited to join the physician who had recently formed the "KS Study Group." There I met and talked with many individuals whose personal and professional lives would be changed by the epidemic. Immediately after the initial meeting, one of the physicians asked me to visit the first U.C.S.F. patient who had been hospitalized with KS. When I went to the oncology unit, I wasn't sure how I would be received; it wasn't one of my assigned units, and Nurse Educators in our setting usually don't have direct patient contact. I initially met with the Administrative Nurse and had the first of many "coming out" talks I would have with professional colleagues over the ensuing years. I had been gradually coming out in social situations since Harvey Milk's death in 1978, but professionally, only in very limited situations. Although I worked at one of the few institutions in the United States where my job was protected regardless of sexual orientation, I was concerned about what people would think. However, I believed then, and still do today, that it is very important for persons with AIDS to know some of their caregivers provide a positive affirmation of their shared lifestyle. I have also come to believe that to fight stereotypes of gay and lesbian people, it is critical that as many of us as possible come out and make our presence known. My personal fear in this process was I might lose the respect and/or peer support of my colleagues, but in reality, it was their support and love which made the process so enriching. Positive self-affirmation was healing. For someone who had spent much of her life hiding from others, being open allowed me to finally be in control of my own life; by sharing my personal perspectives, I made a unique contribution to both patients and staff.

The first time I saw Juan (pseudonym), he was lying quietly in bed. From my discussion with the Administrative Nurse, I knew he was an illegal alien who spoke broken English even though he had been in the United States many years. He was a very private, intensely religious man who had no visitors other than the hospital priest and his brother who came every afternoon. I put on the requisite isolation gown, went in his room and pulled a chair close to his bed. All visible parts of his body—face, hands, and arms—were covered with large purple lesions. "Juan, my name is Angie Lewis. I am a nurse here and I'm also part of a campus association of gay and lesbian people. I want you to know that we are concerned about you and would like to provide any support we can." That statement was the first and last time the words "gay," or "lesbian," or anything similar, were ever mentioned between us. With his agreement, I began a pattern of brief daily visits, most often just 10 or 15 minutes long. I would sit quietly by the bed holding his hand or massaging his feet. Touching is very important for patients who feel so untouchable. I made a conscious decision to not wear gloves, although I always washed my hands very carefully after each meeting. Occasionally he would ask for something—a deck of cards or a magazine—but mostly we just sat quietly. The unit staff was very accepting and supportive of my visits to Juan. As the weeks passed, they began to ask questions about the study group and include me in discussions on Juan's care plan.

By this time I was also visiting a second patient, who presented a distinct contrast to Juan. Patrick was an openly gay white man diagnosed with Pneumocystis carinii pneumonia (PCP). A very articulate individual, he was actively involved in the San Francisco music community and had so many visitors that limits were set so he could rest. Additionally, he had very supportive and loving parents who came from the Midwest to stay with him. When I first met Patrick, he had just been discharged from the Intensive Care Unit where he had required intubation for several days. When I introduced myself to him, his face lit up; he smiled and clasped my hand, saying that although he had several caregivers whom he felt were gay or lesbian, I was the first to acknowledge it. He was obviously pleased and touched by my visit, but because he had strong support systems we both agreed frequent visits were not needed. Also, since we did not yet know how the diseases were spread, I was concerned with possible transmission of infection between Patrick and Juan.

After a brief trip home at Thanksgiving, Juan returned to the hospital for his final stay. With his life and his death, he left a legacy of quiet dignity that remains with those who knew him. He also helped remind many of us that our role as caregiver is to meet the emotional needs of patients as they perceive them, not as we think they should be. Juan had chosen not to talk with his family about his lifestyle. Some staff members felt this reflected "unfinished business," and they wanted to encourage Juan to deal with this issue. Several intense multidisciplinary conferences centered on this topic as staff confronted their fears and feelings related to homosexuality and death. For some staff members who themselves were gay men or lesbians, the dialogue reflected basic questions with which they were struggling. Crucial to the resolution of the situation was the support which was apparent among all of the staff, and their acceptance of a diversity of lifestyles. Their recognition of each person's right to make his or her own choices led to their final decision to not persuade Juan to reveal his lifestyle choices to his family and/or priest. This allowed Juan to die peacefully, content with his decision. Patrick's choices, on the other hand, served a different purpose. For the last few months of his life, he struggled against his disability to complete his musical works and raise AIDS awareness in the musical community. His legacy was the impact he made on others through his music and his willingness to be a "public" person with AIDS.

I was involved in a variety of AIDS activities over the following months. The social work department called asking if the gay/lesbian community had resources for assisting those in need. I made over 50 phone calls in a vain attempt to locate a single lesbian/gay-identified organization that worked with sick persons. In the winter of 1981–'82 few, if any, of the people with whom I spoke had even heard about this new problem! We soon realized that for the time being the traditional agencies, for example, visiting nurses, home health, and so on, would have to suffice. Shortly thereafter, a small group of individuals in the gay/lesbian community, most of whom were involved in health care, held the first meeting of what would evolve into the San Francisco AIDS Foundation. I remember sitting in a school gymnasium leading a small group discussion on provision of patient care services. From that tiny beginning has evolved an organization with over 47 employees and a budget of $2.7 million.

Another major organization, Shanti, which provides counseling and support services, evolved from an agency that had been in quiet existence for many years. In the past, their counseling services were provided to patients and families dealing with cancer, but as needs related to AIDS escalated, they found themselves caring for more and more AIDS patients. Ultimately, they decided to focus all their resources on AIDS patients. As these organizations were evolving, the San Francisco Department of Public Health recognized the need for a coordinated effort to confront the problem, and I became a member of their KS Advisory Committee. In reality, many members of this committee were a core group of people who were providing direct care developing the community agencies, and generally devoting much of their time to the issue of AIDS. The committee facilitated the development of networks among public and private agencies. All of us involved during the early months tried to avoid duplication of services. We attempted to identify the services which were then or would eventually be needed and then determine which organization(s) could logically provide them. We also made very deliberate efforts to include people with AIDS as active participants in all AIDS-related organizations.

As a Nurse Educator, I presented several in-service programs at U.C.S.F. and elsewhere. At the same time, I was also aware of the need to present a broader program for nurses and other health care providers in the community. With the cooperation and hard work of a small, dedicated group of nurses, social workers, respiratory therapists, and nutritionists from U.C.S.F., a multidisciplinary conference entitled, "Kaposi's Sarcoma and Pneumocystis pneumonia: New Phenomena Among Gay Men," was presented in June 1982. We believe this conference, attended by almost 100 participants, was the first all-day program in the nation designed for providers other than physicians. Since then, many other agencies have joined in supporting a series of similar programs addressing the needs of health care providers and community agencies. These programs have now been attended by over 3000 participants.

During the late summer of 1982 I attended, for the first time, the Lesbian and Gay Health Workers National Conference, which was held in Houston. Several sessions were devoted to AIDS, and providers from across the country shared their personal experiences of giving care to persons with AIDS. We spoke of our frustrations in securing not only funding, but basic recognition of the seriousness of the problem. At this point, the term in use was GRID, or Gay-Related Immune Disorder, and at this conference I heard the term AIDS for the first time. One of my most vivid memories from this meeting was helping a friend edit her presentation, and discussing with her our fears and feelings about transmissibility. At that time, no one knew for sure how it was spread; irrational as is seems now, we both hid silent, dark feelings that maybe as lesbians, we were vulnerable. Maybe just because we were one of "THEM" we were destined to get it. I shared with her my experience of awaking with a fever one night, and lying in bed convinced that I was experiencing the first symptoms. Only later was it recognized that while it is possible for AIDs to be transmitted during sexual contact between women, the possibility is far less than for individuals who engage in other types of sexual activity. To date, only two possible cases of sexual transmission between women have been reported in the literature.[1,2]

The early months of AIDS work formed the pattern which I and many others were to follow for several years; AIDS became a driving force in our lives, frequently overshadowing other aspects of our personal and professional responsibilities. Looking back, I can now see that while the work we did was necessary and important, it also dominated my life, sometimes in a negative way. Further, it became the focus of concern for my community; money, time, and energy which previously might been allocated for other gay or lesbian health issues were often directed only to AIDS. Study into less dramatic, but still important health problems such as the Epstein-Barr virus or alcoholism, slowed to a virtual standstill. As the number of those ill or dead increased, funds allocated for lesbian/gay health care from both the public and private sectors excluded other important health areas, especially those related to women. Although each of us realized the crucial significance of the fight against AIDS, there were and still are feelings of frustration. Some lesbians and gay men have expressed anger at the drain on limited resources in order to fight the epidemic. When I consider the future expenditure of America's health care dollars necessary to care for persons with AIDS/ARC, I envision similar anger and frustration in the general society.

Another correlate can be found in the current controversy on sex education in schools and advertising for condoms. In the early years of the epidemic, heated debate in the gay/lesbian community centered on public education and how it should be accomplished. Questions of how much should be revealed publicly about gay sexual activity, how explicit the language should be, and exactly what messages should be given were gradually resolved, although minor areas of disagreement do remain. Some of the experiences of my community during the past five years have served as a portent of what might be ahead for the broader society. What started as a problem perceived to belong only to the gay community has become the nation's number one health concern; every sexually active person is at risk, and all of us who work in health care will feel the effects.

In my AIDS work, I was meeting new friends and colleagues whose support and friendship I continue to treasure, but I also saw and experienced the destruction of other relationships and/or friendships because of my "AIDS obsession." This obsession was heightened as the disease spread; it began to affect each of us more personally as we saw old and new friends get sick and die. The man with whom I had my longest friendship died from PCP; another friend of over 10 years acquired KS and after 4 years of struggling each day to survive, he passed away last month, just 17 days after his lover died; a nurse I hired and supported in his career died during his first hospitalization. Bobbi Campbell, the "AIDS Poster Boy," as he called himself, a new and cherished friend, became an important part of my life; to this day I remember the lapel button he always wore, "I Will Survive." At times it seems it will never end. And regardless of when it does end, I and most people I know will never be the same. Our lives have been profoundly changed not only by the friends and professional colleagues we have met, but most particularly by having experienced the courage and dignity shown by so many of the people with AIDS.

Nursing has played a crucial role in the evolution of a care system for patients with AIDS. Given the fact that no definitive treatment is known, the care required is *nursing care*. It is nurses who offer supportive interventions that improve that quality of life for persons with AIDS and their families, friends, and loved ones. It has often been nurses who have played an instrumental leadership role in the development of educational programs, home care programs, and other creative approaches to provision of care and service. At the bedside, it is the nurse who has been and will be there through the long hours. It is important that we recognize that each of us can make a difference—we can help others look at how "family" is defined in relation to visiting rules; we can be supportive of a diversity of lifestyles; we can be vigilant in relation to confidentiality; and most importantly, we can decrease fear and hysteria by imparting knowledge to others and can help stem the spread of the disease by supporting AIDS education on our jobs, in our community, and in our schools.

REFERENCES

1. Sabatini, M. T.; Patel, K.; Hirschman, R. "Kaposi's Sarcoma and T-Cell Lymphoma In An Immunodeficient Woman: A Case Report." *AIDS Research* 1:135–7 (1984).

2. Marmor, M.; Weiss, L.; Lyden, M.; et al. "Possible Female-to-Female Transmission of Human Immunodeficiency Virus" (Letter). *Annals of Internal Medicine* 105(6):969 (December 1986).

28

Women with AIDS: Sexual Ethics in an Epidemic

Julien S. Murphy

As the number of AIDS cases in the United States approaches 30,000, the threat of AIDS to the public health becomes more ominous.[1] Concern with fighting the spread of AIDS has been shaped by a notion of "public health" entangled in social biases. For instance, "public health" has been historically skewed toward heterosexuality, as indicated by the initial slow responses to the homosexual and bisexual men first diagnosed with AIDS. The concept of "public health" in relation to the AIDS epidemic, however, has initially been biased more toward gay men, exhibiting a gender bias against women as well. That women too are afflicted with AIDS is rarely mentioned. Many people are not even aware that women can be infected with AIDS, and very few know that women with AIDS are not a recent phenomenon, but rather, that women have been afflicted with AIDS since the very beginning of the epidemic.

In the years 1979–1981, when AIDS was called the Gay-Related-Immune-Disorder (GRID), there were 27 cases reported in women. Currently, there have been 1993 cases of women with AIDS in this country with a projection of 18,900 cases in women by 1991.[2] Seventy percent of the current cases of women with AIDS have been diagnosed in the past two years. In addition, there are two classifications in which even more women have been affected: (1) 105,000 asymptomatic women carriers of the AIDS retrovirus; (2) 14,000 women with AIDS-related complex (ARC).[3]

Homophobia and sexism contribute to the lack of public awareness about women with AIDS because the more the disease is stigmatized as a "gay male disease" the more unthinkable it becomes to consider that women may be at risk for AIDS. It has been an invisible fact that women have consistently comprised 7% of the U.S. AIDS cases (9% in Europe,[4] 50% in Central Africa). Women are frequently omitted from AIDS brochures and media coverage, and eclipsed in medical research. Some public health officials would like to hold prostitutes responsible for AIDS in the United States and elsewhere—an unsubstantiated and sexist claim.[5] Even children, who comprise only 1% of U.S. AIDS cases have gotten more media coverage, albeit controversial, and more research attention than women—despite the fact that 75% of pediatric AIDS cases are acquired in pregnancies among infected women.

In general, women with AIDS are made to fit into a male-AIDS-profile which cannot address the central physiological and sociopolitical differences between the sexes, namely, that AIDS, like many sexually transmitted diseases, immerses women in complex fertility and reproductive decisions. As the number of women with AIDS continues to rise, discussion of the ethical dilemmas of fertility and reproduction will become all the more important. It is not known exactly how many asymptomatic HIV carriers and persons with ARC will develop full-blown AIDS or the manifold immune disorders that will be identified before the epidemic is over. In the meantime, we need to shape a notion of public health appropriate to meet the special problems of women with AIDS, a notion that neither regards women and fertility as a disease nor ignores the needs of infected women and their possible offspring.

Ethical discussion of women with AIDs begins with the awareness that, by and large, these women represent the least advantaged groups in society. Women with AIDS are predominantly black (53%), and engaged in the illegal practices of intravenous drug use (51%) and sometimes prostitution.[6] Small wonder, then, that their plight has received so little attention. Nonetheless, women can protect themselves against AIDS. Most women with AIDS (78%) fall into two primary risk categories, both of which can be altered by behavior changes: intravenous drug use (51%) and heterosexual contact with an infected partner (27%).[7] Many of the remaining (22%) cases of women having no known risk factor may be cases of sexual contact with an asymptomatic carrier. Hence, education and behavior changes could greatly diminish the increase in new cases in women and also curb pediatric AIDS. Four major ethical concerns that specifically relate to women with AIDS are the implications of AIDS transmission by intravenous drug use, by heterosexual contact, by prostitution, and by pregnancy.

AIDS AND WOMEN DRUG USERS

One way to curtail the highest risk factor for women with AIDS (intravenous drug use) is instituting a needle exchange program that provides addicts with legal access to sterile drug injection equipment. Such programs are already in successful operation in Amsterdam and Sydney.[8] The first U.S. program is being instituted in New Jersey[9] where one of the largest group of AIDS-infected IV drug users has been found. Although the sterile needle program would, in theory, eliminate AIDS transmission by the sharing of dirty needles among drug users, it has been seen by some as an implicit approval of abusive drug behavior— supplying drug addicts with the means to their illegal habits. However, the punitive attitude towards addicts, presuming that they get the diseases they deserve, cannot be morally justified because the AIDS-infected drug addicts endanger not only their own health but health of their sexual partners and offspring. A needle exchange program with follow-up checks and counseling not only provides a humane attitude toward drug addiction but also an effective AIDS-prevention measure for women drug abusers, their infants, and the women partners of male addicts.

AIDS AND HETEROSEXUAL CONTACT

The major ethical issues of the AIDS epidemic for women concern AIDS transmission by heterosexual contact, the second highest risk factor for women. A discussion of these issues will be useful as well for exploring the implications for fertility and reproduction in sexually transmitted diseases in general. So far, AIDS has not commonly been a bi-directional sexually transmitted disease in the United States. It is highly controversial whether female-to-male transmission of AIDS is anything but an extremely rare route of transmission.[10-14] Of the 566 heterosexual transmission cases in males, 474 of the men's cases are considered heterosexual transmission cases not as a result of direct evidence but because these men had no other identified risks, and were born in countries with high rates of heterosexual transmission. By contrast, 430 of the 545 heterosexual transmission cases in females occurred with women who had heterosexual contact with a man infected with or at risk for AIDS. It has been well-documented that women can be infected by sexual contact with a male partner who has AIDS, ARC, or is an asymptomatic seropositive.[15] Particularly at high risk are women partners of gay or bisexual men, IV drug users, and hemophiliacs. Although the presence of AIDS infection has been found in the vaginal secretions of women with AIDS[16] and seropositive women,[17] there are no documented cases of AIDS transmission between gay or bisexual women.

To safeguard the blood supply, it has been recommended that wives of he-mophiliacs should refrain from donating blood.[18] The same recommendation could extend to sexual partners of all high risk men. Along with protecting the blood supply from contamination by women donors with heterosexually acquired AIDS, we should be concerned with protecting the health of women partners of high risk males.

The ethical issues concerning AIDS are particularly exigent because AIDS is usually a terminal disease. For instance, what are the implications of sexual intimacy when it involves the risk of death? Is there an ethical principle by which women can justifiably refuse unprotected sexual contact with an infected or even a dying partner to whom she has pledged her love "in sickness and in health until death"? Will some women be tempted to ignore the health risks of sexual intercourse with an infected partner just as they neglect contraceptive use? If so, can this choice be justified, or is it irresponsible behavior, or perhaps is it indicative of a larger social ill—namely, that women are socialized to believe they cannot control their own sexual practices for the sake of their own health or desires?

An ethical principle for safe sex would provide justification for women to refuse unprotected sexual contact with an infected or high risk partner. An ethical principle for safe sex claims that: *Any act of sex that undermines the respect and autonomy of oneself or one's partner by endangering the health and livelihood of either or both persons treats persons as mere instruments of but not the proper ends of sexual pleasure.* Hence, to violate the ethical principle for safe sex is to choose to place one's own or one's partner's sexual pleasure above one's own or one's partner's health and well-being. Acts of violent or demeaning sex, as well as unprotected sexual contact with a person infected with or at risk for sexually transmitted diseases including AIDS, would be incompatible with this ethical principle. Similarly, it would be unethical for a woman to knowingly place herself at high risk for AIDS by heterosexual contact even though her love for her partner might be very significant.

A sexual act in violation of this Safe Sex Principle might require a woman to demonstrate her love for her partner by sacrificing her own health as a romantic symbol of commitment. Such an act would be highly exploitative, undermining the woman's integrity and her right to her own life independent of her partner's life. Admittedly, the desire for sexual contact—safe or unsafe—with an infected, at risk, or dying AIDS partner presents an extremely tragic and stressful context for an intimate relationship. Given that women are socialized to self-sacrificing behavior in our culture, the Safe Sex Principle is necessary to protect women's own interests and health. It would unnecessary and horrific if women were to place themselves knowingly at risk for AIDS out of a blind allegiance to their partners. Such a choice, amidst a growing epidemic, could come to epitomize an AIDS suttee—adapting the Indian ritual by which widows willingly were cremated on their husbands funeral pyres to the AIDS epidemic.

The Safe Sex Principle also addresses situations in which a woman feels coerced into sexual contact with an infected or at-risk partner. Such cases combine the act of rape with possible exposure to a terminal disease, posing a double threat to a woman's well-being. There may be other situations that do not qualify as rapes but involve the deliberate failure of an infected or at-risk partner to honor precautions agreed upon in advance of a sexual encounter which both partners desire. Such failure is especially serious in AIDS cases, since the negligent partner, in breaking his agreement, jeopardizes the health of his partner. Slightly less serious is the act of breaking an agreement about contraception—particularly when a pregnancy results. Once again the broken agreement has major implications for the health of the woman partner but does not pose the threat of death that AIDS might. Although it would be unfortunate if it became popular to officially contract out the conditions of sexual contact, what is needed is an increased awareness about risks and responsibilities to one's own health and the health of one's partner, particularly in the AIDS era.

How far should sexual responsibility extend? It is clearly unethical for someone to knowingly infect a sexual partner through deception about one's risk potential or status of health. For instance, the fact that a person is seropositive is no longer a private matter when one is proposing a sexual encounter that would place someone else at risk. But to what extent is the information about AIDS infection a matter of confidentiality? Consider a hypothetical example. If person A knows that person B has AIDS and is not telling sexual partner C while engaging or intending to engage in unsafe sex with C, does A have an ethical responsibility to tell C that B is infected with AIDS? Does it matter if A is B's physician, clergyperson, therapist, grocer, sister, or colleague? Does it matter if that information could have punitive or legal ramifications? In this example, the ethical need for B's sexual responsibility is in conflict with B's right to privacy. Similarly, A's duty to respect the confidentiality of B conflicts with A's duty to protect an innocent person from harm. What are the parameters of respecting information conveyed in confidence when the information is life-threatening to someone else? Clearly, it is not the responsibility of A to correct each and every untruth that B may use in his sexual relationships. Assume B tells A that he lets C believe that he loves her, although he admits he really doesn't. If A were to give C this information, it would be inappropriate, for it would violate B's right to confidentiality and C's right to make sense of her sexual relationships on her own terms. For the sake of C's autonomy and self-respect, it may be appropriate neither to encourage C in her love for B, nor to dash her hopes by divulging a truth held in confidence. However, when information is life-threatening (B is infected with AIDS), B's deception of C places her health and her life at stake without C's awareness. B's right to confidentiality is superceded by C's right to know the state of B's health since C could be infected with a fatal disease.

Particularly because AIDS is a new disease and people are either unaccustomed to or reluctant to incorporate safe sexual practices into their normal sexual behaviors, the obligation to inform someone who might be at risk for AIDS by heterosexual contact is especially crucial. Ideally, B should inform all of his sexual partners of his disease or refrain from activities that would place them at risk. Other people's knowledge of B's health status should not be a "well-kept secret" when there is good reason to believe that B is failing in his responsibility to inform his sexual partners himself. This obligation does not, however, grant people the right to inform anyone besides B's sexual partners. Some proposals to inform persons through premarital blood testing programs are based on this principle.

The obligation to inform sexual partners of people with or at risk for AIDS is most pertinent for safeguarding women from AIDS, since many women simply do not know about all their partner's sexual activities. Also, some AIDS-infected men may practice unsafe sex as a form of denial—rejecting the painful truth of being terminally ill. In any epidemic, and AIDS is no exception, fear runs rampant and along with fear comes denial. Identifying responsible actions that might protect the health of people not yet exposed to AIDS will counter this denial and circumvent the implications of self-deception on the part of the infected.

In many ways, the obligation to inform an unsuspecting sexual partner of an infected or at-risk person makes sex a public matter. Sexual freedom cannot be an absolute right when epidemics of severe sexually transmitted diseases, such as AIDS, are possible. Likewise, the right to privacy about one's sexual contacts cannot be an absolute right, since certain sexual acts may threaten the health of others. Hence public health officials should seek out the sexual contacts of AIDS-infected persons and offer testing and counseling while protecting the confidentially of all persons involved. Because AIDS is a rapidly spreading disease, it is important that possible exposure to AIDS exposure by sexual contact not be completely reliant on the "honor system." However, at the same time, there are justifiable fears that such measures could stigmatize infected men and women in ways that might threaten their professional and private lives. That is why it is imperative that public health policy vigorously promote the rights of persons with AIDS while also ensuring confidentiality in identifying sexual contacts.

Some might argue that the right to privacy in sexual behavior supercedes all other concerns, for it safeguards the freedom of persons to live as they wish. This position opposes state intervention, even in matters of health, and holds each individual completely responsible for his or her own health and for learning about any new health risks. Yet, our society does not really encourage such individual responsibility nor do we have in place the necessary resources that would make self-education possible. The argument assumes that individual freedom, without state intervention in sexual behavior, is more important than the prevention of deaths of people unaware of their exposure to AIDS. In short, it implies that it is better to die free than live with state intervention. Without private education facilities widely available, such a position undervalues the health of persons most vulnerable to AIDS exposure, and is therefore unjustifiable.

An argument may be made that the attempt to diligently inform women who are at risk through heterosexual contact is futile since it has not been established precisely what precautions offer enough protection, nor what the relationship is between being infected and being infectious. In addition, some might fear that assiduous efforts to inform women who are at risk would promote greater sexual panic, perhaps leading to quarantine, and further stigmatization of people with AIDS. These concerns must be addressed in any prevention education campaign. Yet, since certain precautions are indeed possible to reduce the risk of AIDS exposure in sexual contact, this alone merits the identification of sexual partners at risk. Further, there is a larger social end involved—namely, the containment of the AIDS virus.

Although the sexual contact discussion has focused on heterosexual women, lesbians, too, can acquire AIDS through sexual contact, though the risk is much smaller. Some of the 7% of U.S. AIDS cases that are women are lesbians who acquired the AIDS infection through IV drug use, blood tranfusions. or prior heterosexual contact. Although no cases of lesbian sexual transmission have been reported in the United States, it is completely feasible that a woman infectious with the AIDS virus could transmit the virus to her female partner by sexual acts that involve blood-to-blood or vaginal secretions-to-blood contact. As the cases of AIDS in women increase, it is likely that lesbian sexual contact cases will appear, which could constitute a new AIDS risk group. Hence, lesbians, who are not accustomed to deliberating about contraceptive or other precautions before engaging in sex, need to take safe sex seriously by endorsing the Safe Sex Principle so that their health and the health of their partners may be preserved.

Can a sexual ethics in the AIDS epidemic stop short of a sexual moratorium? In cases of AIDS transmission by heterosexual contact would a sexual moratorium be perhaps the "safest" possibility for women with infected partners? It has indeed been suggested that sexual contact with anyone who is at risk or who is infectious should be avoided. However, since it is not known how long an infected person might be infectious, and since more and more people are developing the virus, such a suggestion might bring about the undesirable classification of people into two groups: the infected, sexually active, and the infected, sexually forbidden. This could encourage a desexualization of persons with AIDS, denying these persons one of the most essential expressions of human life.

A more humane response might be to revise the notion of sexual responsibility to include concern for protecting one's own health and the health of one's partner, and to broaden forms of sexual expression so that the most "exciting" sexual acts are not also acts that put one at high risk for AIDS. Sexual activity ought to be in part, a celebration of one's existence, not an endangering of one's health. The right to sexual expressions, assuming they are not health-endangering or exploitive, is a human right and especially necessary in times of epidemic where life seems frail and death pervasive. More than simply limiting current sexual practices to safe sex requirements, we need to discover new sexual practices that can serve as passionate forms of intimacy without the risk of developing AIDS.

AIDS AND PROSTITUTION

A woman's chances of exposure to AIDS are greatly increased by prostitution since prostitution requires frequent sexual encounters with multiple partners.[19] Prostitutes have been considered "reservoirs" for AIDS infection by some AIDS researchers.[20,21] This image of prostitutes as "AIDS reservoirs" suggests that women's bodies are infectious pools of AIDS viruses, storing large quantities of infected liquids, and the source of disease for many. It also implies that men are unsuspecting transmitters of sexual diseases, moving infection from one woman (a prostitute) to another (female sexual partner). The sex bias in this metaphor is apparent. Women are not the orginating cause of sexually trans-mitted diseases. In the case of AIDS, prostitutes may be an infected pool but not necessarily an infectious pool of disease. As many as 40% of prostitutes in some U.S. cities are infected with the AIDS virus,[22] with high rates among prostitutes abroad as well (in Nairobi,[23] Greece,[24] Rwanda,[25] Zaire,[26] Brussels[27]).

It is perhaps idealistic to argue for safe sex measures in prostitution in the United States when prostitution is for the most part illegal and prostitutes subject to arrest. Prostitution continues to be, as Marx stated, an explicit instance of body-enslavement, of "the worker only as working animal—as a beast reduced to the strictest bodily needs."[28] Even where prostitution is legal, such as in Nevada, bordello operators are more concerned with the amount of business a prostitute can produce than with her health. Bordello operators recommend that prostitutes be regularly tested for the AIDS antibody so their customers will be assured the prostitute is "AIDS-free." The same operators do not require screen-ing of clients for AIDS infection, mandatory condom use, nor do they prohibit unsafe sex acts. Some are quick to insist that an infected or seropositive woman be barred from her job without any financial provision for medical care or other needs. The complete expendability of a prostitute's health is made most apparent in the AIDS epidemic where little effort is made to safeguard prostitutes from AIDS.

Given that few economic alternatives exist for women in prostitution, and that prostitution is related to deeper social issues concerning the marketing of sexuality and female bodies, it is difficult to accept the view held by some that prostitutes deserve the diseases they get. It is just as unethical to expose a prostitute to AIDS as it is to expose any person. Simply because the prostitute receives payment for sexual acts does not mean that she warrants less respect or human concern than a person who does not demand payment. Of course, the act of procuring a prostitute is already an act of sexual exploitation and is unethical. The inhumane nature of prostitution suggests that there may be some forms of labor that are neither necessary to society nor consistent with the preservation of human dignity. It might be argued that legalizing prostitution would ensure better health care for prostitutes as well as encourage AIDS pre-vention measures. Yet, legalization of prostitution would also imply a social endorsement of this form of labor. The most effective approach to ending pros-titution would be to institute viable economic alternatives, including job training for the (former) prostitutes and for women who might otherwise resort to pros-titution. At the same time, it is necessary to educate both prostitutes and their customers about safe sex practices.

AIDS AND PREGNANT WOMEN

The problems with women with AIDS sometimes affect not only themselves but also their fetuses. AIDS infection in pregnancy decreases the chances for a healthy infant, and increases the likelihood of the mother developing AIDS symptoms. About two-thirds of the pregnancies of AIDS-infected women result in infected infants, and half of those infants will be affected with the disease within two years.[29] It is possible for the AIDS infection in the fetus to be greater than the level of AIDS infection in the mother. It is not only women with AIDS that give birth to infants with AIDS, but also women with ARC,[30] and even asymptomatic carriers.[31] AIDS in pregnancy in not only detrimental to the fetus, but there is reason to believe that seropositive and ARC women's chances of developing AIDS are increased by the state of being pregnant. Pregnancy seems to accelerate the development of AIDS in seropositive women,[32] and a second pregnancy is even more likely to provoke the presentation of AIDS in seropositive women.[33]

Pregnancy by artificial insemination (AI) can also be a risk for women if the semen donor is infected. Four women have been infected this way.[34] Although little attention is given to births by AI, there are over 10,000 per year in the United States. Hence a large number of women could be at risk for AIDS by AI. Protective measures are needed which would require the systematic screening of all semen donors similar to screening of blood donors.

A key ethical question that arises concerning pregnancies in women with AIDS concerns the right to be pregnant. Does a woman who is seropositive, or has ARC or AIDS have the moral right to choose to be pregnant? Does she have the right to maintain a pregnancy once her disease is diagnosed? Is the right to begin and sustain pregnancy part of women's right to control their bodies, or it the right to pregnancy contingent in part on whether or not it harms the health of the mother and/or the infant? One researcher suggests automatic HIV screening on all antenatal women, irrespective of their consent to such testing.[35] Another suggests that serological testing for AIDS virus antibody prior to issuing marriage licenses.[36] Testing for marriage licenses would give people information concerning the antibody status of their partners only at the time of marriage. However, should marriage licenses be refused to those who test positive on the grounds that refusal would be an effective prohibition against AIDS pregnancies, particularly when it is estimated that there may be as many as 3000 infants and children with AIDS in the United States by 1991? Clearly a measure prohibiting marriage licences for seropositive individuals would be invasive, especially since not all people marry in order to have children. But if this measure is rejected because it violates the basic human freedom to wed independent of procreation, does a woman have the right to begin pregnancy if she knows her husband is seropositive?

Given that the odds are against a healthy pregnancy, and that pregnancy poses a threat to accelerating AIDS infection in the mother, several researchers have recommended abortion of all pregnancies among infected women for health reasons alone, and advised against infected women beginning pregnancy.[37–39] There may be moral grounds as well to prohibit pregnancy when, most likely, the fetus will have a severely damaged immune system and will die within the first two years of life. Given the severity of AIDS, the fact that mothers themselves often die prior to the deaths of their diseased infants, and given the further risk to women's health that pregnancy presents, one might justifiably abort a fetus if one is infected with AIDS provided one believes that every woman has a responsibility, first, to her own health, and secondly, to the health of the fetus, and that the abortion protects the health of the mother and spares the infant AIDS by terminating the fetus. Abortion in this case would not only be consistent with a woman's right to control her body, but would be ethical on the additional grounds of protecting a woman's autonomy through preserving her health and sparing a fetus needless pain and suffering.

Conservatives might argue that every fetus, even a fetus with AIDS, has a right to life, and presumably, a right to an AIDS death. Liberals cite the tremendous drain on medical resources that AIDS infants present, particularly as the numbers increase, and hence, liberals may find abortion of fetuses in AIDS-infected pregnancies warranted. It might be argued that advising against pregnancy and promoting abortion in AIDS-infected pregnancies is a racist tactic since many of the AIDS mothers are women of color. Yet, the appropriate way to address any such racist implications is not to insist that black or brown women with AIDS any more than white women with AIDS terminate their pregnancies, but rather to insist that there be equal access to medical and economic resources for blacks and other minorities.

Perhaps the strongest objection to mandatory abortion measures and advising against pregnancy in cases where women are infected with AIDS is that such measures are a step toward mandatory abortion practices for a wide range of "defective" fetuses: is the fear of a widespread eugenics program. However, there is a major difference in recommending abortion in AIDS pregnancies and recommending abortion for other diseases such as cerebral palsy, or Downs Syndrome—namely, that in AIDS pregnancies the mother herself is already infected with the virus and needs to take every precaution to protect herself from further development of AIDS. Mothers with AIDS might spend their own remaining months of life sustaining a pregnancy that may very well produce an infected infant. One of the dilemmas facing the pregnant woman is the uncertainty of whether the fetus is or is not infected. This is not to say that abortion for pregnancies in which the fetus but not the mother is infected with severe disease would not be morally permissible. It is merely to make the claim that the two situations are quite distinct. Moreover, there may be additional reasons for justifying abortion in AIDS- infected pregnancies including the right not be pregnant if one doesn't choose to be, as well as the right to end a pregnancy because of the psychological stress involved. The constant awareness of a possibly terminally ill fetus in the womb might be a difficult reality to face, especially for a woman who is herself infected. The awareness that the disease might be taking over her body and that her body could be the vehicle by which AIDS is carried into the next generation might be unbearable as well.

The above grounds may justify abortion when a woman has AIDS or ARC, is seropositive, or even is merely exposed to AIDS. But does a woman have ethical grounds, on the other hand, to *maintain* a pregnancy if she is infected with the AIDS virus? The refusal of abortion by infected women could be seen not as a "right" but rather as an act of cruelty for it could result in the suffering of another human entity. What end is being served by bringing an infant into existence that most likely will live in continual pain and suffering? A woman may choose to sustain her pregnancy in hopes that she might still produce offspring, which might give her life meaning. For example, perhaps the woman is asymptomatic and her husband is dying of AIDS. This pregnancy would be their last chance to have a child together, a tangible way for a part of him to live on. A pregnant woman with AIDS might choose to sustain pregnancy as an act of giving life when her own impending death is crowding life out of her.

However understandable these reasons may be, an ethical justification for sustaining pregnancy when it could result in injury and harm to a new human entity must carefully weigh both the mother's right to reproduce and the possibility of an infant born into suffering, disease, and most likely iminent death. In choosing to continue pregnancy, an infected woman is also choosing to further endanger her own health in order to give birth to an infant who might or might not be free of the AIDS virus. She is not choosing to consciously inflict pain and suffering. But, it is very possible that the infant will be born severly infected, and with no legal precedent of infanticide or active euthanasia, the infant would be destined to suffer for as much as two years. This is not to say that choosing to play the odds and go against current medical advice, despite the risk of a negative outcome for herself and her infant, could never be morally justified. But rather, an infected woman should carefully determine if there are any responsibilities she has first to her own body-in-disease.

Clearly everyone owes this to themselves: a meaningful life, and a meaningful death. But how one achieves both amidst a state of bodily infection with perhaps terminal illness must be left to the individual. If an infected woman decides to maintain her pregnancy while fully understanding that it might cause her seropositivity to begin to manifest itself with AIDS symptoms and shortly bring about her death by AIDS, a death that might otherwise not have occurred, she is entitled to respect as a moral decision maker. Conversely, if a woman chooses abortion to avoid becoming an AIDS casualty herself and to avoid giving birth to an infant with AIDS she should not be judged harshly for not self-sacrificing. To seek to enjoy life ever more intensely as AIDS threatens a premature death is also a valid choice—one which is particularly within the moral rights of infected people.

WOMEN AND THE FUTURE OF AIDS

The effects of AIDS on drug use, sexual activity, and pregnancy are the central but not the only implications of AIDS for women. Women will also suffer sex discrimination in access to medical resources and may even suffer a higher rate of incorrect diagnosis.[40] Moreover, given the economic disparity between men and women and the radical biases of our society, women with AIDS will most likely have less access to information and services relevant to their specific needs.

The gender bias of our notion of "public health" needs to be eradicated and the AIDS epidemic could provide the impetus. Public health policy needs to effect the following changes to protect women from AIDS: a broad-based education program on intravenous drug use and drug rehabilitation, including counseling and sterile needle exchange services; the dissemination of safe sex information, an outreach program for testing and counseling prostitutes with a task force for creating alternative income options for them; counseling and medical services for women considering pregnancy or who are already pregnant; free access to abortion for all women; assistance programs for seropositive women who are unemployed; medical insurance for infected women; child care facilities and mother-assistance services for infected women; visitation rights for infected women who may have placed their children in foster care; the adaption of hospice programs to accommodate women with facilities that would enable them to be connected with their children as much as possible if they so choose.

Meanwhile, more of the over 100,000 seropositive women in this country will go on to manifest ARC or AIDS symptoms. More and more relationships, including lesbian or bisexual relationships, will include a seropositive partner and require special care in maintaining the health of each of the partners. There will be more AIDS pregnancies, and more infected infants as well. The hope of a vaccine for AIDS remains a dream. The grim reality of the epidemic is depicted with projections of more than 18,000 women with AIDS in the United States within five years. By 1991, the number of women with AIDS will nearly equal the number of men who have currently been diagnosed with AIDS. It is crucial that the awareness of AIDS and precautions against AIDS be taken seriously now for much can be done. By 1991, AIDS will no longer be some strange virus out of nowhere.. Neither pleas of ignorance nor lack of action will ease the burden of the rising AIDS count. Short of a cure for AIDS, our strongest weapons are education and public policies that seek to preserve the health of all in the community—including women—and compassion in our responses to the epidemic.

We are just now beginning to confront the bleak realities of women dying of AIDS—the multitude of worries they may have about their fate; the children they leave behind; their loss of sexual partners and friends; the anger they may feel toward a sexual partner who may have infected them; the shock and frustration of being pregnant while being gravely ill; the grief at perhaps ending a pregnancy they might have otherwise wanted. Although every death from AIDS is a particularly sad death, women's deaths from AIDS have tragic qualities all their own. Women with AIDS are, in many ways, a spin-off effect of the larger epidemic which has affected predominantly men (93%). Women with AIDS present a new social and ethical dilemma at the intersection of issues regarding sex, fertility, reproductive rights, and economics.

We cannot hope to improve the situations of women with AIDS without openly addressing these issues and thereby formulating policy which will improve the conditions of women in general, and in particular poor women and women of color. We might do well to prepare for these policy discussions by calculating projections for the spread of AIDS in women and to use this devastating information as a motivating force for development of the resources necessary to meet the challenge of AIDS in women.

I thank Alison Deming for her many helpful comments on this paper and John Corcoran for his research and computer assistance.

NOTES

1. All statistics unless otherwise indicated are from the *AIDS Weekly Surveillance Report, Jan. 26, 1987*, Centers for Disease Control, and refer to U.S. AIDS cases only.

2. Projected estimate assumes that 7% of the 270,000 projected U.S. AIDS cases in 1991 will be women.

3. Estimates assume that at least 7% of the estimated 1.5 million seropositive cases of the estimated 200,000 ARC cases are women.

4. World Health Organization, Geneva, Weekly Epidemiological Record. "AIDS: Report on the Situation in Europe." 60:305–312(1985).

5. See Cohen, Judith B.; Hauer, Laurie B.; Cracchiolo, Bernadette, et al., "A.W.A.R.E. A Community Study of AIDS Antibody Prevalence among High Risk Women in San Francisco." Paper delivered at the Annual Meeting of American Public Health Association, Washington, D.C., November 17–21, 1985.

6. CDC *AIDS Weekly Surveillance Report*. op. cit.

7. Ibid.

8. "Jersey 'Willing' to Give Addicts Clean Needles." *The New York Times*, July 24, 1986. See also Burning, E. C., et al., "Preventing AIDS in Drug Addicts in Amsterdam." *Lancet* I(8495):1435(June 21, 1986).

9. Ibid.

10. Polk, F. B. "Female-to-Male Transmission of AIDS" (Letter). *JAMA* 254(22):3177–3178 (December 13, 1985).

11. Haverkos, J. W., and Edelman, R. "Female-to-Male Transmission of AIDS" (Letter). *JAMA* 254(8)1035–1036 (August 23, 1985).

12. Schultz, S.; Milberg, J. A.; Kirstal, A. R.; Stoneburner, R. L. "Female-to-Male Transmission of HTLV-III" (Letter). *JAMA* 255(13):1703–1740 (April 4, 1986).

13. Wykoff, R. F. "Female-to-Male Transmission of HTLV-III" (Letter). *JAMA* 255(13):1703–1705.

14. Redfield, R. R.; Markham, P. D.; Salahuddin, S. E., et al. "Heterosexually Acquired HTLV-III/LAV Disease (AIDS-Related Complex and AIDS): Epidemiologic Evidence for Female-to-Male Transmission." *JAMA* 254(15):2094–2096 (Oct. 18, 1985). See also Redfield, R. R.; Wright, D. C.; Markham, P. D. "Female-to-Male Transmission of HTLV-III" (Letter). *JAMA* 255(13):1705–1706.

15. Vogt, M. W.; Craven, D. E.; Crawford, D. F., et al. "Isolation of HTLV-III/LAV from Cervical Secretions of Women at Risk for AIDS." *Lancet* I(8480):525–527(March 8, 1986).

16. Wofsky, C.B.; Hauer, L. B.; Michaelis, B. A., et al. "Isolation of AIDS-Associated Retrovirus from Genital Secretions of Women with Antibodies to the Virus." *Lancet* I(8480):527–529 (March 8, 1986).

17. Harris, C.; Small, C. B.; Klein, R. S.; Griedland, G. H., et al. "Immunodeficiency in Female Sexual Partners of Men with the Acquired Immunodeficiency Syndrome." *New England Journal of Medicine* 308:1181–1184 (1983).

18. Ragni, J. V.; Rinaldo, C. R.; Kingsley, L., et al. "Heterosexual Partners of Haemophiliacs Must Refrain From Blood Donations." *Lancet* I(8488):1033 (May 3, 1986). See also Jason, J. M.; McDougal, J. S.; Dixon, G., et al. "HTLV-III/LAV Antibody and Immune Status of Household Contacts and Sexual Partners of Persons with Hemophilia." *JAMA* 255(2):212–215 (Jan. 10, 1986).

19. Polk, F. B. "Female-to-Male Transmission of AIDS" (Letter).

20. D'Costa, L. L.; Plummer, F. A.; Bowmer, I., et al. "Prostitutes are a Major Reservoir of Sexually Transmitted Disease in Nairobi, Kenya." *Sexually Transmitted Diseases* 12:64–67 (1985).

21. Redfield, R. R.; Markham, P. D.; Salahuddin, S. Z., et al. "Heterosexually Acquired HTLV-III/LAV Disease (AIDS-Related Complex and AIDS).

22. Vogt, M. W..; Craven, D. E.; Crawford, D. F.; Hirsch, M. S., et al. "Isolation of HTLV-III/LAV from Cervical Secretions of Women at Risk for AIDS.

23. Kreiss, J. K.; Koech, D.; Plummer, F. A.; Holmes, K. K.; Lightfoote, M.; Piot, P., et al. "AIDS Virus Infection in Nairobi Prostitutes," *New England Journal of Medicine* :414–418 (Feb. 13, 1986).

24. Papaevangelou, G.; Roumeliotou-Karayannis, A.; Kallinikos, G.; Papoutsakis, B. "LAV/HTLV-III Infection in Female Prostitutes." *Lancet* II:(8462):1018–1019 (Nov. 2, 1985).

25. Van DePerre, P.; Carael, M.; Robert-Guroff, M.; Freyens, P.; Gallo, R. C., et al. "Female Prostitutes: A Risk Group for Infection with Human T-Cell Lymphotrophic Virus Type III" *Lancet* II(8454):524–52(Sept. 7, 1985).

26. Piot, P.; Quinn, T. C.; Taelman, H., et al. "Acquired Immunodeficiency in a Heterosexual Population in Zaire." *Lancet* II(8394):65–69 (1984).

27. Clumeck, N.; Carael, M.; Rouvroy, D.; Nzaramba, D. "Heterosexual Promiscuity Among African Patients with AIDS." *New England Journal of Medicine* 313(3):182 (July 18, 1985).

28. Marx, Karl. *The Economic and Philosophic Manuscripts of 1844.* International Publishers, 1964, 74.

29. Pinching, Anthony, J. and Jefferies, Donald J. "AIDS and HTLV-III/LAV Infection. Consequences for Obstetrics and Perinatal Medicine." *British Journal of Obstetrics and Gynecology* 92:1211–1217 (1985).

30. Rubinstein, A.; Sicklick, M.; Gupta, A., et al. "Acquired Immunodeficiency with Reversed T4/T8 Rations in Infants Born to Promiscuous and Drug-Addicted Mothers. *JAMA* 249:2350–2356 (1983).

31. Joshi, W.; Path, M. R. C.; Oleske, J. M.; Minnefor, A. B., et al. "Pathology of Suspected AIDS in Children: A Study of Eight Cases." *Pediatric Pathology* 2:71–87 (1984).

32. Gilmer, E.; Fischer, A.; Griscelli, C., et al. "Possible Transmission of a Human Lymphotropic Retrovirus (LAV) from Mother to Infant with AIDS." *Lancet* 1:229–230.

33. Pinching, op cit.

34. Stewart, G. J.; Cunningham, A. L.; Driscoll, G. L.; Tyler, J. P. P., et al. "Transmission of Human T-Cell Lymphotropic Virus Type III (HTLV-III) by Artificial Insemination by Donor." *Lancet* II(8455):581–584 (Sept. 14, 1985).

35. Entwistle, C. C. "Prevention of AIDS." *Lancet*:1364 (Dec. 14, 1985).

36. Lundberg, George D. "The Age of AIDS: A Great Time for Defensive Living" (Editorial). *JAMA* 253(23):3440–3441 (June 21, 1985).

37. Pinching, op cit.

38. Ancelle, P.; Asaad, F.; Borgucci, P. V., et al. *Bulletin of the World Health Organization* 63(4):667–672 (1985).

39. Luzi, G.; Ensoli, B.; Turbessi, G., et al. "Transmission of HTLV-III Infection by Heterosexual Contact." *Lancet* II(8462):1018 (Nov. 2, 1985).

40. Masur, H.; Michelis, M. A.; Wromser, G. P.. et al. "Opportunistic Infection in Previously Healthy Women: Initial Manifestations of a Community Acquired Cellular Immunodeficiency." *Annals Internal Medicine* 97:533–539 (1982).

29

An Ethics of Compassion, A Language of Division: Working Out the AIDS Metaphors

Judith Wilson Ross

THE AIDS METAPHORS

Each new issue in medical ethics produces a near avalanche of journal articles, newspaper editorials, and television appearances by medical ethics specialists, replete with detailed arguments about the right and wrong way to think as well as to act. This hasn't happened with AIDS. There has been much scientific writing and considerable editorial page pontificating, but, until very recently, not much serious ethical analysis, especially from the bioethics community.[1] This reluctance suggests the thorny nature of the ethical problems related to AIDS, particularly those concerning justice and fairness.

What have been proposed, however, are punitive and hostile actions where all the burdens would be borne by one group of people and all the benefits accrue to another group. William F. Buckley's proposal to tattoo all people with AIDS as well as all asymptomatic individuals infected with the human immunodeficiency virus (HIV)[2] is but one example of this kind of thinking.[3] Public opinion polls have reported that a majority of respondents believe that quarantine—even if lifelong—is appropriate for those who have been infected with HIV.[4] This, too, exemplifies an acceptance of actions that are neither just nor fair. The extremity of these proposals—given what is known about the disease and its means of transmission—suggests that the general attitude about AIDS is irrational and not based on ordinary concerns with right and wrong.

Most people receive their information about this disease from the popular literature—TV, newspapers, and the general-circulation weekly and monthly magazines—not from academic journals, CDC (Centers for Disease Control) reports, physicians with practical experience, AIDS education groups, or the AIDS research community. The academic and policy-making communities are both publicly silent about the ethical implications of various actions. Only gay community representatives have consistently addressed ethical issues, but these writers are often seen to be acting solely from self-interest. For the most part, the popular media are setting the terms by which the public perceives this disease.

One need not look at popular media, however, to realize that much of what is increasingly being termed "the AIDS hysteria" is born of fear. Originally, the fear was produced in part from the fact that large numbers of people were dying from an infectious disease that medical science was so powerless to halt. Each year more people die from other diseases than from AIDS. Fifty-four thousand people die in automobile accidents annually—a risk everyone takes each time he or she climbs into a car—but no hysteria drives a public demand for safer cars or lower speed limits. The hysteria generated by AIDS is not just a fear of death. It is also a fear of the unknown.

AIDS is a new disease, at first inexplicable and thus strange. The immediately suggested parallels are historic ones (bubonic plague, influenza epidemics, leprosy). There is no place in our personal memories for these diseases (not, at least, for most Americans under the age of 70) and these historical realities leave little mark beyond linguistic relics ("I'd avoid him like he had leprosy" or "I'd avoid it like the plague"). As a result, AIDS presents itself to this culture as a new phenomenon, not just another difficult disease in a long line of difficult diseases.[5] Its newness means that we have to find a way to conceptualize it. Like the Cargo Cult people who had to create a narrative to explain the existence of World War II planes that dropped industrial world goods into a primitive culture, we need to create a story that explains AIDS to us.[6]

The narrative of a new event is not developed consciously, but coalesces over time as connections (whether accurate or not) are made between known phenomena and the new incident. With AIDS, parallels were promptly drawn in journalistic coverage to plague and leprosy. Beyond this, however, writers frequently adopted a metaphorical style of writing that showed the AIDS phenomenon as part of a more familiar story: AIDS as death, AIDS as punishment for sin, AIDS as crime, AIDS as an enemy occasioning a war, and AIDS as otherness (i.e., a means of dividing the world into two entirely separate segments). Some writers used a single metaphor, others used several, even within one article. The metaphors were common enough and frequent enough to create a single narrative in which AIDS is both a crime against others, a crime deserving punishment, and also a punishment, by death, for those who have divided the civic unity by violating social rules. As Lakoff and Johnson have pointed out, "language is an important source of evidence for what [our conceptual] system is like."[7] In the case of AIDS, these metaphors tell us a great deal about how AIDS fits into our world picture. Within the metaphors lies a fuller justification for many of the actions and policies that have been reported or proposed.[8]

When Susan Sontag analyzed social attitudes toward tuberculosis and cancer in *Illness as Metaphor*, she claimed that discovering the cause of tuberculosis had stripped the disease of its metaphoric existence, with the implication that cancer, too, would lose its metaphors if we understood it better as a physiological phenomenon.[9] This implication has not been borne out for AIDS. Despite the remarkably rapid discovery of the viral etiology and modes of transmission, the metaphors of AIDS have persisted, suggesting an extremely powerful underlying narrative that facts alone will be unlikely to dispel.

It has long been recognized that metaphor is a powerful tool of rhetoric. Metaphor is used to highlight similarities between two otherwise different objects, events, individuals, and so on. Thus, to say that AIDS is a plague or that the person with AIDS is a modern-day leper is to make a statement based on a limited number of parallels between the two. Unfortunately, the metaphor does not include an elaboration of which specific aspects of the two are the same nor how many similar aspects there are. Although the speaker and the audience may agree that AIDS is a modern-day plague, the statement probably has many different meanings to different members of the audience. To illustrate this, let us look briefly at some commonly known and salient characteristics of plague:

it is a disease with a very high death rate; death often occurs very quickly after exposure to the disease; it can spread rapidly—within weeks—throughout a population; because of its contagiousness through casual contact, those with the disease should be avoided; it has existed throughout recorded history, appearing and then disappearing without any explanation for its sudden outbreaks; those with the disease along with their families have been locked up in houses (quarantine and isolation); and its transmission includes insect and animal vectors (rodents, fleas). When the speaker says that AIDS is a modern-day plague, which (if any) of these characteristics does he have in mind? Strictly speaking none is necessarily accurate; the death rate from HIV infection (which is the disease) is high (20–30%, perhaps), but not uniformly fatal, as is often claimed and as pneumonic plague is still likely to be. Death, if it occurs at all, does not occur rapidly. Those with full-blown AIDS live about one to two years after diagnosis.[10] It does not spread very rapidly within a population because it is not spread by casual contact as is plague. Thus, there is no reason to avoid ordinary contact with those who have the infection nor to lock them away in quarantine or isolation. It is apparently a brand new virus and does not appear to involve animal or insect vectors.

When metaphor is used in this unadorned fashion (i.e., without any further clarification as to which aspects of the metaphor source are being isolated and asserted as parallels), the audience is invited to "fill in the blanks," as it were, making as many parallels as seem useful to their personal psychology without concern for factual accuracy. Herein lies the great danger of the metaphor: used casually, as it almost always is, it easily becomes (or, more accurately, is perceived to be) an analogue or a model. The plague, as a metaphor for AIDS, suggests that the two diseases have one or more important things in common. When plague becomes an analogue for AIDS, it is seen as having many, even most characteristics in common. When it is perceived as a model, it is perceived as sharing all relevant features.

AIDS shares a very few important characteristics with the plague or with leprosy, yet both are used so commonly as metaphors and as implicit analogies that it is difficult to recall their many differences. The characteristic that unites the three most strongly is the fear people have of all of them, but the truth of that commonality lies more in human psychology than in the essential nature of the diseases.

When more complex metaphors are used to characterize AIDS, the possibility of more far-reaching misstatements about the disease arises. Thus, although identifying AIDS with plague or leprosy permits a limited number of erroneous implications about the nature of the disease, a metaphor like death, sin, or crime is much more pervasive and much more dangerous.

The metaphor of AIDS as personified death is evoked by those who say they "lost" friends or lovers to AIDS, by those with the disease who ask, "Why did it get me?," by writers who characterize the disease as "striking entire families." This metaphor shows AIDS as a powerful and independent figure choosing its victims. AIDS as death includes a sense of immediateness. As a matter of fact, many people with AIDS live for months and even years, for the most part outside the hospital. Those who are infected by the virus may never be ill or may develop chronic illness that is not fatal. Yet to have AIDS or to have the AIDS virus is equally to be claimed by death within this metaphor. The metaphor of AIDS as death permits us to dismiss all of those who have been infected by HIV, whether they have AIDS, ARC, or are asymptomatic presumed carriers; they are dead to us. When this metaphor is filled out, it tells us that we need not worry about the feelings of those with AIDS or HIV when deciding how to act toward them because they are effectively, if not actually, dead.

The metaphor of AIDS as death contributes to and coexists happily with the metaphor of AIDS as punishment for sin. When Death comes to look for victims, it must have some principle of choice. We are uncomfortable with death as a random event. Those whom death has chosen to visit (or their families, or even perfect strangers) may ask "Why was I (or he/she) chosen? What have I (or he/she) done to deserve this?" The personified death that chooses its victims is seen within this metaphor/narrative as a punisher. The punishment is Death's choice itself: death is the punishment for sin. Those who are chosen look to see what sin they have committed that justifies this selection; those who have not been chosen look to see what they have *not* done in order to understand why they have been spared. The metaphor does not permit a description of death from disease as an individual-neutral event. It does not encompass the notion that a virus will flourish if it finds itself in conditions that permit it to do so. HIV does not flourish because it finds itself in homosexual relationships, in multiple sexual partnerships, in IV drug users, or in illegal activities. It is simply a virus doing its job. Because it is a virus doing its job, anyone who comes into contact with the virus may find him/herself suffering the effects of the virus's "job."

As Susan Sontag noted in *Illness as Metaphor*, metaphor permits and even encourages giving "disease a meaning—that meaning being invariably a moral one."[11] The metaphor of sin says that those who are infected have the virus *because* they were engaged in specific activities of which many people do not approve. They are, thus, "responsible" for their disease: they "deserve" it. The disease is *their* problem, not the problem of those who do not take part in the disapproved behavior (be it drug use, homosexual acts, or "promiscuous sex," whatever that may mean to the disapproving individual). In addition, the AIDS story created by Death as Punishment for Sin means not only that those who have the virus deserve their fate but also that those who have not engaged in the disapproved behavior are safe from the disease. Death does not visit the righteous. Hence this narrative achieves a double purpose for those who are not infected: they may safely abjure responsibility or concern for those who are infected (because it is their own fault) and they need not worry about their own health.

AIDS as crime is presented in two ways: first, the disease itself is a crime that must be solved. This aspect of the metaphor concentrates on researchers as detectives looking for clues to solve the mystery of AIDS. The AIDS story in this metaphor takes the standard form of the detective story in which the good guys track down the bad guys to stop the continuing crime. The reality of HIV infection doesn't fit this metaphor well and leads to a confusion between whether the "bad guy" is the AIDS virus or the person who carries the virus. The infected individual becomes not only justly punished for his behavior but justly hunted down by others because of his infected status.

The second aspect of the metaphor of AIDS as crime is the disease as supercriminal, a serial murderer who embarks on intercontinental killing sprees.

This kind of criminal is so threatening that only the most extreme methods can be used to defeat it. If this disease is a crime, only something bigger, more aggressive, and more powerful than it can be expected to defeat it. Finally, it means fighting crime with crime. Although not referring to AIDS, the advertising campaign for Sylvester Stallone's 1986 movie, *Cobra*, captures the heart of this metaphor/story: "Crime is a disease and Cobra [that is to say, more crime] is the cure." When AIDS is seen as a major crime, it is easy to accept that only a bigger criminal and greater violence can defeat it. Thus, punitive and hostile actions appear to be justified and even necessary in "tracking down" and "defeating" the disease (and its carriers).

The metaphor of medicine as war is so common that we can scarcely imagine any other way of talking about how health care providers deal with diseases and patients. It is commonly said that medicine's job is to fight disease (as opposed to preventing illness). When the practice of medicine becomes war (and the phrase "the war against AIDS" is perhaps the most common metaphor used in the popular press), then the patient becomes the battlefield. When transmission of disease involves an infected carrier, especially an infected asymptomatic carrier, then the metaphor-become-analogue/model of AIDS as war makes the carrier a spy and a traitor. Traitors and spies are internal enemies for whom capital punishment is justified. The enemies are now clearly identified: the virus is the external (foreign) enemy, the carrier the internal (traitorous) enemy. Defeating or capturing one enemy also involves defeating or capturing the other one. Ordinarily we don't worry much about the civil rights of foreigners or enemies and, in time of war, there is certainly no room for such concerns.

The final AIDS metaphor, the metaphor of otherness, is perhaps less an independent metaphor than the result of the previous four: those who are dead, those who are sinners, those who are criminals, and those who are enemy-harboring traitors. These are "the others," outside the general population, as so many speakers and writers have commented.[12] The sense of otherness is demonstrated in the way in which people talk about what "we should do about them" (i.e., those who are infected by HIV). The constant use of the terms leper and leprosy in referring to HIV infection and people with AIDS continually reinforces this sense of otherness, for the leper is perhaps the most persistent and widespread instance we have of human exile. The leper is traditionally outside the human community, both physically and spiritually. He/she is truly seen as something different and "other" than us, for the life of isolation with the sole prospect of slow death has deprived the leper of relationship—that which defines the human community. By enclosing people with HIV infection firmly in the story of otherness and of leprosy, we can treat them less generously, less compassionately, and less fairly. In the same way that foreigners—a different kind of "other"—are seen as ineligible for the constitutional protections guaranteed to American citizens, those with HIV infection can be denied more basic rights derived not from law but from the requirements of human decency.

Metaphors and their encompassing analogue narratives do not merely play themselves out in journalism and dinner table conversation; they play themselves out in real life, in actions that affect other people. The stories on AIDS and HIV infection that hold our attention can influence our thinking and our actions. All five of these metaphors encourage a denial of respect for persons, the single most important principle upon which our ethical analyses are based. Whether the issue is caring for patients with AIDS and ARC, supporting seropositives who are asymptomatic, or providing HIV testing, metaphors that characterize an individual as apart, guilty, and as good as dead will encourage unethical responses; the person is not, in reality, different, guilty, or dead.

THE METAPHORS IN PRACTICE

Care of Patients with AIDS and ARC

The vast number of health care providers who work with AIDS patients have undoubtedly given the best possible care to their patients, which was especially commendable during that period when it was not clear whether the health care worker was at substantial risk of contracting the disease from the patients. Nevertheless, beginning around 1983, there have been numerous stories of failure to provide appropriate care for patients with AIDS because of their perceived difference. Hospitals have refused admission to people with AIDS or shipped them unceremoniously to other hospitals; anesthesiologists have been unwilling to administer anesthesia to them; surgeons have refused to perform lung biopsies; nursing and dietary aides have refused to enter patients' rooms; patients have been unnecessarily isolated within hospitals; nurses have refused to care for them; pathologists have refused to perform autopsies; hospital staff members have insisted upon wearing extraordinary amounts of protective equipment; internists have refused to perform endoscopies; unwritten hospital policies have denied ICU care; AIDS patients have borne the burden of cost constraints by being denied expensive care since they are expected to die anyway; dialysis has been denied for patients with both acute renal failure and chronic end stage renal disease; information about AIDS patients has been bandied about the hospital and beyond its confines as choice gossip; and, most recently, medical students have begun to shy away from internships and residencies at hospitals where there is a substantial AIDS patient census. These responses are all encouraged and even made sensible by the divisive metaphors of AIDS.

Repeated studies have demonstrated the minimal risk that patients with AIDS pose to health care workers if the providers take appropriate protective steps.[13] AIDS and ARC patients are, of course, entitled to all the care and services necessary for their illness and one can hope that as information about the minimal risk permeates the health care professions instances of inappropriate denial of treatment or provision of uncaring treatment will disappear. Staff education, however, tends to be provided at a technical level and is unlikely to alter the intense emotional holding power of the metaphor/narratives that the media have furthered. Most hospitals have had little experience with AIDS patients and thus there is no great impetus for providing any education. Furthermore, many hospitals report that when AIDS education programs are given, few attend.

Hospital ethics committees are increasingly concerned about how to deal with ethical questions surrounding treatment of patients with AIDS, ARC, or positive antibody results. It is not clear what role committees can play in addressing the issues when there are so many conflicting messages being sent. What, for example, is the ethics committee to say about the commitment to confidentiality when every employee is insisting upon knowing which patients are HIV positive and which are not? Should hospital employees be expected always to use appropriate protective measures when exposed to patient secretions and body fluids? Or must the patients submit to the release of antibody status information, regardless of how stigmatizing it may be, so that the health care workers need only use protective measures when they know they may be at risk? The metaphors that reduce the patient's entitlement to rights leave ample room for insisting that the patient take the risk of stigmatization while the health care provider accepts the benefits of increased convenience and reduced personal anxiety.

Beyond the question of risk to health care providers, however, there are a number of difficult ethical issues that education alone cannot solve. The question of how much treatment the AIDS patient should receive is not limited to medical/technical analysis. Policies—personal or institutional, written or unwritten—that deny ICU care to all AIDS patients are ethically questionable. The metaphor of AIDS as death encourages this view since, the unspoken argument goes, a patient who is as good as dead need not be treated. The President of the Society for the Right to Die, Mrs. A. J. Levinson, was recently quoted in *The New York Times* as saying that "The only good thing to come out of the AIDS epidemic is that many more doctors are thinking twice before doing everything they can to, for instance, cure pneumonia in an AIDS patient. Do these patients want to be cured of pneumonia now so that they can certainly die of AIDS next year?"[14] It would certainly seem more than possible that *even* AIDS patients might like another year of life, especially when that year will probably be spent, for the most part, outside the hospital. There is still a real possibility for what is increasingly being called "quality life." Levinson, however, appears to regard those with AIDS as already dead; the metaphors sustain her attitude.

In a similar vein, R. M. Wachter, a resident at San Francisco General Hospital, reported that AIDS patients were increasingly refusing intensive care and respirator care.[15] He believed that they were being encouraged to do so by physicians who had become seriously depressed by the prospect of so many young patients dying. As a result, housestaff were, perhaps, endorsing patient's refusal of life-prolonging treatment in order to "get it over with quickly."[16] But Wachter, unlike Levinson, sensed that there was something wrong with this, that it was not a celebration of the right to die.

In another San Francisco-based study, clinician-researchers Steinbrook, Lo, Tirpack, and associates, found that people with AIDS significantly over-estimated the effectiveness of ICU care in saving the lives of patients with Pneumocystis carinii pneumonia.[17] Yet, they too claimed that more and more patients were refusing life-sustaining care. This apparent contradiction may have a reasonable explanation—for example, those with AIDS may believe that ICU care will prolong their lives but don't want their lives extended because they believe the quality of their lives is too poor. It is also possible, however, that patients are being implicitly or explicitly discouraged from requesting or consenting to life-prolonging treatment (including treatment available in the ICU) by someone else's judgment that their quality of life is not worth maintaining or that the financial cost to the hospital is too high. Since they are as good as dead, since we owe them nothing, there is no need to prolong their lives, suggest the metaphors.

Fortunately, in California, the legislator has provided a solid mechanism by which the patient can control his medical care even when he is no longer competent. Because AIDS involves a considerable risk of central nervous system involvement and thus possible dementia and incompetence, the Durable Power of Attorney for Health Care is an important tool for the patient. In addition, because so many of the AIDS patients are gay men living in nontraditional family arrangements, it is particularly important for them to name the person whom they wish to make decisions for them. Nevertheless, Steinbrook, Lo, Noulton, and associates, found in a second study, that many physicians are not discussing this issue with their patients, even though the patients would like to discuss it.[18] Many patients have not signed durable power statements, perhaps because they do not know about them. Initiating discussion of this issue is extremely difficult, of course, and it appears that such discussion may be avoided unless conscious steps are taken. San Francisco General Hospital has a policy that requires discussing the durable power of attorney with all AIDS patients within 48 hours of their initial admission.[19] Other hospitals, however, are not as aggressive in pursuing this problem. Physicians are frequently reluctant to discuss the use of advance directives such as living wills, natural death acts, or durable powers of attorney with any patient, but this reluctance is so overwhelming with AIDS patients that there must be some deeply seated emotional pull that keeps them from doing so.

Providing or foregoing life-sustaining treatment for AIDS patients has all the ordinary difficulties involved in making such a decision with the added problems of the patient's mental competence to make decisions, and potential conflicts between the patient's family and lover or friends about what the patient would have wanted. The metaphors make it easier for families and caregivers to reject treatment. Although that may be what the patient too, would have chosen, without clear evidence we will only be guessing or imposing our own preferences. To circumvent these problems, hospitals may have to provide special training for certain employees, to ensure that advance directives are discussed with AIDS patients.

Advice to Individuals Who Are Seropositive and Asymptomatic

Asymptomatic seropositive individuals are currently presumed to be infectious (although they may not be) and this presumed infectiousness is thought to be a permanent condition. Issues of particular concern to health care workers with respect to asymptomatic seropositives include: what advice should be given to seropositive pregnant women, to seropositive women who may wish to become pregnant, and to seropositive individuals in general; what responsibilities does the physician have for protecting sexual partners of those who are seropositive; and should some kind of restrictions be applied to seropositive health care providers?

The problem of pregnant seropositive women is not entirely new as there are substantial parallels in genetically transmitted diseases. The infant of a pregnant seropositive woman will not inevitably have AIDS. Assuming that abortion is an ethically acceptable choice, standard ethical analysis would not maintain that abortion was obligatory or even necessarily appropriate since there is some possibility that the abortion will be performed on a fetus that does not and will not have the virus or ensuing disease.[20] Nevertheless, many public health officers and physicians have suggested that seropositive women should not become pregnant, implying that *they* perceive the risk of the child's contracting AIDS too great to be taken.[21] It would logically follow, then, that abortion would be the appropriate response to pregnancy in these circumstances, and a San Francisco Health Commission Task Force (chaired by pediatrician Moses Grossman) recommended "encouraging abortion for newly pregnant women infected by the AIDS virus."[22] Influenced as we all are by the images the metaphors encourage, it may be difficult to be neutral. We may agree that no one should risk giving birth to a child with AIDS, for it would be like giving birth to a nonhuman. Health care providers may make recommendations against pregnancy and for abortion and sterilization rather than provide information that would allow women to weigh the risks and benefits and to make their own, informed choices.

The physician's responsibility for protecting third parties—especially sexual partners of seropositive individuals—is a very thorny issue. The legal parallel is the *Tarasoff* duty to take appropriate steps to protect known, threatened third parties from dangerous patients in pyschotherapy. If a physician knows that a seropositive patient is not informing his/her sexual contacts of the risk, does the physician have a duty to inform that person(s)? Several writers maintain that there is such a duty but suggest that the duty may be met by informing public health authorities.[23] However, if it is generally known that the public health authorities are not conducting contact-tracing, does that end the physician's duty? This issue is going to become increasingly troublesome, but the AIDS metaphors will advise always acting to protect others—the third parties. That is because, within the metaphors, the patient with HIV does not merit consideration; his/her responses, needs, and concerns are not relevant, given the underlying fault/guilt and the need to stop the disease/crime.

The Public Health Service has issued recommendations for counseling individuals who are asymptomatic but seropositive.[24] They include informing past and future sexual partners of seropositive status, informing medical and dental workers of seropositivity, refraining from donating blood, and using "safe sex" practices.[25] There is relatively little disagreement about these recommendations but it may be unrealistic to expect people who are already deeply distressed by their seropositive status to respond affirmatively to these guidelines. Paul Volberding, one of the most experienced clinicians in the country with respect to AIDS, has said that informing a patient that he or she is seropositive is as anxiety-provoking as telling him/her that he/she has AIDS.[26] Given the enormous impact of this information, how will the individual respond to the advice that is given? Telling others of seropositive status—whether professionals, acquaintances, friends, family members, or lovers—risks extraordinary ostracization. Furthermore, the news will almost inevitably be circulated to yet a broader group people. One may expect confidentiality to be honored within the medical field (even if practice does not meet expectations), but no such expectation exists in the social environment. Very little is known about how to provide these recommendations in a way that will encourage and support compliance. Not much attention has been paid to the inevitable psychological denial that will accompany the receipt of such devastating news. There is, somehow, the assumption that "they" will behave as "we" want them to, even though "we" do not think too much about what sacrifices and burdens that behavior entails.

Seropositive health care workers are not usually seen to pose a particular threat to patients because the primary modes of transmission are sexual intercourse and blood exchange. However, some writers have argued that seropositive health care providers should not be permitted to conduct invasive procedures if there is *any* risk of blood contamination. Health care providers' desire to know about patients' positive antibody status is mirrored by the less-discussed issue of whether patients have a right to know about the positive antibody status of their physician, nurse, or technician. As to the former, there are several pieces of legislation that have recently been introduced in California that would allow all those directly involved in the patient's care to have access to antibody status information. As to the latter, patients will probably not be able legally to have access to information about their health care providers. Nevertheless, the ethical dimension of this question remains and one could surely speculate about whether the metaphors of AIDS, focused as they now are around IV drug users and gay men, will spill over to health care workers who are seropositive, even if they are not members of high risk groups. Recent reports of an unusual delay by the CDC in issuing guidelines about health care providers who are antibody positive and their obligations to their patients suggest that this may already be happening.[27]

Providing HIV Testing

When the HIV antibody test was introduced in March 1985, there were widespread announcements that the function of the test was to screen blood, not persons. However, the test is being increasingly used or recommended for screening people. Currently, the following groups of people are being screened: all members of the military, all military applicants, U.S. military academy students, all blood and plasma donors, all organ and tissue donors, all sperm donors, and in Nevada, Colorado, Iowa, and Missouri, prisoners.[28] In addition, the following is but a partial list of groups who have been suggested as appropriate for either mandatory screening or routinely recommended voluntary screening: health care workers, health care workers who perform invasive procedures, dialysis patients, pregnant women, patients in hospitals, applicants for marriage licenses, children placed for adoption or foster care whose mothers may be in high risk groups, college students, all members of high risk groups and their sexual partners, hemophiliacs and their sexual partners, candidates for organ transplant, prisoners, prostitutes, patients in chemical dependency hospital units, attendees at sexually transmitted disease clinics, applicants to drug diversion programs, transfusion recipients (prior to March 1985), all women with more than one sexual partner, and health and life insurance applicants.

The public policy issue of testing revolves around weighing the benefits gained by individuals' knowing their antibody status and the risks of that information being used against them. So far little is known about what happens to individuals who are asymptomatic and antibody positive: that is, what benefits accrue to others if the seropositive person chooses "alternative behaviors" to prevent spread of infection, and what social and psychological disadvantages accrue to the individual from knowing their status. As previously noted some physicians have reported that telling a person that he/she is antibody positive is even more psychologically distressing than telling a patient that he/she has AIDS.[29] The general failure in the United States to provide adequate counseling and strong guarantees of confidentiality for those who are found to be seropositive will surely contribute further to this distress. The public fear of anyone who is "tainted" with AIDS may also lead to measures that are extremely harmful to the person who is antibody positive. The benefits from this testing are naturally assumed to be for others, who will then be able to avoid exposure to the virus.

The debate on this issue—which is extremely intense—focuses on whether the burden of preventing the spread of infection should be placed on those who are seropositive or on those who are not. Should those who are presumed to have the virus protect others by changing their sexual behaviors and informing their prospective sexual partners of their antibody status, or should those who are presumed not to have the virus protect themselves by changing *their* sexual behaviors and not engaging in practices that will put themselves at risk? Do you have a duty to find out whether you are seropositive and, if you are, to then take on the burden of protecting others? Or do you have a duty to take on the burden of protecting yourself from risking infection, from becoming seropositive? The divisive metaphors of AIDS make it easy to place the burden of knowledge, stigmatization, and significantly altered behavior exclusively on the "others," on those who are separate and different and who have, in the language of the metaphor, placed "us" at risk because of their sinful and criminal activities. Thus, many health care providers are much more interested in finding out patients' antibody status than in insisting that everyone practice appropriate infection control procedures.

RESOLVING THE METAPHORS

If we are to think what is just and what is fair in dealing with the complex public and personal issues that the human immunodeficiency virus brings to us, it is necessary first to clear our minds and our language of the metaphors that so easily lead to punitive actions at the individual, the professional, and the government level. Justice and fairness require that if there are to be burdens and benefits, they should be distributed evenly—not all the burdens for those who are seropositive and all the benefits for those who are seronegative.

The metaphors tell a different story, of course. Because they are inherently divisive, they suggest that burdens should be placed on to the guilty, while benefits should go to the innocent. The metaphors emphasize protection of the public health at the expense of the public good. It must be remembered that we are all—sick and well, infected and uninfected—members of that public. The metaphors deny that we live in a human community in which all need to be protected and care for. A culturally accepted story that says one group of people embodies death, sin, crime, war, and otherness is powerful information that suggests that we are not all in this together. Despite the widespread acceptance of these metaphors, they are not necessarily true. Those who are carriers of the HIV virus need to care about and to protect those who are not; those who have not been exposed need to care for and to protect those who have been. It is not that some of "us" need protection and some of "them" need to sacrifice their rights; that some belong to death while others embrace life, that some are righteous and others are sinners; that some are criminals and others their victims; that some are enemies and others loyal and deserving citizens; that some may be cast out, while others are kept securely within. We are all in this together; we are all innocent. Surely those who have been exposed to AIDS have enough to suffer without being victimized by metaphorical myths.

Disease, especially disease that may lead to death, always takes on a dramatic quality. Drama encourages elevated language. A brief stroll through the *Reader's Guide* listings under AIDS will demonstrate the drama that aids has provided for readers in the past few years: "Now No One Is Safe," "Battling AIDS," "The Plague Years," "AIDS Panic," "Public Enemy #1," "Death After Sex," "Homosexual Plague Strikes New Victims." The moral meanings of these headlines (and hundreds more) and the metaphors they enclose are shaping public response to this disease. It is giving this disease, as Sontag warned, a moral meaning, but that morality is in our minds not in the disease. If ethical judgments about caring for patients, about restricting viral carriers, and about providing HIV testing are to be based on positive, humane attitudes, it is time to confront the inner meanings our language betrays and then to rid not only our speaking and writing but also our thinking of these metaphors. We cannot begin to consider ethically appropriate responses until we firmly fix in our minds that the over 70,000 Americans with AIDS, the unknown numbers with ARC and lesser illnesses, and the over 1 million currently asymptomatic seropositive individuals are not someone unknown, different, foreign, or alien. They are our friends, our brothers, our sisters, and our children. They are a part of us and, as members of our human community, they *are* us.

NOTES

1. The first articles to deal with ethical issues in a substantial way include *The Hastings Center Report's* Special Supplement, AIDS: The emerging ethical dilemmas, August 1985; and June Osborn's The AIDS epidemic: Multidisciplinary trouble. *New England Journal of Medicine* 1986:314(12):779–782.

2. HIV (human immunodeficiency virus) is the name chosen by the International Committee on Taxonomy of Viruses to replace the previously used and increasingly confusing names of HTLV-III, LAV, and ARC. See Coffin, J., et al. Human immunodeficiency viruses. *Science* 1986:232:697.

3. Originally published in *The New York Times* and reprinted in the *Los Angeles Daily Journal*, 3/21/86, p. 4.

4. See, for example, the *Los Angeles Times* poll, 12/19/85, §1, pp. 1, 30. Other polls (*Newsweek, Time*) have shown similar results.

5. The slowness of perceiving the disease in Africa may, in part, be attributed to the greater prevalence of untreatable disease there, making AIDS just another difficult disease among an abundance of disease.

6. For a discussion of the way in which narratives structure our ethical choices, see Hauerwas, Stanley. *Truthfulness and Tragedy*, University of Notre Dame Press, 1977, especially Chapter 1, "From system to story: an alternative pattern for rationality in ethics."

7. Lakoff, George, and Johnson, Mark, *Metaphors We Live By*, University of Chicago Press, 1980, p. 3.

8. For a fuller discussion of the AIDS metaphors and their sources, see Ross, J. W., Ethics and the language of AIDS, in *AIDS: Ethics and Public Policy*, edited by Pierce and vanDeVeer, Wadsworth, in press.

9. Sontag, S. *Illness as Metaphor*. NY: Vintage Books, 1979.

10. Figures on survival after diagnosis vary somewhat depending upon category patient group, and date selections. For example, San Francisco General Hospital reports a survival time of 21 months from time of diagnosis for those with Kaposi's sarcoma (*Medical Tribune* 1985 July:26(19)3, whereas Landesman et al., report a figure of 224 days for the date of first hospitalization with opportunistic infection (Landesman, S. H.; Ginzburg, H. M.; Weiss, S. H. The AIDS epidemic. *New England Journal of Medicine* 1985:312(8):521–524).

11. Sontag, S. *Illness as Metaphor*.

12. Margaret Heckler was the first to receive wide publicity for using this aspect of the metaphor when she said that "we must conquer [AIDS] as well before it threatens the health of our general population." As quoted in *Journal of the American Medical Association (AMA)* 1985:253(23):3377. Subsequently, it has been commonly used by many speakers and writers.

13. For a discussion of risk to health care providers, see McCray, E. Occupational risk of the acquired immunodeficiency syndrome among health care workers. *New England Journal of Medicine* 1986 April 24:314(17):1127–1132.

14. The *New York Times*, 3/17/86, pp. 1, 13.

15. Wachter, R. M. The impact of the acquired immunodeficiency syndrome on medical residency training. *New England Journal of Medicine* 1985:314(3):177–179.

16. Wachter is not the only one to express this concern. Susan Light, M.D., discussing her feelings about forgoing treatment (for patients other than those with AIDS) as a house staff physician, comments that "I wanted it [i.e., their death] to be over so I would not have to be faced daily with our 'failure' and the visible grief of the family." Letters, *Journal of the AMA*. 1986:255(22):3113.

17. Steinbrook, R.; Lo, B.; Tirpack, J., et al. Ethical dilemmas in caring for patients with the acquired immunodeficiency syndrome. *Annals of Internal Medicine* 1985:103(5):787–790.

18. Steinbrook, R.; Lo, B.; Moulton, J., et al. Preferences of homosexual men with AIDS for life-sustaining treatment. *New England Journal of Medicine* 1985:314(7):457–460.

19. Wachter, R. M. The impact of the acquired immunodeficiency syndrome on medical residency training.

20. Risk figures are reported from 0% to 65%. Recommendations for assisting in the prevention of perinatal transmission of HTLV-IIIg/LAC and AIDS. *Morbidity and Mortality Weekly Report* 6 Dec 1985:34(48):722.

21. The Centers for Disease Control states that "infected women should be advised to consider delaying pregnancy. . . " Ibid., 725.

22. *Los Angeles Times*, 1/6/86, §1, p. 2.

23. See, for example, Mills, M.; Wofsy, C. B., Mills, J. Infection control and public health law. *New England Journal of Medicine* 1986:314(14):931–936.

24. *Morbidity and Mortality Weekly Report* 1985:34:1–5.

25. Centers for Disease Control. Additional recommendations to reduce sexual and drug abuse-related transmission of human T-lymphotropic virus Type III/lymphadenopathy-associated virus. *Morbidity and Mortality Weekly Report* 1986:35(10):152–155.

26. Norbert Rapoza, reporting Volberding's comments, *Journal of the AMA* 1985:253(23):3463–3465.

27. Newsline. *Physician's Management.*, May 1986:26(5):15.

28. Glasbrenner, K. Prisons confront dilemmas of inmates with AIDS. *Journal of the AMA* 1986:255(18):2399–2400, 2404.

29. See, for example, the *Los Angeles Times*, AIDS testing dilemmas: To know or not to know, 4/1/86, pp. 1, 10.

30

Risk and Obligation:

Health Professionals and the Risk of AIDS

Erich H. Loewy

AIDS has become the feared epidemic of our times. For a variety of reasons AIDS has been seen as a threat by the professional as well as by the lay public out of proportion to its current reality. The public, fearful of risking AIDS by contributing blood, has curtailed blood donations.[1-3] Some health professionals, fearful of contracting the disease, have hesitated to perform patient care, even care that carries only the most remote risk.[4] At times, physicians have refused to take care of AIDS patients, surgeons have refused to operate, and pathologists to autopsy them.[5] Fears associated with "catching AIDS" have varied from the slight, albeit realistic, fear of direct inoculation with blood to the more fanciful notion that AIDS can result from merely touching such patients.

AIDS and the response to it have often been compared to other historic epidemics, especially to the "Black Death" of the 14th century. The analogy is apt, not because AIDS today carries the same threat that the medieval plague did yesterday, but because our panic and fear of an "unknown" scourge perceived then and now by many as God's punishment seems to have the same flavor. During those times and during other epidemics, physicians and other health professionals had to confront their fears in a similar milieu.

This essay will examine the obligation of health professionals in the face of fear in general and AIDS in particular. The problem will be explored from the following perspectives: (1) a historical introduction probing past epidemics and the behavior of professionals in confronting them; (2) an analysis of fear and courage in the medical setting; (3) differing views of community, justice, and social contract; (4) notions of professionalism and obligation in the context of history and community; and (5) practical consequences of these views.

HISTORICAL CONSIDERATIONS

The question "Do most physicians assume the obligation to treat patients despite personal risk?" is not one for which an immediate answer, shrouded as it is by time, is readily available. Before using epidemic disease as a paradigm for this examination, we must be sure that what we now recognize as transmittable disease (and transmittable by personal contact) was likewise recognized as transmittable through contact during the time examined. Further, we must seek confirmation or refutation of the thesis that physicians cared for their patients despite risks in indirect sources such as chronicles, municipal records, and the literature of the time. Poetry, stories, and sagas are illustrative not so much in that they provide facts as in that they supply a feeling for tacit expectations. Whether physicians who fled were viewed with scorn or their fleeing was considered to be a societal norm suggests the prevalent attitudes toward their obligation.

There is sound evidence that the principle plagues were recognized to be contagious. Thucydides in the 5th century BC seems well aware of this and mentions the disproportionate number of physicians who, during the Plague of Athens, died taking care of patients.[6] Despite the fact that until about the 16th century physicians were not expected to treat the irreversibly sick,[7] Hippocrates (460–370 BC) gives careful instructions for the purification of air during epidemics and implies that physicians must stay, help their patients, and guard themselves against infection. During the second century of our era, Galen fled Rome during the Antonine Plague. He feared that Marcus Aurelius, who was his patient, might have him returned to Rome in chains and found it necessary to develop an intricate series of excuses and apologies. The defense of Galen (that, in fact, he did not desert when it clearly seems he did) for what was obviously viewed by himself and others as "wrong" has survived until today.[8]

The Plague of Justinian, which was undoubtedly what we call "plague" today (i.e., caused by *Yersinia pestis*[9,10]), lasted from circa 540 to 590 and in its bubonic and pneumonic forms ravaged the Western world. Procopius, who not only gives a beautiful account of the times and their social mechanisms but who also supplied us with an excellent clinical description, speaks of "physicians examining the bodies of the dead."[11] Despite the disastrous consequences of the plague on Justinian's plans for a Byzantine Roman Empire,[12] the internal life of Byzantium, although severely strained, continued. Physicians, Procopius implies, stood by their patients.

The "Black Death" swept Europe from 1348 to 1350, killing between one-third and one-half of the population.[13] In its wake, repetitive pulses of plague scourged Europe until the 17th century, when, for reasons that are not entirely clear, it disappeared.[14] There is a relative wealth of both historical and literary material available for this period.[15–18] Social effects were devastating: children abandoned parents and parents children, husbands and wives deserted each other, prayer vigils alternated with or encompassed orgies,[19] flagellants roamed the streets, further aggravating the ongoing pogroms[13,20]; society was maddened.[21] Famine and the failure of the dead to be buried added to the hysteria. But societal dislocation was less complete then once thought: magistrates continued to perform their duties, and when they died, other took their place; wills were written and probated; priests gave last rites; physicians made their appointed rounds.[22,23] The social fabric, badly strained, held enough so that change of existing institutions, rather than complete anarchy, resulted. Although many magistrates, priests, and physicians may have run away, many more stayed and often died, enabling moral continuity and the preservation of an implicit social contract.[24] In Perugia, Gentile de Foligno methodically autopsied victims, eventually falling prey to the plague. Guy de Chauliac, whose works have come down to us and who was physician to Pope Clement VI, stayed but was sorely afraid: "And I, to avoid infamy, dared not absent myself but with continual fear preserved myself as best I could."[24] His "fear of infamy" tends to support the notion that physicians who fled were not the norm and incurred communal disapproval.[25,26]

Europe continued to suffer sporadic epidemics of plague until the late 17th century. During this time, some municipalities passed laws forbidding physicians to leave during epidemics, and some hired special "pest doctors" who, although there were earlier examples, foreshadowed the public health physicians of today. During the Great Plague of London in the summer of 1665, a meeting of the Royal College was adjourned because of the epidemic.[27] Most physicians, like Glisson and Wharton, stayed; occasionally one, like Sydenham,[28] fled but felt the necessity of explaining his failure to stay: many such physicians treated mainly upper-class patients who generally fled, and so, in a sense, they fled with and not from their patients.

In more modern times, during the yellow fever epidemics of 18th-century Philadelphia, physicians, notably Benjamin Rush, stood their ground. Later, during the great influenza pandemic, whose mortality was far from negligible, physicians did not flee. They remained, worked, and often died, as did those caring for persons with tuberculosis and polio in more recent times. The message seems clear: throughout history society expected its functionaries to continue their duties in good times and in bad.[25] The fear of infamy and their perception of duty led most physicians to take the risk and to stay with their patients.

FEAR AND COURAGE IN THE MEDICAL SETTING

Hopes and fears share a common meeting ground in being future-directed. Both have a stake in the unknown and, therefore, in what cannot be proved. We fear and hope for what has not happened, and often we balance fears and hopes in determining our actions at least as much as we predicate such actions on purely rational grounds. That is not to say that hopes and fears are, of necessity, unrealistic, but they share an element of the mystic with the empirical in different degrees. No wonder, when it comes to hopes and fears, irrational as well as unreal elements may enter. My fear of being electrocuted if I touch a live wire is quite rational (even if unreal in the sense that many things could interfere); my fear of developing AIDS by shaking a patient's hand is irrational as well as unreal. In dealing with fears, the irrational as well as the unreal deserve to be considered.

Fear will be defined as a sensation or feeling of anxiety caused by a realization, perception, or expectation of impotency in the face of perceived or expected danger or evil.[29] It subsumes qualities of dread, awe, and other emotive and aesthetic elements. Courage is defined as "disposition to voluntarily act, perhaps fearfully, in a dangerous circumstance . . . "; its "essence is the mastery of fear for the preservation of a perceived good against dangers."[30] Courage, then, enables action in the face of fear; duty, courage, and fear are inextricably linked.[29]

Fear, however, does not necessarily oppose duty. Rather, the fear of not doing what is perceived to be one's duty, the fear of censure, the fear, as it were, of "infamy" may help to overcome the fear that cautions against risks. Furthermore, emotive, symbolic, and aesthetic elements enter into a decision to act or not. Fearing to be shocked by an electrical device at the bedside, I may nevertheless overcome this fear; yet if the same instrument is covered with slime or vomitus, I may not do so. Disgust and fear here are mutually reinforcing and may preclude action. Courage is needed to overcome fear as well as revulsion.

In dealing with infectious disease, physicians have generally felt themselves disposed to assume the risks and to stay with their patients, and so in more recent times have other health professionals. When contagion is unassociated with other strong repulsive qualities, physicians in general have suppressed their fears and, in spite of their anxieties, have treated.

AIDS is subtly different. Its history, shrouded in mystery in the eyes of many, is nebulous: Haitian, African, a reservoir in monkeys, an entirely new disease. All these endow AIDS with an air of the arcane which both appeals to and repels superstitious persons. It affects the "immune system," which, unseen and not concrete, as are other body systems, only heightens the mystery. Further, its mode of transmission, in the eyes of many, places it in the category of "sin" rather than disease. It is believed to be "venereal" and "venereal" under what are generally held to be especially repugnant circumstances. That illicit drug users are also likely to be affected only strengthens the feeling that "sin" is somehow involved: AIDS represents the just wages of sin. Homosexuals and drug users are "deserving" of God's punishment. That some transfusion recipients and many hemophiliacs inexplicably share in this "punishment" is often conveniently ignored.

Physicians and other health professionals are shaped, conditioned, and nourished by their culture. As any other group within a society, they share prevalent attitudes, values, and fears with other members of their community. Values, fears, and attitudes are not different in kind but rather are abstracted, and modified, from those prevalent in the community. Persons inclined toward the health professions have only a somewhat different hierarchy of values and fears. Medicine's aims and moral views differ in emphasis and detail, but they cannot differ substantially.[31] The attitudes of health professionals in dealing with AIDS patients reflect community values as well as the medical ethos.

COMMUNITY, JUSTICE, AND SOCIAL CONTRACT

The way we look at the ontology, structure, and relationship within a community presages the attitudes we adopt toward justice, social contract, and the "natural lottery." This, in turn, will profoundly affect our private and professional concept of obligation and duty.

Community, on the one hand, can be seen as a group of individuals bound together merely by duties of refraining from harm to one another.[32] In such communities, freedom is seen as the necessary condition of morality (a "side constraint"[33]) rather than as a fundamental value. Freedom is endowed with an absolutist ring and cannot be negotiated.

On the other hand, communities can be seen as being bound by more than these "minimal conditions."[34] These are, of course, the minimal conditions, which, while necessary, are insufficient to describe community in the way we usually think of it. In communities united by more than minimal conditions,[11] freedom becomes a value. In their definition, such communities include the more imperfect, and more discretionary, Kantian duties of charity, beneficence, and fellow-feeling.[35]

Communities not united by certain ways of behaving toward each other cannot long endure.[36] Individuals must refrain from injurious acts to each other. Refraining from such harm to another enables coexistence. But this alone fails to describe most people's notion of community. Communities demand a commons in which members work toward their own as well as toward their neighbor's good. Community, as ordinarily conceived, is cemented by the inclination of its members toward each other's good. In such communities, freedom of necessity has a fundamental value, but freedom, in such communities, is viewed as one value among others and not as the condition for such values. The difference is profound: communities united only by duties of refraining may regard benevolent acts as laudable (and then would be hard pressed to say why benevolence should be laudable rather than merely a matter of taste) but not as obligatory and will not permit communal decisions that take from one (no matter how well off) to give to another (no matter how much in need).[37] Taxation for welfare, for example, would not be allowed. Communities that consider the welfare of other members critical to their own definition of themselves will, to the best of their ability, try to assure a decent minimum standard for all members and will not hesitate to infringe some of its members' freedoms (by taxing them, for instance) to achieve that end.[38]

Persons' views of justice flow from their conception of community. The ancient formula—that justice is giving to each his due[39]—leaves that which is due undefined. A view of community predicated only on duties of refraining from harm one to another would find that "what is due" is individual noninterference. On the other hand, a view of community as cemented by duties of beneficence would see in "what is due" entirely different things. The particulars of such beneficence, then, become a social construct over time and place. Men who perceive freedom to be a fundamental value but a value, nevertheless, will negotiate and steer between the Scylla of absolute freedom (leaving many of their poorer fellows at the mercy of individual caprice) and the Charybdis of totalitarian control (leaving themselves with essentially no viable choice).

Both those who believe in a justice based only on duties of noninterference (autonomy-based justice) and those who take a wider view of community (beneficence-based justice) will honor and enforce contracts made between autonomously consenting members of the community. But contracts in autonomy-based justice are not subtended by a desire for each other's good. In such a system, beneficence is reduced to strictly stipulated and stipulatable conditions beyond which no further duty exists. Physicians' relationships with their patients, then, need only to follow a strictly contractual model.

Social contract, the tacit understanding among members of a community that enables communal cohesion and function, emerges from the view of community among its members and, in turn, shapes the individual's point of view. This dynamic interaction not only enables communal function during a given period of time but also permits the evolution of the communal ethos. Social contracts have historical roots. Physicians as individuals, and physicians as a professional group, are entwined in their own historical ethos and in the social contract that cements their greater community. Within the confines of that contract, there is the understanding that actions will be congruous with the contract and that the profession as a group and the professional as an individual will be bound by it. No contract is for life. Contracts, shaped by the context in which they are embodied and modified by changing circumstances, are dynamic instruments of function. But contracts cannot justly be abrogated unilaterally, privately, or capriciously; there has to be mutuality, agreement, and due process.

Views of what has been called the "natural lottery"[40] are intertwined with our notions of community as well as of justice. By the natural lottery is meant "chance" or "luck" which distributes poverty or wealth and beauty or ugliness as well as health or disease. Some will subdivide this further into a "natural" and "social" lottery, but emphasis here is on a lottery concept in which the "luck of the draw" determines an individual's fate. All those things not directly attributable to the individual's doing or clearly caused by another are viewed in this way. There are three basic ways of looking at the natural lottery:

1. The outcome of the natural lottery is no one's fault and therefore does not confer obligation on anyone or on the community. Plainly speaking, the outcome is "too bad." In the words so often used by the law or by insurance companies, these are "acts of God." (The peculiar viewpoint of God which informs such opinions is another matter.)

2. The outcome of the lottery, while not anyone's fault, is more than just "too bad." In the sense that the recipient of fate's largesse has done nothing to deserve it, adverse outcomes are not only unfortunate but are, in fact, quite unfair. Based on beneficence, such a viewpoint may entail an assumption of obligation.[41,42]

3. The result of such a lottery can be viewed in yet another way. Events and social goods are not generally as simple as being struck by lightning or slipping on a banana peel. When we are born to wealth or poverty, crash our car, or succumb to a heart attack, there is more than chance alone at work. The conditions that create, aim, and hurl lightning are as yet out of human control; the conditions that create, perpetuate, and ignore poverty, build cars, control highways, or are implicated in disease are, at least in great part, a social construct. Over and over again, health and disease have been shown to be intimately linked with poverty and other clearly social conditions.[43-47] In this view, many of the outcomes of such a "lottery" are far more than unfortunate: they are unjust, because innocent persons have drawn the short lot in a lottery which, at least in part, is of our own communal making. This, by virtue of communal liability as well as beneficence, confers duties of aiding those who have drawn the short lot.

If community is viewed as united by more than the duties of refraining, victims of the natural lottery are likely to be viewed and treated far differently from otherwise. Justice, which gives to each his due, will feel that such "due" not only includes leaving the victims alone to fend for themselves as best they can but also enjoins members of such a community to come to their help. Coming to their help now is more than just a "nice thing to do"—by definition it is seen as an essential function of community and, in that sense, a duty.

PROFESSIONALISM AND OBLIGATION

The words profession and professionalism have been much bandied about until today every activity would have itself a profession. Profession has been variously defined.[48] At its core are such concepts as specialized knowledge, prolonged training, and service to the community.[49] Profession in the medical context has been characterized by autonomy through a process of political negotiation and persuasion.[50] In popular understanding, however, profession, in addition to this, implies dedication to an ideal which transcends the technical activity itself and in so doing subserves a moral end. This definition, much the same as the distinction between art and craft made by Plato, would have a craft using technical means for material ends and an art using technical means for a moral end.[51] Medicine professes the ability to perform "a good act of healing in the face of the fact of illness."[52] That act, technical in its nature, is aimed at a moral end: the "good" of the patient, however defined.

In professing the ability to perform a "good act of healing," professionals not only proclaim technical expertise, they tacitly profess willingness to use their expertise for the patient's good. Willingness makes technical skill operative: without it, skill is socially useless. In testing skills, willingness is presumed. Willingness to perform a technically good act of healing involves technical and moral choices: choices of what is "good" and what is "bad." Such choices are a composite of intermeshed facts and values among which hope and fear play a role. Choice relies, in part, on implicit social contract.

Physicians, professing willingness to exercise expertise in their field of health care, are bound to the promise of competence and willingness by an obligation rooted in an implicit covenant and social contract. Communities are secured by social contract, a tacit understanding among its members that underpins their function.

Communities organized only about duties of refraining, if such really exist, will have a social understanding secured by a tacit contract much different from those united by duties of coming to each others' aid. Communities of the first sort will rely on explicit contract between healer and patient or on explicit contract between the community and the physician. They will not expect physicians or other members of the community to transcend the immediate contract. However, communities that define themselves as dedicated to their members' "good" will understand such contracts in other ways. Beneficence and caring will be the tacit accompaniment of all freely entered associations or covenants within their confines. Without such tacit understanding, enforced here and there by law,[53] such communities would be disrupted. Such contracts do not always operate smoothly, and they are often ignored: the affluent industrialist in ignoring social conditions, the wealthy nation glutted with food amidst world hunger, ignore these at ultimate peril.

Physicians, like all groups of persons, view their professional obligations in the light of historical precedence and communal expectations. The backbone of medical professionalism—the willingness to exercise technical skills in pursuit of moral ends—implies three obligations: (1) the presence and maintenance of skills; ((2) a conception of the moral end; and (3) a willingness to make a moral choice and to engage in the activity appropriate to that choice.

Willingness to perform a task implies the realization that some negative element, be it obstacles, fear, or pain, may be associated with the task. To be willing to do a given thing without any, no matter how remotely perceived negative elements is almost tautologous.[29] To be a will, the will must potentially be disposed to pit itself against trouble in the discharge of its task. An assumption of risk, no matter how remote or how little, is implied in "being willing."

PRACTICAL CONSEQUENCE

Physicians and other health professionals are members of a community. Individuals within that community generally share in its precepts and are united by the social contract in which all share. They expect their functionaries, be they policemen, carpenters, teachers, or doctors, to perform their duties in good times and in bad. The obligations assumed and the risks taken are not without their compensation: physicians have been blessed with immense privileges, prerogatives, and power as well as abundant material reward.

Individuals are not expected to pit themselves against certain death, and they are not expected to assume risks forever. There are "reasonable" risks, and there are acceptable ways of terminating professional obligation no longer suitable to person or condition. "Reasonable" risks are reasonable within the historical context of the community and the social contract that underpins them. Professional obligations, in turn, can be abrogated by physicians or others within a just community. Abrogation or termination of such obligations, however, must be done without ripping the social fabric. Just as physicians may specialize and, therefore, be expected to treat some things but not others, and just as physicians may wash their hands of the entire enterprise by retiring or by changing their occupation, physicians may refuse to care for any disease or condition of their choosing. This must, however, be done in a timely fashion, publicly and with due notice. Violations inevitably result in censure, stigma, and, in some parts of the world, legal action.

AIDS, while often perceived as different, is an infectious disease, transmittable only under certain well-specified circumstances and conferring an apparently very small risk on care givers. It differs from other infectious disease in that (1) once transmission has occurred, the certainty of clinical infection is questionable; (2) once the actual disease is diagnosed, it appears to date to be almost universally fatal; and (3) it carries with it a stigma. Except for the last point, it is similar to other historical epidemics in their time. Factually speaking, the risk assumed by care givers is minimal. It is far less than was assumed by our historical forebears and is certainly not greater than that assumed by functionaries in other fields. The stigma carried by AIDS, the mystique and aura of "sin" surrounding it, adds to our fears.

Our fears and our sense of duty are modulated by all these considerations as well as by the changes community has undergone in recent times. No longer are we the "tight little island" of yesteryear.[5] Our society has become egocentric, hedonistic, and less community-oriented; we are dedicated to personal advantage, comfort, and gain. Moral expectations for others have grown, and expectations for ourselves have been attenuated. "Rugged individualism" is extolled; social action is looked at as curious. Running risks for social benefits sits poorly with us. Also, we physicians have been spoiled: when we deal with contagion, we are used to curing. We do not expect to be infected, and, when we are, we expect to be cured. AIDS not only disgusts us, it reminds us that our "invincibility" is hubris, that we too are mortal. And we, great men and women that we are, don't like it.[5]

If one (1) holds that the definition of community entails not only duties of refraining from harm one to another but likewise powerful obligations of aid one to another, (2) feels that this definition is cemented and secured by an enduring and slowly evolving social contract that binds one to another, (3) believes that a historically grounded professional ethos commits professionals within such communities to obligations of willingness to use their requisite skills for moral ends, and (4) affirms that justice, in giving to each his due, commits professionals as part of the larger community to render their peculiar services to their fellows, one will inevitably concede that physicians and other health professionals are obligated to have the courage to take reasonable risks in the face of their fears of contagion.

REFERENCES

1. *New York Times*: Fear of AIDS cancels blood drive on Coast, p a11L; 11 January 1985

2. Engel M: Fear of AIDS limits blood donations: *Washington Post* V109; p WH 15; 15 January 1986

3. Scott EP, Therkelson DJ, Siess JM: Effect of acquired immune deficiency syndrome (AIDS) on blood transfusion and donation patterns in state of Minnesota. *Minn Med* 68(9):665–669, 1985

4. Engel M: Rescuers balk at moving body of AIDS victim. *Washington Post* V109; p A1; 6 February 1986

5. Loewy EH: AIDS and the physicians fear of contagion. (Editorial.) *Chest* 89(3):325–326, 1986

6. Jonsen A: Made personally available.

7. Amundsen DW: The physicians obligation to prolong life: A medical duty without classical roots. *Hastings Ctr* 8(4):23–31, 1978

8. Walsh J: Refutation of charge of cowardice against Galen. *Ann Med Hist* 3:195–208, 1931

9. Bratton TL: The identity of the Plague of Justinian. *Trans Stud Coll Phys Phil* 3(2):113–124, 3(3):174–180, 1981

10. Russel C: That earlier Plague. *Demography* 5:179–184, 1968

11. Procopius: *History of the Wars; Secret History; Buildings* (Transl: Williamson G). New Haven, CT: Twayne Publishers, 1967

12. Cameron A: *Continuity and Change in Sixth-Century Byzantium*. London: Variorum Reprints, 1981

13. Marks G: *The Medieval Plague*. New York: Doubleday, 1971

14. Sigerist HE: *Civilization and Disease*. Chicago: University of Chicago Press, 1943

15. Boccacio G: *Decameron* (Transl: Muso M, Bondanella P). New York: New American Library, 1982

16. Cipolla CM: *Cristofano and the Plague*. Los Angeles: University of California Press, 1973

17. Bullein W: *A Dialogue Against the Fever Pestilence*. Oxford, U.K.: Oxford University Press, 1888 (1931)

18. Tuchman BW: *A Distant Mirror*. New York: Ballantine Books, 1978

19. Deux A: *The Black Death 1347*. London: Weybright-Tolley, 1969

20. Nohl J: *The Black Death*. San Francisco: Harper and Bros, 1961

21. Langer WL: The Black Death. *Sci Am* 210(2):114–121, 1961

22. Emery EW: The Black Death of 1348 in Perpignan. *Speculum* 42(4):511–623, 1967

23. William D: *The Black Death: The Impact of the 14th Century Plague*. Binghampton, NY: Mediaeval and Renaissance Texts and Studies, 1982

24. Campbell AM: *The Black Death and Men of Learning*. New York: AMS Press, 1966

25. Rath G: Ärztliche Ethik In Pestzeiten. *Munch Med Wochenschr* 99(5):158–162, 1957

26. Amundsen DW: Medical deontology and the pestillential disease in the late Middle Ages. *J Hist Med* 32:403–421, 1977

27. Defoe D: *A Journal of the Plague Year*. Oxford, U.K.: Basil-Blackwell, 1928

28. Veith I: Medical ethics through the ages. *Ann Bull NWU Med Sch* 31:351–358, 1957

29. Loewy EH: Duties, fear and physicians. *Soc Sci Med* 22(12):1363–1366, 1986

30. Shelp EE: Courage: A neglected virtue in the patient-physician relationship. *Soc Sci Med* 18(4):351–360, 1984

31. Loewy EH: Introduction. In Loewy EH (ed): *Ethical Dilemmas in Modern Medicine: A Physician's Viewpoint*. Lewiston, NY: Edwin Mellen, 1986, pp. 1–15.

32. Loewy EH: Communities, obligations and health care. *Soc Sci Med* 25(7): 783–791, 1987
33. Nozick R: *Anarchy, State and Utopia*. New York: Basic Books, 1974
34. Callahan D: Minimalist ethics. *Hastings Ctr* 11(5):19–25, 1981
35. Kant I: *Foundations of the Metaphysics of Morals* (Transl: Beck LW). Indianapolis: Bobbs-Merrill, 1978
36. Reeder JP: Beneficence, supererogation and roles duty. In Shelp EE (ed): *Beneficence and Health Care*. Dordrecht, Holland: D. Reidel, 1982, pp. 83–102
37. Englehardt HT: Rights to health care. In Englehardt HT (ed.) *The Foundations of Bioethics*. New York: Oxford University Press, 1986
38. Rawls J: *A Theory of Justice*. Cambridge, MA: Harvard University Press, 1971
39. Aristotle: *Nichomachean Ethics*. (Transl: Ostwald M.) Indianapolis: Bobbs-Merrill, 1962
40. Englehardt HT: Health care allocations: Responses to the unjust, the unfortunate, and the undesireable. In Shelp EE (ed): *Justice and Health Care*, pp 121–137. Dordrecht, Holland: D. Reidel, 1981
41. Outka G: Social justice and equal access to health care. J Religious Ethics 2(1):11–32, 1974
42. Outka G: Letter to the editor. *Perspect Bio Med* 19(3):449–452, 1976
43 Kosa J, Zola IK: *Poverty and Health: A Sociological Analysis*. Cambridge, MA: Harvard University Press, 1975
44. Hearings Before Subcommittee on Oversight and Investment: *Infant Mortality Rates: Failure to Close the Black-White Gap*. Washington: U.S. Government Printing Office, 1984
45. Fuchs VR: *Economic Aspects of Health*. Chicago: University of Chicago Press, 1982
46. U.S. Department of Commerce: *Social Indicators*. Washington: U.S. Government Printing Office, 1980
47. U.S. Department of Health and Human Services: *Health Characteristics According to Family and Personal Income*. Washington: U.S. Government Printing Office, 1985
48. Cogan MI: Toward a definition of profession. *Harvard Educ Rev* 23:28–39, 1953
49. Goode WJ: Encroachment, charlatanism and the emerging profession: Psychology, medicine, and sociology. *Am Sociol Rev* 25:902–914, 1960
50. Freidson E: *Profession of Medicine*. New York: Harper and Row, 1970
51. Plato: *Gorgias* (Transl: Woodhead D). In Hamilton E, Huntington C (eds): *Plato: The Collected Dialogues*. Princeton, NJ: Princeton University Press, 1978
52. Pellegrino ED: Toward a reconstruction of medical morality: The primacy of the act of profession and the fact of illness. *J Med Phil* 4(1):32–56, 1979
53. D'Irsay S: Defense reactions during the black death 1348–1349. *Ann Med Hist* 9:169–179, 1927

31

Creative Acceptance:
An Ethics for AIDS

Rev. Bernard Brown

Current ethical principles seem to be inadequate for the problems associated with AIDS. Perhaps a simple, new structure of hope is needed—an ethic in which the person with AIDS creatively accepts himself[1] as still growing; moreover, the larger community actualizes its integrity and its bonding by accepting and supporting the persons with AIDS. Searching the past Christian experience in providing hospitals for the dying, the new ethics described here proposes two points of acceptance useful for all people willing to move beyond denial and to spark concrete ethical progress.

TWO ETHICAL PRINCIPLES OF ACCEPTANCE: PATIENTS ACCEPT DEATH; OTHERS ACCEPT THE PATIENT

This twofold acceptance is a key to enriched ethical action in the AIDS crisis. The principle that the AIDS patient realistically admit his condition requires true acceptance of self as the patient really is: sick and certain to die too soon, but accepting this dying as a process of moving toward a completion of one's life. The patient simultaneously knows and accepts himself as living, growing, worthy, with more love yet to expend, and hopeful of available holistic support.

The second principle is that the larger society grow to become so creative in its thinking that it can accept with new insight these brothers and sisters who need our care. Our growth through the challenge of their presence requires of us true acceptance of our AIDS-infected neighbors as they really are: not essentially different from the rest of us who will also face death; still growing creatively in their human virtues, but lonely and needing whatever physical, emotional, or spiritual hope we can give.

Two Christian Culture Points Facilitate Acceptance

An ethics for AIDS is best based on an actual working *ethos*, a successful cultural pattern that for 20 centuries has helped millions in their sufferings. Such a Christian *ethos* has been a successful ethics model both in earlier plague and leprosy times and for modern AIDS. Just as the denial problems coalesce around the patient and society, the acceptance reasoning will follow two corresponding basic points of Christian vision: (1) The terminal patient's actions and decisions can create maximum fullness of personality development and some will envisage graduating into a new and better life-after-death, with consequent new hope and nobility, and (2) society recognizes our bonding as brothers and sisters forming one organism which Christians, echoing Paul, call "the Body of Christ." This is but an escalation of the Jewish heightened consciousness of the clan and our shared fate within it.

A Mystical Examination

These two roots flowered to produce new insights in Christianity. The mystic kernel of these tenets–that the patient who accepts dying grows into eternal life, and that society grows by accepting brotherhood with the sick—unfolds as follows.

Graduating into the community of eternal life. "De subitanea et improvisa morte, libera nos, Domine." This supplication, chanted through some 15 centuries of Christian prayer in the Litany of the Saints, "From a sudden and unprovided death, do deliver us, O Lord," expresses a considered and stable value with which Christians have preferred to approach death—as a final occasion of personality growth with time enough to prepare themselves. Until a medical cure is available, most persons with AIDS know that they face death—all too soon, but with time to prepare. Where some see in this imminent death cause for despair, deeper Christians among them see a boon and a blessing: growth time to prepare for the most important event of conscious life. Such is the vision of achieving final affirmation of one's basic inner goodness and worth, then moving on gracefully, with the hope of eternal life. The Christian model of a good death includes dignity and the peace of mutual forgiveness, love, and support.

The dying patient's assurance of eternal life after death makes a difference in his present life and in his ethical decisions and actions. Countless dying people have found that the hope of continuity into eternal life validates efforts toward personal development, since one's unique personality will be forever dynamic and operative among all the others in the community of heaven. This New Testament-based vision[2] guarantees the promise of the last wrapping-up moments of one's life and helps avoid the suicide of despair by showing that in the period of suffering one's personality growth is finally forged.

Motivation for compassionate AIDS outreach. The first Jewish Christians envisaged themselves as a people together who formed a fabric, a moral entity, a community here on earth which *is* the divine reality called "Christ"—the "mystical body of Christ." Jesus, who had explicitly identified with the poor, the suffering, the sick, the imprisoned, the leper, the outcast, the dying, said that in reaching out compassionately to such persons, his followers would find and be kind to *him.* Today one enacts this Christic love in caring for the person with AIDS. This collective human moral action is identified as the "corporate Christ"; it *is* the salvific *reality*, for it constitutes the Christ-reality of the twentieth century.

Acceptance in History

Hospitals and Nursing: Dedicated Healers

Precisely in such compassion for the poor and for persons with AIDS is the collective salvation, that is, the corporate health and nobility of the whole people.

If a culture is judged by how it cares for its weakest members, the Western culture of early Christian Europe up through the Middle Ages gradually grew to find its soul and its success as a human society. Historically, it has been those formally dedicated to following Christ—the monks and nuns of the 10 centuries after the fall of the Roman Empire—who out of their vision of Christic love pioneered working in the contagion of the charnel houses. Perhaps the most glorious (because both visionary and successful) chapter in history is that of the religious origins of today's Western hospital and nursing system. The vision, Christ-seen-in-the-poor, was translated into the reality of ethical action also in times of plague and leprosy. This was the successful vision in which both the healthy helpers and the poor and sick found their nobility; from such a powerful principle of ethics their actions and decisions flowed—to the benefit of all around them.

Leprosy: A Parallel in Denial and Acceptance

For centuries, leprosy was more persistent and feared than any other plagues in Europe. It established a pattern of how Christian people acting as the corporate Christ would respond to plagues like the Black Death. Some good did come from the tragedy of leprosy: there were heroes among civilized Christians who learned not to run away from leprosy in denial, but to accept lepers as part of the body of Christ.

An important question from the leprosy experience that applies to the AIDS crisis is, how did pre-Medieval Christian Europe act? First, with great psychological distancing and denial (just as we do). They echoed the Jewish biblical precepts of thorough precaution before contagion of all sorts. But in Europe, caution led to such extreme measures as ostracizing lepers from towns, even from roadways. Some "Dark Age" Christians were even known to perform the complete funeral service over a leper, stand him in a grave, and take all his property because he was declared "dead" and probably was being punished by God. The healthy ritualized the lepers' banishment from human society as much as possible. Harbinger of our hospital warning signs, a rattle was given to the leper to forewarn all of his tainted presence. In just such a milieu, however, some of these same people found their Christic roots and provided care for the lepers. In spite of all the stories about decadent clergy in the Dark Ages,

> the fact remains that it was through the brave and unceasing labors of the priesthood that leprosy was finally stamped out in Europe. At a date when the ominous sound of a leper's rattle sent most scurrying, the early monks rallied together and converted their houses into leper hospitals and lazar houses. In France, during the thirteenth century, it is recorded that no less than *two thousand* of these institutions existed and in England at the same period there were two hundred founded, of which the majority were controlled by the ecclesiastics.
>
> "All guests who come shall be received as though they were Christ" was the rule of the lazar houses and it was a rule that was faithfully observed. Nobody, in those times of famine and pestilence, cruelty and persecution, was ever turned away and the same hearty welcome and treatment was accorded all, regardless of rank. . . . For the first time in history consideration was shown the leper; he was well fed . . . a roof was over his head and his spiritual needs were attended.[3]

A major strength of Christianity throughout history has always been its slow but eventual ability to identify unerringly the principle of Christ in the outcast.

NEW ETHICAL PRINCIPLES APPLIED TO THE PERSON AND SOCIETY

Now that we have seen the Christic motivation that can spark acceptance, how might it open to all people some of the helpful ethical possibilities based on the twofold vision of acceptance of growing-towards-death and acceptance of the neighbor?

Actions of the Person Accepting Self as Dying

Telling Others

For persons with AIDS courageously to decide to be honest with others who might be endangered by continued high risk behavior involves a basic acceptance-versus-denial issue; it requires one to accept the truth of one's own predicament. The experienced counselor appreciates the difficulty with which personal acceptance of the AIDS diagnosis is achieved, the necessary first step before being able to tell others. One man came home from the doctor and showered for hours, as if he wanted to scrub out that damned spot of archetypal uncleanness. All libido is said to be immediately lost in certain people upon learning of their AIDS diagnosis. This further weakens a self-image that will have to be stronger than ever, for courage before the community posits a new challenge to one's honesty in self-revelation.

Should a person with AIDS tell friends? Why should they know if there is no danger to them? After all, does he not have a right to the privacy of his own body? Not in an absolute sense. The collectivity of the community in this situation is even more important, even holy. Both an ethics of acceptance and honest, mature relationships help the person with AIDS and friends and family members to face the facts. They might all learn to live more truthfully and interact more openly through the difficult process of knowing, accepting, and dealing with such a threat to their friendship.

Should the person who has AIDS tell his employer when the danger to others is little or none? Suppose he knows the employer would summarily fire him? With mounting medical bills, the AIDS victim cannot afford to lose his job and health insurance. For the sake of both dignity and finances, he needs to work and should be allowed to do so. An ethics of acceptance finds it vitally important for these people to keep their jobs, for reasons of human dignity, productiveness, and sense of community. Some AIDS counselors list workplace continuance as the number one priority both in chronology and in importance.

Personal Desires versus Public Safety

The San Francisco *cause célèbre* of gay bathhouse closings is an excellent example of the conflict of personal desires and the common well-being.[4] In this case there were indeed personal rights at stake which the gay community was loathe to surrender, but such rights do not constitute an absolute in ethics, where personal rights often must be relinquished to maximize public safety. Disregard for others' health has no defensible ethical position in our responsible acceptance of each other. On metaphysical grounds, the collective health of the corporate group comes much closer to being an absolute compared to individual rights; the health of the whole might be called holy. In Christian language, when there is true conflict the formation of the corporate Christ is more important than the desires of the individual.

Suicide: Denial of Life or Acceptance of Death?

Suicide by terminal AIDS patients is a serious problem.[5] This phenomenon reflects the cumulative sense of suffering from pain, of being a burden to others, of having no future, as well as the shame that society heaps upon both the homosexual and the intravenous drug user with AIDS. In addition, the strain of repeated hospital stays and multiple treatment regimens, none of which produce a cure, adds to the stress. The patient may know that there is organic brain damage with consequent dementia that will worsen. All these factors contribute to a questioning of life and death. Even the standard Christian counseling that encourages personal growth and nobility right to the natural end may seem pointless in the face of dementia or coma (which restrict any growth)—and many persons with AIDS are certain of that prognosis. With such a future, those who had enjoyed higher self-esteem, but who now lack the adaptation techniques gained from earlier suffering, and who lack strong systems of support, are more likely to commit suicide.[6]

Passive suicide is more common than active suicide in this population.[6] One medical doctor who had AIDS-related violent diarrhea and vomiting deliberately did not seek help. Evicted from his former residence for "health reasons," he did not even unpack his boxes in his new apartment, but expressly let himself go into extreme dehydration and death. Beyond questions of responsibility to the community, the main ethical issues of autonomy were freedom of choice and personal control over one's destiny. To other persons with AIDS with such dismal medical prognoses, theoretical distinctions between active and passive means to achieve the end (death) more quickly are viewed as invisible boundaries. Did this doctor exhibit a stoic acceptance of what life had to offer? Was the giving up positive or negative? Did he have a further vision that made letting go a constructive act?

During times of crisis there is an increased need to not sidestep the life/death issues but to make those difficult decisions and make them in a more practical way than past ethical theories anticipated. With the increase of older sick people, this society was already heading toward a moral crisis over the permissibility of voluntary euthanasia and assisted suicide. But suddenly AIDS appeared and exacerbated the need to examine the question of the right to choose the timing of one's own death.

For many people, norms for suicide often mean "permission," as they might wish to seek some assurance of freedom from guilt. A patient-centered practical conclusion, drawn from many larger systematic philosophies of death and suicide,[7] finds the real impetus against suicide is actually love of life, not the classic theoretical textbook *reasons* prohibiting suicide which may be inapplicable or meaningless in many cases. No doubt most involved in caring for the seriously ill at the bedside day and night agree that in certain grievous cases there is no persuasive reason which would convince the person to go on living. But as recent cases in the Netherlands and Florida show, a major ethical problem exists: no one seems to know how to formulate any generalized rule against suicide, valid for all cases, which would also allow greater understanding of the extreme sufferer needing unusual compassionate "permission" (to assure freedom from guilt) for going against this rule about suicide. Society's hesitancy here stems both from fear of slippery-slope misuse (by which society begins to slip into letting the single exceptional suicide become the norm), and from the fact that in such an intimate area every case is unique and must be handled individually. The harsh realities call more for society's helpful care than for suicide guidelines. From a patient-centered practical viewpoint, the following ideas are important in an ethics of acceptance.

Peace of mind and freedom from guilt. As hospital chaplains and counselors of the dying can attest, both ethics and religion are truly concerned about norms for achieving peace of mind and for freeing from guilt. If some norms steer one away from certain types of actions (suicide), it is societal wisdom which speaks for one's emotional peace and freedom from future guilt, both of which are crucial not only for the patient, but also for the survivors. A classic example is that guilt-reducing staple of death-and-dying ethics, voiced yet again in the official assurance of Pope Pius XII:[8] don't feel guilty about not using extraordinary means to keep someone alive; be at peace, it's okay for them to die when nature's timing has come. While everything about death is touched by ambiguity ("it could have been different") and even by the mystery of eternity, the clearest possible assurances and norms are necessary because so many people do feel a vague spontaneous guilt before the mystery of death.

There are three groups of people to be considered in a suicide: the survivors (be they family or friends), the possible facilitator of an assisted suicide, and, most importantly, the patient near death contemplating the necessity to end the pain. For the survivors, understanding the uniqueness of another's pain and limitations and why the suicide happened, is the necessary first step before consolation and healing can develop in the grief process. So much of grief is love unfinished, and one often has cause to feel guilty about that incompleteness. An important and creative antidote, good for Christians and so many others, is that the love is so dynamic that it *will* go on for all eternity, that one can look forward to rejoining the beloved in that community of perfect love where there is no more pain nor prejudice.

The surviving family will, for their own peace of mind, grasp at the thought that the suicide victim saw no other viable alternative. A criterion from the lore of the moralists is helpful for an ethics of suicide: When dealing with a genuine dilemma, the most important question is, What is the *viable* alternative? This brings us to the awareness that real dilemmas are not a choice between good and evil, between what to do and not to do on the basis of what is good, but rather are usually a reluctant choice between the lesser of two relative evils, one of which must be humanely chosen. Suicide is always an evil when evaluated against personal and community love and growth issues, but it is sometimes perceived as the lesser of two evils by those involved when compared with dementia or such great pain that one can neither grow with it nor profit from human contact. On the other hand, the surviving family may feel that there clearly would be more peace and less guilt if the patient had persevered in giving to and receiving from others the growth and love still available in the unfinished business of life.

The assistants in a potential suicide may take their first ethical cue from the person dying, who may insist that suicide is a better or necessary choice. However, if they truly want to be helpful in a work of charity and comfort, this question must be considered: Can they not find yet new ways to make this life not only endurable but worthwhile for their friend? If the dying one sees suicide as ethical and necessary, the potential facilitator, with different ideals, may or may not be ethically able to assist in good conscience. Because most ethical people are so oriented toward the positive, they will normally stand against suicide. The danger when persons with AIDS "accept death" by contemplating suicide is that their "acceptance" can go too far and disguise a despairing life-rejection which aborts the available hope and growth life still has to offer.

But what about voluntary euthanasia by the patient near death who views his living in pain or dementia as futile or even impossible? Can the proposed suicidal action of a living person be construed as constructive and consistent with the life values for which this person and this life have stood or have yet to stand? For we do presuppose that a certain common level of aspiring to be constructive and to make a good impression is true of human nature. Is suicide a disappointing undoing of those very values within that individual?

How then do we deal with the pressures pushing some persons with AIDS toward suicide? Our clear norm in the face of suicide is to accept life and growth for all they are worth.

Making life worth living. The underlying acceptance and valuing of life, seen by some as a gift from God, is no doubt the fundamental reason for opposing suicide. If this is so, then society must realistically raise the quality of life for its weaker members instead of simply rejecting the concept of suicide. Too often it is as if we hear society and the court telling the Elizabeth Bouvias[9] of the world, other sufferers in intractable pain, and persons with AIDS alike, "We the healthy find life worth living, or at least we can accept our relatively comfortable lot in life; therefore thou shalt also accept thine."

Rev. Harold Burris,[6] who arranges housing and care for homeless AIDS patients in Washington, D.C., said that none of his charges have committed suicide. His network, which provides companionship, recreation, all types of caring, even feeding for those who cannot feed themselves, and a clean and dignified place to live, seems to make the difference between hope and despair. This practical example of the ethics of helping the neediest of the sick and, therefore, of accepting the other is so successful that the stickier questions of suicide are obviated.

The real issue then for the counselor helping the patient to grow is how to make hope accessible. If the patient can be energized to pursue inner growth even through pain and suffering in the final days and to surmount the temptation to despairing suicide, a sense of personal dignity will surely follow. More important, such personal internal growth and its consequent ethical sense also contribute to the whole community's goodness and peace.

The natural fruition of human nature is to approach death in its natural biological timing, perhaps because one loves this life, this growth, these people, enough to stay here as extensively and as intensively as humanly possible. The principle of acceptance keeps even sick and weak patients accepting more life and growth here and now, doing something positive and creative with life's darker moments.

Actions of Others Accepting the AIDS Patient

Medical and Religious Idealism and Denial

Many doctors and nurses, clearly overburdened, are doing all they possibly can for AIDS patients; they are genuinely courageous and dedicated to improving the quality of individual life.[10] After the families and the medical community, the religious community is perhaps the next most vitally interested and caring group—witness Mother Teresa's newest home for homeless terminally ill AIDS patients in Washington, D.C. And yet, in the psychodynamics of denial and acceptance, because acceptance is so difficult to attain, these three groups (families, medical, and religious communities) with most at stake are, not surprisingly, also the first *loci* of predictable denial.

Institutional idealism (we see a ready example in the church) by its very nature will predictably deny the individuals ill with AIDS in its own ranks—idealistically they don't exist. Perhaps more surprising than the natural first stage of institutional denial is the often unfounded presumption that the dedication and idealism of caregivers (clerics or physicians, for example) should make them immune to the deviations from monogamy or celibacy that increase the risk of AIDS. In the real-life contradictions that exist, there is a logical and necessary distinction between the universal *ideal* with the limitations in its stance and its language on the one hand, and the individual members, some of whom will engage in less than ideal behavior on the other hand. It is helpful to see the moral failings behind personal cover-ups or denials of AIDS that occasionally occur among doctors or clergy for what they are: personal failures to live up to an ideal and not therefore an issue of ethics, assuming that this individual is not infecting or influencing others. In every individual case known to this writer and his sources, personal affliction renders that doctor or cleric more compassionate and helpful, a better ethical person who reaches out to help others.

Public Policy and Sex Education: Acceptance of Basic Realities

Taking the truth—and the facts of life and death—in stride seems not yet possible in our puritanical society that is not mature enough to deal openly with the sexual education of its youth. How, then, will society deal with the challenge presented by Surgeon General Koop who proposes,[11] among other things, a more frank and thorough sexual education of school youth to help prevent the further spread of AIDS? What value is to be put upon the personal prudishness and reluctance to speak of such sexual facts to one's children when society is faced with a deadly unchecked epidemic? Embarrassment or squeamishness about the *education* regarding sexual *facts* and practices has little religious standing or moral valence when measured against the "principle of the common good," the overwhelming religious imperative of charity and courage involved in protecting a population from a deadly virus. But lest the specter of sex (including use of condoms) education in public schools loom too large on the horizon as the only means necessary to reach the Surgeon General's health goals, there must also be opportunities for, as well as respect for, the classic involvement of parents in instilling their personal values which foster abstinence and monogamy. Both public and parental education are types of acceptance (as opposed to denial) of sexual truth, an acceptance into which this society has yet to grow. By comparison, children of many other cultures, in past and present history, sleep in one room with parents, witness childbirthing, and know more about the facts of life and death and, consequently, cope more naturally and healthily with these realities than American youngsters. Future generations might well credit the AIDS epidemic with finally ending the puritanical period of this country in this one regard.

Families and Churches

Families sometimes dispossess their own members because of AIDS. Counselors find an interesting pattern among family members of male homosexuals with AIDS. Blood sisters of persons with AIDS are the all-time winners for loyalty in visiting their sick brothers. Next, it is the lovers and friends who remain steadfast. In the middle range are the patients' mothers. Male family members have the most severe reactions against homosexually transmitted AIDS; the fathers and, least supportive of all, the blood brothers are too often found to be most devoid of sympathy and understanding.

Churches are like families in their idealistic rejection patterns. One interpretation says that those Christian churches with a history of rejection or fear of sex outside its traditional place in marriage have been the slowest to come forward in activating their theories of Christian charity. It is no paradox that their rigid human morality inhibits their human charity. To their shame, Christian churches still drag their feet today in proportion to the sexual connotations associated with AIDS. An ethics of acceptance would rise above any putative sexual origins of AIDS (which in any event is not true for increasing numbers of cases of infected needle, blood transfusion, or perinatal transmission). Why or how someone became sick is completely beside the point of their needing care. Assuming punishment and guilt as an explanation of misfortune is a throwback to a theology outmoded by the Book of Job; it is misguided and found incorrect by Jesus (John IX, 3). Especially in a Christian system proclaiming brotherhood, only compassion and holistic healing are to the point.

Schoolchildren seem to be in less danger from infected children than is indicated by the intense response of emotional parents ignorant of the medical facts about AIDS. The very atmosphere and purpose of a school is precisely for absorbing basics of science and ethics and learning how to cope wisely and successfully with the realities of life, which may include such serious medical (and other) difficulties. An ethics of acceptance envisions a society, beginning in our elementary schools, that is wisely aware of AIDS and how to avoid its dangers; a society that is helpful, holistic, and hospitable; a society that insists on accepting reality by living and coping, facing and mastering it.

"But I Might Catch It!"

We who are the "others," the caretakers, fear becoming the newest persons with AIDS; hence our hesitancy in working with or accepting these sick individuals into our lives. An ethics of acceptance has a two-pronged response: information and inspiration.

First, to allay fear, one will seek wisdom and information. Media reports about AIDS are usually our most frequent sources of information (or misinformation) about this epidemic. Ethical problems immediately arise since the very nature of much of the media seeks sensationalism. We, the public, should be aware both of the media's shortcomings and of accurate medical facts. With an ethics of acceptance, we want the whole truth.[12]

Second, as a people valuing this gift of struggling humanity, we remind each other of one of our culture's true heroic stories. Exactly one century ago Damien de Veuster, the Belgian priest who volunteered to live forever with the lepers of Molokai (Hawaii), began his famous sermon with "We lepers . . . " He was stricken with leprosy only after some 20 years of serving in utter poverty, lacking even simple hygiene. Sister Marianne and her followers who continued Damien's work determined that they would take hygienic precautions; not one of them ever caught leprosy even though they served as nurses for decades. Damien remains for both the medical and the religious communities an outstanding historical and psychological study of creative acceptance leading to personal peace and dignity.

AN ETHICS OF ACCEPTANCE: A SUMMARY

WHAT To Do?

Ethics is, in part, about actions—thoughtfully chosen, value-laden actions that we *do*. For a terminal patient, there is the serious work of acceptance—or preparing for death—by coming to peace with oneself and one's family and friends. For society, there is holistic healing to be done and loving care to be given to the sick and dying patients. A nonmoralizing stance is essential for communication between the person with AIDS and the caregiver. Both can then become more creative, exploring a vision for filling the time remaining. Thus patient and society can strive together to maximize the peace, love, and hope in each other. While these endeavors have been often based in visionary ideals found in religious models, the actual implementation is in reality, as always in ethics, going to admit of a yet broader range of thoughtful ethical choices.

WHOM To Care For?

Those who see themselves committed to new personal and societal growth through such an ethics of acceptance would care, in whatever ways needed, for *everyone*, no illness excluded. To put it more strongly: We reach out to care, not in spite of the nature of AIDS, but precisely because the very need attracts such caretakers. Since religions are institutions of idealisms, the "official church position" on how one views AIDS patients is known more accurately from its charter documents and its macro-history than from any individual deviants. Thus any classical Christianity—and certainly its ancient Catholic core (occasional uninformed or insecure bishops and priests notwithstanding)—firmly repudiates the recent fundamentalist cant of looking down on the homosexual as having incurred a punishment from God in the form of AIDS. Although a large group of sincere Christians do espouse this "punishment" explanation of AIDS, the most basic law of universal charity and their own scriptures make an even more fundamental demand: "Do not judge lest you be judged." Another older Christian approach drew a distinction between the sin (to be rejected) and the sinner and his sickness (to be accepted and cared for). An even more basic distinction is shown in the adage, "Love the sinner but hate the sin." Doing this demands some creative growth in society, and will lead to the necessary distinction whereby one can choose to reject the homosexual lifestyle, neither encouraging nor condoning it, and at the same time mercifully accept and tend to the sick person.

Priests and ministers have expressed fears of status loss if they even mention AIDS from the pulpit in any compassionate way. They fear for their jobs and their respect, as if they might be thought to "condone the sinner," when they really mean to encourage imitating the mercy of Jesus the Healer.

Christianity has sometimes been called a study in the history of heresies, better known for its aberrations from its idealism than for its excellent fulfillment. Perhaps the AIDS crisis shows society's latest insecurity (before both the gay lifestyle and the disease), an imbalance that results in harsh treatment of the sick. To better buttress ourselves in the Christic courage to care for all the sick, it should be remembered that Jesus was harsh on only one type of sinner—the Pharisee who in his righteousness was harsh on others. Preferring mercy, Jesus refused to be led into conversing about any individual's sin as he always denied any consequent punishment by calamity,[13] unlike so many of his followers who become eloquent about the sins of others and conclude by punishing them.

Those of good will who may have hesitated to reach out in caring to the homosexual person with AIDS should be reassured by the knowledge that Jesus (see John IX, 3) rejected the claim that misfortune (of the blind man in this case) is punishment for sin, saying that such infirmity is there "so that the glory of God might be revealed," which occurs whenever we step in with healing and compassion to create new hope and new life.

WHO Does The Caring?

Everyone who can does the caring, as the recent hospice movement of putting patients back into the homes also shows. Within Christian ethics, when patience grows thin and there is temptation to give up, the caring person ideally is transfused with a renewed awareness and motivation of vitally functioning in the community of the corporate Christ. At this moment of weakness, some are strengthened by identifying themselves as Christic caretakers, doing what Jesus would do, thereby etching out further delineations of their own heaven-bound personalities.

WHY?

Why does one accept the AIDS patient and do so with such a creative acceptance that leads to caring? In Christian traditions there are three reasons: (1) self-transcendence in (2) an archetypal truth and (3) a great history proving the first two. Throughout history, religious motivation has proved to have a very firm constancy and resolve. For centuries, thousands of hospital nuns consistently kept at their loving care when few others would, creating the first international system of hospices, and giving witness to what a powerful ethic human nature can indeed achieve. Small wonder that mainly those with heroic or supernatural motivation would do this work, for the nature of the medieval contagions often meant that the caretaker had to be ready to die with her patient. Their self-transcendence was two-fold: it's worth it to die because there is heaven beyond death and because this patient here before me participates in being not just a mere individual, but is bonded to that vital organism which achieves its heights in the "body of Christ." Both caretaker (facing possible infection and death altruistically) and patient fit into the archetype of Christ on the cross. Patients frequently approach death with the perennial question, "Why must one go through this?" They are helped to transcendence by an archetypal model ("Christ showed that the normal way to glory is through such suffering"). This simple vision sparked tremendous creative growth in self and in caring for the neighbor: the truth and work of the universal Crucifixion goes on day by day—that is, the ongoing necessity to help others (and self) live and die well on the way to eternal life with God and community.

CONCLUSION: A CONSCIOUSNESS OF COMPASSION

Acceptance is a concrete structure of hope. What we have experienced with AIDS is only the tip of the iceberg—not just in the quantity of cases, but also in the nature of the challenges facing hospitals and hospices, the caring and acceptance structures in the future. A qualitatively different energy based in greater love, humanity's strongest point, will be asked of all members of human society.

What can we hope for? An ethics of acceptance gives a consciousness of compassion that can always transcend the fear of communicability of disease. Like Elisabeth Kübler-Ross struggling to care for AIDS children today, so too were Damien of Molokai and Mother Teresa moved by a qualitatively different love, an I—Thou energy of caring which inspired each with a vision whereby nothing could be more important than compassionate solidarity with the afflicted. They lived out an ethics, a principled thoughtfulness guiding their actions, tapping a deeper energy that changes the world.

Persons with AIDS rely on this compassionate energy. This spiritual energy becomes an ethical principle from which creative actions flow. Acceptance is the first step in actualizing our vision, the ground of our being who we most deeply are. Holistic healing of both patient and society is then the goal of an ethical principle of acceptance.

Ethics, as well as the whole human race, will have failed in its ideals if science alone vanquishes AIDS while strong and healthy persons ostracize and neglect their weak and ill fellow beings. There is every hope that, with an ethics inspiring so many caretakers to stay by the bedsides, the sick, in their hour of growth and of need, will find us truly brothers and sisters, truly ethical and creatively accepting.

NOTES

1. Our focus here, unlike the empathic *Newsweek* article cited in 10., which centered on a lovable, innocent female social worker and mother with AIDS, will be primarily on the more typical AIDS patients whom society blatantly rejects on the basis of homosexuality. Although this writer subscribes to nonsexist language, since virtually all AIDS patients referred to in this chapter are male, it will be both accurate and efficient to refer to them with masculine pronouns. We will also be focusing on the United States.

2. Cf. Hellwig, Monika. *What Are They Saying About Death and Christian Hope?* NY: Paulist, 1978 and Teilhard de Chardin, S. J., on how a mystic views his own death in *The Divine Milieu.*

NY: Harper & Row, pp. 89–90. See also Karl Rahner, S. J. *On the Theology of Death*. NY: Herder, 1961.

3. Farrow, J. *Damien the Leper*. NY: Doubleday Image, 1954, pp. 97–98.

4. Fitzgerald, F. "A Reporter at Large: The Castro-II" *The New Yorker*, July 28, 1968, pp. 44–63.

5. Conference with Joseph Izzo, M.S.W., Whitman Walker Clinic, Washington, D.C.

6. Conference with Rev. Harold Burris, Whitman Walker Clinic, Washington, D.C.

7. Beauchamp, T., and Perlin, S. *Ethical Issues in Death and Dying*. Englewood Cliffs, NJ: Prentice Hall, 1978; Hellwig, M. *What Are They Saying about Death and Christian Hope?* NY: Paulist, 1978; Maguire, D. *Death by Choice*. NY: Doubleday, 1974; Lebacqz, K., and Englehardt, H. T. "Suicide and the Patient's Right to Reject Medical Treatment." In *Death, Dying, and Euthanasia*, edited by Horan, D., and Mall, D., Frederick, M.D.: University Publications of America, 1980, pp. 669–705.

8. *Acta Apostolicae Sedis* 49 (1957), pp. 1031–1032.

9. Elizabeth Bouvia is the name of the quadriplegic women in southern California who petitioned the courts (at first unsuccessfully) to discontinue her forced feeding and to allow her to die of the natural consequences of her MS by which she could not feed herself.

10. See the inspiring story by Goldman, P., and Beachy, L. "The AIDS Doctor," *Newsweek*, July 21, 1986, pp. 38–50.

11. *Journal of the American Medical Association* 256 (Nov. 28, 1986), pp. 2784–2789.

12. The broader range of journalistic ethics is well described in Check, W. "Public Education on AIDS: Not Only the Media's Responsibility." *Hastings Center Report*, August 1985, Special AIDS Supplement, pp. 27–31.

13. John VIII, 6; John IX, 3; Luke VII, 39; Luke XV, 32; Luke XIX, 7.

32

Literature and AIDS:
The Varieties of Love

Laurel Brodsley

INTRODUCTION

AIDS is a frequently lethal disease, usually sexually transmitted. By its very nature, it raises a fundamental question. When the most intimate act of sexual expression becomes deadly, how can people, using our common phrase, "make love"?

Recently, a series of stage, television, and film dramatizations have helped us understand how our definitions of love are challenged by AIDS. In *An Early Frost*, parents reestablish loving support of their son suffering from AIDS. In *As Is*, an infected man confronts the loss of his promiscuous sexuality and learns to accept a monogamous and nurturing relationship. *The Normal Heart* portrays a leader in the battle against AIDS who loves truth but lacks political tact. In *Parting Glances*, the AIDS patient weighs his love for life against the inevitable anguish of a miserable death. In the Los Angeles-based theater-piece, *Aids/Us*, AIDS patients, their partners, parents, children, and counselors, voice their individual response to the nature of love under the challenge of this condition. Through these and other works, authors are sharing with all of us the special nuances of love among people suffering from AIDS.

We also have another source to help us understand our feelings, behavior, and alternatives when faced with this terrible disease. Our legacy of great literature offers examples of delicate and insightful explorations of every parameter of human relationships. While the original topics could not be AIDS, throughout history people have battled terminal illness, confronted handicaps, withstood terrible plagues, and come together to weep and to celebrate.

Literature can offer immense comfort. Dr. Gerald Friedland, the leader of the AIDS treatment team at the Montefiore Medical Center in New York, mounted on his office wall a quotation from Camus' great novel, *The Plague.*

> So that he should not be one of those who hold their peace but should bear witness in favor of those plague-stricken people; so that some memorial of the injustice and outrage done them might endure; and to state quite simply what we learn in a time of pestilence: that there are more things to admire in men than to despise. He knew that the tale he had to tell could not be one of a final victory. It could be only the record of what had had to be done, and what assuredly would have to be done again . . . by all who, while unable to be saints but refusing to bow down to pestilences, strive their utmost to be healers.[1]

[1]Reprinted with permission from Albert Camus: *The Plague*, p. 278, Stuart Gilbert, Trans. Copyright © 1972, Alfred A. Knopf, Inc.

Dr. Friedland placed it near his desk, he told reporters from *Newsweek*, as a credo, "a rationale for carrying on a struggle whose only outcome for doctors was burying the dead" (Goldman and Beachy 1986). The journalists' description of Dr. Friedland's work, his patients, and his staff, is permeated with echoes from Camus, whose great work can give shape and meaning to our responses to AIDS.

I will discuss how three works of art portray love under tragic circumstances analogous to those of AIDS. In Shakespeare's sonnet #71, "That Time of Year . . .," a dying man enjoins his lover to see his illness and death clearly, and through this process of honest perception, enhance their love. John Milton's religious poem, "When I Consider How My Light Is Spent," addresses the crisis of a sudden and devastating loss of physical function and its effects on his secular commitments and his love for God. Camus' *The Plague* demonstrates, among so many other insights, how men can express love for each other, their community, and God, through their dedication to conquering disease. Great literature can help us understand the meaning of relationships when our sexuality and our very survival are threatened by AIDS.

WILLIAM SHAKESPEARE'S SONNET #71, "THAT TIME OF YEAR"

Shakespeare's sonnet "That Time of Year" is a love poem spoken by a dying man physically ravaged by disease. Terminally ill, yet possibly quite young, he addresses his beloved, a woman or a man, who has known his past glory and stands by him at his final demise. Aware of his condition, the speaker expects no pity; instead, he simply requests that his beloved accept and understand his condition, and through this act of perception, their love will be increased.

SONNET #71 (ca. 1595)

That time of year thou mayst in me behold
When yellow leaves, or none, or few, do hang
Upon those boughs which shake against the cold,
Bare ruined choirs where late the sweet birds sang.
In me thou see'st the twilight of such day
As after sunset fadeth in the west,
Which by-and-by black night doth take away,
Death's second self that seals up all in rest.
In me thou see'st the glowing of such fire
That on the ashes of his youth doth lie,
As the deathbed whereon it must expire,
Consumed with that which it was nourished by.
This thou perceiv'st, which makes thy love more strong,
To love that well which thou must leave ere long.

This poem, in itself, is especially poignant for AIDS victims and loved ones. The speaker, like so many victims, is a man of talent and accomplishment, for his body, now a "bare ruined choir" was one "where late the sweet birds sang." His time on earth has been reduced from the promise of a full life to one of a season, or a night, or the last moments of a brief and dying fire. Yet, in the midst of his disease and its inevitable conclusion, his beloved has remained at his side, a witness to both his earlier glory and his present decay. The poem's mood radiates a sense of tenderness, beauty, and compassion, as the two partners mutually accept their terrible plight and comfort each other through the power of their love.

The reader is immediately moved by the poet's evocation of visual beauty, even while describing illness and decay. The opening four lines, with their description of autumnal trees, has an elegance not unlike a Japanese print. The bough, the few, lightly tinted leaves, the entwining patterns of the bare branches, create a pattern which is permeated with light and space. The analog of ruined choirs evokes a glimpse of historical ruins with their rich suggestion of past civilization and glory. The sweet birds who once sang recall the poet's earlier productivity and art. Thus even as his illness wastes his frame, it also reveals more ancient, and essential, contours of his body and spirit, through space and time.

The poet then compares death to sleep, his passing to a sunset. Yet the sunset which fades in the west points to the black night which will come, reminding us also of the day we enjoyed. Death itself, while sealing us off from life, also brings rest.

In the comparison of life to a fire, the speaker delineates the paradox of death-in-life and life-in-death. The fire, even as it consumes him, glows with vitality. The ashes which now snuff out his life were the product of his former glory. His very illness, like that of AIDS, was a product of his youthful energy, vigor, and love.

The final couplet reaffirms the poet's relationship with his partner. Their love grows in inverse proportion to the decay of his flesh, almost as if it were purified through the falling away of the dying man's earthly existence.

Shakespeare's sonnet exquisitely transforms the agony of decay into an intensity of love, through the power of perception, understanding, and truth. As such, it can act as an inspiration and model for AIDS patients and their companions, for they too seek to understand, accept, and maintain their love through the ravages of this disease.

Shakespeare also hints at another aspect to this relationship. The speaker, with his emaciated body, fragile flesh, and shaking limbs, is a dying man. The beloved, who sees, perceives, and finally, must leave, is intact. Together, they are maintaining a bond within the constraints of this tragedy. The beloved is staying by his lover, nurturing him, caring for him until the end when he must relinquish him to death. In this tender relationship between the weak, dependent patient and his strong, able caretaker, both accept the harmony and appropriateness of this bond—the dying man without shame, the beloved, without qualms. Hence this pem offers a model for loving care by those confronted with AIDS. The beloved honestly perceives the frailty and needs of his or her partner; the partner, in truthful assessment of this disease, welcomes the concern, care, and compassion of the companion.

Shakespeare's theme of nurturance is being explored anew by contemporary writers on AIDS. *As Is* portrays the challenge of two lovers renegotiating their relationship from one of sexuality to nurturance. in *AIDS/US* one speaker describes his loving care for his partner and how, a year later, a vision of this bond formed during his caretaking becomes a spiritual epiphany which helps him to accept this disease.

Thus, as we see in both Shakespeare's poem and many patients with AIDS, partners are accepting the responsibilities of a nurturing kind of love. They maintain an unconditional acceptance of their weakened partners. And the patients learn to accept this care, without resentment or shame. As Shakespeare reveals through his verse, honesty, autonomy, and maturity are possible even within a physically unequal relationship. It is not sexuality, but compassionate perception and acceptance of the truth of the disease, "which makes thy love more strong."

JOHN MILTON'S "WHEN I CONSIDER HOW MY LIGHT IS SPENT"

Shakespeare speaks of the loving companionship between partners, even as one of them is dying. Milton, in his religious sonnet "When I Consider How My Light is Spent," questions the personal meaning of an illness and its devastating psychological, political, and spiritual effects. Reason and logic cannot provide meaning for such a catastrophe, but an understanding of God's love for all men, including those stricken by disease, can help us accept our condition and survive.

WHEN I CONSIDER HOW MY LIGHT IS SPENT (1655)

When I consider how my light is spent
 Ere half my days, in this dark world and wide,
 And that one talent which is death to hide,
 Lodged in me useless, though my soul more bent
To serve therewith my Maker, and present
 My true account, lest he returning chide;
 "Doth God exact day-labor, light denied?"
 I fondly ask; but Patience to prevent
That murmur, soon replies, "God doth not need
 Either man's work or his own gifts; who best
 Bear his mild yoke, they serve him best. His state
Its kingly. Thousands at his bidding speed
 And post o'er land and ocean without rest:
 They also serve who only stand and wait."

As the poem opens, Milton attempts to comprehend, through the use of logic, the meaning of his terrible disease. Yet as his "considers" his predicament, he faces a paradox. His worth, as an individual and within the scheme of God and his country, resides in his capacity to share his talents with the world. Without sight, unable to read or write, his life seems devoid of meaning. How could God both demand that he express his genius, yet deny him the health to do so?

Milton's question is shared by most patients suddenly overwhelmed by a catastrophic accident or disease: "Why did I get this disease?" For many AIDS patients, the answer is painfully clear: they engaged in "unsafe" practices which transmitted the HIV virus. But for others—wives of hemophiliacs, partners of IV drug users or bisexuals—their only "fault" was to "make love." Logic and reason cannot bring meaning to Milton's blindness nor to the disease of AIDS.

As the poet refers to his own life, a deeper significance is suggested. For Milton, the foremost spokesman for a revolutionary government, the question "Why me?" refers not only to his personal but his public achievements. He had devoted his life to defending a political and ethical system which was anathema to other nations. If his work was curtailed by his blindness, all that was gained by his efforts might be destroyed and his society might return to its previous oppressive practices. Handicapped by disease, his work would stop, and the promise of his achievements would come to naught.

The analogy between Milton and leaders in the AIDS support community is painfully apt. So many have devoted years to freeing homosexuality from cultural and legal restraints and are now dedicating their lives to battling AIDS. This virus is killing some of its most prominent and talented members, and as more and more people die, both the individual achievements of gay leaders and the acceptance of the gay community itself are threatened.

In his poem, Milton perceives that reason alone is impotent. Through the intervention of Patience he turns to the wonder of faith. God does not value men only for their work or their talents; people have worth simply by being themselves. Milton accepts God's love, which he will receive even if he cannot live according to the tasks God had decreed for him. Likewise, he must learn that God accepts all men, no matter what kind of life they have led.

Similarly, some AIDS patients are realizing that their lives are not valuable only because they do important work or serve a fine cause. Merely being human is good enough. Many are learning to accept themselves, even with their disease. And others, empowered through the ordeal of their illness, are discovering a higher power which sanctifies their lives.

Milton reveals a man confronting the personal, political, and spiritual consequences of his unexpected and devastating disease. He found solace through his acceptance of God and his faith that patience and love would be sufficient. He coped successfully with his blindness, and years later produced one of the greatest poems in English canon, the religious epic, *Paradise Lost.*

At this point in the AIDS crisis, the homosexual community as well as the nation at large cannot know the outcome to this terrible epidemic. Milton reminds us, however, that the group, if not the individual, has the power to survive. New leaders will arise: some will defend homosexual rights, others will develop new treatments or perhaps discover a vaccine or cure for AIDS-related disorders. As Milton says, there are thousands who will accomplish the necessary tasks. For those who cannot, "They also serve who only stand and wait." We must have faith in our love for God and in His love for us. Strengthened by this spiritual relationship, we can overcome the challenge of AIDS.

ALBERT CAMUS' *THE PLAGUE*

Camus' *The Plague* (1947) portrays a world devoid of Shakespeare's intimate love or Milton's spiritual commitment. The town of Oran is ugly and materialistic, concerned only with the immediate gratifications of money and pleasure. Its citizens lack any values that would give meaning to illness and death. For Camus, the plague, as horrible as it is, will offer this community an opportunity to transcend its petty existence. Through men's honesty in the face of terror, their compassionate moral choices, and, finally, their commitment to their fellow men, they will achieve a new awareness of the meaning of life and love.

In a curious way, the havoc wrought by our modern-day plague, AIDS, is forcing our culture also to redefine its values, behaviors, and ethics. Oran is not unlike our own towns and cities. We also have refused to face the devastations of sickness or the trauma of death. Camus' plague-ridden world speaks directly to us.

The abrupt quarantine of Oran initiates the process of the citizens' redefinition of love. Husbands are separated from wives, parents from children, lovers from their partners. In a chapter of exquisite lyricism, Camus describes how the townspeople suffer with their terrible sense of loss. As the support and comfort normally available through family and intimate friends are withdrawn, the people are left desolate and alone. As the memories of their beloveds fade, their sense of the past, their hopes for the future, and their very identities wither and die. Bereft of intimate relationships, they feel like the living dead. Some even welcome infection by the plague as a reprieve from their meaningless lives.

Although we do not have a formal quarantine system in America, we do have intense, informal pressures which isolate people with AIDS from the support normally granted to people with handicaps, illness, or terminal disease. Despite the fact that AIDS is not generally contagious, except through the exchange of body fluids, its victims may be shunned as if they were pariahs, denied the rights of education or employment, armed service or the sacrament. Our culture has not yet come to understand how isolation affects our capacity as individuals or as a community to love.

In the circumstances of a plague, people must create new patterns of love. For Camus, alternative forms are neither religious, as for Milton, nor private, as for Shakespeare. Instead, Camus suggests a more abstract kind of devotion: a commitment to truth, compassion, and moral action. Camus' words for these types of love, "abstraction" and "friendship," refer to the love of truth and love for one's fellow man. They do not relate to individual benefit but to public good.

Our American culture, with its focus on individual rights and repressive moralistic policies, inhibits the development of programs to serve the greater community. Educational programs on AIDS transmission and prevention, which must reach a broad spectrum of our citizens, are attacked by clergy and politicians for their content, values, and advocacy of the use of condoms. Mass screening for AIDS is seen as a violation of individual rights of privacy. Distribution of sterile needles is rejected because this may seem to "condone" illegal intravenous drug abuse.

Our model of private health care and insurance, which is dependent upon the individual or his employer's ability to pay, is threatened by the growing number of AIDS/ARC patients. When people who are seropositive are denied coverage and public health care funding is tight, AIDS/ARC patients may find that—in a country which prides itself on its health care—they cannot receive medical services at all (Oppenheimer and Padgug 1986).

The process of shifting health care from individual patients to the group is a difficult task. In *The Plague*, when Dr. Rioux identifies the obscure disease as the plague and suggests public health measures, he is faced with general denial and rage. Recognition of the disease and implementation of essential measures would bring severe economic and political consequences for the town. In the face of this criticism, Dr. Rioux insists that public officials must sacrifice private needs and act out of a love for truth to best serve the needs of the town.

Similarly, the homosexual community was initially reluctant to face the truth of AIDS, its mode of sexual transmission, and the identification of gays as the primary high risk group. In both Oran and our own cities, only after intimate friends had died from the disease did people accept the necessity of public, rather than private, responses. Ironically, as AIDS now moves into the IV drug user and heterosexual communities, we are again resisting what needs to be done.

An honest perception of the truth is only the first step in our confrontation with a plague. Camus demands that individuals must next make a moral decision to act. In his novel, each character, finally acknowledging the lethal nature of the disease, nevertheless dedicates himself to serving his community. As individuals, they do not even consider themselves heroes. Dr. Rioux narrates, "It's a matter of common decency . . . It consists of doing my job." This commitment to acting for the common good is even more powerful than the ties of romance. Rambert, who must choose between his mistress and the town, discovers that men may not be capable of dying for love, but can be fully prepared to die for an idea. Panaloux, the priest who initially preached that the plague was God's punishment for the town's sins, now has a vision of God's love, and dies, dedicating himself to helping his fellow man.

Camus insists that love demands a total surrender to the service of others in the face of this terrible disease. Cottard, the only "villain" in the book, seeks selfish rather than communal ends. His behavior is presented not as evil, but as lacking Camus' moral values of "abstraction" and "friendship." Cottard had "an ignorant, that is to say, a lonely, heart."

In America, we are coming to recognize the importance of community services for AIDS. In the major cities, men and women are creating humane educational, support, and treatment programs to serve the needs of seropositives, ARC and AIDS patients, and their loved ones. Some medical centers are shifting from expensive and private health care plans to ones which can satisfy both individual and community needs. AIDS patients themselves are sacrificing their precarious health status to work on hot-lines, serve on counseling groups, give public performances, and participate in medical experiments, so they can help others who may now or in the future have AIDS. Slowly, policies based on love rather than fear are helping AIDS sufferers, homosexual and heterosexual alike.

Camus, like Shakespeare, also demonstrates that "Agape," love for our fellow man, as well as "Eros," or sexual desire, can be expressed through individual and communal relationships. Dr. Rioux and his helper Tarrou, through their discussions and actions, demonstrate their love for the truth and for their community. As they combat the plague together, they also become intimate friends. Near the end of the story they take a few hours off from their work. Together, they wander to the beach, then, wordlessly, swim into the sea. Here, in a passage of lyric beauty, Camus portrays the loving intimacy of the two men. Soon afterwards, Tarrou succumbs to the plague and Dr. Rioux nurses him throughout his illness and stands by him at his death. His grief for Tarrou is intense: the loss of a true friend is irreparable.

Dr. Rioux's and Tarrou's model for intimacy was not a romantic, sexual, or sacred union, although their vision of peace touched upon spiritual revelation.

In its quiet intensity, their love is closest to the acceptance and comfort a mother gives her child, or in Shakespeare's sense, a beloved gives his partner. True friendship transcends the fear of personal death. It supports the partner through every ordeal, nurturing him when he is sick and comforting him in his dying. This love is beyond words; it is a silent devotion.

From Camus, we can learn that in the crisis of a fatal disease like the plague or AIDS, romantic and sexual love become less relevant. Instead, an opportunity arises allowing men and women to achieve a higher kind of intimacy and meaning through their selfless commitment to the welfare of others. From this communal interaction comes a love for the truth, for moral action, and for spiritual peace that directs and enriches our lives shattered by crisis, disease, and death. Of all actions, the most exquisite, intense, intimate, and painful, is the loving care of a dying friend.

BIBLIOGRAPHY

Camus, Albert. *The Plague* (1947). Translated by Stuart Gilbert. New York: Vintage Books, 1972.

Goldman, Peter, and Beachy, Lucille. "One Against the Plague." *Newsweek* 115:3, July 21, 1986, pp. 38–50.

Hoffman, William A. *As Is*. New York: Vintage Books, 1985.

Katz, Michael, *AIDS/US*. Unpublished play, Los Angeles, 1986.

Kramer, Larry. *The Normal Heart*. New York: New American Library, 1985.

Oppenheimer, Gerald M., and Padgug, Robert A. "AIDS: The Risks to Insurers, The Threat to Equity." *Hastings Center Report* 16:5, October 1986, pp. 18–22.

33

The Malignant Metaphor:
A Political Thanatology of AIDS

Michael A. Simpson

In that country if a man falls into ill health or catches any disorder or fails bodily in any way before he is seventy years old, he is tried before a jury of his countrymen and if convicted is held up to public scorn and sentenced more or less severely as the case may be. But if a man forges a check, or sets his house on fire, or robs with violence from the person, or does any such things as are criminal in our own country, he is either taken to a hospital and most carefully tended at the public expense, or if he is in good circumstances he lets it be known to all his friends that he is suffering from a severe fit of immorality, just as we do when we are ill, and they come and visit them with great solicitude—for bad conduct, though considered no less deplorable than illness with ourselves, and as unquestionably indicating that something is seriously wrong with the individual who misbehaves, is nevertheless held to be the result of either pre-natal or post-natal misfortune.

Samuel Butler was writing in Erewhon,[1] over one hundred years ago, of a mythical land where criminal behavior is seen as sheer bad luck, while illness is wicked and deserves punishment. The tendency to cossett criminals, and to view them as "sick" rather than conceivably ever "bad," has increasingly been built into many legal systems, especially the American. Now the second part of the prophecy is coming true.

AIDS has become the most political of diseases: a contagion within a stigma within a prejudice. Just as OPEC ended the era of cheap energy, AIDS has ended the era of cheap sex.

With this incurably fatal disease doubling its victims every six months, alarmed projections point out that if it continued at such a rate, it would within a decade kill everyone in the USA, and in a further decade would kill everybody on earth ten times over. Since the age of nuclear weaponry and planned megadeath, such projections look less fanciful than they might have, once.

The other image that recurs in recent writing is the medieval Great Plague. In many historical records, the period of the Black Death, especially from 1348 to 1352, is simply a blank. Monastic chronicles tend to pause at the same point. If any entry appears for the year 1349 it tends to be the same words: *Magna mortalitas.*

Such colorful images are understandably popular in the purple prose[2] that has accumulated in recent years—for sheer vividness they effectively stimulate the sense of *Schadenfreude*, the sheer "isn't it *awful*" titillation enjoyed by those who enjoy the horror of others.

Susan Sontag[3] has written vividly and effectively of the metaphorical uses of illness—and AIDS has the perfect characteristics to make an especially powerful metaphor. It is intractable, incurable, deadly, when Medicine is supposed to be

397

able to cure or control everything. It is insidious, sneaky, implacable, ruthless; the secret agent that lurks within, biding its time before it strikes; a wicked, all-powerful predator.

Such diseases, as Sontag emphasized, "will be felt to be morally, if not literally contagious." How much more powerful the literally contagious disease, so closely identified with morally controversial causes, seen as arising from morally condemned activities, and arising from body parts and actions embarrassing for society to acknowledge! AIDS has followed the course Sontag delineated for such conditions, "awash in significance." The disease becomes identified with "the subjects of deepest dread"—decay, pollution, death, weakness, corruption—and then itself becomes a metaphor. Then it is used as a metaphor, to describe and typify the horror of other matters. "The disease becomes adjectival" in Sontag's fine phrase. "Something is said to be disease-like, meaning that it is disquieting or ugly." So it has been with AIDS—it makes its appearance in bad jokes ("What's the hardest thing about having AIDS? Trying to convince your Mom you're Haitian"), then, literally, in the writing on the wall. Next it is used in popular speech ("Why are you all avoiding him? Anyone would think he had AIDS!"); and finally in literature.

Pollution and stigma are related so much more to some causes of death than to others. AIDS joins a robust heritage of horrors. Tuberculosis used to be thought to be caused by "too much passion, afflicting the reckless and sensual." Others through that its successor, cancer, was a disease "of insufficient passion," arising in those who are sexually inhibited, repressed, inactive. The tuberculous were sexy, as the Romantics exploited the aesthetics of cruelty, and the beauty of the morbid as Mario Praz[4] so eloquently described. Tuberculosis, however, gave a spiritual, ethereal, redemptive death—even to the morally questionable. Victorian literature is teeming with the tidy, peaceful, good deaths of the tuberculous, especially the pure and pious children. Syphilis, on the other hand, was a morally polluting disease that could give a dirty death even to noblemen.

We have grown unused to the experience of major epidemics not amenable to technological control. In 1983 (oddly ignoring AIDS) William McNeil[5] wrote that a major difference between us and our ancestors, profoundly different from earlier ages, "is the disappearance of epidemic disease as a serious factor in human life. Nowadays, if a few score of people die of an infection, officials declare an epidemic." If the male chauvinist ignores the woman's point of view, here is the voice of the Western chauvinist. Though it accurately reflects a popular point of view in the West, it is inaccurate. In the unheard Third World, what the West would consider epidemics are part of the routine burden of the people. Even in the West, new diseases aren't a novel experience—Burkitt's lymphoma, Legionnaire's disease, Toxic Shock syndrome, Congo Fever, Lassa Fever, O'nyong nyong fever—have all emerged in recent decades. Those most Westernly in their impact, like Toxic Shock syndrome and Legionnaire's disease, were quite rapidly brought to heel. This century has seen a similar scale of afflictions, even in the USA. In 1918, Spanish flu killed 400,000 Americans, with an average age of 33 years. The polio epidemics throughout the fifties struck down large numbers of the young, too, and similarly led to anxious scrutiny of self and loved ones for the stigmata of the peril.

There has often been international political chauvinism in the naming of such afflictions—Spanish Flu, Asian Flu, Mao Flu. The English disease Syphilis has been, in its time, called the French Pox (Morbus gallicus), and the Spanish, Portuguese, Italian, Neapolitan, Burgundian, German, and Polish disease, and so on. AIDS hasn't yet been given a clear nationality. Haiti was damaged by a reputation for harboring it, and African nations have been keen to avoid being blamed for its origins. Black[6] has perceptively pointed out how "Americans take perverse delight in being proud of their flaws; and many in the United States have adopted AIDS as the national disease. If it's a terrible plague, it must be ours." The Russians were reputed to like to think they invented things first (though they have notably failed to lay claim to AIDS); Americans like to think that their version is bigger, better, more awful, more something or other, than anyone else's.

There are marked similarities between the ways in which society responded to previous plagues and pandemics, and the way in which modern society is reacting to AIDS; and much may be learned about potential future social developments by a study of the past. A neglected area of study has been how some epidemics have been clean of metaphorical contamination and moral contagion. Some pandemics—Malaria, Yellow Fever, Diphtheria, Polio—have been relatively unencumbered by such muddling excess baggage. But others have aroused responses familiar to the AIDS crisis.

Plague itself, which became an immortal metaphor for contagion,[7-20] showed three great waves of infection and death—around the sixth century A.D., in the fourteenth century, and in the late nineteenth century through to the Second World War (the latter mainly in China and Asia, though it also became endemic among rodents in the Western USA during that time). The plague's early symptoms—fever, malaise, fatigue, large glands, other infections—were not unlike those of early AIDS, and were similarly perfect material for hypochondriasis and panic—sweats, dry cough, skin blotches—all are easy for almost anyone to perceive and fear that they are infected. Self-scrutiny and monitoring for the fatal stigmata are and were common, just as in the 1950s the child who had "overexerted" himself and had a headache, gave rise to fears of Polio. But Bubonic Plague killed within one to five days, unlike the stealth of AIDS.

The first pandemic, Justinian's plague, led to what contemporary sources and historicans including Gibbon considered to be 100 million deaths. Modern historians estimate a lower total—but, still, the death of 20–25% of the population. With accompanying diseases, social disruption, and wars, the population in many parts of Europe fell by 50% between the sixth and eighth century. Arab sources describe major outbreaks in the seventh century. The Moslem religious leaders at the time saw the plague as sent by God as a mercy and martyrdom for the faithful, a direct invitation to Paradise. (For the infidel, it was merely a horrid death with no consequent benefit.)

The second great pandemic, the Black Death, has led to controversy over its origins, similar to that over the roots of AIDS.[21] An early outbreak among Tatars besieging a city illustrated the political uses of infection—they used catapults to lob the corpses of plague victims over the citadel walls, leading to the plague spreading to the Christians within (an early example of the use of germ warfare and of lethal missiles!). Around 25–30% of the population of Europe died; in some cities 50–60%, though the Pope received a curiously exact report that 47,836,486 had died in Europe! There were recurrent outbreaks in succeeding centuries, often (as in the Great Plague of London in 1665) affecting individual cities catastrophically. A Papal Bull of 1348 proclaimed that the Black Death was "the pestilence with which God is afflicting the Christian people" (though medical opinion at the time favored an astrological explanation), a sign of God's displeasure with the extent to which people were ignoring His commandments.

One writer[22] has suggested a connection between social reactions to the Black Death and the emerging hostility towards homosexuality within the Middle Ages. The early history of prejudice is not well documented,[23] but a major historian of this field, Boswell,[24] considers that the homophobic hostility arose well before the fourteenth century plague. Early psychology at times favored the view that suppression of desires was dangerous. Kant, in *Anthropologie* (1798)[25] wrote that "The passions are . . . unfortunate moods that are pregnant with many evils," and that "He who desires but acts not, breeds prestilence." In the late sixteenth and seventeenth centuries it was popularly believed that "the happy man won't get plague." Latterly, it seems, the gay man can.

There certainly was a connection between the Plague and anti-Semitism. As has so routinely been the case in epidemics, "people blamed their enemies for propagating it,"[26] and blamed those marginal in society. Very early in the cycle, lepers had been blamed for poisoning the wells. The lepers blamed the Jews. From around 1348 in France, a wave of anti-Semitism, with the extermination of Jews in over 350 individual massacres in Europe, spread widely; the waves and ripples of that orgy of anti-Semitism have not yet stilled.

The Black Death led to a useful stress on cleanliness and hygiene, and a social move towards the restraint of passionate excess. There was also a desperate search for wierd and complex treatments. The class bias was opposite to that of AIDS—the well-to-do were less afflicted, being less crowded and more able to avoid infection.

Leprosy was another instructive example.[27] It actually had a relatively low mortality and was not as highly infectious as popularly believed. But its cruel capacity to cripple and disfigure lead to a disproportionate degree of horror and social scapegoating.

One explanation for the expulsion by Rameses II of 90,000 Jews from Egypt was that they harbored "a disgraceful disease," probably leprosy. Leprosy, too, was seen as a corruption, the consequence of sin, unclean and wicked. Lepers lost the right to marry, to inherit, to protection, to religious participation. They were segregated to colonies or lazarettos, and had to be marked by special clothing, and to warn others by sounding bells or clacquers. There was the "Leper's Mass"[28] in which the leper was declared "dead among the living," the subject of a form of requiem mass, and symbolically buried alive, while socially dead. Saul Nathaniel Brody wrote eloquently in *The Disease of the Soul*[29] that "The leper was by turns the object of vilification and of sympathy. A physician could assure the leper himself that his disease was a sign that God had chosen to grant his soul salvation, but he might simultaneously include in his diagnosis that his patient was morally corrupt." The Church might similarly decree that leprosy was a gift of God, but its bishops and priests would nonetheless use the disease as a metaphor for spiritual degeneration. The leper was seen as sinful and meritorious, as punished by God and as given special grace by Him.

In fact, the Church seems less simultaneously ambiguous than Brody depicts. The Church appears to have played a leading part in the exclusion and stigmatization of the leper until the Crusades. Once Crusaders began to return with what appeared to be leprosy, contracted in the Holy Land, the Church began to recall Christ's Compassion, and converted leprosy into a holy disease, and the lepers into "Christ's poor." The "Leper's Mass" ceased.

Cholera[30-33] was pandemic in the nineteenth century, and millions died from it. It, too, was seen as the result of the commonness of sin in society. The rich feared the poor, who in turn felt Cholera to be an agent of oppression, even a conspiracy to destroy them. Riots and social turmoil accompanied earlier epidemics, even in Paris, London, and New York.

But before AIDS, no major disease has so richly and obviously linked sex and death and personal behavior as *syphilis* (before antibiotics).[34] Syphilis, too, arrived as a mysterious epidemic, previously unknown, spreading rapidly while physicians could do nothing to cope with it. Wide epidemics were seen in Europe in 1494–1497. A popular theory claims that the sailors with Columbus brought it back from the Carribean. Reports of no signs of syphilis in old world skeletons prior to 1493, but in Amerindian skeletons 500 years earlier, would support this view. Like AIDS, syphilis may indeed have been a donation from the Third World to the Old World. As we've seen, the nations of Europe hastened to name it and blame it on each other. It was, obviously, seen as a punishment "on the parts of shame" for dissolute excess; and the Emperor Maximilian I of the Holy Roman Empire declared that it was Heaven's punishment on blasphemers, reminding us that even where the sexual connection with the disease was fairly obvious, its moral meanings were seen as even wider and more serious.

Some writers[35] have claimed that widespread outbreaks of syphilis in Renaissance Europe were an important influence in the rise of Puritanism. The career of epidemic syphilis, like AIDS, has shown the typical pattern—the "moral panic," the shift from seeing the unfortunate events as a threat towards stereotyping victims as moral monsters, not worthy of human considerations, leading to an escalation of the perceived threat and to absolutist positions and postures, the popularity of extreme and repressive "solutions," and the compassionless moral burlesque of cruelty in the name of the compassionate Christ.

Syphilis accumulated a typically heavy accretion of metaphorical meanings as the grimmest of gifts—yet its uses as metaphor were slightly limited, as it wasn't seen as especially mysterious. Trotsky spoke of the syphilis of Stalinism, and there's a grisly harping on syphilis in *Mein Kampf*. The fears of "bad blood" and contamination have been revived by the risk of AIDS transmission by blood transfusions. Like the Jews and lepers accused of poisoning the wells, there have been wild rumors of people with AIDS deliberately contaminating blood supplies, and of "call-boys of death" in London, bitter at their fate, deliberately trying to infect as many people as possible.

The same proud persecuting prejudice has reared up with the AIDS epidemic as it did among the religious bigots who hunted the lepers, the plague victims, and the others. A shameful editorial in the *Southern Medical Journal* wrote with questionable medical ethics of the disease as "a fulfillment of St. Paul's pronouncement," and of its victims as suffering "the due penalty of their error." A self-congratulatory fundamentalist has complained of the spending of tax dollars to "allow these diseased homosexuals to go back to their perverted practices without any standards of accountability." Popular, snide jokes are, as ever, highly indicative of the slavering prejudices that underlie them. One refers to the disease as WOGS—the Wrath of God Syndrome. Another says "It affects homosexual men, drug users, Haitians, and hemophiliacs—thank goodness it hasn't spread to human beings yet." Black[36] quotes interviews, with one respondent saying "It's having a good effect on homosexual behaviour, causing them to be—um." (Interviewer: "Less promiscuous?") "No—Dead." And then there are those who say that they hope for a cure—but not too soon.

When one observes the relish with which the pious celebrate the suffering of the impure as divine retribution, one wonders what may be the divine punishment for heartlessness.

It is surely ironical that the perfect Right-Wing virus, with its fortuitous preference for stigmatized victims, made its appearance in the West at a time of Conservative government policies (Reagonomics, Thatcherism). Their support was in part a reaction to the "permissive" trend of the 1960s and 1970s;[37] their policies (slashing health and welfare spending) impaired the ability to respond to the new agent. Society's own "immune system" was impaired. During the search for the causative agent, for instance, biased thinking may have delayed progress. Early victims were identified as homosexuals, rather than according to what their actual behavior was, and a gay drug addict was usually listed as gay rather than as an addict. There is little doubt that had AIDS first become recognized in the USA as a plague exclusively killing Fundamentalist born-again WASPs, the response in terms of research funding and care programs for people with AIDS would have been very different.

Some have emphasized the novelty of the AIDS epidemic in the modern experience (in the West at least) as a cause of the selective death of large numbers of young men without the ideological justifications of war or church. But such a distribution of deaths is not unusual in this century, and Vietnam gave us the experience of a war lacking a consensus of justifying ideology and widely perceived as meaningless. Elliot[38] estimates that there have been some 100 million man-made deaths in the twentieth century. Admittedly, manmade death has tended to replace epidemics as the cause of megadeath. Back in 1972, Elliot commented drily that, "To this day there survives, amongst some of the well fed and cared for, a nostalgia for the slums of disease." That nostalgia has, by now, surely been fully indulged.

AIDS is as yet a long way from matching the carnage of the First World War. In Britain, some 6 million men fought, over half the adult male labor force—and 1 in 8 were killed, a further 1.5 million disabled. The war deaths, too, were concentrated in younger age groups. Of men 20–24 in 1914, 30.58% were dead; of those 13–19, 28.15%.[39] One calculated that if the British Empire's war dead marched four abreast down Whitehall, it would take them three and a half days to pass the Cenotaph that was their memorial. There are relatively few serious studies of the consequences of such patterns of mass death,[40,41] but they are very relevant when we consider the potential impact of AIDS. The war dead included a high proportion of the talented. The birthrate went up immediately afterwards, making good the losses numerically, before returning to its routine rate (an unconscious community healing effect, also seen following disasters like Abervan); but of course the qualitative loss was not so promptly recoverable. Will the AIDS losses prompt some similar increase in the otherwise wide trend towards lower birthrates in the West?

There is also a potential not only, as had already been demonstrated,[42,43] for a change in sexual behavior towards monogamy and more traditional forms of expression, but also towards less loving behaviors, if the projected high death rates occur and last. The historical experience has been that where mortality is high, there is reduced emotional involvement. As Aries said[44] in his study of the history of childhood, "People could not allow themselves to become too attached to something that was regarded as a probable loss." Stone, in a more formal study of the family, sex, and marriage in England 1500–1800[45] noted that "It is fairly clear that the reactive lack of concern for small infants was closely tied to their poor expectation of survival, and that there is on the average a rough secular correlation between high mortality and low gradient affect." Macfarlane[46] has suggested further ways to study this effect.

The First World War was followed, as AIDS was preceded, by a wave of interest in Spiritualism, with great popularity of books like *Life Beyond Death With Evidence*, just like the *Life After Life/Before/Between Lives* genre of the 1970s and 1980s which followed the Vietnam experience. The wide range of modes of public acknowledgment of the reality of the deaths and of their scale, was matched by private denial. Before World War I, spiritualism was diffuse and ineffectual. But influential figures like Sir Arthur Conan Doyle and the scientist Sir Oliver Lodge (both of whom had lost sons in the war) encouraged intense "scientific" interest (which was not scientific at all) in parapsychology.

There are other consequences of national consciousness of large-scale losses. After the First World War, detective novels became far more violent, bloody, and murderous—as did movies after Vietnam. Indeed, the extent of such effects of the AIDS pandemic may be less perceptible only because we are still seeing similar effects from Vietnam.

The constant relationship of death and sex shows in other ways, too. It has been argued that the more active sexual freedom of the 1920s was a response to the death of the earlier generation, and part of the drive behind the sexual hedonism of the 1960s to the 1980s may have had similar roots. The "Make Love, Not War" slogan of the Sixties has almost, in the Conservative Eighties, become "Make War, Not Love."

The relationship is an ancient one[47]—that soldiers, the more they feel close to the threat of death, feel driven into sexual activity. Julius Caesar flogged soldiers with symptoms of gonorrhea; Richard III had soldiers with "pox" hung. Promiscuous French soldiers under Louis XIII in Italy in the fifteenth century busily spread the new horror—the French evil, *il morbo Gallico*—syphilis. Wars have always needed busy anti-VD campaigns, stressing the mortal danger of sex. A notable British wartime poster showed a skull wearing a woman's exotic hat and orchid, saying "Coming *my* way?" and added "The 'easy' girlfriend spreads Syphilis and Gonorrhea which, unless properly treated, may result in blindness, insanity, paralysis, premature death."

Whatever the roots of the Sexy Sixties and Seventies, the Anxious Eighties might engender in some quarters the opposite of the safe monogamy advised just *because* of the very real risk of death. Costello[47] cites a G.I. saying "the typical soldier gives himself up for dead before he ever sees combat . . . so every woman might be his last . . . imagine what its like to make love while assuming that tomorrow you'll be dead." He also quotes a celebrated Madam during the

First World War as saying "I've noticed it before, the way the idea of war and dying makes a man raunchy, and wanting to have it as much as he could. It wasn't really pleasure at times, but a kind of nervous breakdown that could only be treated with a girl and a set-to."

The homosexualization of AIDS, and its stigmatization has had an obvious impact in slowing the extent and efficacy of our response to it. The happenchance that it first became noticeable among homosexuals led to an excessive focus on the search for uniquely homosexual causes for it, including what Jacques Leibowitch[48] called the "Sodom and Gonococcal" theory of causation. The overlapping complexities have been ignored: homosexuals who are addicts; the high incidence of prostitution and unsafe sex in addicts; the high incidence of addiction in prostitutes.

Spending on research was niggardly. The Centers for Disease Control (CDC) budget for AIDS in 1982 was $2 million. Yet in 1976, for the ludicrous "Swine Fever" fiasco, $135 million was hurriedly spent in order to fail to prevent a nonexistent epidemic of a very minor disease with a campaign which killed well people! But then Swine Fever was expected to have much more decent and vote-earning victims. The journal Science[49] complained petulantly of an "unprecedented spending spree" on AIDS research, due to the power of the U.S. gay community—contriving to be inaccurate, prejudiced, and unscientific, all at once.

As in previous major epidemics, bizarre conspiracy and "plot" theories have arisen, blaming AIDS on a chemical agent sprinkled on bathhouse floors, or added to KY jelly; or to a germ warfare agent that may have gone astray (or may even have achieved its intended purpose). Though obviously farfetched, one doesn't have to travel so far to farfetch something these days. We do now know that for two decades, the U.S. Army did explore the practicality of germ warfare by releasing what they thought to be harmless germs in U.S. cities, airports, and subways.[50]

As with other sexually related studies, there have at times been hints almost of jealousy and awe, as inhibited scientists and epidemiologists encountered the promiscuous and active. The virgin scientist encountering a group with a median of 1160 different sexual partners may have difficulty in comprehending the alternative lifestyle ("When do they have time to get sick?" asked an epidemiologist).

In Russia and Eastern Europe, where AIDS is considered a symptom of Western decay, there has been similar reluctance to admit to the potential extent of the problem. In December 1985, Prof. Victor Zhdanov in Sovietskaya Kultura admitted to ten cases in the Soviet Union, and an official estimate of 60 cases by the first quarter of 1986 is quoted. Sixty cases out of some 400 million people may represent an underestimate. Unofficial reports of AIDS death in Czechoslovakia have appeared, and in Hungary, antibody screening of blood donors, homosexuals, and drug addicts seems to have been in operation since January 1986. Again, an isomeric politicization of AIDS, identifying it with foreign decadence, may hamper the response to a biological Chernobyl.

The promiscuous were already well familiar with sexually transmitted diseases and infections—proctitis, urethritis, amoebae, hepatitis, shigella, worms, gonorrhea, syphilis, herpes, even lymphogranuloma venereum were accepted risks.

But "For those doing a sexual high-wire act, medicine was a safety-net."[51] Everything was felt to be already or imminently curable. Until AIDS, which rekindled the deadly risk of sex that had haunted us in previous centuries. The age of safe danger had passed.

I have written elsewhere in early work[52,53] towards a feminist thanatology, of the nearly universal and persistent relationship between women, sex, and danger. Over the ages, there was a persistently prejudicial emphasis on Woman as the historic cause of misfortune and mortality, the danger being ascribed to her insatiable, irresistible, but deadly sexuality and guile. Belief in the evil of woman was sustaining to the development of an all-male Establishment, and the long litany of lethal ladies popularly reinforced the message—Eve, Pandora, Salome, Jezebel, Lucrezia Borgia, Lilith, Kali, Astarte, Medea, Messalina, Circe, Delilah, and other grisly girls.

The association between sexual pleasure and danger is new to men (except for the Mors Syphilitica which was always blamed on the women); similarly new is the association between male sexuality and danger to men. Women[54] have long been subject to dangerous sex—the risks of pregnancy, childbirth, abortion, miscarriage, and the puerperium have limited woman's potential across the centuries. Heterosexual AIDS, the form which dominates the picture in Africa, may radically affect attitudes. Gay sex has been more experienced at encompassing dangers, with the risks of violence, police intervention, blackmail, and betrayal having been especially real in earlier decades. As there was some diminution in those risks, almost as if there had been some habituation to the added spice of danger and related condiments, there seems to have been a move towards higher risk sexual forms—promiscuity, physically hazardous acts, fantasized, simulated, or real sadomasochism. The risky and the risqué became blurred.

This sex/death margin remains barely explored. The Victorians, despite public ostentation in the matter of death and grief, had not, so the quieter and more intimate documents of history reveal, successfully come to terms with these eternals in their private lives. Similarly[55,56] they showed public prudishness and private prurience. But the popular view has persisted, as Cannadine has expressed it[57] of the "beguiling and nostalgic progression from obsessive death and forbidden sex in the nineteenth century, to obsessive sex and forbidden death in the twentieth." And just when we contrived in Western society to frankly rediscover death while still freely dealing with sex, what arrives? Lethal sex and sexual death.

The forbidden and dangerous can have a powerful appeal, as Nietzsche noted in the Wanderer and His Shadow[58]: "A prohibition, the reason for which we don't understand or admit, is almost a command not only for the stubborn but also for those who thirst for knowledge: we risk an experiment to find out *why* the prohibition was pronounced." The complex lifestyles of gay sex and of the intravenous drug addict have elaborately evolved, and maybe in some forms they have done so not despite the dangers, but in part because of the danger.

Behaviors that were proscribed and forbidden became politicized as acts of defiance against a resented repression. To some, it seemed important not just to have won the right to behave as one wished, but to exercise that right as frequently as possible, as if the more it was exercised the more free one was. In the original sense *Carnivals* were occasions to celebrate the temporary flesh while it still exists; *carne vale*, "farwell, meat." They could represent, as Black[59] has said, not just the orgy preceding the asceticism of Lent, but "Saturnalia before the endless abstinence of death."

Intravenous addicts have contrived to ignore their high-risk profession as effectively as men who work high on steel scaffolding or high-risk hobbyists like free-fall parachutists. The risk may have become not a barrier to overcome before deciding to take part, but a primary reason for doing so. Gay sex may come to incorporate premature death within the lifestyle, as black ghetto life has had to—for young black males in America, murder or drug overdose have been leading causes of death for some time. Gay culture has long included a powerful interest in eroticism and death—as seen in the works of Thomas Mann, Genet, Mishima, and Fassbinder.

Black[59] quotes a report that some sadomasochists are already eroticizing AIDS, viewing it as "the ultimate S-M trip: the thought that one might be pumping one's 'lovers' full of death . . . is considered 'hot.' " The same respondent claims that medical "scenes" during sex play have increased. So an alternative to abstinence or monogamy for some might become the deliberate seeking of the danger, gaining thrills by copulating on the brink of eternity. Apocalypse Wow!

Clearly, the epidemic will give life to both amateur and professional prejudices. It fits so well with the popular contagion theory of homosexuality and of drug abuse—the idea that social "deviants" somehow "recruit" or infect otherwise straight people, as if homosexuality or addiction were themselves viruses which could be "caught" (premises which the pro-censorship lobby would seem to inhabit.)

Just as one saw in the responses to previous plagues and epidemics, there are very serious threats to liberty. In various countries there have been instances of great risk to civil liberties: a man refused treatment unless he listed the people with whom he'd had sex; refusals to serve on a jury because the defendant had AIDS; police objecting to give breathalyser tests; patients being neglected in hospitals. There have been proposals to restrict international travel; to ban people with AIDS from airline flights; to forcibly administer tests for AIDS; enforced isolation of possible carriers; compulsory hospitalization. There's a report[60] that in New South Wales, Australia, it has been made a criminal offense "to knowingly infect someone with HIV."

As Black has said, perceptively,[61] "Draconian laws to control the spread of AIDS, which violate basic civil rights, may be more dangerous to the community than the disease itself." AIDS is being used by many as an excuse for a sexual counterrevolution, to discard not just unsafe behaviors, but as many as possible of the other changes wrought in the sixties (and somewhat overwrought in the seventies). Black sees the issue very clearly. "How one reacts to AIDS is a measure of what one believes about sexual pluralism—and, even more importantly, what one believes about the individual's freedom in all ways, not just sexual, to be different. AIDS tests how a society balances the rights of the few with the good of the many."

There are many similar issues bound up in these affairs. Black is brilliantly incisive in analyzing the Western scene in a rather Americo-centric way. In Africa, AIDS is not a minority problem, not a disease of the "others," of those already marked out for misfortune—it afflicts the majority.

Another issue, intertwined, is that of self-inflicted disease. Some argue that public monies should not be spent on people with AIDS, because "they brought it on themselves," because it is the direct result of something they chose to do, of their own free will. The issue of "free will" in relation to some of the behaviors involved is debatable. But there are entire specialties like Sports Medicine, with expensive facilities, devoted entirely to self-inflicted disease and self-inflicted injury. There has not been any serious protest against the gigantic cost to society of the disease caused by cigarette and tobacco addiction, and little concern with the high costs of alcoholism and recreational drug abuse.

Indeed, there has been a long tradition of allowing people to die in pursuit of fun. America even has a constitutional devotion to protecting life, liberty, and the pursuit of happiness—not the limitation of risk. And *their* pursuit of happiness, even if in ways that wouldn't make me happy, does not threaten my life or liberty. Unless I have sex with them or exchange blood with them, people with AIDS don't endanger me—unlike the smoker who pollutes my lungs and specifically damages my health, or the drunken driver who kills others. Analogous to the principle of informed consent to treatment or research, it would be preferable that people could make informed dissent, to make a behavioral choice fully informed as to the risks (especially when the benefit may be immediately obvious, and the risks late and hidden).

It is odd that societies that encourage the sale and promotion of death on the installment plan in cigarettes and alcohol, and prefer the sale of cars that operate most efficiently at illegal and dangerous speeds, should be so selectively interested in controlling other people's sexuality, whether or not it may limit a risk to themselves or others. Smokers know exactly what risk they are taking; people with AIDS are generally suffering the results of a risk undertaken when no one knew that the risk existed.

A Director of the National Institute for Human Sexuality in South Africa, Dr. L. I. Robertson, has reported an increasing number of inappropriate referrals from psychologists and physicians suggesting aversion therapy to "convert" homosexuals to heterosexuals, to "save them" from the risk of AIDS. To propose that people should fundamentally alter their sexual behavior is a far more major undertaking than giving up smoking or drinking. If one doubts that, it may be a homophobe response, assuming that an "abnormal" sexual identity is easy to give up, especially if it's good for one to do so. If a heterosexual finds (as many in Africa have) that this form of sex life is dangerous, how quickly and easily could they adapt to life as a homosexual? or a celibate? or switch to zoophilia? When syphilis made heterosexuality dangerous, very few people gave it up.

In fact, a surprising degree of adaptation seems to be taking place, with dramatic changes in sexual behavior recorded. As early as 1983 there were reports of a sharp decline in the number of partners and in the incidence of high-risk activities, and in the incidence of VD in various cities. In the 1960s a humorous magazine set a competition to define a new erogenous zone—and there wasn't a single response. Yet recently there have been trends towards nongenital stimulation, and an eroticization of nipples, massage, and condoms. Masturbation is showing a rising popularity and is less abused. The large U.S. sex industry seems to have shown some responsibility towards encouraging safer practices—certainly it has shown far more social responsibility than the tobacco industry has ever shown, anywhere.

Quite apart from civil liberties issues, there is the question of whether drastic legal responses actually help to control disease. Throughout history, governments have tended to fight epidemics with legislation and information.[62] Quarantine tactics across Europe did help to control the bubonic plague, from Medieval times. As recently as the turn of the century in San Francisco, a detention center was set up for plague victims, and there was talk of isolating or even burning Chinatown.[63] During the Cholera pandemics of the nineteenth century, emergency laws allowed for the compulsory isolation of victims and controlled burials, despite protests about the erosion of personal liberty. Compulsory admission to hospitals was enacted for infectious diseases. Some of the laws are still unrepealed in many states.

The Contagious Diseases Acts in mid-Victorian Britain (trying to avoid a defeat of the British Army by VD) allowed the authorities to detain any woman suspected of prostitution, and allowed compulsory medical examination and enforced treatment. But apart from their obvious appeal to those who like to feel that complex social problems can be forcibly solved, such measures have not been effective. It perverts the doctor-patient relationship when doctors must become informers and enforcers. It drove those most in need of help (for everyone's benefit) to avoid it rather than seek it. The Contagious Diseases Acts were a failure, and had to be repealed.[64] As Porter[65] has written in a wise summary of the experience of medical history, "If we begin to treat victims like criminals we alienate those whose co-operation is most needed and encourage them to behave like criminals; not least, we risk turning doctors into gaolers."

There is even room for an elegantly unpleasant interplay between the stress of a population being discriminated against, and the likelihood of contracting an infection and of succumbing to it. As I have shown in my review of behavioral microbiology[66] stress, especially if poorly coped with, can lead to changes in immunity, increased vulnerability to infection, and a potentially worse outcome of the disease. These effects are clearly demonstrated chemically and at a cellular level. It is still not clear why some people exposed to the virus develop an infection and others do not; or why only some of those infected by the HTLV-III virus develop AIDS. It is expected that numerous co-factors will be identified as contributing to the development of AIDS infection. Early studies of people with AIDS are beginning to suggest that they may indeed have suffered particularly stressful life events in the year before diagnosis and may express more guilt and unease about their sexual behavior (though it is far from clear that the latter is not an effect of the diagnosis, rather than its cause).

Clearly AIDS is likely to change the way we look at life. A generation or two had the easy illusion of safe sex. The general impression was that there were drugs to cure syphilis and gonorrhea, and Herpes didn't kill; the Pill seemed to be a safe way to avoid pregnancy. Drugs could be thought of as brave ways to explore one's inner self, and their risks due only to bad luck or carelessness. Though each of these beliefs were only partly true and often dangerously untrue, the drive towards finding completion in some substance or somebody external to oneself, was powerful. There was something as heady as any drug in the sharing of sex; something sexual in the insertion of shared needles. But the searches for completion now, more clearly than ever, can lead to dissolution and disaster instead.

As Porter has said:[67] "In contrast to smallpox, it takes two consenting partners to spread AIDS. The days of sex without responsibility are over. Responsible sex infringes no person's liberty. It is our only practical option."

REFERENCES

1. Butler, S. *Erewhon*. Harmondsworth: Penguin, 1970.
2. Britton, A. AIDS—Apocalyptic metaphor. *New Statesman*, March 15, 1985.
3. Sontag, S. *Illness as Metaphor*. New York: Farrar, Straus & Giroux, 1978.
4. Praz, M. *The Romantic Agony*. 2d ed. New York: Oxford University Press, 1951.
5. McNeil, W. *The Plague of Plagues*. The New York Review of Books, July 21, 1983.
6. Black, D. *The Plague Years: A Chronicle of AIDS, the Epidemic of Our Times*. London: Pan Books, 1986.
7. Webster, C., Ed. *Health, Medicine & Mortality in the Sixteenth Century*. Cambridge: Cambridge University Press, 1979.
8. Slack, P. Mortality Crises and Epidemic Disease in England, 1485–1610. In *Health, Medicine & Mortality in the Sixteenth Century,* edited by C. Webster. Cambridge: Cambridge University Press, 1979.
9. Gottfried, R. S. *Epidemic Disease in Fifteenth Century England: The Medical Response and the Demographic Consequences*. Rutgers, NJ: Rutgers University Press, 1978.
10. Rosebury, T. *Microbes and Morals*. New York: Viking, 1971.
11. Slack, P. *The Impact of Plague in Tudor and Stuart England*. London: Routledge & Kegan Paul, 1985.
12. Alexander, J. T. *The Bubonic Plague in Early Modern Russia: Public Health and Urban Disaster*. Baltimore: Johns Hopkins University Press, 1980.
13. Dols, M. W. *The Black Death in the Middle East*. Princeton, NJ: Princeton University Press, 1976.
14. Gottfried, R. S. *The Black Death: Natural and Human Disaster in Medieval Europe*. New York: Free Press, 198.
15. Pollitzer, R. *Plague*. Geneva: World Health Organization, 1984.
16. Ziegler, P. *The Black Death*. New York: Harper & Row, 1971.
17. Williman, D., Ed. *The Black Death: The Impact of the Fourteenth-Century Plague*. New York: Medieval & Renaissance, 1982.
18. Mullett, C. F. *The Bubonic Plague and England: An Essay in the History of Preventive Medicine*. Philadelphia: Porcupine Press, 1977.
19. Dyer, A. D. The influence of the bubonic plague in England. *Journal of the History of Medicine and Allied Sciences* July 1978, 308–376.
20. Schrewsbury, J. F. D. *A History of Bubonic Plague in the British Isles*. Cambridge: Cambridge University Press, 1971.
21. Norriss, J. East or West? The Geographic origin of the Black Death. *Bulletin of the History of Medicine* 51:1 (1977).
22. Lancaster, R. What AIDS is doing to us. Christopher Street (New York), 1983, no. 75.
23. Gerard, K., and Hekina G. eds. *The Pursuit of Sodomy in Early Modern Europe: Male Homosexuality from the Renaissance through the Enlightenment*. New York: Haworth Press, 1986.
24. Boswell, J. *Christianity, Social Intolerance and Homosexuality*. Chicago: University of Chicago Press, 1980.
25. Kant, I. *Anthropologie*. In *Kant Werke: Akademie Textausgabe Preussiche Akademie der Wissenschaft*. Hawthorne, NY: De Gruyter, 1986.
26. McGrew, R. E. *Encyclopedia of Medical History*. London: Macmillan Press, 1985.
27. Dols, M. W. Leprosy in Medieval Arabic medicine. *Journal of the History of Medicine and Allied Sciences* 34:314–333 (July 1979).
28. Simpson, M. A. Thanatology, Death & the Middle Ages. Keynote address, Durban Conference, Medieval Society of South Africa, July 7, 1986.
29. Brody, S. N. *The Disease of the Soul*. Ithaca, NY: Barker, 1974.
30. McGrew, R. E. *Russia and the Cholera, 1823–1832*. Madison, WI: University of Wisconsin Press, 1965.
31. Pollitzer, R. *Cholera*. Geneva: World Health Organization, 1959.
32. Morris, R. J. *Cholera: Eighteen Thirty-Seven*. New York: Holmes & Meier, 1976.
33. Delaporte, F. *Disease and Civilization: The Cholera in Paris, 1832*. Cambridge, MA: MIT Press, 1986.

34. Crosby, A. W. *The Columbia Exchange. Biological and Cultural Consequences of 1492.* Westport, Ct: Greenwood Press, 1972.

35. Lancaster, R. *What AIDS Is Doing to Us.*

36. Black, D. *The Plague Years.*

37. Moorcock, M. *The Retreat from Liberty: The Erosion of Democracy in Today's Britain.* London: Zomba Books, 1983.

38. Elliot, G. *The Twentieth-Century Book of the Dead.* London: Allen Lane, 1972.

39. Winter J. M. Some aspects of the demographic consequences of the First World War in Britain. *Population Studies* XXX:541 (1976).

40. Winter, J. M. Britain's 'Lost Generation' of the First World War. *Population Studies* XXXI:450 (1977).

41. Cannadine, D. "War and Death, Grief and Mourning in Modern Britain." In Whaley, J. (Ed.) *Mirrors of Mortality*: *Studies in the Social History of Death,* edited by J. Whaley. London: Europa Publications, 1981.

42. Burton, S. W.; Burn, S. B.; Harvey, D. et al. AIDS information in Scotland. *Lancet* 2:1040–1041 (1986).

43. Judson, F. N. Fear of AIDS and gonorrhoea rates in homosexual men. *Lancet* (1983).

44. Aries, P. *Centuries of Childhood.* New York: A. A. Knopf, 1962.

45. Stone, L. *The Family, Sex and Marriage in England, 1500–1800.* London: Weidenfeld & Nicholson, 1977.

46. Macfarlane A. "Death and the Demographic Transition: A note on English Evidence on Death, 1500–1750."In *Mortality and Immortality: The Anthropology and Archaeology of Death,* edited by S. C. Humphreys and H. King. New York: Academic Press, 1981.

47. Costello, J. *Love, Sex and War, 1939–1945.* London: Pan Books, 1986.

48. Leibowitch, J. *Un Virus Etrange Venu Diailleurs.* Paris: Grasset, 1983.

49. Kolata, G. Congress, NIH open coffers for AIDS. *Science* July 29, 1983, 436.

50. *Washington Monthly,* July-August 1985. Cited by Black, D. *The Plague Years.* London: Pan Books, 1986, pp. 174–175.

51. Altman, D. *AIDS and the New Puritanism* London: Pluto Press, 1986; Altman, D. *AIDS in the Mind of America.* New York: Anchor Press/Doubleday, 1986.

52. Simpson, M. A. Death and Ideology: Political Thanatology and the "Femme Fatale" Syndrome. Monograph, Seminar in Contemporary Cultural Studies, 6-CCSU, University of Natal, Durban, South Africa, October 1985. (ISBN 0-86980-474-x).

53. Simpson, M. A. *Femme Fatale.* London: Quartet. 1988, in press.

54. Shotter, E. *A History of Women's Bodies.* London: Allen Lane, 1983.

55. Harrison, B. Understanding the Victorians. *Victorian Studies* X:239–262 (1966–1967).

56. Pearsall, R. *The Worm in the Bud: The World of Victorian Sexuality.* London: Penguin, 1983.

57. Cannadine, D. War and death, grief and mourning in modern Britain.

58. Nietzsche, F. "The Wanderer and His Shadow." In *Complete Works,* by F. Nietzsche. New York: Gordon Press, 1974.

59. Black, D. *The Plague Years.*

60. Porter, R. History says no to the policeman's response to AIDS. *British Medical Journal* 293:1589–1590 (1986).

61. Black, D. *The Plague Years.*

62. Porter, R. History says no to the policeman's response to AIDS.

63. Trauner, J. The Chinese as medical scapegoats in San Francisco, 1870–1905. *California History,* Spring, 1972.

64. McHugh, P. *Prostitution and Victorian Social Reform.* London: Croom-Helm, 1980.

65. Porter, R. History says no to the policeman's response to AIDS.

66. Simpson, M. A. Stress and Infection—Towards a Behaviorial Microbiology. *Infection Control,* August 1986, pp. 8–9.

67. Porter, R. History says no to the policeman's response to AIDS.

VII

AIDS AND THE COMMUNITY

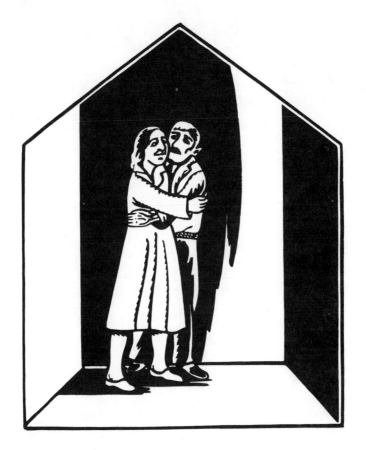

AIDS and the Community
A care giver embraces a person with AIDS.

34

AIDS and Public Health

John C. Moskop

INTRODUCTION

Just 2 years after its first identification in 1981, acquired immune deficiency syndrome (AIDS) was declared the No. 1 priority of the U.S. Public Health Service.[1] Dr. Mervyn Silverman,[2] former San Francisco director of health, has called AIDS "the most complex health problem of the century" (p. S22). One would have to have been a very well isolated hermit over the past 5 years not to have some awareness of the tremendous public concern about AIDS. This paper will give an overview of public health issues surrounding this disease. First, at the risk of belaboring the obvious, it will very briefly offer several reasons why AIDS poses both serious and complex public health problems. Second, it will review a number of public health measures that have been adopted or proposed and comment on their moral dimensions.

A SERIOUS AND COMPLEX PROBLEM

Let us recall why AIDS is both a serious and a complex public health problem. A disease becomes a public health issue when it poses a serious threat to a whole community or society. To pose such a threat, the disease must have at least the potential to be both severe and widespread (we do not adopt significant public health measures against acne or athlete's foot, despite their prevalence, or against very rare but fatal genetic diseases, despite their severity). AIDS easily satisfies both of these conditions. Ongoing research efforts have not yet produced an effective therapy or vaccine, and thus the case fatality rate for AIDS remains virtually 100%,[3] with a mean survival time after diagnosis of 13 months according to one study.[4] Furthermore, human immunodeficiency virus (HIV), the virus that causes AIDS, has been widely disseminated across the United States since its introduction in the late 1970s. Some 50,000 AIDS cases had been reported to the Centers for Disease Control (CDC) by the end of 1987, and more than half of these patients have died. This is only the tip of the iceberg, however, since approximately 250,000 suffer from AIDS-related complex (ARC), and 1–1.5 million Americans have HIV infection. By 1991, the cumulative number of AIDS patients is expected to reach 270,000.[5] Finally, the annual cost of medical care for AIDS patients is expected to rise from $1.6 billion in 1986 to $10.8 billion in 1991.[6] Although this figure still represents only a small percentage of total U.S. health care costs, the rapid increase in the cost of caring for AIDS patients will put a significant strain on major public and teaching hospitals, which care for a large percentage of AIDS patients.[7] It will also, of course, be a financial catastrophe for patients without adequate health insurance.

These facts should persuade us of the seriousness of the AIDS problem and justify the common use of terms like "public health emergency"[8] and "epidemic"[9] to describe it. They also suggest reasons for the complexity of the problem. Most importantly, because we lack the "easiest," most effective methods for controlling the virus, namely a vaccine or cure, we must rely almost entirely on measures designed to modify personal behaviors that are likely to transmit infection. For AIDS, as for every public health problem, there exists a range of possible measures that extend from encouraging voluntary behavior changes to imposing rigid control over behavior. Although effective voluntary programs are clearly preferable, many have questioned whether efforts to promote voluntary changes in high-risk behaviors alone can bring this "public health emergency" under control.

Some have recommended additional measures that would limit personal privacy and individual freedom of action. However, such measures are problematic from a moral point of view, because they require the subordination of one set of fundamental values—individual privacy and freedom—to another—public health and safety. Moreover, because 90% of current AIDS victims are gay men and intravenous drug abusers,[10] the major burden of invasive or coercive public health measures against AIDS would fall directly on them. Such measures could significantly worsen the serious problems of discrimination and stigmatization they already face. In a recent article in the *New England Journal of Medicine*, Mills et al.[11] argue that "AIDS poses the most profound issues of constitutional law and public health since the Supreme Court approved compulsory immunization in 1905" (p. 931).

PROPOSED PUBLIC HEALTH MEASURES

We move now to a review of specific measures that have been adopted or proposed to control the spread of AIDS. Included are programs or proposals in the following eight general areas: (1) public education; (2) distribution of sterile needles; (3) screening and treatment of blood, blood products, and other tissues; (4) voluntary and mandatory screening of persons for evidence of infection; (5) reporting; (6) contact tracing; (7) isolation or other restrictions on freedom of movement or association; and (8) physical marking of persons with AIDS. These areas will be discussed in order, roughly, of decreasing justifiability, although significant moral issues arise within each one.

Public Education

By providing a good understanding of what AIDS is, what it can do, and how it is transmitted, education seeks to encourage people to change their behavior so as to minimize the risk of acquiring or transmitting the disease. Like informed consent to health care, public education about AIDS can achieve the praiseworthy goal of enabling individuals to make important life choices based on adequate and accurate information about the consequences of those choices. Almost no one denies the value of AIDS education, but differences of opinion do exist about *who* should be educated and *how* such education should be provided.

The most obvious candidates for educational programs are those who are at highest risk of acquiring the infection—gay and bisexual males, hemophiliacs, intravenous drug users, and sexual partners of members of these groups. Health education programs designed for specific groups have been developed in San Francisco, New York, and other cities, often through the cooperative efforts of public health departments and gay-rights organizations. Disputes have arisen, however, over both the content and format of such programs. Consider, for example, the following exchange in the *American Journal of Public Health*. Citing the high percentage of infection among gays in several cities and the resultant probability of exposure to the virus conferred by even a few high-risk sexual contacts, Handsfield, of the Seattle-King County Department of Public Health, argues that "gay men should be advised to abstain from all but monogamous sexual activity in permanent, committed relationships. 'Safe sex' guidelines, for new or casual partnerships should be presented only as a distinct second choice."[12]

McKusick and colleagues of the University of California at San Francisco reject this proposal as unrealistic and argue instead for less stringent recommendations, which gays are more likely to carry out successfully.[13] Which is preferable—recommending strict limitations on sexual activity to which most gays will not conform, or recommending behavior changes more likely to be adopted but less likely to prevent infection? The answer will presumably depend on the actual number of persons whose behavior is changed in the recommended way by each approach and the actual risks of the recommended behaviors. It may, however, be very difficult to gather that information.

Some have opposed sexually explicit AIDS education materials on the grounds that they condone morally repugnant behaviors such as homosexuality, prostitution, and IV drug abuse. This position may provide a kind of moral satisfaction, but the fact that many will continue to engage in these practices suggests two serious drawbacks. First, condemning high-risk individuals and abandoning them to ignorance about how to protect themselves suggests a lack of compassion for the potential victims of a devastating disease. Second, this approach will likely fail to bring the epidemic under control.

Perhaps even more controversial is the role of AIDS education for low-risk groups, such as students and the general public. Because many students will confront decisions about sexual activity and drug use during school years or shortly thereafter, classroom teaching offers an opportunity to inform them of the foreseeable consequences of those decisions. Recent reports by the Institute of Medicine and by Surgeon General C. Everett Koop have emphasized the need for sex education that includes information about AIDS in elementary and secondary schools.[13,14] Many others, including Secretary of Education William Bennett, are much more reticent about providing such education in schools, presumably on the grounds that it will encourage sexual activity and drug use among young people.

Finally, what about AIDS education programs for the general public, like the National AIDS Test broadcast in October 1987 on network television? Given the current extent of infection, such programs may make only a modest contribution to preventing the spread of the disease, but they may also perform several other valuable services. In particular, they may allay the unfounded fear that AIDS is transmitted through casual contact and thus help to counteract widespread misinformation in the popular press. Laying such irrational fears to rest may help to reduce the ostracism, discrimination, and stigmatization suffered by AIDS patients, infected persons, and, to a lesser extent, all gays and IV drug users.

Distribution of Sterile Needles

Despite its obvious importance, however, education alone may not be able to change high-risk behavior enough to bring the AIDS epidemic under control. One population that may be very difficult to reach by means of educational campaigns is intravenous drug users, since many members of this ill-defined group have dropped out of the mainstream of society to pursue their illegal habit, and drug addiction may impair their ability to understand or respond to educational appeals. Thus, public health authorities in New York have proposed a different kind of preventive measure for drug users, namely, programs for the exchange of sterile needles and syringes for used and possibly contaminated equipment, since this is thought to be the major vehicle of transmission of HIV in this group. Questions can be raised about both the efficacy and justifiability of this approach. It will be effective only if easier access to needles motivates users to change established needle-sharing practices. Three countries, the Netherlands, the United Kingdom, and Australia, have reported initially encouraging results with limited needle exchange programs.[16] A more serious objection to providing access to sterile needles is that it will encourage drug abuse, a hazardous and criminal activity. This is a real danger, but in view of the rapid spread of infection among drug users and the potential for further spread of the virus from this group via sexual and perinatal routes, providing sterile needles may still be justifiable as an emergency measure. Just as important, it should be noted, are increased efforts to prevent addiction and to treat all those addicts who desire to overcome their habit.

Screening of Blood, Blood Products, and Other Tissues

The development of screening tests and other measures that can prevent the spread of virus through transfusion and transplantation represents the first important success in the control of AIDS. Because current screening methods identify the presence of antibodies to HIV and these antibodies do not appear until several weeks after infection, there is still a minute risk of being infected by a blood transfusion.[17] For this reason, blood banks have continued their practice of asking that individuals in high-risk groups refrain from donating blood.

Although screening tests were first used primarily for the protection of the nation's blood supply, they also provided information about the infection status of each individual donor. Thus, screening undertaken to identify infected blood and testing to determine the infection status of individuals are really two sides of the same coin.

Voluntary and Mandatory Screening

As the new screening tests were about to be released to blood banks early in 1985, many persons barred from donating because they were members of high-risk groups voiced a desire to find out their infection status. Under pressure from these groups, the federal government provided funding for alternative testing sites across the country to provide testing apart from blood donation.[2] Current CDC guidelines stress the importance of counseling all those tested to ensure that they understand the implications of both positive and negative results.[18] A highly controversial issue for these voluntary screening programs, however, is whether to provide screening anonymously. This is current practice in several states, including California, but not in other states, which require identification but promise confidentiality. Only if those tested are identified can they be contacted for follow-up. Public health officials argue that such follow-up contacts are essential for providing new information, gathering epidemiological data, and, if appropriate, pursuing contact tracing.

The value for epidemiology of data from follow-up contacts with the relatively small, self-selected group of persons seeking voluntary testing will be quite limited. Moreover, as I will argue shortly, contact tracing is probably not a justifiable practice in this context. Most importantly, requiring identification may greatly inhibit high-risk individuals from seeking testing, despite their desire to know their infection status. Gays, especially, have voiced their fear that despite promises of confidentiality, positive test results may come to be used against those tested. Unfortunately, the explicitly homophobic attitudes of a number of public officials lend at least some credence to gays' mistrust of government intentions toward them. Kenneth Wing, for example, has suggested that recent enforcement of laws against sodomy may be a harbinger of increasing legislative and judicial attacks on sexual privacy.[19] The U.S. Supreme Court has recently confirmed Wing's prediction by upholding a Georgia law that makes sodomy a crime.[20] The Court ruled in this case that the constitutional right of privacy does not apply to homosexual activity. In the wake of this major setback for gay rights, public fear of AIDS may easily serve as a rallying point for further legal attacks on gays. Thus, no matter how it occurs, breach of confidentiality resulting in public dissemination of a positive test result is likely to have dire consequences for the person tested, including loss of job, loss of health insurance, and social stigmatization. Perhaps very strong guarantees of confidentiality can minimize these risks, though it may be difficult to convince lawmakers to provide such guarantees or to convince individuals at risk that confidentiality will be maintained.

If nonanonymous *voluntary* screening is difficult to justify, the prospects for justifying mandatory screening must be much bleaker. Nevertheless, in his first major speech on AIDS, delivered in May 1987, President Reagan called for mandatory testing of federal prisoners and immigrants and routine testing of applicants for marriage licenses.[21] By routine testing, Reagan meant a general practice of premarital testing which strongly opposed individuals could decline without legal penalty. State legislatures are very interested in premarital HIV testing; as of July 31, 1987, 79 bills on the subject had been introduced in 35 states.[22] Three states, (Illinois, Louisiana, and Texas) have already enacted statutes concerning premarital screening, and another state, Utah, prohibits marriage to a person who has AIDS.

The effectiveness of such mandatory and widespread screening programs in curtailing the spread of AIDS, however, has been widely challenged by public health scholars. In a recent study in *JAMA*, for example, researchers projected the consequences of a policy of universal mandatory premarital screening in the United States.[22] They concluded that such a policy would require annual screening of some 3.8 million people, at a cost of $100 million, to detect 1219 HIV-infected persons, less than 0.1% of those infected in the United States. Moreover, because of limitations of the tests, some 130 infected persons would be told that they were not infected, and almost 400 persons without HIV infection would be told that they probably were infected. That is, one in 10 infected persons would not be identified by the tests, and one in four persons who test positive would not be infected. Moreover, at least some of the 1200 infected persons correctly identified by the tests would already have transmitted the virus to their partners. This study concludes that compulsory premarital screening for HIV does not appear to be a sensible allocation of resources.

Similar problems—high costs, low yield, and high false-positive and false-negative rates—will afflict other mandatory HIV screening programs for low-risk populations. The prospects for compulsory screening of high-risk groups are no more attractive from a moral point of view. Despite their potentially higher yield, screening programs for these groups are likely to subject individuals at risk to increased discrimination, force them to go underground to avoid testing, and discourage voluntary behavior changes.

Some insurers now require HIV screening as a condition for obtaining health or life insurance. If this is required for health insurance, seropositive individuals, their families, and ultimately public support programs like Medicaid will bear the entire financial burden of their health care. If this information is available to others, such as employers offering a group health plan, these individuals will also risk loss of their jobs and other sources of financial support. In view of these grave risks, insurers' efforts to identify AIDS risk should be no greater than their attempts to identify those at risk for other prevalent life-threatening illnesses. Moreover, screening should not be required unless test results can be kept confidential. As private insurers become less able to bear the growing financial burden of health care for AIDS patients, new federal initiatives may be needed in this area.[23]

Finally, at least one political organization, Lyndon LaRouche's National Democratic Policy Committee, advocates mandatory screening of the entire population and isolation of all infected individuals.[24] The LaRouche forces backed an unsuccessful referendum on this issue in California in 1986. Their idea, presumably, is to achieve a "final solution" of the AIDS problem; I use that term advisedly, in view of the massive coercion their plan would require.

Reporting

Early in its history, AIDS was added to a long list of infectious diseases whose diagnosis must be reported to public health authorities. The rationale for such reporting is clear—information about who has a disease and what risk factors they exhibit is essential for drawing conclusions about how the disease is transmitted and how transmission can be prevented. Reporting may also enable specific infection control measures such as contact tracing. Thus, since the discovery of AIDS, the federal Centers for Disease Control has been a major source of epidemiological information about the disease. Based on this rationale, however, if some information is good, more information is presumably better, and in fact, CDC has recommended that states consider making HIV infection, as determined by antibody testing, a reportable condition.[18] Six states already require reporting of this condition.[25] As noted earlier, however, the epidemiological value of these additional data may be limited. Unlike AIDS patients, only a small, relatively nonrepresentative group of infected persons would be reported—blood donors, military recruits and personnel, prisoners, and those who voluntarily seek testing. Some individuals will receive false-positive results and be incorrectly reported as infected. Others will avoid voluntary testing out of fear of breach of confidentiality and its subsequent ill effects.

Contact Tracing

Attempting to identify, notify, and treat the sexual contacts of diseased individuals is a common method for controlling sexually transmitted diseases such as syphilis. Several authors have recommended this approach for controlling the heterosexual transmission of AIDS.[26,27] Tracing is thought to be cost-effective for heterosexual but not homosexual contacts because of the lower prevalence of the disease among heterosexuals and the presumed smaller number of sexual contacts. Because the virus can be carried for a long period of time, however, members of either group may have had many sexual contacts. Notifying a few of these may have little overall effect on the spread of the virus. Contacts identified could, of course, be tested and counseled but, unlike syphilis patients, not cured. Another major difference between syphilis and AIDS is that syphilis does not confer the same stigma today as AIDS. Notification of contacts severely compromises the confidentiality of a diagnosis of AIDS or HIV infection, since fearful or angry contacts may have no compunctions about spreading this information within the community. Like mandatory reporting, therefore, contact tracing may be a powerful disincentive to seeking voluntary testing. If this is the case, the anticipated benefits of contact tracing of heterosexuals, including reduction of AIDS in children, may not be realized. Even if HIV transmission could be prevented in some cases, it is not clear that this would justify the concomitant loss of confidentiality and the subsequent risk of serious adverse consequences. A more effective approach may be to urge infected persons themselves to inform their contacts and to be sure that testing and counseling are available for those contacts.

Quarantines and Other Restrictions

Proposals in this area have taken several forms, including the closing of establishments in which high-risk behaviors occur; the barring of AIDS patients or infected persons from schools, jobs, and other environments; and the enforced detention or isolation of infectious persons. Despite the often drastic nature of these restrictions, they have received a great deal of attention and support; for example, millions have followed the struggles of AIDS patients like Ryan White in Indiana and the Ray children in Florida to return to public schools.

There is, of course, moral and legal precedent for restricting personal freedom on public health grounds in both the control of infectious disease and the involuntary commitment of the mentally ill. For a particular restriction to be justifiable, however, it should satisfy at least the following four conditions: (1)

the person or place to be restricted poses a demonstrable threat to the public health; (2) the magnitude of the threat, as determined by its probability and severity, is greater than the harm threatened by the proposed restriction; (3) the proposed restriction *can* significantly lessen the threat; and (4) there are no less restrictive or intrusive means available to accomplish this goal.

The recent controversy over San Francisco's bathhouses illustrates the difficulty of satisfying all these conditions. Closing the bathhouses arguably satisfies the first three conditions—that is, it is probably an effective, but not unduly harsh, method of lessening the demonstrable threat of anonymous sexual contact with multiple partners. A less restrictive approach, however, in the form of regulations forbidding sexual contact in the baths and requiring the posting of educational and warning signs, was initially adopted by the San Francisco authorities.[11] The Health Department later ordered the closing of particular bathhouses found to be violating these regulations. The California Superior Court, however, did not uphold this order but instead imposed further measures to inhibit sexual practices such as requiring removal of cubicle doors and expulsion of patrons observed to be engaging in high-risk sexual activities. The problem with the Court's measures, however, is that they, too, may prove to be ineffective.[11] Thus, the least restrictive *effective* means of addressing this threat may in fact be closing the offending establishments.

Most proposals to bar AIDS patients or infected persons from schools or jobs fail to satisfy one or both of the first two conditions mentioned above. For example,[28] most school children with AIDS pose no demonstrable threat to classmates, because there is no evidence of viral spread through casual contact, the chance of parenteral exposure to infected body fluids is minimal, and, even if such exposure should occur, the risk of transmission of virus through a single limited exposure is very small (pp. 45–55). Moreover, being barred from attending school is obviously a major hardship for these children. For similar reasons, the CDC[25] has recommended that health care workers who do not perform invasive procedures, personal service workers such as barbers and manicurists, and food service workers not be restricted from work on the basis of HIV infection (p. 693).

Perhaps the most difficult problems in this area are raised by proposals to isolate or incarcerate infectious individuals, especially those who continue to engage in high-risk activities. Such behaviors are known to transmit the virus, but how serious a threat each *particular* individual poses may be more difficult to demonstrate, since some AIDS patients and antibody-positive individuals are not or are no longer sexually active, and some exposed individuals may not develop the disease. Moreover, if a threat can be demonstrated, will it always outweigh the severe hardship of enforced detention or isolation? Such individuals would presumably have to be detained as long as they are infectious, perhaps for the rest of their lives. Even if the threat is serious enough to justify detention, will the isolation of a few individuals significantly lessen it, or will wholesale detention of infectious individuals be necessary? Since 1–2 million Americans may already be infected, wholesale detention evokes, in my mind, the very negative images of the internment of Japanese-Americans during World War II.

Finally, are there less restrictive alternatives to imprisonment or isolation? Mills et al. report a case of a Florida prostitute with AIDS who was confined to her home and ordered to wear a monitor that signaled the police if she strayed more than 200 feet from her telephone.[10] This alternative is somewhat less restrictive than jailing, but there is some question whether it is effective. Was surveillance also necessary to ensure that this person was not practicing prostitution at home? Supposing surveillance did provide evidence of continuing prostitution, would we then need to use spying devices to determine whether the customers were using condoms? Although the reasons for wanting to protect others against persons who will not modify high-risk behaviors are clear, effective measures to accomplish this goal will need to be either highly restrictive or highly invasive. Any systematic attempt to implement such measures will pose difficult practical problems and be extremely costly.

Physical Marking of Persons with AIDS

Finally, let us consider one last proposal which some may find less restrictive than isolation. This proposal was offered with apparent seriousness by William F. Buckley in a 1986 op-ed article in the *New York Times*.[30] Buckley suggests that "everyone detected with AIDS should be tattooed on the upper forearm, to protect common-needle users, and on the buttocks, to prevent the victimization of other homosexuals." This proposal invites comparison with Nathaniel Hawthorne's infamous scarlet letter. Buckley, in fact, acknowledges the analogy with the scarlet letter, pointing out that the scarlet letter was designed to stimulate public condemnation, whereas the AIDS tattoo is designed for private protection. The intentions may well differ in the two cases, but the consequences—shame, violation of bodily integrity, stigmatization, and discrimination—are likely to be quite similar.

CONCLUSION

In summary, then, this paper has argued for the seriousness and complexity of AIDS as a public health problem and reviewed specific public health measures ranging from the urgent to the controversial to the ominous. Although reasoned conclusions about specific programs may differ, the fundamental values at stake demand that we undertake a careful evaluation of our public health options. In general, we have seen that more invasive and coercive public health measures like mandatory screening, contact tracing, and isolation are not justifiable in view of their limited effectiveness, high cost, and serious potential for stigmatization, discrimination, and other harms. If that is the case, we must redouble our efforts both to encourage healthy behavior through education and voluntary screening and to find an effective treatment and vaccine for this dread disease.

REFERENCES

1. Brandt, E.N. (1983). The Public Health Service's number one priority. *Public Health Reports, 98*, 306–307.

2. Silverman, M.F., & Silverman, D.B. (1985). AIDS and the threat to public health. *Hastings Center Report, 15*(4), S19–S22.

3. Krim, M. (1985). AIDS: The challenge to science and medicine. *Hastings Center Report, 15*(4), S2–S7.

4. Rivin, B.E., Monroe, J.M., Hubschman, B.P., & Thomas, P.A. (1984). AIDS outcome: A first follow-up. *New England Journal of Medicine, 311*, 857.

5. Barnes, D.M. (1986). Grim projections for AIDS epidemic. *Science, 232*, 1589–1590.

6. Scitovsky, A.A., & Rice, D.P. (1987). Estimates of the direct and indirect costs of acquired immunodeficiency syndrome in the United States, 1985, 1986, and 1991. *Public Health Reports, 102*, 5–17.

7. Andrulis, D.P., Beers, V.S., Bentley, J.D., & Gage, L.S. (1987). The provision and financing of medical care for AIDS patients in U.S. public and private teaching hospitals. *JAMA, 258*, 1343–1346.

8. Batchelor, N.F. (1984). AIDS: A public health and psychological emergency. *American Psychologist, 39*, 1279–1284.

9. Landesman, S.H., Ginzburg, M.H., & Weiss, S.H. (1985). The AIDS epidemic. *New England Journal of Medicine, 312*, 521–525.

10. Centers for Disease Control. (1986). Update: Acquired immunodeficiency syndrome—United States. *Morbidity and Mortality Weekly Report, 35*, 17–21.

11. Mills, M., Wofsy, C.B., & Mills, J. (1986). The acquired immunodeficiency syndrome: Infection control and public health law. *New England Journal of Medicine, 314*, 931–936.

12. Handsfield, H.H. (1985). AIDS and sexual behavior in gay men. *American Journal of Public Health, 75*, 1449.

13. McKusick, L., Coates, T., & Horstman, W. (1985). Response from McKusick et al. *American Journal of Public Health, 75*, 1449–1450.

14. Norman, C. (1986). $2 Billion program urged for AIDS. *Science, 233*, 661–662.

15. Koop, C.E. (1987). Surgeon General's report on acquired immune deficiency syndrome. *Public Health Reports, 102*, 1–3.

16. Walters, L. (1988). Ethical issues in the prevention and treatment of HIV infection and AIDS. *Science, 239*, 597–603.

17. Centers for Disease Control (1986). Transfusion-associated human T-lymphotropic virus type III/lymphadenopathy-associated virus infection from a seronegative donor—Colorado. *Morbidity and Mortality Weekly Report, 35*, 389–391.

18. Centers for Disease Control. (1986). Additional recommendations to reduce sexual and drug abuse-related transmission of human T-lymphotropic virus type III/lymphadenopathy associated virus. *Morbidity and Mortality Weekly Report, 35*, 152–155.

19. Wing, K.R. (1986). Constitutional protection of sexual privacy in the 1980s: What *is* Big Brother doing in the bedroom? *American Journal of Public Health, 76*, 201–204.

20. *Bowers* v. *Hardwick*, 106 S. Ct. 2841 (1986).

21. Boffey, P.M. (1987). Reagan urges wide AIDS testing but does not call for compulsion. *New York Times*, June 1, pp. A1, A15.

22. Cleary, P.D., Barry, M.J., Mayer, K.H., Brandt, A.M., Gostin, L., & Fineberg, H.V. (1987). Compulsory premarital screening for the human immune deficiency virus: Technical and public health considerations. *JAMA, 258*, 1757–1762.

23. Oppenheimer, G.M., & Padgug, R.A. (1986). AIDS: The risks to insurers, the threat to equity. *Hastings Center Report, 16*(5), 18–22.

24. Petit, C. (1986). California to vote on AIDS proposition. *Science, 234*, 277–278.

25. Gostin, L., & Ziegler, A. (1987). A review of AIDS-related legislative and regulatory policy in the United States. *Law, Medicine and Health Care, 15*, 5–16.

26. Echenberg, D.F. (1985). A new strategy to prevent the spread of AIDS among heterosexuals. *JAMA, 254*, 2129–2130.

27. Marmor, M., Lyden, M., & Grossman, R. (1985). Containing the AIDS epidemic. *JAMA, 254*, 2059.

28. Centers for Disease Control. (1987). Recommendations for prevention of HIV transmission in health-care settings. *Morbidity and Mortality Weekly Report, 36*, 35–185.

29. Centers for Disease Control. (1985). Summary: Recommendations for preventing transmission of infection with human T-lymphotropic virus type III/lymphadenopathy associated virus in the workplace. *Morbidity and Mortality Weekly Report, 34*, 681–686, 691–695.

30. Buckley, W.F. Jr. (1986). Crucial steps in combating the AIDS epidemic: Identify all the carriers. *New York Times*, March 18, p. A27.

35

Public Schools Confront AIDS

Elizabeth P. Lamers

INTRODUCTION

The acquired immune deficiency syndrome (AIDS) was not immediately identified as a separate disease when it first appeared in the United States. Initially,
a sharp rise in the incidence of Kaposi's sarcoma, a rare and usually fatal type
of cancer, was noticed, especially among homosexuals. This was later associated
with a rise in the number of cases of *Pneumocystis carinii* pneumonia in the
same population. When the disease now known as AIDS was identified in 1981,
it was not thought to be contagious. What had been called the "gay epidemic"
and the "Haitian disease" was finally named acquired immune deficiency syndrome, or AIDS, in 1983.

AIDS initially appeared to be limited to homosexuals and intravenous drug
users. However, when AIDS appeared among hemophiliacs and recipients of
blood transfusions, the general population began to feel vulnerable. By Sept.
12, 1988, 72,766 cases of AIDS had been diagnosed, and 41,064 deaths (56%
of the total number of cases) had occurred. A plague mentality arose; amid
fearfulness, misinformation, and overreaction to the disease, some in society
looked for a scapegoat. Even though scientific knowledge and understanding of
the virus and resulting pathology developed rapidly, AIDS patients and their
families nonetheless became the new untouchables. Legislators in California,
Texas, and Ohio introduced bills to segregate persons identified as AIDS infected
from the general population. Some fundamentalist ministers preached that AIDS
is divine retribution for living an unnatural (i.e., homosexual) life style. In May
1983, Patrick Buchanan, former Director of Communications at the White House,
wrote in a syndicated column in a style reminiscent of a fire-and-brimstone
preacher that "[homosexuals] have declared war on nature, and now nature is
exacting an awful retribution."[1] Attributing blame for a new and unexplained
disease is not a new phenomenon. Cotton Mather (ca. 1663–1728) stated, "Sickness is in fact the whip of God for the sins of many".[2]

When AIDS first appeared, scientists observed patterns of association of the
disease with particular segments of the population but only subsequently demonstrated the mechanism of transmission of the virus. Journalists used terms
such as "sexual contact" and "sharing of bodily fluids" in reporting on AIDS,
leaving many people with little idea of how AIDS is spread. Even the literature
from the Centers for Disease Control and other health authorities has perpetuated some of the misunderstanding, with polite terms such as "intimate contact"
used to describe the method of transmission of the AIDS virus. A poll conducted
by the *New York Times/CBS News* in September 1985 showed that nearly half
of those polled thought they could catch AIDS by sharing a glass with an AIDS

patient, although it was documented by epidemiologists and other scientists that AIDS could be transmitted only by sexual contact or by exposure to infected blood, including maternal-fetal transmission. The fact that AIDS had been transmitted by blood transfusions led a number of people to mistakenly assume that it was therefore unsafe to give blood.[3]

Both *Newsweek* and the *Washington Journalism Review* criticized media coverage for being less than explicit about the mode of AIDS transmission.[1,4] Some reports actually suggested that casual contact could spread the disease. Others resorted to exaggeration, for example: "Now No One Is Safe From AIDS"— *Life*, July 1985; "School Cook Dies of AIDS: He Chopped Green Beans & Roast Beef"—*New York Post*, September 12, 1985; "AIDS Child Bites Classmate, Now Both Are Doomed"—*Weekly World News*, November 12, 1985. The fact that the medical community has stated that it considers AIDS a relatively difficult disease to contract for those who are either celibate or monogamous has not been totally reassuring. In fact, *Newsweek* reported that physician attempts at reassurance about AIDS has caused some people to distrust doctors. An example of this distrust was shown by a New York City mother who said she was keeping her child out of school because "We are afraid our children will catch the disease even if those so-called, quote-unquote experts say it is impossible."[3]

HISTORICAL OVERVIEW

The public health aspect of classroom education has an interesting, if brief, history. Children were first educated at home by their parents. Gradually, small informal groups (e.g., cousins or neighbors) were educated in a specific home. Eventually these small groups evolved into formal schools, the precursors of our current school systems. As the number of children in a classroom increased, the chances of infectious diseases spreading from child to child also increased.

Even today, during the first year of a child's schooling, parents often notice an increase in the frequency of infection in their child. Some parents may wonder if school is really worth the risk of illness. However, the frequency of infection usually decreases after the first year of school as children develop a broader immunity to viral respiratory infections and as they receive the formal and informal instruction in personal hygiene which in itself reduces transmission of many microorganisms. Viral diseases are spread not only from child to child; child-to-parent transmission has also been confirmed. The *New England Journal of Medicine* recently reported that children in day care centers had transmitted cytomegalovirus (CMV) to their parents.[5] This is especially serious for pregnant women, because CMV can be passed to the fetus. It has been demonstrated that CMV infection in pregnant women has resulted in a 10% increase in the rate of birth defects. A significant literature has developed surrounding infectious disease control in school-based settings.[6] The public health implications of viral infections acquired in a classroom setting are more complicated than was formerly thought.

Serious infectious diseases that once were a part of childhood are now largely eradicated owing to immunization, antibiotics, and improvements in sanitation. Schools generally require that all entering students provide evidence of having been inoculated against diphtheria, tetanus, pertussis, measles, mumps, rubella, and polio. Some school districts also require testing for exposure to tuberculosis. In California, children whose parents have personal or religious objections to inoculations may enter school without the usual medical certificate of inoculations. The parents of these children must sign an affidavit that they are opposed to inoculations on personal or religious grounds and that they (the parents) understand that in the event of an outbreak of a contagious disease, their children will be excluded from school until the outbreak has subsided.

Until the current AIDS crisis, epidemics in Western society were largely a thing of the past. The annual recurrence of influenza is usually described as an "outbreak" rather than an epidemic. Polio, the last epidemic, when considered retrospectively infected relatively few, but affected many in terms of the fear of death or disability associated with the disease. Between 1915 and the introduction of the Salk vaccine in 1955, over 500,000 persons contracted polio. Fifty-seven thousand (11%) died, and many others were left with residual paralysis.[3] This statistic helps to put into perspective the current AIDS epidemic wherein 41,064 (56%) have died as of September 12, 1988.

During the 1940s entire towns were sprayed with DDT in an effort to kill flies despite a lack of evidence that the polio infection was transmitted by insects. Because most polio cases occurred in late summer, many school openings were delayed. Milwaukee in 1944 declared a citywide quarantine, prohibiting children from leaving their own yards during the season of peak polio contagion.[7]

DISEASE AND THE CLASSROOM

Ever since children have been brought together for public education, the classroom has served as an arena for resolving larger issues. The conflict between scientific Darwinism and religious creationism escalated from the classroom to the famous Scopes "monkey trial."[8] The social issue of integration versus segregation was played out in classrooms in the South in the 1950s.[8] The religious issue of prayer in the classroom became a major political issue in the early 1960s. The educational issues surrounding AIDS have already attracted the attention of parents and religious groups who have strong feelings about what subjects may be taught in the classroom.[9]

The basic conflict involved is one of rights and responsibilities. The rights of the individual must be preserved. The rights of society must be protected. The school has the responsibility to educate and must operate in the public interest. The school also makes educational decisions on behalf of the parents (in loco parentis).

AIDS is a public health issue. The school as a representative of the public interest has a responsibility to teach the facts necessary to reduce the spread of AIDS. To teach these facts properly, the school must present information that some parents find objectionable on moral and religious grounds.

For example, education about AIDS requires that children be taught the basic facts about sex, birth control, and drug abuse. It is apparent that the most effective approach is to present this information before the children become involved in sexual activity and drug abuse. It is not enough for schools to support sexual and drug abstinence. Children need to know the facts so that over time they can make decisions based on sound knowledge. If this were a perfect society, moral persuasion would be sufficient to reduce the spread of AIDS. The teenage pregnancy rate shows, however, that this is not a perfect society. Public health issues demand a broad, reasoned, educational approach to AIDS. The general adult tendency to want to shield children from unpleasant realities must, in this instance, yield to the imperative of providing children with life-saving information. Rabbi Steven Robbins of Temple Emanuel in Beverly Hills, California, has stated the problem even more bluntly: "If you have any problems about talking to your child about AIDS, it may come down to a condom or a casket for your child."[10]

For 20 years the classroom has been relatively free from public health concerns. Immunization against polio eliminated the last major epidemic among school-age children. The development of effective treatment for tuberculosis meant that schoolchildren who formerly were isolated in sanatoriums could now attend school, once they were past the infectious stage of the disease. The availability of safe and effective immunization against diphtheria, pertussis, tetanus, measles, rubella, mumps, and polio has made the classroom a relatively safe gathering place for children.

One major medical development of the past two decades that has affected the classroom environment for many children has been improvements in treating childhood cancer. Because of new therapies, children with cancer who formerly left school, never to return, are now able to experience remission or even complete cure. Children now return to the classroom during the maintenance phases of treatment. As childhood cancer has become treatable, it carries less of a stigma. But some parents still fear their child can "catch" cancer from a schoolmate with the disease. Classroom teachers have learned to cope with the child with cancer returning to the classroom. Courts have frequently upheld the rights of children with disabilities to remain in the classroom and to receive the necessary assistance to obtain an education.

AIDS presents a challenge to schools for several reasons. The classroom has been relatively "safe" for over two decades; that it is presumed not to be "safe" any longer is itself a threat to some parents. The mortality rate for those with AIDS exceeds that associated with polio or cancer. The mechanisms of AIDS transmission raise moral, religious, and sexual connotations that are threatening for many adults. This presents an added dimension to the challenge facing teachers and school boards to design educational programs that provide the information and motivation necessary to eliminate the further spread of the disease. The fear of their children "catching" AIDS from an infected classmate has caused parents to question recognized medical authorities.

It is known that the AIDS virus is not a stable virus like the polio virus. The human immunodeficiency virus (HIV) mutates rapidly. Given our present knowledge and technology, one-time immunization against HIV seems an unlikely method of effective prevention. The current lack of any immunization against or effective treatment for AIDS raises the specter of an epidemic threat to all segments of the population for years to come.

SCOPE OF THE PROBLEM IN SCHOOLS

Because AIDS is transmissible and thus far incurable, school boards have had a difficult time deciding whether or not to admit a child with AIDS. The *Harvard Medical School Health Letter* points out, "There appears to be no cogent reason for excluding such children (with AIDS) from the classroom, unless they have behavior problems, such as habitual biting, that could lead to transmission of the virus."[11] The same letter recommends the establishment of local task forces to conduct confidential case-by-case reviews. Articles in the *New England Journal of Medicine* state that the AIDS virus is not transmitted by casual contact, even within a family unit in which there is close contact with the infected person (sharing household items or household facilities, washing items used by AIDS patients, or hugging or kissing them).[12,13] In a recent study designed to determine routes of transmission, the AIDS virus was isolated from only one of 83 saliva samples, although the virus was detected in 28 of 50 blood samples from the same population.[13]

The American Medical Association has suggested that preschoolers with AIDS not be admitted to day care centers, because they might bite or scratch other children and may not yet be completely toilet-trained. The AMA suggests that these factors might contribute to the spread of the virus. However, physicians emphasize that school-age children do not pose a health threat to their classmates and should be allowed to participate in the same activities as healthy youngsters.[14] Although the child with AIDS does not pose a contagious threat in the classroom, the natural progression of the disease leads to a point where immunosuppression in the ill child causes the classroom to become a threat. The immunosuppressed child cannot tolerate viral and bacterial organisms that pose no threat to healthy classmates. At this point the child with AIDS should be removed from the classroom to a setting (e.g., home) where there is limited exposure to pathogenic organisms.

The Education for All Handicapped Children Act of 1975 (Public Law 94-142) was enacted to ensure that all children, handicapped or not, receive an education. Therefore the question is not "Should the child with AIDS be educated?" but "How and where should the child with AIDS be educated?" There are various ways of educating handicapped children within the educational system. Some can be educated in classrooms within hospitals; others, in segregated classrooms within regular schools or in segregated classrooms in schools for handicapped children. Still others can be educated at home, either by a home teacher or with a video link to the classroom. Although educating a child in a special class or at home may satisfy PL 94-142 and the educational needs of the child, these solutions do not necessarily satisfy the child's social and psychological needs. It has long been recognized by educators that schools impart more than book learning. School boards that have segregated handicapped children have been challenged by parents who claim that the social and psychological dimensions of a regular classroom are as important as the instruction received.

Different school boards have handled the problem of the student with AIDS in different ways.[15-20] Most school boards have not taken any action until faced with a student or teacher with AIDS. Some boards (e.g., Beverly Hills, CA) have set up panels of medical experts to review cases as they arise.[20] In certain situations, the question of admitting a student with AIDS to school could not be resolved by the school board and has been referred to a local court.[21] A decision by the courts in favor of admitting the child does not necessarily resolve the matter. For example, when a Kokomo, Indiana, court determined Ryan White had the right to return to class, parents of his schoolmates raised a $12,000 bond to continue their fight to exclude him.[22] In other school districts, parents have withdrawn their children rather than have them attend classes with a student known to have AIDS. Not only have AIDS patients been barred from attending school, but there have been instances of children or siblings of AIDS patients being barred from school until proved to be uninfected.[15-17]

The case of "Mark" in Swansea, Massachusetts, has unfortunately been the exception rather than the rule.[19] Mark has AIDS and has been allowed to attend public school largely through the efforts of the school superintendent, John McCarthy. McCarthy learned the scientific facts about AIDS and educated the community by arranging for physicians to meet with teachers and parents. McCarthy had more credibility in his community than do many superintendents. He has been a teacher and administrator in Swansea for three decades, and he has taught or coached several of the town's school board members. Nonetheless, his judicious approach to obtaining the pertinent information and providing the appropriate resources serves as a model of enlightened leadership.

Teachers as well as students can become infected with the AIDS virus. As yet, there is no clear pattern of how school boards handle the problem of a teacher with AIDS. The National Education Association (NEA) opposes mandatory testing of teachers for AIDS and has stated that teachers with AIDS should be permitted to keep their jobs. In Orange County, California, a teacher with AIDS was offered an alternative job to classroom teaching. He filed papers with the U.S. District Court in Los Angeles seeking a declaration of his rights.[23] The Court (9th Circuit Court of Appeals) upheld his right to return to the classroom, and he was reinstated as a classroom teacher. This is the highest legal application to date showing AIDS as a protected handicap.[24]

School boards must also consider the economic implications of the decisions regarding the education of the child with AIDS. Will a school board's decision result in a costly lawsuit? If it is decided that the child with AIDS should be placed in a special education class, will the cost be borne by the school or district, or can the expense be covered by a state or federally funded program? The majority of the monies a school district receives from the state is determined by the daily attendance of students. By admitting a student with AIDS, a district may risk losing income if other students refuse to attend out of fear or in protest. In many school districts, multiple and prolonged withdrawals would constitute a financial hardship.

School districts must also consider the possibility of a future lawsuit if another child becomes seropositive and the infection can be traced to the readmitted student with AIDS. Because at present there is no cure for AIDS, some school boards are reluctant to tell parents that their children are safe in a classroom with a child with AIDS. The long incubation period of the AIDS virus (months to years) compounds the uncertainty. The current epidemic demands that school boards act now, although the consequences of their actions may not be known for years.

At present, school-age children with AIDS were infected either in utero or by later transfusion with AIDS-contaminated blood or blood products. The number of children infected by contaminated blood is expected to decrease as methods of processing blood extracts improve, as new means of screening donors are utilized, and as methods are refined to test blood for the presence of the AIDS virus. The majority of children infected in utero are the offspring of intravenous drug users. Some of these children, ill at birth, never leave the hospital. Of those that do go home, most do not survive to school age.[17] At present the number of children infected antenatally with AIDS is increasing. An education program for IV drug users could decrease this figure, even though this population is notoriously difficult to change (see Chapter 11). Dr. Rubinstein, professor of pediatrics at New York's Albert Einstein College of Medicine, has stated, "These [the infants known to have AIDS through maternal transmission] are the very sick children. A much larger number are infected but not very sick yet. Nobody knows how to label them. We are talking about maybe 2000 children."[17]

EDUCATION IN THE CLASSROOM

Education regarding behaviors to prevent the spread of the AIDS virus offers the greatest hope of containing this epidemic. Students must be taught the basic facts about the transmission of AIDS. Dr. Edward Gomperts, director of the hemophilia center at Children's Hospital in Los Angeles, states the need: "Imagine the scenario of high schools with sexually active kids hooked on drugs and infected with AIDS. We could have a generation of infected kids."[17] Dr. C. Everett Koop, Surgeon General of the United States, has asked for AIDS education to begin in elementary school. This poses a problem to some school districts, since effective education about AIDS requires discussing subjects previously considered "taboo" in elementary classrooms: homosexual practices and birth control.

To be effective in combating the spread of AIDS, educational materials must be clear and explicit. Parents who have been reluctant to allow heterosexual sex education in schools may be even more resistant to allowing their children to be exposed to concepts of homosexuality and the use of condoms. To eliminate any discussion of homosexuality and "safe sex" would be to ignore important parts of the problem and solution. The Los Angeles Unified School District has developed a new curriculum on AIDS and sexually transmitted diseases for junior and senior high school students. By the end of the 1986–87 school year, this new program will be extended to sixth-grade students. A number of other school districts across the country are also developing comparable courses designed to halt the spread of AIDS.

As more persons with AIDS return to school, students need to learn how the AIDS virus can and cannot be transmitted. They need to know that persons with AIDS can be touched and hugged without fear of becoming infected. They must learn that the AIDS virus cannot be transmitted to uninfected members of the same household in the course of ordinary day-to-day living. Students also need more than facts, however; they need time to discuss their fears and feelings with teachers who have been properly educated regarding the social, psychological, physical, and public health aspects of this unique disease.

When a student dies of AIDS, his or her classmates will need support in dealing with their feelings of loss and grief. They will have questions about AIDS, death, and grief that require answers. They will need encouragement to verbalize their feelings as well as support to attend funeral services and to convey condolences to the bereaved family.[25,26] Teachers must become familiar with the mechanisms of grief. They need to know that some students may become more aggressive and outspoken while others may cry, withdraw, or even develop (transient) exemplary behavior.[25,26]

Ideally, students, teachers, and parents will work together to meet the challenges presented by AIDS. If the problems are faced openly, creative solutions supportive of social and psychological growth can replace some of the early reflexive adjustments made out of fear and misunderstanding.

AIDS AND THE NEWS MEDIA

The projected morbidity and mortality resulting from the AIDS pandemic mandates the development of coordinated educational and social approaches to provide all people with basic factual information about the disease, its mode transmission, and methods to reduce the risk of infection.

The news media (press, television, magazines, radio, videotapes) have a significant place in the lives of students. It has been estimated that the average elementary or secondary school student spends 6 h per day watching television and considerable other hours watching videos, reading magazines, or listening to the radio. Sexually oriented advertising is commonly used to market a variety of products, from automobiles to music and clothing. Sexual themes play a central role in the entertainment industry. Popular songs frequently contain references to overt sexual activity. There is evidence to suggest the existence of a strong "copy cat" phenomenon in adolescent behavior.[27] Does the same sort of imitative behavior pertain in sexual matters? And if so, does it represent a public health threat in terms of the transmission of AIDS?

Media programming supportive of casual sexual involvement would undoubtedly dilute the effectiveness of instructional programs designed to foster abstinence, restraint, and "safe sex." Planning for and implementation of instructional programs to reduce the transmission of AIDS should include a review of media impact on the behavior of those for whom the courses are designed. Current evidence of government concern for monitoring the content of radio programming has recently appeared.[28]

Since release of the Surgeon General's report on AIDS, sex education and the use of condoms have gained wide exposure in the media. Discussion in the media regarding the use of condoms has suddenly weakened the taboo against advertising birth control devices on television and in newspapers. The major networks, once reluctant to offend a substantial segment of their audience, have used concern about AIDS as a means of justifying the acceptance of condom advertising. The networks also continue to offer many hours each week of sexually provocative programming with no more than a disclaimer that "the material in the following show may be offensive to some."

Newspapers, like television, have appeared to operate under a double standard: while refusing to accept advertising for birth control devices, they have continued to allow the use of sexually provocative material to market a wide variety of products. The AIDS crisis appears to have allowed both television and newspapers to accept advertising for condoms on the basis that their use will reduce the transmission of AIDS. But it is doubtful if the media will spontaneously reexamine their attitude toward accepting and programming sexually provocative material. It is unlikely, also, that newspapers and television will make the quantum leap from mentioning the term "safe sex" to accurately describing safe sex practices.

CONCLUSION

AIDS presents a complicated social, psychological, and public health challenge to educators and school boards. Resolution of the problem will depend on learning the medical facts about AIDS, developing effective strategies for educating students with AIDS and their classmates, and developing educational programs designed to reduce the transmission of the AIDS virus.

In the absence of any effective treatment for AIDS and with no immediate prospect of the development of a vaccine, education offers the only hope of limiting the spread of this dangerous disease. It has been predicted that tens of millions of people will die of AIDS worldwide during the next 10 years. The number of people of any age who contract the virus can be influenced by the development and implementation of effective educational programs. Content aimed at understanding and preventing this devastating disease through the assumption of appropriate preventive behaviors on the part of the individual and the community is essential to the well-being of all. Public schools play a significant role in preserving the health of all members of society and in assuring the vitality of future generations.

REFERENCES

1. Alter, J. Sins of omission. *Newsweek*, Sept 23, 1985, 25.
2. Morrow, L. The start of a plague mentality. *Time*, Sept 23, 1985, 37.
3. Adler, J., Greenberg, N.F., Hager, M., McKillop, P., Namuth, T. The AIDS conflict. *Newsweek*, Sept 23, 1985, 18–24.
4. Diamond, E., Bellitto, C. M. The greatest verbal coverup. *Washington Journalism Review*, March 1986, 38–42.
5. Pass, R.F., Hutto, C., Ricks, R., Cloud, C.A. Increased rate of cytomegalovirus infection among parents of children attending day-care centers. *New England Journal of Medicine*, 1986, *314*(22), 1414–1423.
6. Articles such as those reviewed in *Reviews of Infectious Diseases*, 1986, *8*(4).
7. Leerhsen, C. Epidemics: A paralyzing effect. *Newsweek*, Sept 23, 1985, 23.
8. Court decisions: *Brown* vs. *Board of Education*, 347 U.S. 483 (1954); *Scopes* vs. *State*, 154 TNN. 105, 289 S.W. 363 (1927); *Engel* vs. *Vittale*, 370 U.S. 421 (1962).
9. Gillam, J. Group seeks ban of "obscene" AIDS material in schools. *Los Angeles Times*, Apr 22, 1987, Part 2, 3.
10. Personal communication, March 1, 1987.
11. *Harvard Medical School Health Letter*. AIDS update (Part II), 1985, *11*(2), 2–5.
12. Friedland, G.H., Saltzman, B.R., Rogers, M.F., Kahl, P.A., Lesser, M.L., Mayers, M.M., Klein, R.S. Lack of transmission of HTLV-III/LAV infection to household contacts of patients with AIDS or AIDS-related complex with oral candidiasis. *New England Journal of Medicine*, 1986, *314*(6), 344–349.
13. Sande, M.E. Transmission of AIDS. *New England Journal of Medicine*, 1986, *314*(6), 380–382.
14. McAuliffe, K. Health/medicine. *U.S. News & World Report*, June 30, 1986, 63.
15. Barber, J., Luckow, D. An epidemic of fear. *Maclean's*. Sept 23, 1985, 61, 62.
16. Cimons, M. Loved ones latest victims of AIDS discrimination. *Los Angeles Times*, June 2, 1986, Part I, 1, 12, 13.
17. Dobbin, M., Kyle, C. The youngest victim of AIDS. *U.S. News & World Report*, July 7, 1986, 71–72.
18. Johnson, L. Kindergarten suspends AIDS victim, 4. *Los Angeles Times*, Sept 11, 1986, Part I, 3, 34.

19. Kirp, D. Commentary: AIDS victim. *San Francisco Examiner*, July 16, 1986, Section A, 11.

20. Mitchell, J. Beverly Hills School Board calls for creation of medical advisory panel to review AIDS cases. *Los Angeles Times*, Mar 2, 1986, Part W, 1, 13.

21. Overend, W. Judge orders return to class for AIDS boy. *Los Angeles Times*, Nov 18, 1986, Part I, 1, 22.

22. *Los Angeles Times*. Group raises cash in fight to bar AIDS victim from class. Mar 3, 1986, Part I, 14.

23. Billiter, B. AIDS victim sees fight to teach again as rights case. *Los Angeles Times*, Aug 12, 1987, Part I, 3.

24. Personal communication with David I. Schulman, Deputy City Attorney, Special Operations Division, AIDS Ordinance Enforcement Unit, Los Angeles, April 11, 1988.

25. Lamers, E.P. The dying child in the classroom. In Paterson, G., Ed., *Children and Death*. London, Ont.: King's College Press, 1986.

26. Lamers, W.M. Jr. Helping the child to grieve. In Paterson, G., Ed., *Children and Death*. London, Ont.: King's College Press, 1986.

27. Gould, M.S., Shaffer, D. The impact of suicide in television movies: Evidence of imitation. *New England Journal of Medicine*, 1986, *315*, 690–694; Ostroff, R.B., Behrends, R.W., Lee, K., Oliphant, J. Adolescent suicides modeled after television movie. *American Journal of Psychiatry*, 1985, *142*, 989; Correspondence, *New England Journal of Medicine*, 1987, *316*, 876–878.

28. McDougal, D. Shock radio crackdown jolts industry. *Los Angeles Times*, Apr 18, 1987, Part 6, 1, 11.

36

Hospice and Home Care for Persons with AIDS/ARC:
Meeting the Challenges and Ensuring Quality

Jeannee Parker Martin

INTRODUCTION

Every community is or will be faced with the challenge of caring for individuals with acquired immune deficiency syndrome (AIDS) and AIDS-related complex (ARC). We are reminded of this daily by newspaper and television reports of the millions of people who have been exposed to the AIDS virus, by scientists who inform us that AIDS is directly related to sexual behavior and intravenous drug use, and by large cities that report the increasing impact of persons diagnosed with AIDS/ARC on health care and social service systems already stretched to their limits. It is the responsibility of every community to review its resources and prepare for an increase in the number of AIDS/ARC cases. Without such preparation, hospitals will become overcrowded, home health and hospice programs will be inadequately utilized, and long-term care facilities will remain inaccessible.

In most communities in the United States, home health care is an existing alternative to hospitalization. Unfortunately, many home health agencies feel inadequately prepared to care for persons with AIDS/ARC. Other home health agencies feel that the physical and psychosocial needs of the person with AIDS/ARC will drain already limited resources. Another barrier to home care is the hospitals' fear of discharging a severely or terminally ill patient. Hospital discharge planners are often concerned that the patient's problems will be too complex for home management. Finally, patients may be reluctant to go home, and friends or family members may fear they cannot provide the intensive care that will be required as the patient's status deteriorates.

These barriers are not insurmountable. As demonstrated by the community's response in San Francisco, careful planning, cooperation, and education reduce the barriers to access and allow persons with AIDS/ARC to receive care at home or to identify alternatives when home care is no longer an option.[1] This article identifies the challenges that administrators and staff face in keeping the terminally ill individual with AIDS/ARC at home. It offers suggestions to best meet the needs of the person with AIDS/ARC living at home, and it suggests alternatives when home care is no longer an option. The experience of the AIDS Home Care and Hospice Program of the Visiting Nurses and Hospice of San Francisco is referred to throughout this chapter. This program was the first of its kind in the world, and it has developed an innovative approach to home and hospice care for persons with AIDS/ARC.

A CHALLENGE TO THE MULTIDISCIPLINARY
APPROACH

Caring for the person with AIDS/ARC is an unprecedented challenge for those providing home hospice care. Not only do those with AIDS benefit from the multidisciplinary approach (Fig. 1) adopted by most hospice programs, but the physical and psychosocial complexities of AIDS *require* this sensitive and humane approach. To address these complex needs, home hospice programs are being constantly challenged to provide more patient care services from all members of the multidisciplinary team. These members include attendants (homemakers/home health aides), nurses, physicians, social workers, therapists, volunteers, clergy, and other liaisons. However, reimbursement restrictions and staff limitations mean that, although the need for care is great, the available resources are few.[2]

The traditional patient referred for in-home care has only one or two physical and social complications. These usually require intervention on an intermittent basis. In contrast, the person with AIDS/ARC usually has three or four opportunistic infections, a complicated social history, and extensive psychological needs. This individual requires intensive intervention by all members of the multidisciplinary team from the outset of care.

Even the most experienced hospice home care team will have difficulty with the problems related to AIDS/ARC. Planning interventions early to meet the patient's physical, emotional, psychological, and spiritual needs prevents barriers to home care later. Although many factors influence the composition of the multidisciplinary team, every home health agency should try to use the following health care providers. If these providers are not available internally, it is important to identify other resources in the community to assist the home care team.

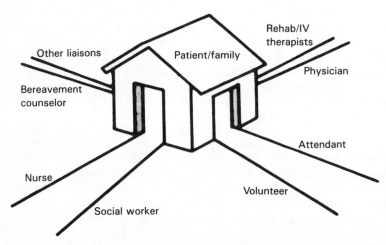

Figure 1.   The multidisciplinary team model used by the AIDS Home Care and Hospice Program in San Francisco. (Used with permission of the Visiting Nurses and Hospice of San Francisco.[10])

Attendant Care

Meeting the patient's practical needs is essential if the person with AIDS/ARC is to remain at home. The attendant (homemaker/home health aide) is the primary team member to intervene with the patient on a daily basis. The care provided by the attendant may include assisting with bathing, toileting, eating, walking, light housework, and other activities related to personal care. Complicated physical and neurological changes often make it difficult for the person with AIDS/ARC to carry out routine tasks. In fact, because of symptoms such as weakness, memory loss, confusion, and diarrhea, most persons with AIDS eventually need assistance with all activities of daily living. Since many persons with AIDS/ARC live alone and do not have family and friends available to help on a daily basis, they may require care by the attendant around the clock. The Visiting Nurses and Hospice of San Francisco's AIDS Home Care and Hospice Program provides an average of 8 h of attendant care per day to each patient in the program.

Resources for attendant care may be limited. Therefore, careful planning for attendant care should begin before the patient is discharged from the hospital, and it should be reassessed frequently once the patient is at home. As the patient begins to deteriorate and require more assistance, creative planning may be necessary. Attendant care may be provided by a combination of paid staff, volunteers, friends, and family members. Sometimes family members only need a break on weekends. In these circumstances, arranging for 24-h respite coverage may enhance the friends' or family members' participation in care giving at other times.

Some attendants may be willing to "live in" with the patient. When attendants live in, they are expected to be *available* 24 h a day, but they are not expected to work constantly throughout the day. Live-in attendants are paid for 8 h of work per day, and they are provided free room and board by the patient. This arrangement may be particularly appealing when the individual lives alone or when family members work and are not available 24 h a day.

Another option may be to consolidate attendant care into a group living situation. This option entails several persons with AIDS/ARC moving into a house that functions as a residential care facility. One attendant can care for two or three patients, allowing each of them to receive care around the clock. A ratio of one attendant for every three patients is adequate in most situations. However, the extent of physical and neurological complications must be considered when such assignments are made.

One example of consolidated attendant care is Coming Home Hospice, a program of the Visiting Nurses and Hospice of San Francisco. Coming Home Hospice is a 15-bed licensed residential care facility. Its goal is to provide 24-h care and supervision to terminally ill patients with AIDS/ARC and other terminal diseases. The on-site staff include a residence manager, cook, and maintenance crew. Twenty-four-hour attendant care and other hospice services are provided by the staff of the AIDS Home Care and Hospice Program or Traditional Hospice Program of the Visiting Nurses and Hospice. This humane and cost-effective alternative opened in early 1987. It is the first of its kind in the United States and serves as a model approach for consolidating home care services.

Nurses

In most home health agency or hospice programs, the nurse is the case manager and the team member who must assess the patient's physical condition, provide interventions, and communicate with the physician about changes in the patient's status. The nurse also educates other team members about infection control precautions, pain and symptom management, and other comfort measures. In the AIDS Home Care and Hospice Program, nurses makes an average of two scheduled home visits per week to each patient under their care. The unpredictability of the patient's status makes it important that a nurse also be on call 24 h a day to assess changes and suggest interventions to care givers staying with the patient. This degree of availability and flexibility for making home visits may prevent unnecessary trips to the hospital and may allay anxieties as the patient's condition deteriorates.[3]

Schietinger[4] describes a continuum of disability for the person with AIDS/ARC. This continuum includes individuals who are *apparently well*, *acutely ill*, *chronically ill*, and *terminally ill*. It is a helpful model in describing the varying degree of involvement of the home care nurse as the patient's condition changes. (Other team members also are involved as the patient's status requires their interventions.) As the person with AIDS/ARC progresses along the continuum of disability, the nurse is the team member who most frequently assesses the patient. Initially, for example, the person with AIDS may be *apparently well*. The apparently well individual may require intermittent visits by the nurse to evaluate the patient's condition after an initial diagnosis of, for example, Kaposi's sarcoma (KS). The person may receive several weeks of chemotherapy or radiation therapy to alleviate the symptoms of KS. As the patient's condition stabilizes, he or she may require education and instruction related to the early signs and symptoms of common opportunistic infections. During this stage, the patient may improve and may regain a preillness level of functioning.

The same individual may experience an *acute illness* caused by another opportunistic infection, such as *Pneumocystis carinii* pneumonia (PCP), several months later. At this point, the patient may require home intravenous antibiotic therapy, oxygen therapy, and frequent evaluations of symptoms related to PCP. This individual may require ongoing home nursing intervention as his or her status deteriorates, education related to energy conservation, and instruction about early signs and symptoms of a recurrent episode of PCP. Returning to a preillness level of functioning may be an unrealistic goal at this time.

As the person enters a state of chronic illness related to yet other symptoms of disease, the nurse will become more involved in the home care plan. It is likely that the *chronically ill* person with AIDS will experience irreversible complications, such as retinitis related to cytomegalovirus infection. The nurse regularly assesses the patient's symptoms, evaluates for signs of new disease, monitors medications, and implements other therapeutic regimes that will keep the patient comfortable.

The *terminally ill* person with AIDS/ARC has a prognosis of 6 months or less. This individual may have severe irreversible physical complications as well as neurological impairment. The hospice nurse makes frequent home visits to ensure the patient's optimum level of comfort during the final weeks or days of life. The nurse provides education and support to all care givers regarding symptom relief, comfort control, and signs of impending death.

Social Workers

The role of the social worker in caring for the person with AIDS/ARC is as varied as the psychosocial problems that affect AIDS/ARC patients. These psychosocial problems are often the most challenging to the home care plan. The social worker intervenes with financial planning, housing concerns, emotional support, funeral planning, and bereavement follow-up. In the AIDS Home Care and Hospice Program, the social worker makes an average of one visit per week to meet the needs of the patient and family. The social worker may provide counseling to patients and to their lovers, friends, and family members to help them cope with the diagnosis of AIDS/ARC.

The psychosocial concerns of persons with AIDS/ARC are multiple and complex. Issues may vary depending on the patient's coping mechanisms and the support the patient receives from friends and family members. Some issues identified include the lack of traditional support systems, lack of financial resources, loss of housing, loss of control over legal matters, and bereavement concerns related to the issues of multiple loss.[5] These may greatly influence the patient's, friends', or family's ability to accept or provide support as the patient's status deteriorates. The social worker becomes intimately involved in assisting the patient, friends, and family in identifying resources to help resolve conflicts created by these issues.

The social worker may be involved at any time on the continuum of disability described above. In fact, the need for social work intervention may be greatest at the onset of the illness, when the patient must sort through complicated financial matters and begin to address the issues related to death and dying. The social worker may be the front-line person to identify alternative resources in the community as the patient's status fluctuates early in the illness. As the person progresses along the disability continuum, the social worker may become less involved until the patient is in the terminal stages of the illness. At this time the social worker may assist the patient, friends, and/or family with tasks related to final arrangements and funeral planning, or may counsel them about dying and bereavement follow-up after the death occurs.

Volunteers

Volunteers are valuable staff extenders, particularly when reimbursement sources are limited. They are able to provide patient care support, such as assisting with respite for personal care givers; practical support, such as running errands and providing transportation to clinic appointments; massage therapy, to help decrease physical and emotional discomfort for patients and friends or family members; emotional support, such as counseling the patient and friends or family members to help them cope with the illness; and bereavement care, such as facilitating support groups or providing one-to-one counseling for friends or family members after the patient has died. The ways to utilize volunteers are unlimited. The volunteers will offer more ideas for intervention as they become familiar with the complex physical and psychosocial problems of persons with AIDS/ARC as well as the demographic characteristics of the patient population.

Every hospice program must evaluate its volunteer resources to adequately meet the needs of persons with AIDS/ARC. All communities have access to a wide range of volunteer resources. Volunteers may be available through church groups, senior citizen groups, civic organizations, high schools, colleges, university programs for nurses and social workers, gay and lesbian organizations, local cancer societies, minority groups, and other organizations. No group should be "avoided" for fear they may not want to work with persons with AIDS/ARC. Volunteers benefit from educational forums that help to allay their anxieties about direct patient care contact. Other volunteers may prefer to run errands or assist with office work. The value of volunteers must not be underestimated as home hospice programs attempt to provide extensive care to allow persons with AIDS/ARC to live in peace, comfort, and dignity at home.

Rehabilitation Therapists

Although the person with AIDS/ARC may be in the terminal stage of the illness when he or she enters a home care or hospice program, gaining the maximum level of independent functioning is always the goal. For many hospice patients this may simply mean eating a meal without assistance or sitting in a chair for a few minutes at a time. Rehabilitation therapists, such as occupational, physical, or speech therapists, are a key component of the multidisciplinary team. The occupational therapist may be able to assist the family in rearranging furniture for the patient whose vision is impaired because of cytomegalovirus retinitis to instruct in energy conservation techniques for the patient whose pulmonary status is compromised owing to *Pneumocystis carinii* pneumonia. The physical therapist may assist the patient with range-of-motion exercises that help strengthen weakened muscles. The speech therapist may assist the patient with swallowing techniques that improve food and fluid intake. A liaison therapist to the multidisciplinary team may help other team members recognize problems early, when the patient and family derive maximum benefit from such interventions.

Physician Consultant

The physician consultant assists all team members. The physician participates weekly in patient care conferences and is available at other times to answer questions. In the AIDS Home Care and Hospice Program, the physician consultant is not the primary physician for patients admitted to the program. Rather, the patient's own physician remains the primary physician and directs the patient's plan of care. The physician consultant does make recommendations, either to team members or to the primary physician. The physician consultant also plays a major role in educating the staff and serving as a community liaison to physicians in the community to encourage the use of home hospice care.

Pharmacist

Because of the multiple physical and neurological complications, most persons with AIDS/ARC take a number of medications. Side effects and interactions between these medications may be confusing to the nurse responsible for administering them. A pharmacist may help interpret proper dosing and response to medications as well as potentially dangerous synergistic effects. A pharmacist may also be familiar with new indications for medications that may successfully control symptoms to opportunistic infections. The pharmacist does not make home visits but, rather, attends the weekly patient care conferences to educate staff in the administration of medications.

Clergy/Spiritual Counselors

Although some patients have a priest, minister, or other designated person to assist in meeting spiritual needs, most do not. A pastoral care counselor helps staff identify impending spiritual needs as the person is approaching death and identifies available clergy or spiritual counselors in the community who are available to visit the patient. If a pastoral care counselor does not attend weekly patient care conferences, a list of counselors should be available so that the social worker can assist the patient or family member in locating an appropriate counselor.

Other Consultants

At times, other expertise may be required to develop the plan of care for the person with AIDS/ARC. In every community, many individuals are available to assist the multidisciplinary team. These may be substance abuse specialists at alcohol and drug rehabilitation centers, infection control experts at the local hospital, or epidemiologists at the local or state health departments. It is important to seek out these individuals to assist staff in providing appropriate care at home.

Patient Care Conferences

It is important to provide a regular forum for all members of the multidisciplinary team to discuss the home care plans. This provides them with an opportunity to discuss problems and identify ways to keep the person with AIDS/ARC at home. Other community representatives may provide valuable information about resources to aid in a particular situation. This may even benefit other patients receiving home care. Joint problem solving will assist staff members to intervene appropriately when other patients experience the same problem and provide team members with support regarding patient care decisions.

Team Support

It is difficult to overlook the team's own need for emotional support. As staff members provide assistance to patients who are dying from AIDS/ARC, their own concerns arise. Staff in any hospice program explore their own vulnerability to illness and the associated issues related to death and dying. In dealing with persons with AIDS/ARC, staff experience the frustration and hopelessness related in the treatment of the disease. Some team members may be in an identified risk group and may be concerned that they will be diagnosed with AIDS/ARC. Others may have friends or family members diagnosed with AIDS. All team members experience the loss and grief as patients die of AIDS/ARC.[6]

Administrators must be acutely aware of the staff's own need for regular emotional support. Providing time for formal support and informal support is essential. Time for support groups, patient care conferences, leave time off, bereavement counseling, and positive reinforcement and recognition for their work helps prevent unnecessary burnout. Staff turnover will decrease if team members feel the manager's sensitivity to the difficulties incurred by the provision of patient care. Managers will be saved countless hours in recruitment if staff are supported in their work.

BEREAVEMENT SUPPORT

Until recently, the full impact of multiple AIDS/ARC deaths was not clearly understood. However, as thousands of people die in communities around the country, it is clear that support and guidance are needed long after the death occurs. Family and friends may seek out the support of the social worker and/ or trained bereavement counselors. Group support for lovers and friends may provide a forum for mutual sharing and time for grief. Additional groups geared toward parents and siblings may allow them to work through difficult psychosocial concerns, life-style issues, and grief. Often family members fear they will not receive support from friends because of the nature of the illness and life-style issues involved. If the family is returning to a small rural community where myths about AIDS/ARC are perpetuated, support from friends or relatives may be minimal, perhaps nonexistent. Referring these family members to local hospice programs may provide them with necessary additional counseling or bereavement follow-up.

The bereavement concerns required by those grieving the loss of the person with AIDS/ARC often go beyond the normal grieving process. The bereaved individual may have lost many other friends and relatives to this devastating illness and may be unable to cope with one more loss. This same individual may be facing the diagnosis of AIDS/ARC. This complicated bereavement process requires a sensitive approach by social workers and bereavement counselors to allow the person time to process the death and accept the loss.

ENSURING REIMBURSEMENT

Most home health agency and hospice programs are eligible for reimbursement from a variety of third-party payer sources. These include Medicaid (Medi-Cal in California), Medicare, Department of Social Service Title XX, private insurance, and other local resources for individuals who are disabled and/or terminally ill. The AIDS Home Care and Hospice Program generates approximately 56% of its funding from these sources and private donations. The remaining 44% is received through a grant with the City and County of San Francisco and the California State Department of Health Services (Fig. 2). Since local and state resources vary, home health agencies and hospice programs must rely more heavily on reimbursement from private resources.

Between mid-1984 and mid-1988, the AIDS Home Care and Hospice Program cared for more than 2000 persons with AIDS/ARC at home. Of these individuals, approximately 60% were eligible for Medicaid (Medi-Cal), 35% for private insurance, and 2% for Medicare; 2% paid out of pocket, and 1% were no-fee patients. These 700 patients each received the full range of multidisciplinary team services described above. The average patient received two nursing visits

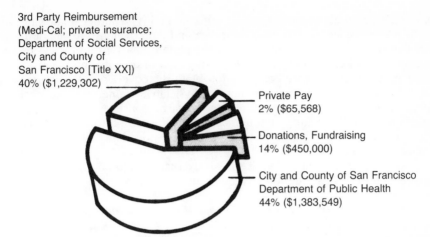

3rd Party Reimbursement
(Medi-Cal; private insurance;
Department of Social Services,
City and County of
San Francisco [Title XX])
40% ($1,229,302)

Private Pay
2% ($65,568)

Donations, Fundraising
14% ($450,000)

City and County of San Francisco
Department of Public Health
44% ($1,383,549)

Figure 2. Projected revenue sources for fiscal year 1989 for the AIDS Home Care and Hospice Program. (Used with permission of the Visiting Nurses and Hospice of San Francisco.[10]

per week, one social worker visit per week, 6 h of volunteer assistance per week, and 8 h of attendant care per day. The average length of stay was 57 days from the start of care at home until discharge, which for 80% of all cases was death at home.

Despite the magnitude of services provided, the average cost per patient-day was $100. This compares with an average local hospital cost of $773 per day.[7] Many persons cared for at home require 24-h assistance by attendants because of severe physical and neurological complications. If considered on an individual basis, the cost for only those needing round-the-clock care is still less than $300 per day.

This cost information is important for several reasons. First, many private insurance companies are interested in implementing cost-saving measures and are willing to negotiate a waiver in their client's existing policy. If the home care agency is able to present convincing evidence of cost savings, the insurance provider is likely to adjust their client's policy. The client's policy, which may have had limited home care coverage, now may be adequate to allow for the full range of home care services for an unlimited period. The insurance company realizes a savings of thousands of dollars due to the home care agency's interest in keeping the terminally ill person with AIDS/ARC at home. The home care agency may be able to establish a new precedent for services with the insurance provider. Not only will this precedent help others with AIDS/ARC, but such waivers may be obtained for non-AIDS/ARC patients who require 24-h home care assistance.[8]

To obtain maximum insurance coverage, it is important to remember the following points, as outlined by Steven Zembo,[9] when negotiating with private insurance representatives:

1. Obtain complete referral information specifying types and level of home care services needed; reason for hospital admission; whether the diagnosis is

acute, chronic, or terminal; prognosis; self-care ability; whether home care is in lieu of prolonged hospitalization; insurance and employment information.

2. Contact the employer by phone if the patient has a group policy through the employer. Then, confirm in writing a summary of the information provided.

3. Contact the insurance company to obtain the coverage information.

4. Obtain a letter from the patient's physician documenting the need for service. This letter is always required and must be consistent in specifying the services needed. Therefore, communicate this information to the physician.

5. Identify an individual to assume financial responsibility for the balance of the cost not reimbursed.

6. Assist clients in negotiating for an extension of their medical leave of absence to ensure continuation of their insurance policy.

Information on cost savings is also important for changes in public policy. Legislators are keenly aware of the costs of health care (usually hospital), but few have accurate information about the costs of long-term care, including home care. It is the responsibility of home health agency administrators to share information on cost savings with local, state, and federal legislators. Doing this may lead to improved accessibility and availability of home care services to persons with AIDS/ARC.

WHEN HOME CARE IS NO LONGER APPROPRIATE

Some persons with AIDS/ARC require long-term care that cannot be provided at home. Patients with chronic physical debilitation or severe neurological impairment may not be able to receive care at home because they need 24-h care and supervision. Neither public nor private insurance providers are likely to provide unlimited 24-h care coverage. When the patient's resources are exhausted, alternative placement outside the home must be identified.

In most communities, options for the long-term care of individuals with any chronic illness or disability are limited. Identifying alternatives for persons with AIDS/ARC is even more difficult because of fears and concerns about infection control precautions and life-style issues. It may take special educational forums and community pressure before the person with AIDS/ARC obtains access to limited skilled, intermitent, or extended-care beds. It is essential that every community begins early to explore its options and begin the long process of education to allay anxieties related to the care of persons with AIDS/ARC.

Residential Care Facilities

Residential care facilities, or board-and-care facilities, provide an ideal setting for individuals with AIDS/ARC who are able to carry out personal-care activities but who require supervision around the clock owing to neurological impairment. As the person becomes less ambulatory, the residential care facility should be able to increase assistance for personal-care activities.

This setting provides a low-cost housing alternative for persons who may be homeless or whose home environment is no longer appropriate for home care. Some facilities may be able to care for several persons with AIDS/ARC at the same time. Since home care is provided by an outside home health agency in most board-and-care facilities, these services may be consolidated for two or three patients at the same time. In this way, a more cost-effective approach to care is instituted. If the patient requires a higher level of care, arrangements for transfer are made by the residential care operator or the home care team.

Adult Day Care Centers

Some persons with AIDS/ARC may need supervision during the daytime while family members work or take a break from care giving. Care around the clock at home may be unnecessary. Adult day care centers may be an appropriate setting, since their staff are accustomed to providing care for persons with personal care needs as well as neurological impairment.

These centers are an untapped resource for the care of AIDS/ARC patients. Staffing patterns to accommodate the physical and neurological complications encounters must be explored. Education to others using the facility must also be provided to answer questions and allay fears about AIDS/ARC. Adult day health centers may provide an ideal setting for patients who cannot be left unsupervised at home. This alternative should be explored in every community as an additional resource along the long-term care continuum for the person with AIDS/ARC.

Skilled Nursing Facilities

Skilled nursing facilities offer yet a higher degree of patient care than either residential care facilities or adult day care centers. These facilities are appropriate for individuals who have complex physical and neurological complications requiring intervention by a licensed vocational nurse or a registered nurse throughout the day. Patients admitted to skilled nursing facilities may need monitoring 24 h a day with medications, wound care, intravenous therapy, or other interventions.

Like other facilities, skilled nursing facilities have remained untapped for several reasons. In some communities, skilled nursing beds are limited. Waiting lists for admission to a facility may be many months and sometimes more than a year. In other communities, the staffs of skilled nursing facilities have not been properly educated about AIDS/ARC. The staffs are often confused or frightened about patient care needs. Finally, the reimbursement available for skilled nursing facilities is often limited by both public and private resources. The inadequate reimbursement offers little incentive for operators of skilled nursing facilities to consider the admission of AIDS/ARC patients.

Nonetheless, skilled nursing facilities may be the most valuable resource in every community. Patients increasingly require experienced professionals for ongoing physical care and neurological support that cannot be well managed at home. Educating the staff of skilled nursing facilities about the care requirements will minimize their fears and provide a supportive long-term care environment. Encouraging legislators to increase reimbursement levels will maximize access to skilled nursing facilities, since operators will have more incentive to accept AIDS/ARC patients.

One single option for care is inadequate in any community. Rather, long-term care administrators and legislators together must explore every alternative.

Options that are not currently available must be explored. Education must be provided to the staffs of these facilities so that the first admission will receive compassionate and supportive care. If these options are not explored, patients will stay in acute-care settings longer, taxing both the financial and the personal resources in the community.

CONCLUSION

Providing hospice care to individuals with AIDS/ARC at home is challenging in the best of circumstances. As patients experience physical debilitation and severe neurological complications, the multidisciplinary team approach of most hospice programs is ideal to meet the needs of patients with AIDS/ARC, their friends, and their family members. This sensitive and humane approach offers support from early in the disease process, to assist patients as they struggle with difficult treatment decisions, until long after the death occurs, to enable friends and family members to cope with the loss of a loved one.

Administrators must prepare their staffs for admissions of individuals with AIDS/ARC. They must review all policies and procedures, such as admissions criteria and infection control policies. Administrators must arrange for regular in-service education for their staffs to ensure understanding about AIDS/ARC and quality patient care services. In this manner, the skilled and compassionate care required by individuals with AIDS/ARC will be anticipated and provided from the outset. It is our responsibility to ensure that home care and hospice services are available to all persons with AIDS/ARC and that when home care is no longer a viable alternative, other long-term care options are available.

REFERENCES

1. Foster J, Hall HD. Public health and AIDS. *Caring* 1986;5(6):4–11, 73–78.

2. Martin JP. The AIDS home care and hospice program: A multidisciplinary approach to caring for persons with AIDS. *American Journal of Hospice Care* 1986;3(2):35–37.

3. Martin JP. Ensuring quality hospice care for the person with AIDS. *Quality Review Bulletin* 1986;12(10):353–358.

4. Schietinger H. A home care plan for AIDS. *American Journal of Nursing* 1986;86:1021–1028.

5. Schoen K. Psychosocial aspects of hospice care for AIDS patients. *American Journal of Hospice Care* 1986;3(2):32–34.

6. Beresford L. The hospice team, stress, and staff support. *California Hospice Report.* San Francisco: Northern California Hospice Association, 1986;4:1–5.

7. Scitovsky AA, Cline M, Lee PR. Medical care costs of patients with AIDS in San Francisco. *JAMA* 1986;256:3103–3106.

8. Martin JP. Challenges in caring for the person with AIDS at home. *Caring* 1986;5(6):12–20.

9. Zembo S. Insurance negotiation. *AIDS Home Care and Hospice Manual.* San Francisco: VNA of San Francisco, 1987;159–160.

10. Hughes A., Martin JP, Franks P. *AIDS Home Care and Hospice Manual.* San Francisco: VNA of San Francisco, 1987.

37

Housing for People with AIDS

Helen Schietinger

INTRODUCTION

Since the beginning of the AIDS epidemic, people with AIDS have been shunned and feared irrationally. As a result of this fear as well as other problems, a disproportionate number of people who are HIV-positive or who have AIDS or ARC have lost their housing.

There are a number of reasons for loss of housing, a major reason being rejection based on fear of contagion. The tremendous fear of contagion surrounding AIDS has caused many family members, roommates, and lovers to refuse to live with someone who is diagnosed with AIDS or who has a positive HIV antibody test. Even neighbors have rejected people with AIDS. Sally, for example, was living in a low-cost housing project. When her children's friends discovered that she had AIDS, she was harassed by her neighbors, forcing her to move.

The second reason people with AIDS need new housing is rejection based on fear of the dying process. We live in a society that fears death, and many people will abandon friends or loved ones rather than assist them as they deteriorate and become dependent. When Bob was admitted to the hospital with a diagnosis of *Pneumocystis carinii* pneumonia, his roommates said he could not return to the apartment, because they did not think they could care for an "invalid." They quickly moved his belongings into storage and found someone else to move into the apartment.

At times the people with whom a sick person is living are looked to for the provision of care when the person is discharged from the hospital. Often home care services are inadequate, and when those sharing the responsibility for care can no longer do so, they may not allow the person with AIDS to return to their house, feeling that was their only option. When Peter was readmitted to the hospital, his lover, who had been caring for him at home by himself, said he could no longer cope with the strain of being up all night and trying to go to work during the day. He requested that Pete not be discharged home again, even though Pete did not want or need to stay in the hospital.

The third reason that people with AIDS lose their housing is the financial devastation that accompanies the illness. When people are diagnosed with AIDS and become disabled, they are often no longer able to work. Thus they lose their source of income, which causes a dramatic change in economic status. Many people with AIDS who have been accustomed to a comfortable standard of living find themselves unable to pay the rent or mortgage. Jose lost his job when illness that was a consequence of ARC resulted in too many days away from work. He and his wife had a house full of furniture when they were evicted for not paying their rent. They were forced to sell or give away most of their furnishings, because there was no place for storage. Their small residence hotel room cost nearly his entire Social Security check, and whatever money remained was needed to pay for food.

Among the growing population of the urban homeless there is a subset of individuals who have AIDS and ARC. Homeless prior to becoming ill, their suffering is increased because they are weak and vulnerable. In at least one city in the United States, the shelter program for the homeless has refused to provide shelter to anyone whom it discovers to have AIDS. Even those who are able to secure shelter at night must leave in the morning and wait in line again in the evening for a cot.

HISTORY OF THE PROBLEM IN SAN FRANCISCO

The Shanti Project was the agency in San Francisco that responded immediately to the AIDS crisis. For nearly 10 years this private, nonprofit agency had trained and supported volunteers in providing emotional support to people who were experiencing life-threatening illnesses and to people who were grieving the loss of a loved one. Shanti volunteers made themselves available to the first people suffering from AIDS in San Francisco. They shifted their focus entirely to people with AIDS when it became clear that the numbers were reaching epidemic proportions and that other community resources were often not available to these people because of the public's fear to contagion. As volunteers became involved in the lives of people suffering from AIDS, they also became aware that a high proportion of their clients had difficulty in maintaining themselves in the community. Disability often prevented persons with AIDS (PWAs) from carrying out basic functions such as shopping or doing laundry. PWAs frequently became transient as they lost their homes because of fearful roommates or inability to pay rent. The Shanti Project responded to the situation in 1983 by applying to the city for special funding to develop two new programs for PWAs. The Practical Support Program trained and supervised volunteers to provide services such as cooking, shopping, errands, etc. The Shanti Residence Program established housing for PWAs who had no place to live. Although each of these programs operates separately, the services provided by the support program are integral to the housing program.

THE SHANTI AIDS RESIDENCE PROGRAM

The Residence Program is structured to provide independent housing in small group-living situations. Shanti leases apartments throughout the city. Each of the apartments is owned by a private property owner, and Shanti holds the lease, but receives funding from the city to pay the rent. As of February 1987, Shanti had 12 such apartments providing housing to a total of 47 residents at any given time. Each apartment had three to six bedrooms. The residents share the kitchen, living room, and bathroom and have their own individual bedrooms. The common areas are generously furnished through donations from the community, and the bedrooms are either furnished by the individual resident or by Shanti, according to need. Most of the apartments are large Victorian flats with spacious rooms, and they are all tastefully furnished and homey. Even though there are special items such as a pay phone in each kitchen, the apartments do not have an institutional feeling about them. Each house has its own individual character and is home to those who live there.

Requirements for admission to the Shanti Residence Program are that a person have a CDC-defined diagnosis of AIDS, be in need of housing, be a resident of San Francisco, and be able to live cooperatively with others. The application process usually takes up to 2 weeks, and there is always a waiting list which averages 15. Residents are charged rent at a rate of 25% of their income or disability benefits.

The Residence Program began in May 1983 with a staff of one (the director) and has expanded to include the equivalent of 7.5 full-time positions. As new houses have been opened, determining the appropriate level of staffing to maintain the program has been a challenge. An adequate number of paid staff has been vital to the success of the program. Volunteer support from the Shanti Practical Support Program has also been an integral part of the program since its inception, and more recently, volunteer clerical support in the office has been essential to the maintenance of the program.

The office staff consists of a director, who administers the program and provides liaison with other agencies; an administrative assistant, who coordinates the application process and office operations; a half-time secretary; and volunteer clerical support. The director is a nurse with administrative experience.

The maintenance staff provide physical maintenance of the houses, clean the rooms when someone dies or moves out, furnish the rooms for new residents, and orient them to their new home when they move in. A staff person cleans and disinfects the bathrooms weekly, and volunteers provide weekly house-cleaning services.

The social work staff (who are called residence advocates) function basically as case managers. They interview and screen applicants, facilitate group harmony through weekly house meetings in each house, and monitor residents' physical and emotional status, referring people to community resources for services such as home care or emotional support as needed. The two full-time advocates who have master's-level social services education are essential to assure the well-being of the people living in the houses.

No staff members live in the houses. After 5:00 p.m. and on weekends, the people who live in the Shanti residences are expected to function independently. The advantages of this model are that no licensing is required and that people who live in the houses have a tremendous amount of flexibility and independence, which helps them maintain their dignity and sense of autonomy. The addresses are kept confidential to assure that each house is a private residence, not a facility open to the public.

The staff of the residence program become intensely involved in the lives of the people they house despite the limits of staff participation in the houses. When a person applies to the program, filling out the paperwork with the administrative assistant and the intake interview by the residence advocate are situations that evoke the story of that person's struggle with AIDS. Providing emotional support and counseling are appropriate and essential at this time. The maintenance staff are in and out of the person's home and often become an important mainstay of emotional support for the person. The average length of stay is 3–4 months, with most people living in the houses until they die. Obviously, staff members experience loss continuously as the 47 people for whom they provide housing move through the process of becoming debilitated and dying. The weekly staff support group in which the staff members process their grief and anger is a critical component of the Residence Program.

There are four types of licenses that must be considered in establishing the guidelines of a housing program for people with AIDS. In San Francisco, if more than six unrelated adults live in one building, a hotel license is required. In California, if a program provides meals and personal care to people, or if the residents' money is being managed by the program, a residential care license is necessary. If mental health or substance abuse services are being provided, a residential treatment facility license is required. If skilled nursing care is provided by the program, a skilled nursing facility license is required. The Residence Program only provides housing and refers residents to other community services when needed. Thus, it avoids the restrictions imposed by these other licensed facilities. This allows a tremendous amount of flexibility in the kind of living situation that can be available to a person.

The Residence Program has provided stability to people whose lives have been disrupted by a diagnosis of AIDS. In the first 3 years of the program, over 200 people benefited from living in a Shanti residence. For many, the most immediate benefit lies in not having to pay almost their entire Social Security disability income for a dismal hotel room with no kitchen facilities. Another obvious benefit for people who are physically capable of maintaining the activities of daily living is that they can live in a Shanti residence without having to give up any of their independence, including buying and cooking their own food and having their own guests. People with AIDS struggle to maintain as much control as possible over their lives, as demonstrated by the fact that most residents choose not to share cooking with their roommates.

One touching example of what is possible in a Shanti residence happened when a Latino man whose primary language was Spanish was discharged from the hospital back to the residence in which he lived. His family lived in a Latin American country and could not obtain visas to visit him, but his small evangelical church community became his family. They were able to visit him, in the privacy of his own room, and provide support he would not otherwise have had.

Social interaction is facilitated by the shared living space, and the advocacy arm of the program provides a range of support with the possibility of rapid intervention if services are needed. Because AIDS is a chronic, debilitating illness, it is clear that nearly all residents will face the need for supportive services at some point. When individuals deteriorate physically and want to remain in their home environments, volunteer and licensed home care services become essential. In San Francisco when the Residence Program first opened, attempts were made to enable people to remain at home by utilizing the traditional home care system, the In-Home-Support-Services system of the Department of Social Services (DSS), and volunteers from the Shanti Practical Support Program. It was soon evident that these services were inadequate when a person reached a certain stage of disability and that the home care services provided by hospice home care agencies were then necessary to maintain people at home.

Through a special attendant care program for people with AIDS, the San Francisco Hospice Program was able to provide 24-h home attendant care for people who elected to remain at home even into the terminal stages of the illness. This became the AIDS Home Care and Hospice Program. Usually, only one person in a household would deteriorate at any given time. The other residents would continue their activities while their roommate received care from the hospice team.

The reactions of the residents have been uniformly supportive of housemates who do not want to return to the hospital to die, despite the emotional stress it poses for them. For some people it has been the anticipated loss of a housemate that has precipitated their asking for a Shanti emotional support volunteer. House meetings, facilitated by the residence advocate, normally retain a focus on living even when there is an undercurrent of anger and grief about an ill or dying housemate. The residence advocate facilitates the sharing of all of these feelings in the supportive environment of the house meeting. Residents move in and out of confronting feelings about having a life-threatening illness, a healthy coping mechanism familiar to those working with dying people.

As the number of people with AIDS in San Francisco escalated, the needs outgrew the attendant care resources, and it became less and less possible for the hospice program to enable people with AIDS to die at home if they needed 24-h attendant care (unless they could pay for most of the care themselves or had insurance that would do so). Even with a specially funded AIDS home care program, services were limited by the resources of the program.

In response to this problem, the AIDS Home Care and Hospice Program collaborated with Shanti to meet, on an interim basis, the need for 24-h care by providing ongoing home attendant care in two of the 10 Shanti residences, each housing five people. Only people who required 24-h care were accepted into these houses. If a person reached the point of being unable to remain safely in his or her home (or Shanti residence) without 24-h care, these houses provided another option within the community where more personal care was possible than in a hospital setting. This community-based 24-h care situation has been transferred from Shanti housing to a more appropriate facility. In March of 1987 the San Francisco AIDS Home Health and Hospice program opened a residential care facility with a capacity for 15 people, at least 10 of whom are people with AIDS. This new facility, called Coming Home Hospice, utilizes the same model of 24-h home care attendant services. The board-and-care model provides more efficient consolidated services than are possible in the individual Shanti residences.

The Shanti AIDS Residence Program model has proved itself successful in providing excellent housing for certain groups of people with AIDS, often enabling them to establish a quality of life and level of security they had lost following diagnosis. The Shanti model is not the answer to the housing needs of all people with AIDS and does not, even in collaboration with intense hospice services, fill the desperate need for 24-h care for debilitated people with AIDS. However, it has met a tremendous need, and it has been used as a model for AIDS housing programs in many cities across the country.

PROBLEMS IN PROVIDING HOUSING

Usually a person with AIDS needs a variety of services, and often the lines between these needs become fuzzy. Many people with AIDS need housing, but many others would not need accommodations if adequate home care were available where they were living. Some people do not need housing or home care but instead need intermediate care in a facility in which there are round-the-clock supervision and care. A person with AIDS may be in denial about his or her level of debilitation, insisting that he or she only needs housing and refusing to admit a need for personal care. Often is is difficult to recognize physical debilitation in the protected hospital environment. A person may be discharged home, only to return shortly because of lack of such care. It is important to recognize that PWAs do not require housing alone. A variety of volunteer and home care and hospice services as well as social services must also be provided to maintain debilitated people with AIDS in the community. One of the problems that arise in providing housing to PWAs is associated with inadequate community-based home care services.

Another problem posed to agencies providing housing PWAs is that the person must be willing to accept care. Many people with AIDS are fiercely independent; they are young and they have difficulty accepting the dependence forced on them by their illness. They often refuse to be hospitalized or to accept nursing care at home. This leaves them isolated without adequate assistance, and at best they have poor nutrition and poor hygiene as they become less and less able to meet their own daily needs.

A compounding problem occurs if PWAs are cognitively impaired and confused, as is often the case when there is extensive neurological involvement. Such individuals may become a danger to themselves and others. For example, they may forget to turn off stove burners, or they may wander out of the house without knowing where they live. Both of these examples have occurred more than once in the experience of the Shanti Residence Program, and they point to the difficulty is assuring an appropriate transition between one level of service and another.

The worst-case scenario occurs when a person becomes mentally incompetent and has designated no one or has no next of kin to make health care or financial decisions. One way of possibly avoiding this problem is by initiating discussion with PWAs early in the course of the disease regarding the assignment of medical and durable power of attorney to a family member, lover, or trusted friend. The desire to assist the person in maintaining as much dignity and automony as possible and the need to protect his or her safety and that of others are often in conflict. The process of determining that a person is incompetent and requires involuntary hospitalization or conservatorship is traumatic and cumbersome. Establishing conservatorship is a (necessarily) time-consuming legal effort that is traumatic to the individual but something that needs to be addressed in long-term planning for incompetent individuals who have no family or friends designated to assume that role.

In short, the agency that assumes responsibility for providing housing to people with AIDS often finds itself in the position of dealing with physically and mentally debilitated people who are not able to make good decisions for themselves and who may be mentally incompetent. Many people with AIDS who need housing also have no significant others or family members nearby to take over the decision-making processes for them. This can place the agency in a difficult position, even if there are adequate community services available to meet the person's needs.

MODELS OF HOUSING NEEDED

People with AIDS who are homeless vary tremendously in their socioeconomic status, in their life styles, and in their living situations. Different models of housing are needed for different populations of people with AIDS.

Independent Group Living

Most people with AIDS are individuals who have been functional in society prior to their illness and are used to living independently. These people would be appropriate for the independent group living model, in which people with AIDS share a kitchen, bathroom, and living room but have individual bedrooms. This shared-living situation with no supervision enables the person to reestablish his or her unique personal surroundings and maintain individual cooking and social contacts as desired.

The Shanti AIDS Residence Program in San Francisco was the first program of this kind, and most of the housing programs for people with AIDS in major cities in the United States are based on this model. AIDS residence programs have been set up in Boston, Washington, D.C., and New York City, for example. The model assumes that the person is capable of living cooperatively with other people in a group living situation, a factor that is usually assessed on intake interview or through landlord and other references. The concept of independent group living sounds deceptively simple to manage. In reality, however, taking responsibility for housing people with AIDS is a tremendous responsibility. For example, ensuring the safety of the physical facilities requires constant vigilance, as people who are debilitated often cannot attend to details (such as whether cardboard boxes are placed against the gas water heater or whether a space heater has been plugged into an inadequate extension cord). Providing housing also requires monitoring the physical and emotional status of residents. This includes being available to access health care when necessary and to mediate in disagreements among housemates. Staff must be able to distinguish between these normal disputes and inappropriate behavior by a resident, and they must be prepared to deal with behavior that endangers or humiliates another resident. Obviously, this type of program requires a trained and very dedicated staff and well-supervised volunteers.

Residence Hotel

There are people who were socially marginal prior to their illness who are unable to live cooperatively with others. This group includes many of the homeless, the mentally ill, and the chemically addicted. These people's lives are often chaotic and disorganized, and they are unaccustomed to negotiating and maintaining social contacts within an unstructured atmosphere of mutual respect. Thus, they would not be appropriate for an unsupervised group living situation. They need a more structured housing situation in which there can be constant supervision of the premises by someone in authority to monitor behavior and to assure that those who are debilitated are protected from the actions of those who might be disruptive. The model would most appropriately be a hotel in which people have individual rooms but share a common kitchen, common dining room, and bathrooms. Another excellent model would have individual efficiency apartments. In either case the advantage is in having a hotel manager on the premises 24 h a day who is responsible for the facility. A social services component is essential to assist individuals whose difficult lives have been even more disrupted by the diagnosis and symptoms of AIDS. These are people who will require close medical and nursing monitoring, good home care, and case management, as their health needs are complex and they have difficulty negotiating the health care system.

Family Housing

Another group of people who need housing are families: people with AIDS who live with significant others and people with AIDS who have dependents. Examples are people with AIDS who have lovers or spouses, any man or woman who has children, and children with AIDS who have a family. Having a family creates a much more complex need for housing than single people have, and neither independent group living nor individual hotel rooms may be appropriate. In the Shanti AIDS Residence Program, it is challenging enough for three to six unrelated adults with AIDS to live within one household. To add family members or significant others to this configuration is a level of complexity with which people with AIDS haven't the 'energy to deal and invites chaos in the living situation. For the same reason, children would be too potentially disruptive to residents other than their parents. Practically speaking, Shanti found it impossible to justify providing subsidized housing to the significant other as well as the person with AIDS, because the resources are so desperately needed by other people with AIDS.

Low-income public housing would seem to be the solution for the homeless family. However, one case has already been cited of a woman who was ostracized from the housing project in which she lived with her children. Even if the residents of existing housing programs were to accept the PWA and his or her family, it is common to wait for years before a space becomes available. Thus, the person who becomes homeless after a diagnosis of AIDS may die before traditional public housing becomes available.

A model that would best serve the needs of families would be a building with studio and one- and two-bedroom apartments so that each family could have its own living quarters. The staff needed to manage the program would probably be similar to that of the Shanti Residence Program, except that a strong child care component would also be necessary to provide support for debilitated parents.

Foster Care

Children with AIDS may also need housing or, more specifically, foster care. There are children with AIDS whose parents have died of AIDS or who have been abandoned by their parents. Many of these children do not need to be in hospitals but require foster care in order to be discharged into the community. This becomes a very difficult placement issue, particularly in areas such as New Jersey and New York, where there are large numbers of foster children with

AIDS. It is difficult enough to provide a normal environment to a child who faces the stigma our society places on having AIDS. Consider the instances in which parents have removed their children from school rather than allow them to attend school with a child who is HIV antibody-positive or who has AIDS. However, it is almost impossible to provide the usual opportunities for growth and social development to an infant or child with AIDS who has no family and who is a ward of the court. The foster home systems in most cities are not prepared to address the issues that arise regarding confidentiality of diagnosis and fear of contagion when dealing with children who are HIV-seropositive or those with AIDS or ARC. Staff within the system, the public, and potential foster parents must all be educated to the desperate need for care and the low risk for contagion so that the growing number of parentless babies and children who are HIV-seropositive or have AIDS can find homes in the community.

SUMMARY

The tragic physical and emotional effects of HIV infection are compounded by the often detrimental economic consequences for and negative social reactions to the person with AIDS, ARC, or HIV seropositivity. Loss of housing as a result of an AIDS diagnosis or HIV seropositivity is a problem poorly resolved by the traditional social service system. It has become clear that people with AIDS require different types of housing according to their social and physical situations.

The model of small independent group living situations has been developed and is successful with a particular group of people with AIDS, given a well-organized home care program in the community. Other models need to be developed for other populations of people with AIDS, particularly given the continued increase in numbers among women and children.

CASE STUDY

When Richard came into my office for the first time, he was wearing a clean, freshly pressed shirt and pair of slacks that were now two sizes too big for him. He had two Kaposi's sarcoma lesions on his face which were only discernible to my practiced eye, as they were carefully covered with makeup. He sat down and apologized for taking so much of my time on the phone the day before. He had called from the Social Security office, where he had just been told that even though his paperwork had been completed 3 months ago, his claim would not be processed and finalized for 2 more months. He had used up all of his state disability and his savings in the intervening months, and now he was desperate. He owed next week's rent for the residence hotel he was living in and had no money. I referred him to the social services department of the San Francisco AIDS Foundation for advocacy within the Social Security system (hopefully to speed up the process of securing his benefits) and for obtaining emergency assistance. The social workers at the AIDS Foundation would provide him with emergency housing, give him access to the food bank, and help him apply for General Assistance for the intervening months until his Social Security check arrived. I also made an appointment for him to come in and apply to the Shanti AIDS Residence Program.

As we talked in person, he described his relief that the social worker had been able to see him yesterday. He had 3 more days at his hotel, and after that he was going to be able to move into the emergency housing of the AIDS Foundation while he applied to the Shanti Residence Program. Richard began to relax as I described to him the way the Residence Program works—how the houses are set up, what the application process is like, and so forth. He asked the typical questions, such as, "What are the other people like who live there?" and "How much does it cost?" He admitted he had almost canceled the appointment because he was afraid that living with other people with AIDS would be depressing, but my description of the general attitudes and situations of the residents made him feel better. He realized that the sliding rent scale made this housing affordable even with his small Social Security income, and he also looked forward to having a kitchen again, after living for a month in a hotel room. It was important to him to be reassured that he could buy and cook his own food and that he would have his own room. He finally concluded, "I've lived by myself all of my adult life, and I don't look forward to having roommates, but I guess having my own room will be enough privacy."

In my interview with Richard, I discovered that his parents had moved from Mexico to Los Angeles when they were first married and that he had been born in Los Angeles, the first of four children. He lived at home while attending college, but when he got his first job as an engineer, he moved into his own apartment. He remained close to his family, frequently going to Mass with them on Sunday. He had several close friends at work, all of whom were heterosexual. Richard was bisexual and had never intimated to any of his co-workers or his family that he had sexual relationships with men. When he was diagnosed with KS, he quit his job and left town immediately, traveling to Europe, where he lived in a monastery in a life of meditation and contemplation. After 6 months he realized he had to return to the United States because his health was failing. He decided to come to San Francisco to ensure that none of his friends or family from Los Angeles would discover that he had AIDS. He was convinced that all his close friends, especially those with children, would be horrified to discover that he had AIDS and would assume that the reason he got AIDS was that he was homosexual. In fact, he had misgivings about moving into a Shanti Residence because of the implications about his sexual orientation. I questioned whether *he* had prejudices against homosexuality that would make if difficult for him to accept and respect his housemates, all of whom at that time would be gay men. I did assure him that the policy of the program was to accept any adults with AIDS regardless of sexual orientation or gender. I got my first laugh out of Richard when he told me he would actually enjoy being among gay men, where he would not have to be on guard for once about the "other half" of his social life.

Richard went on to say that when he had arrived in San Francisco, he established himself in a small residence hotel. He continued to depend on his state disability checks, which would last a year from the time be began receiving them. He made no friends, but he contacted his family to tell them where was. He spent most of his time in his room, having only enough energy to go to a restaurant for one or two meals a day and to the library once a week. He saw no need to be followed by a doctor, as he was physically stable except for his skin lesions and his malaise. The world did not crash around him until his money ran out and he found himself literally destitute for the first time in his life. He was too proud to ask for help until he was desperate, and he had considered the act of calling Shanti a personal defeat.

I finished my interview with Richard and helped him begin filling out the paperwork of the application. A week later the paperwork was complete, and a date and time were set for him to move into one of the Shanti residences, assisted by the maintenance specialist. The morning he moved in he called me in tears. He wanted me to know that he was overwhelmed with gratitude at how welcomed he felt by the staff and his new housemates and at how comfortable and homey the house was. He had felt isolated and alone for so many months, and here people seemed to really care about him. He had experienced so many blows to his self-esteem as he lost his income, his status as an engineer, his beautiful apartment, his physical stamina, his youthful physical attractiveness, and his friends and family. He had expected this transition to be another step down from the dingy but clean hotel he first found when he moved to San Francisco. Instead, here was a tastefully furnished apartment with a well-appointed kitchen, and his room was large enough to spend lots of time in without feeling hemmed in. The first thing he did was put the easy chair beside the window so he could have plenty of light for reading.

Two months went by uneventfully for Richard. He was quiet and kept to himself most of the time, but he showed concern for his roommates. When Bob became short of breath, he accompanied him to the emergency room in a cab so that Bob would not have to negotiate the medical system alone. In weekly house meetings, Richard was a mediator, using gentle confrontation rather than joining Bob and Andy in getting angry at Paul for leaving the kitchen in a shambles. He had a friendly, easygoing way about him which generated a sense of family among the four of them. They all bought separate groceries, but once or twice a week made a meal and had a dinner together. Richard insisted on doing his own grocery shopping rather than asking for a practical support volunteer for help, despite the fact that the trip exhausted him for 2 days afterward. He had a sense of self-sufficiency and independence, because he could take care of all his own needs and also help Bob a little.

Richard continued to take meticulous care to apply makeup to his face before seeing anyone in the morning. As the weeks went by, however, the lesions on his face spread and became more prominent. Makeup was needed all over his face and neck, and his shirt collar often rubbed away the makeup on his neck within a short time, revealing a blotchy purple ring at his throat. One afternoon on the bus, some schoolchildren noticed the lesions and taunted him publicly for having AIDS. The humiliation hurt him deeply, and he decided to ask for a volunteer to drive him to the store from then on. He called the house his haven—the only place in the world where he felt safe and accepted. He knew that here anyone he encountered—Shanti staff, volunteers, roommates' visitors—would be able to handle his physical appearance.

At a certain point, Richard's legs began to swell, and his face became puffy and edematous, which meant that the KS was spreading to his lymph nodes and blocking fluid drainage from his legs and face. He walked noticeably more slowly. At weekly house meetings, comments from his roommates suggested that he was becoming limited in his ability to bathe and carry out other activities of daily living. I suggested to him privately that it might be useful for a home care nurse to visit him and assess his physical situation and his nutritional level. Perhaps he or she could recommend assistive devices such as a shower chair and a cane, or a home health aide to help with a bath and a meal. He was adamant that he did not want a nurse to visit him and that he could take care of himself. I told him that if he changed his mind, or if he became weaker, he could call me and I would seek a referral for him. In the meantime, he agreed to let the maintenance specialist bring a hassock to his room so that he could elevate his legs while sitting in his chair. At a certain point he asked his practical support volunteer to make his bed, but he insisted on continuing to do his laundry himself (there were a washer and dryer in the house, but the activity exhausted him). He struggled to maintain his independence while he deteriorated physically. He spent so much of his limited energy carrying out basic activities that he rarely had the stamina to do things such as go to the library.

It was Andy who called the office one morning to say that Richard had fallen trying to get to the bathroom during the night, and they had found him sleeping on the floor in the morning. He was short of breath and could not bear his own weight, and they had dragged him back to bed. I contacted his physician, who hospitalized him and diagnosed *Pneumocystis carinii* pneumonia. His roommates as well as the residence program staff visited him in the hospital, bringing him books and pictures for his bedside table. At this point he asked for an emotional support volunteer.

He and Janet immediately became close. During this hospitalization, he decided to contact his parents and tell them he had cancer. He had a hard time convincing them not to come to San Francisco to be with him, because they were extremely concerned about him. He began to make plans to draw up a will, although he jokingly said the only thing he owned was debts.

Richard was discharged home to the residence with care from the San Francisco AIDS Home Care and Hospice Program. A nurse stayed in close touch with him, and he had an attendant three times a week to cook some meals and help him with personal care. He gradually regained enough strength to be out of bed most of the day but never lost the need to use a walker. After 2 months, the KS invaded his left lung. Continuous oxygen kept him fairly comfortable, and with 4 h of attendant care a day, he was able to remain at home. Bob and Paul had both become very weak and also had home care. Among the three of them, the home care program consolidated the attendant care, providing 12 h daily. Andy complained at times about the loss of privacy caused by care givers' being in the house all day but said he would rather have his roommates at home with him than in the hospital.

When Richard became terminally ill, he was calm and resigned to dying. He had accepted his increasing level of dependence but was now dyspneic and in pain almost constantly, despite taking oral morphine. He decided that he needed to tell his family that he was dying, even though it would mean disclosing his diagnosis. He wanted them to come to see him before he died. His mother arrived the day after he called, and his father flew up on the weekend. They rented a hotel room nearby, but the maintenance staff brought a cot over to Richard's room from the storeroom so that they could take turns staying with him at night. It seemed as though a steady stream of sisters and brothers and nieces and nephews visited Richard for the next week. Two couples with whom he had been close friends at work flew up to see him. Several people were visibly shaken when they saw Richard's physical condition, and his emotional support volunteer and the hospice nurse spent a great deal of time in the living room listening to them.

The last time I spoke with Richard, he told me that it had been very important for him to find the safety of the residence program. He had first sought refuge in a monastery in Europe, which was where he faced the reality of his diagnosis. But it was in the Shanti residence that he found that he still had a life to live, after fleeing from everything and everyone who had meant anything to him. People let him live in dignity here when he had thought that he should be ashamed of accepting help. He was thankful that he had gotten over being afraid of being disowned by his family and friends, and in fact said he owed them an apology for disowning *them*.

Richard died quietly in his own bed in a Shanti residence, surrounded by those who loved him and whom he loved. He is not forgotten by the staff and volunteers at Shanti and the AIDS Home Care Program, whom he touched very deeply in his quiet, unassuming way.

VIII

AIDS AND THE PROFESSIONAL

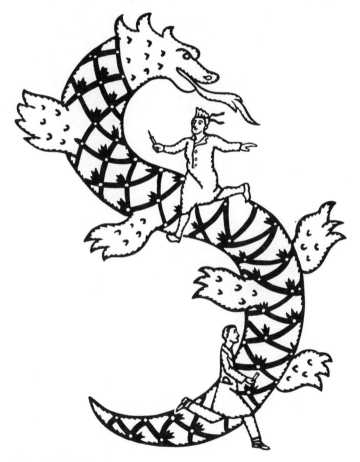

AIDS and the Professional
Care givers strive to vanquish the dragon.

VIII

AIDS AND THE PROPER SIGNAL

38

AIDS: A Special Challenge for Health Care Workers

Linda Hawes Clever

INTRODUCTION

AIDS (acquired immune deficiency syndrome) is a multisystem disease. It affects many organs and personal support systems of patients; it also affects the health care system. This paper will focus on the latter. Its special objective is to review and make recommendations about the human immunodeficiency virus (HIV) and its profound effects on health care workers. Note should be made, however, of the pervasive consequences of AIDS and its attendant horrors for health care institutions. For example, health care policy, financing, politics, planning, research, and training have been influenced. Facilities, public health and public education measures, and rehabilitation programs have been developed or modified. But the heart of any system is its people. This review therefore concentrates on the nurses, physicians, social workers, therapists, and support personnel who are faced with the daily challenge presented by AIDS. Topics include infection control, risk of contagion, ethical and legal considerations, beliefs and behaviors, and emotional reactions. Recommendations are made regarding the development of policies and educational programs.

INFECTION CONTROL

One of the earliest responses to AIDS was from the Centers for Disease Control (CDC) and pertained to occupational safety for health care workers.[1] The CDC and other organizations have continued to publish useful guidelines ever since.[2-9] Basically, since HIV is transmitted by blood, blood products, and blood-contaminated tissue fluids, infection control advice parallels guidelines for the hepatitis B virus. The "body substance isolation"[10] approach encompasses these precautions and is being incorporated into many hospitals' policies and procedures. The philosophical underpinning is that any patient may be infected with any agent and that thought, caution, and protection are required in all patient care activities. Gloves and gown are recommended if blood, mucous membrane, or secretion/excretion contact may occur. Eye protection and mask are indicated if airborne debris may be encountered during patient care activities. Needle punctures and other wounds must be avoided. Hand washing is essential; education must be perpetual. Personnel should recall that human tuberculosis is an increasingly recognized complication of AIDS[11] and take appropriate precautions. Severe diarrhea may require enteric precautions. Cleanup of rooms and equipment is surprisingly easy since HIV, although vicious, is highly vulnerable.[6] Commonly used mycobacterial germicides, heat, and ethylene oxide all kill the virus.

RISK OF CONTAGION

There has been substantial interest in the health of health care workers involved in the care of HIV-infected patients. Although some workers are HIV antibody-positive, with very few exceptions these findings have been attributed to life style or characterized by inadequate epidemiological data or absence of specific occupational exposures.[13] Dr. Julie Gerberding has followed nearly 1000 employees at San Francisco General Hospital for 4–5 years. All work with AIDS patients, and over half have had specific exposures. Only one of the physicians, dentists, nurses, or laboratory or housekeeping personnel with negative life-style risk factors has seroconverted (J. Gerberding, personal communication, July 15, 1988). A CDC study of 938 significantly exposed health care workers found no signs or symptoms of AIDS; only 2 out of 451 tested had a positive antibody.[14]

Unfortunately, a handful of HIV parenteral exposures has resulted in well-documented, work-related conversions of HIV antibody from negative to positive. According to an early report, a British nurse did not have an "ordinary needle stick . . . a small amount of blood may well have been injected" from an arterial line of an AIDS patient.[15] Later, an American nurse received an intramuscular bloody injection with a 1.67-mm-diameter needle during an emergency procedure.[16] The incidents were unusual, since they involved deep injections of contaminated blood; they were not simply needle sticks or splashes. But it is now clear that typical needle sticks and other parenteral exposures can cause acute HIV illness and seroconversion.[17,18]

HIV remains extremely difficult to transmit in health care settings, however. (It should be noted in passing that there is no evidence of HIV transmission in more "ordinary" workplaces.) In addition, caring for AIDS patients at home is also very low risk. Many AIDS patients in the United States have received home care from family members. To date, only one of the care givers (excluding those in a sexual or IV drug relationship) has developed a positive antibody.[19] In this instance, the mother of a child with a congenital gastrointestinal malformation was heavily exposed to his blood and feces. She did not wear gloves; she did not wash her hands regularly. Her antibody converted about 1½ years after her son was given contaminated blood.

Recent reports of work-related HIV seroconversion in health care workers give cause for reflection. Utilization of common and reasonable infection control guidelines has prevented most viral spread to health professionals, yet accidents do happen. These accidents reinforce the imperative for safe work practices and equipment. They raise questions of career choice and ethics; they also raise the specter of fear.

ETHICAL/LEGAL CONSIDERATIONS

Fear and loathing can lead to unfortunate circumstances. The news media have reported exclusions of AIDS children from school, firing or shunning of workers with AIDS, and reluctance of some health personnel to care for AIDS sufferers. Plumeri[20] points out that, from a legal standpoint, refusal to care for an AIDS patient is not classified as *abandonment* unless there is a failure to arrange for alternative services. According to AMA ethical standards, there is no obligation to care for any patient except in emergencies. On the other hand, a recent AMA Council on Ethical and Judicial Affairs wrote, "A physician may not ethically refuse to treat a patient . . . solely because the patient is seropositive."[20a] Conte et al.,[3] Burrow,[21] and the American College of Physicians[22] have taken firm stances in favor of providing "competent and humane care" to all patients including HIV-infected persons.[23] These authors and organizations make a strong case for acknowledging that health care workers have always assumed risks when caring for patients, and that AIDS patients are no different. Zuger and Miles[24] and Pellegrino[25] analyze various ethical rationales: patients' rights, physicians' knowledge, and professional moral obligations. The consensus is, "The denial of appropriate care to patients for any reason in unethical."[23]

BELIEFS AND BEHAVIOR

It has been hypothesized that fear of AIDS contagion is greatest where there is the least clinical experience of it.[26] Additionally, in the absence of vigorous and continuing professional education, opinions of health personnel may correspond to those of the general public. Two Gallup polls, one done in New York City and one in the United States as a whole, showed that between 10% and 39% of adults and teenagers either did not know or were wrong about important AIDS facts.[27] For example, about 19% of teenagers did not know or were incorrect about the association between IV drug abuse, needle sharing, and AIDS. About 18% of those in the study groups did not know whether or thought that a person could get AIDS by casual contact. Prejudice and homophobia as well as ignorance may determine beliefs and behavior. Twelve percent of nurses and 3% of physicians at a large urban teaching hospital with many AIDS patients felt that "homosexuals who contract AIDS are getting what they deserve."[28]

Two other studies used a mock vignette describing a gay male with AIDS or a straight male with leukemia with identical jobs, recreations, symptoms, and feelings.[29,30] Both physicians and nurses had more a negative attitude toward the gay AIDS patient. Both groups felt that the gay patient was more responsible for and deserving of his illness; both groups were less willing to interact socially with the AIDS patient. Fortunately, both groups also felt that the AIDS patient deserved sympathy and understanding, albeit not as much as the leukemia patient did.

Whatever the cause, there have been reports of legal action or neglect in the care of AIDS patients. An HIV antibody positive British psychiatric patient, known to be avoiding arrest, was turned over to the police after he cut his hands and smeared blood on himself and his room and ward. He had broken a behavioral contract, and his blood was judged to be a risk to staff and patients.[31] In another instance psychiatric staff members ignored an AIDS patient, allowing him to elope.[32] Others have not encouraged AIDS patient participation in a therapeutic milieu.[33] Concerns have sometimes been voiced (" 'It did bother me just to breathe the air' in Mr. D's room").[34] Sometimes, there has been quiet, passive resistance. On the other hand, an untold number of physicians, nurses, social workers, researchers, counselors, and others have sought the challenge of AIDS and have worked past exhaustion. Others, even with concerns and reservations, have not asked for transfers and have stretched their minds and souls to help deal with the problem.

Beliefs and behaviors of health professionals and the way these can be altered provide fertile research opportunities.

EMOTIONAL REACTIONS

Experience with AIDS has inevitably led to emotional consequences. The situation can be likened to wartime—but there is no victory in sight. The health care "soldiers" are under attack from the front, flanks, and rear. They are fighting a pernicious enemy, HIV. They have inadequate knowledge and resources. They are being asked unanswerable questions about research results, specific prognosis, and epidemiology ("How can you be so sure that AIDS isn't spread casually?"). They face dissatisfied patients and families and probes from the news media. There is little enough time for rest and recreation. They may neglect their own families and friends—and themselves. They are beset by fatigue and may have their medical training skewed and constricted.[35] They are being forced to ask uncomfortable questions and struggle with issues such as confidentiality versus public health.[22] They may be overly optimistic or pessimistic, isolated, and resentful of workload.[36]

Horstman, in McKusick, studied 82 physicians in San Francisco who had worked with AIDS patients for an average of 3.2 years and who, on average, spent nearly one-half of their time with HIV-affected patients.[37] Fifty-six percent reported that they were experiencing more stress than ever before in their careers; almost half responded that they had never had more anxiety or fear of death. Gay health professionals had an intensified fear because of their life style (which often underwent dramatic changes, but perhaps too late).

Fear is not protective, of course, and health care professionals do get HIV illness. A 1986 survey found that at least 60 health care workers in 11 San Francisco hospitals have developed AIDS or related conditions secondary to life style (Dorothy B. Nielsen, personal communication). They face the same stigmatization, isolation, guilt, remorse, pain, discomfort, suffering, and loss of income and status as other AIDS patients.[38,39] Lastly, all health workers may share physicians' reactions to their patients' serious illness, dying, and death. Guilt, anger, failure, and above all, grief sweep over them in the midst of the "battle."[40] The self-image changes from healer to helpless.

The experience of caring for AIDS patients is not all negative, however, especially if the goal is changed from "seeking cure" to "assuring safe passage." Intellectual stimulation is enormous: as far back as 1984, both the number of medical publications and the reported number of new AIDS patients grew exponentially.[41] Working with and deriving support from a multidisciplinary team of colleagues can be satisfying. The opportunity for academic advancement and/ or public recognition can be gratifying. The swapping of "war stories" can be heady. On a more profound level, many health professionals examine their personal goals and faith and develop a sense of mission. They may also broaden their understanding and respect for human strengths, weaknesses, wisdom, wit, and warmth. They may come to grips with their own limitations.

RECOMMENDATIONS

It is imperative to write policies covering infection control, research, and personnel practices that are data-based, fair, and practical. These policies are sure to change as knowledge increases. Infection control policies should cover patient care, universal precautions, and cleanup. Concern about HIV must not divert attention from hepatitis B virus, which causes far more illness and death. These hepatitis complications are almost wholly preventable, however, when effective vaccination and postexposure policies are enforced. Postexposure HIV antibody testing and counseling should be performed if confidentiality can be maintained. Decisions should be made about special policies, if any, for pregnant health care workers. Research protocols should be established that protect research and cleanup personnel and the environment. Available NIH guidelines may be helpful in this respect.[42] Return-to-work and work assignment policies for health professionals with HIV-associated conditions should be established. Institutions should consider these employees case-by-case, using criteria established for any competence-threatening or life-threatening illness.

Educational programs must be developed for health personnel and for the community. Facts are accumulating and knowledge is changing rapidly; misinformation is screamed in headlines; questions arise; panic swells. Constant education oriented to many levels is essential. Written material is important, but small group presentations accompanied by question-and-answer sessions are often resoundingly successful. Training programs should be well rounded and not overwhelmed by HIV-related problems. Floor nurses need information, as does the nursing leadership. The latter group especially may escape routine educational programs but *must* be up to date on AIDS; special, even mandatory, programs may be necessary.

Housekeeping and maintenance personnel have significant concerns that need addressing. Board members and administration should also understand AIDS in detail because of their responsibilities for policy formulation and for internal and external communications. Finally, health professionals have an uncommon obligation at this time to educate the public and counteract hysteria. We must ceaselessly talk with groups ranging from schoolchildren to elders about the ethical, humanitarian, scientific, infection control, and public health issues of AIDS.

In addition to internal and external educational programs, support services for grieving, exhausted, troubled, fearful employees must be established. Caring for dying patients can be overwhelming and debilitating,[43,44] and interventions must be designed to help distressed health professionals cope. A multidisciplinary approach is useful and may include medical, nursing, chaplain, and counseling staff.

CONCLUSION

HIV presents unrelenting challenges. One way or another, it is affecting virtually every adolescent and adult in the United States and indeed the world. Research is burgeoning. Attitudes, sexual beliefs and practices, and drug use are being reexamined. Educational programs for professionals and the public are becoming more widespread. Public health policy, the law, human rights, science, and ethics face new challenges as pockets of hysteria, judgmentalism, and ignorance flourish. Feelings run high in patients, their friends and families, the public, employers, and health professionals. Emotional and physical consequences are pervasive and devastating. Health care institutions and health workers must rise to the occasion. Sound and effective approaches to the workplace threat of HIV have been developed and implemented. These measures, coupled with continuing education and emotional support for health care professionals, will help assure workplace safety and health in the AIDS era.

REFERENCES

1. Centers for Disease Control (CDC). Acquired immune deficiency syndrome (AIDS): Precautions for clinical and laboratory staffs. *M.M.W.R. 31*:577–80 (1982).

2. CDC. Acquired immunodeficiency syndrome (AIDS): Precautions for health care workers and allied professionals. *M.M.W.R. 32*:450–1 (1983).

3. Conte, J.E. Jr., W.K. Hadley, M. Sande, et al. Infection control guidelines for patients with the acquired immunodeficiency syndrome (AIDS). *N. Engl. J. Med. 309*:740–4 (1983).

4. CDC. Recommendations for preventing transmission of infection with human T-lymphotropic virus type III/lymphadenopathy-associated virus in the workplace. *M.M.W.R. 34*:681–6, 691–5 (1985).

5. CDC. Recommendations for preventing transmission of infection with human T-lymphocyte virus type III/lymphadenopathy-associated virus during invasive procedures. *M.M.W.R. 35*:221–3 (1986).

6. Martin, L.S., S. McDougal, S.L. Lososki: Disinfection and inactivation of the human T-lymphotropic virus type III/lymphadenopathy-associated virus. *J. Infect. Dis. 152*:400–3 (1985).

7. Valenti, W.M.: AIDS update: HTLV-III testing, immune globulins and employees with AIDS. *Infect. Control 7*:427–30 (1986).

8. Editorial. Dentists found at small risk to AIDS: L.A. task force. *Am. J. Orthodont. 89*:82 (1986).

9. Howland, W.S.: AIDS and the anesthesiologist. *Hosp. Physician 22*:17–24 (1986).

10. CDC. Recommendations for prevention of HIV transmission in health care settings. *M.M.W.R. 38*(2S):3S–18S (1987).

11. CDC. Diagnosis and management of mycobacterial infection and disease in persons with human T-lymphotropic virus type III/lymphadenopathy-associated virus infection. *M.M.W.R. 35*:448–52 (1986).

12. CDC. Update: Prospective evaluation of health-care workers exposed via the parenteral or mucous-membrane route to blood or body fluids from patients with acquired immunodeficiency syndrome—United States. *M.M.W.R. 34*:101–3 (1985).

13. CDC. Update: Evaluation of the human T-lymphotropic virus type III/lymphadenopathy-associated virus infection in health care personnel—United States. *M.M.W.R. 34*:575–8 (1985).

14. McCray, E., et al. Occupational risk of the acquired immunodeficiency syndrome among health care workers. *N. Engl. J. Med. 314*:1127–32 (1986).

15. Anonymous. Needlestick transmission of HTLV-III from a patient infected in Africa. *Lancet 2*:1376–7 (1984).

16. Stricof, R.L., D.L. Morse. HTLV-III/LAV seroconversion following a deep intramuscular needlestick injury. *N. Engl. J. Med. 314*:1115 (1986).

17. Oskenhendler, E., M. Harzic, J. Le Roux, C. Rabian, J.P. Clauvel. HIV infection with seroconversion after a superficial needlestick injury to the finger. *N. Engl. J. Med. 315*(9):582 (1986).

18. CDC. Update: Human immunodeficiency virus infections in health care worker exposed to blood of infected patients. *M.M.W.R. 36*:285–9 (1987).

19. CDC. Apparent transmission of human T-lymphotropic virus type III/lymphadenopathy-associated virus from a child to a mother providing health care. *M.M.W.R. 35*:76–9 (1986).

20. Plumeri, P.A. The refusal to treat: Abandonment and AIDS. *J. Clin. Gastroenterol. 6*:281–4 (1984).

20a. AMA Council on Ethical and Judicial Affairs. Ethical issues involved in the growing AIDS crisis. *J.A.M.A. 259*(9):1360–1 (1988).

21. Burrow, G.N. Caring for AIDS patients: The physician's risk and responsibility. *Can. Med. Assoc. J. 129*:1181 (1983).

22. Health and Public Policy Committee. Acquired immunodeficiency syndrome. *Ann. Intern. Med. 108*:460–9 (1988).

23. *Ibid., 108*:460–9 (1988), p. 462.

24. Zuger, A., S.H. Miles. Physicians, AIDS, and occupational risk. *J.A.M.A. 258*(14):1924–8 (1987).

25. Pellegrino, E.D. Altruism, self-interest, and medical ethics. *J.A.M.A. 258*(14):1939–40 (1987).

26. Glazer, G., H.A.F. Dudley, G. Ayliffe, et al. AIDS and the health professions. *Br. Med. J. 290*:852–3 (1985).

27. CDC. Results of a Gallup Poll on acquired immunodeficiency syndrome. New York City, United States. *M.M.W.R. 34*:513–4 (1985).

28. Douglas, C.J., C.M. Kalman, T.P. Kalman. Homophobia among physicians and nurses: An empirical study. *Hosp. Commun. Psychiatry 36*:1309–11 (1985).

29. Kelly, J.A., J.S. St. Lawrence, H.V. Hood, et al. Nurses' attitudes toward AIDS. *J. Cont. Ed. Nsg. 19*:78–83 (1988).

30. Kelly, J.A., J.S. St. Lawrence, S. Smith Jr. et al. Stigmatization of AIDS patients by physicians. *Am. J. Publ. Health, 77*:789–91 (1987).

31. Thompson, C., G. Isaacs, D. Supple, et al. AIDS: Dilemmas for the psychiatrist. *Lancet i*:269–70 (1986).

32. Cummings, M.A., M. Rapaport, K.L. Cummings. A psychiatric staff response to acquired immune deficiency syndrome. *Am. J. Psychiatry 143*:682 (1986).

33. Polan, J.J., D. Hellerstein, J. Amchin. Impact of AIDS-related cases on an inpatient therapeutic milieu. *Hosp. Commun. Psychiatry 36*:173–6 (1985).

34. *Ibid.*, p. 175.

35. Wachter, R.M. The impact of the acquired immunodeficiency syndrome on medical residency training. *N. Engl. J. Med. 314*:177–80 (1986).

36. Steinbrook, R., B. Lo, J. Tirpack, et al. Ethical dilemmas in caring for patients with the acquired immunodeficiency syndrome. *Ann. Intern. Med. 103*:787–90 (1985).

37. L. McKusick. (Ed.). *What to Do about AIDS: Mental Health Professionals and Physicians Discuss the Issues.* Berkeley: University of California Press (1986).

38. Morin, S.F., K.A. Charles, A.K. Malyon. The psychological impact of AIDS on gay men. *Am. Psychol. 39*:1288–93 (1984).

39. Rosner, F., S. Shapiro, L. Bernabo, et al. Psychosocial care team for patients with AIDs in a municipal hospital. *J.A.M.A. 253*:2361 (1985).

40. Tolle, S.W., D.E. Girard. The physician's role in the events surrounding patient death. *Arch. Intern. Med. 143*:1447–9 (1983).

41. Bender, B.S., T.C. Quinn: Medical response to AIDS epidemic. *N. Engl. J. Med. 310*:389 (1984).

42. Richardson, J.H., W.E. Barkley. *Biosafety in Microbiological and Biomedical Laboratories*, 1st Ed., pp. 1–23, 37–40. Washington, D.C.: DHHS Publication No. (CDC) 84-8395 (1984).

43. Artiss, K.L., A.S. Levine. Doctor-patient relation in severe illness: A seminar for oncology fellows. *N. Engl. J. Med. 288*:1210–4 (1973).

44. McCue, J.D. The effects of stress on physicians and their medical practice. *N. Engl. J. Med. 306*:458–63 (1982).

39

Health Care Professional Education and AIDS

Harvey S. Bartnof

INTRODUCTION

The epidemic of AIDS and other infections due to the human immunodeficiency virus (HIV) presents specific problems in educating physicians and other health care providers. When these problems are addressed and overcome, health care providers will be better prepared to deal with HIV-infected patients, their families, and their communities. In turn, this will maximize the care of the patient; allow for a smoother transition through dying for the patient; mitigate negative reactions from family, friends, and the community; and decrease the number of persons who might otherwise become infected with the virus. Thus the health care provider–patient relationship will be optimized, and inroads toward limiting the spread of the epidemic will have begun.

Specific problems encountered in educating health care providers include (1) phobias surrounding AIDS, including death and dying; (2) the traditional role of physicians and other health care providers in providing health information; (3) new concepts in pathobiology relevant to HIV infection; and (4) occupational stress and anxiety in treating AIDS patients. These problems will be discussed sequentially in this chapter.

PHOBIAS SURROUNDING AIDS

Health care provider phobias surrounding AIDS mirror those of the lay public. Initially, most information on AIDS is presented to all individuals, including health care providers, by the news media. After denial, fear of AIDS is the initial reaction in lay persons and health care providers. The level of fear is similar to the societal reaction to the syphilis epidemics in Europe that began in the 1490s.[1] Thus, fear of AIDS is a normal human emotional reaction to contagion and death and is not entirely caused by the news media. After becoming educated about AIDS, particularly the evidence for noncasual transmission, most individuals' fears and phobias yield to understanding. However, phobic blocks for both the practitioner and the patient preclude this transition from fear to understanding. Such phobias include:

1. Phobia of death and dying.
2. Phobia of premature death—i.e., dying young.
3. Phobia of a protracted wasting state culminating in death.
4. Phobia of contracting a new infectious disease that has no prevention or cure. This includes fear by health care providers for themselves and their family

members or friends by the psychologic mechanisms of projection, transference, or countertransference.

5. Phobia of disfigurement—e.g., the skin lesions of Kaposi's sarcoma.

6. Phobia of diminished life qualities—e.g., loss of mental capacity, loss of body control, loss of ability to generate income—and phobia of social isolation.

7. Phobia or disapproval of sexuality or sexually transmitted diseases with the concomitant avoidance by physicians of obtaining a sexual history as part of the medical history.

8. Phobia, disapproval, or prejudice against homosexuality, its life style and universality. Male homosexual activity accounts for the highest proportion of AIDS cases in the western world, and AIDS cases have been reported from every state in the United States and in 74 countries.[2,3] Kalman et al., in surveying 37 medical house officers and 91 registered nurses in a New York City hospital, found that nearly 10% of respondents agreed with the statement, "Homosexuals who contract AIDS are getting what they deserve."[4]

9. Phobia, disapproval, or prejudice against intravenous drug users, prostitutes, and prisoners. These groups engage in behaviors that many consider to be taboo or immoral, and certainly illegal.

10. Phobia or prejudice against ethnic minorities.

11. Phobia of uncertainty or perceived unknowns relevant to the HIV epidemic.

12. Phobia of disclosure or censure. The diagnosis of AIDS assumes an identity of homosexuality or intravenous drug usage.

13. Phobia of helplessness with secondary depression in health care providers. Just 50 years ago, physicians were able to provide few cures, some diagnoses, and much psychologic support. Then the era of antibiotic "magic bullets" enabled them to provide many cures. With AIDS, medicine has returned to the earlier era; i.e., health care providers are helpless to cure the primary HIV infection and often feel therapeutically impotent.

Education about AIDS must include information on these phobias and pretest scales that enable health care providers to identify their specific phobias and the mechanisms that will enable them to resolve the phobias, clearing the pathway for unbiased patient interactions. This transition is not always possible. Until the transition is made, clinical judgment, patient care, and routine hospital functioning may be impaired. For example, surgeons have refused to perform biopsies or surgeries because the procedure was "not indicated"; nurses have called in "sick" when it was their turn to care for the AIDS patient. This transition is less likely to have taken place before a hospital's first AIDS patient and is more likely to have taken place after a hospital has admitted several AIDS patients. In general, phobia of AIDS decreases when knowledge of AIDS increases.

TRADITIONAL ROLE OF HEALTH CARE PROVIDERS

Traditionally, physicians and other health care providers have been reliable sources of health and medical information. As the field of medicine continues to develop increasing amounts of scientific data (some of which is relevant to clinical practice), it has become increasingly necessary for those in clinical practice to stay current with such information. This allows practitioners to provide optimal care and advice for their patients, although the task is not easy for clinicians who work 60–80 or more hours per week.

The task of remaining current is also compounded by the presence of the news media, which report the latest medical information and breakthroughs on the evening television news or newspaper headlines days to months before the practitioner is able to receive the relevant information by mail in the appropriate medical journal. Undoubtedly this occurs before the clinician learns about the subject at a medical conference. Indeed, a practitioner who desires preparedness for the day's patient questions is best served by reading the morning newspaper.

In addition, we live in an age of consumerism, whereby the patient may not readily accept the physician's opinion as the ultimate authority. Patients today increasingly and appropriately may ask, "Why?" and want a second or third medical opinion. Older practitioners may perceive this as an erosion of their once-held authority-figure status.

These three factors—increasing rate of medical information accumulation, the immediate vigilant eye of the media, and a tendency toward patient consumerism—have made the physician's traditional role as a medical health resource a difficult one. This is especially true with the AIDS epidemic. Practitioners unarmed with basic current medical information on AIDS are ill equipped to be providing AIDS information to their patients and communities, much less making clinical decisions.

NEW CONCEPTS IN PATHOBIOLOGY

HIV represents a new human pathogen. It is the cause of AIDS and related infections that first manifested in the middle to late 1970s by retrospective examination of the clinical data.[5] There is much epidemiologic[6] and clinical[7] evidence to support this. Just as syphilis was unknown to European doctors in the 1490s, when syphilis first appeared in epidemic form, AIDS and other HIV infections would be unknown to modern-day practitioners who completed their medical training in the early 1980s or earlier.

Several pathobiologic concepts of HIV infection are new, and the vast majority of those completing their training prior to 1985 would be unfamiliar with these concepts. These health care providers are otherwise intelligent, accomplished, and competent clinicians whose knowledge must constantly be updated. With the AIDS epidemic, not only is new information being produced, but new concepts of pathobiology have been introduced which dramatically change the way we understand this chronic retroviral infection. Such pathobiologic concepts related to HIV infection include:

1. A several-years' antibody-positive, often virus-positive, yet asymptomatic carrier state. The blood and genital secretions of these individuals are potentially infectious to others. These asymptomatic individuals have normal physical examinations, so their infected contagious state would otherwise be unknown to their clinicians and sexual partners.

2. A positive antibody state that does not necessarily confirm immunity.

3. A tendency that is not absolute for asymptomatic carriers to manifest clinical or symptomatic HIV disease, including AIDS, which increases over time.[7]

These concepts are more readily understood by health care providers well versed in the viral immunology of other chronic viral infections—e.g., chronic hepatitis B, herpes simplex, and varicella zoster. Because knowledge of the natural history of HIV infection is incomplete (we are less than a decade into the effects this pathogen has on humans), not even university-affiliated AIDS researchers can know or predict the long-term natural history of this retroviral infection. Similarly, doctors in the 1490s could not have known of the tertiary stage of syphilis. Because HIV is a new pathogen, new concepts in pathobiology and drug treatment protocols are evolving all the time. These factors also present problems in health care provider education about AIDS.

OCCUPATIONAL STRESS AND ANXIETY

Occupational stress initially is related to phobias of death and contagion, as discussed previously. But a few points are important to emphasize. After the initial phobias are alleviated, the finite albeit small risk of nosocomial (hospital)-acquired HIV infection remains.[8] There are four cases in the world literature of documented health care provider, hospital-acquired HIV infection from accidental needle sticks.[8] Fortunately, the risk of this occurrence per needle stick is less than 1%, compared to a 5–33% risk for acquisition of hepatitis B virus under similar circumstances.[9] If no percutaneous exposure occurs, the risk of hospital-acquired infection for health care providers is essentially zero. This assumes that appropriate infection control guidelines are followed and that no sexual activity or drug abuse with needle sharing occurs in the hospital setting.

Fear of contagion is not new in the field of medicine. In fact, only in the last three decades have health care providers incurred a relatively low risk of nosocomially acquired infections. Even today the incidence of tuberculosis among physicians is higher than that of the general population.[10] Perhaps medical and nursing school applications should include "informed consent" explaining the risk of occupationally acquired infections including tuberculosis, hepatitis B, and, although less likely, AIDS. Often, health care providers are concerned about non-needle-stick hospital exposure to the AIDS virus. As of May 1, 1986, 3.7% (34/922) of health care providers with AIDS had a risk category that was "undetermined."[11] This proportion does not differ significantly from the 2.8% of AIDS patients with "undetermined" risk among non-health care providers.[11] Of those 34, two are still under investigation, and information was incomplete for 15 because of the patient's death or refusal to be interviewed.[11] Educating health care providers on these studies tends to diminish, though not eradicate, some of the occupational stress of working with AIDS patients.[14]

A recent study by Gordon et al. examined the knowledge, behavior, and attitudes toward AIDS of over a thousand hospital workers.[12] Over two-thirds believed that AIDS is easily transmitted by a needle-stick injury. Fifteen percent believed AIDS is more common among hospital workers than among other non-high-risk persons. Over half stated they would wear a gown or mask in a room with an AIDS patient. One-third felt they should be permitted to refuse to care for AIDS patients. About half indicated they spent less time with AIDS patients. One-third actively avoided involvement with AIDS patients. One-fourth of the hospital workers expressed extreme anxiety in dealing with AIDS patients. Accurate knowledge about AIDS and its transmission was highly significantly correlated ($p < .0001$) with low anxiety, a willingness to work with AIDS patients, and appropriate professional behavior toward AIDS patients. This study documents suboptimal knowledge about and behavior toward AIDS patients and suggests that in-service education and counseling providing accurate knowledge about AIDS may result in less anxiety and more compassionate and appropriate patient care.[12]

McKusick et al. recently surveyed 150 San Francisco Bay Area physicians (82 of whom responded) who had been working with AIDS patients for an average of 3.2 years. Since working with AIDS patients, 36% experienced more depression, 34% more anxiety, 46% more stress, and 36% more fear of death.[13] Physicians who were gay-identified were more likely than heterosexual physicians to have experienced increased anxiety, depression, stress, and fear of death since first taking care of AIDS patients. The authors determined that the different psychologic response was related to gay physicians' perceptions of their nonprofessional risk for AIDS. In this study, 63% stated they were gay or bisexual, and 33% stated they were heterosexual.[13]

Stress reduction and burnout avoidance are key issues in health care provider education about AIDS. These issues can be mitigated by education, multidisciplinary patient care rounds, and ongoing stress reduction groups.[14] The nurse turnover rate at ward 5A, the inpatient unit at San Francisco General Hospital designated for AIDS patients, has been significantly lower than that of all other wards owing to mutual support groups.[15] Other reports of regular small-group mutual support discussions of physicians' subjective experiences and case management have helped maintain the physical and emotional stability of those physicians.[16]

SPECIFIC EDUCATION FOR HEALTH CARE PROVIDERS

Education about AIDS (and related HIV infections) for physicians and other health care providers is available and accomplished by new and established routes of continuing education. These include hospital in-service continuing education programs, outside institute continuing education programs, government-sponsored education programs, national and international conferences on AIDS, medical and other journals, specialized AIDS newsletters, computer on-line services, texts, and lay newspapers and magazines.

Hospital in-service continuing education on HIV includes both basic and advanced AIDS education. Basic AIDS education is commonly referred to as "AIDS 101." This has been accomplished at university-affiliated and community medical centers and hospitals after AIDS patients were admitted. Basic AIDS education must include the following topics: transmission routes; risk to health care professionals; infection control; evidence for noncasual transmission; and social/psychosocial issues including AIDS phobias and confidentiality. All hospital and clinic personnel (including ward clerks, secretaries, housekeeping personnel, and volunteers) should receive the education in "AIDS 101." Furthermore, all hospital personnel should be able to achieve a passing score on an AIDS prevention and knowledge scale such as the AAPK—Advanced AIDS Prevention and Knowledge.[17]

Advanced AIDS education for health care professionals includes the following topics: U.S. and African epidemiology; clinical manifestations; hospital, hospice, and home infection control; prevention; spectrum of HIV infection; neurologic manifestations; pediatric manifestations; virology; immunology and laboratory tests; hemophiliac and transfusion issues; psychiatric/psychosocial issues; ethical and legal issues; and other social issues including confidentiality and death and dying. As the epidemic spreads, most U.S. hospitals will have AIDS patients, necessitating the need for widespread, in-house advanced AIDS education. Documentation of assimilated knowledge by health professionals who treat AIDS patients is accomplished by achieving a postcourse passing score on an AIDS prevention and treatment scale such as the AAPKT—Advanced AIDS Prevention, Knowledge, and Treatment.[17]

The American Hospital Association has specifically advocated in-house AIDS education for all physicians and is implementing a plan to do so. Bellevue Hospital in New York City has video-based staff education and stress reduction programs for their professional staff.[18] Memorial Sloan-Kettering Cancer Institute has developed staff education that includes formal psychoeducational meetings between patients, physicians, and other health care workers. This has strengthened the physician-patient relationship and informs physicians about patient's perspectives and concerns, thereby diminishing mutual distrust and suspicion.[19]

Several institutions provide hospital on-site AIDS education for health care professionals. These include the California Nursing Association, Professional Symposia International, and AVERI (the AIDS Virus Education and Research Institute).

National and international symposia on AIDS have enabled researchers and clinicians involved in many different aspects of AIDS patient care and research to exchange clinical data and experiences. Such symposia include NYU Medical Center (March 1983), Atlanta (April 1985), Paris (June 1986), Washington, D.C. (June 1987), and Stockholm (1988).

Medical student courses on AIDS can be very helpful as a university-based means of HIV education. A trial elective course chaired by this author in the spring of 1986 at the UCSF School of Medicine led to an enrollment of over 250 students from the Schools of Medicine, Nursing, and Pharmacy. Ten 1-h lectures over 10 weeks were expanded to eleven 1-h lectures and two 1-h discussion panels for the winter quarter, 1987,[20] through the auspices of the AIDS Professional Education Project under contract from the National Institute of Mental Health. Feedback, measured by evaluations and comparisons of pre- and postcourse knowledge and attitudes, indicated improved knowledge on HIV, less fear in dealing with AIDS patients, and an overall excellent rating of the course.[21] Topics included in the course, "AIDS-HIV 1987: Overview and Update," were as follows:

Overview and Introduction
Epidemic Perspectives and Treatment Issues
Virology and Vaccine Horizons

Immunology, Lab Tests, and Autoimmunity
Clinical Manifestations of AIDS
ARC
Neurologic Manifestations
Oral Manifestations
Transfusion and Blood Banking
Pediatric HIV Infections
Hemophiliacs and AIDS
Psychiatric/Psychosocial Issues
Women and AIDS
Ethnic Minorities and AIDS
Health Care Provider Issues
Infection Control
Public Policy
Ethics
Legal Issues
Panel: Persons with AIDS and ARC
Panel: San Francisco Systems of Care

They provide for an excellent multidisciplinary survey course that addresses the needs and interests of medical and nursing students. The unfortunate fact that San Francisco has the highest density of AIDS cases of any U.S. city has allowed for a wealth of clinical expertise by UCSF and community health care providers. This in turn has allowed us to call upon the experience of 19 UCSF clinicians and researchers to lecture for the course.

The lecture titles and subjects were derived from a needs assessment completed by students and the experience of many UCSF AIDS clinicians and researchers. I will review the scope of the subject material at this point.

The "Overview" lecture presented by this author is necessary to provide a framework of the varied biomedical and psychosocial AIDS topics and a reference for the remaining topics in the course. In addition, the Overview lecturer introduces each subsequent topic's relatedness immediately prior to each lecture to allow for maximal course cohesiveness.

"Epidemic Perspective and Treatment Issues" was presented by Paul Volberding, M.D. Having been involved with AIDS patients since the first reports in 1981, Dr. Volberding is able to provide a unique perspective from 6 years of clinical experience. Jay Levy, M.D., discoverer of the AIDS-associated retrovirus, discussed "Virology" of HIV infection with implications for vaccine development. The significance of a lifelong retroviral HIV infection incorporated into human DNA of different cell types has far-reaching implications. Daniel Stites, M.D., discussed "Immunology, Laboratory Tests, and Autoimmunity." Present knowledge of human immunology relevant to HIV infection indicates that we still have much to learn. A discussion on diagnostic tests provides an understanding of the terms "screening test," "confirmatory test," "ELISA," "Western blot," and "false-negative" and "false-positive antibody tests." Evidence of autoimmune dysfunction are present in patients with AIDS, and inclusion of this topic enables a more complete understanding of the scope of clinical manifestations of HIV infection.

"Clinical Manifestations of AIDS" was delivered by Harry Hollander, M.D., and "ARC" (AIDS-related complex or conditions) was discussed by Donald Abrams, M.D. With an increasing awareness of primary HIV infection of the brain, spinal cord, and nerves (without CDC-defined AIDS), Robert Levy, M.D., Ph.D., discussed "Neurologic Manifestations." Since the first manifestation of AIDS or ARC may present in the mouth, Deborah Greenspan, B.D.S., presented "Oral Manifestations." Coincident with the persistent erroneous public perception of risk of AIDS by blood transfusions and other relevant issues, Herbert Perkins, M.D., discussed "Transfusion and Blood Banking Issues."

Groups at higher risk for AIDS than the general population were discussed by Peggy Weintraub, M.D. ("Pediatric HIV Infections"), and Marion Koerper, M.D. ("Hemophiliacs and AIDS"). Jay Baer, M.D., in discussing "Psychiatric/Psychosocial Issues," covered the relevant topics of delirium, dementia, death and dying, life adjustment reactions, health care provider anxiety, and the "worried well."

With an increasing number of U.S. women affected by HIV, Constance Wofsy, M.D., discussed "Women and AIDS" and included prevention issues. The next wave of AIDS patients in California is expected to occur in ethnic minority groups including intravenous drug users; hence the topic "Ethnic Minorities and AIDS" was delivered by Amanda Houston-Hamilton, D.M.H.

Since health care professionals have concerns of acquiring a nosocomial HIV infection, Julie Gerberding, M.D., discussed "Health Care Provider Issues," and Mary Anne Johnson, M.D., elucidated "Infection Control."

No health care professional can be divorced from the social implications of the epidemic; hence Philip Lee, M.D., addressed "Public Policy" issues including economics, and Albert Jonsen, Ph.D., discussed "Ethics" topics including the right of confidentiality, the right of privacy, the rights of the public, quarantine, and power of attorney. "Legal Issues," including discrimination, civil liberties, and issues surrounding the use of the HIV antibody test, were addressed by Ben Shatz, J.D.

Two panels were held. The first included persons with AIDS and ARC, who discussed their personal experiences with their disease and highlighted both positive and negative experiences with health care providers. A question-and-answer period was included. The second panel took advantage of the many community-based AIDS service agencies that have provided the backbone of San Francisco's model for AIDS care. Panel members included representatives from the following: San Francisco General Hospital's outpatient ward 86; San Francisco AIDS Foundation, which provides education, social services, and a food bank; Shanti Project, which provides practical and emotional support for persons with AIDS and their families and loved ones; Hospice of San Francisco; and the UCSF AIDS Health Project, which administers the Alternative Test Site Program (to describe the clinical experience surrounding anonymous and confidential HIV antibody testing).

The American Medical Association, in recognizing the need for physician education on AIDS, has formed regional pilot education programs in 1986 and will expand these programs for all physicians.[22] The National Institute of Mental Health and the Department of Health and Human Services are currently funding many institutions to provide education on HIV and AIDS for health care professionals throughout the United States.

The U.S. Public Health Service, through the Centers for Disease Control

(CDC), provides a 2-day seminar on AIDS education for physicians and other health care providers. The nine sexually transmitted disease prevention and training centers are jointly sponsored ventures among state and local health departments, selected medical schools, and the CDC. Topics in the 2-day seminar include epidemiology and medical aspects; clinical screening and laboratory diagnostics; clinical identification; infection control; psychosocial issues; homosexual life styles; AIDS prevention; death and dying; and community networking for maximal resource utilization.[23]

Less efficient although more traditional means of physician education on HIV include the medical and other journals with original research or letter/editorial contributions. Journals tend to be less efficient owing to (1) lag times until publication; (2) busy clinical schedules, which may preclude reading of journals; (3) relative inaccessibility of journals (i.e., reader location); and (4) the lack of an appropriate framework or reference for the clinical material. Such journals include the New England Journal of Medicine, the Lancet, the Journal of the American Medical Association, Science, Nature, the British Medical Journal, the Annals of Internal Medicine, Morbidity and Mortality Weekly Report, and various specialty/subspecialty journals. In spite of the fact that AIDS is perceived as a disease to be cared for by specialists in infectious diseases or oncology, the treatment of persons with AIDS and ARC is best accomplished by primary care providers using subspecialty/specialty consultation and a multidisciplinary approach. Thus the subspecialty and specialty journals will have abundant information on HIV. The range of journals include neurology, neurosurgery, pediatrics, radiology and imaging, dermatology, pathology/laboratory medicine, psychiatry, virology, immunology, and the medical subspecialties of hematology/oncology and gastrointestinal and pulmonary medicine.

Other AIDS newsletters and journals have emerged that may summarize, outline, or editorialize articles from standard journals and other AIDS news. These include AIDS Alert, CDC AIDS Weekly, AIDS File, Focus, AIDS Medical Update—CIRID, and AIDS Newsletter London. Original contributions on AIDS and related topics are found in AIDS, an International Bimonthly Journal (Gower); AIDS Research and Human Retroviruses (Liebert); Focus (UCSF); and AIDS File (UCSF).

A few texts on AIDS have been printed, whereby one or more editors oversee chapters written by specialist or subspecialist AIDS researchers.[24-26] These texts tend to be biomedical in their scope, whereas this text is more multidisciplinary.

Computer on-line services allow individuals with a computer terminal and modem to access medical information on AIDS from various medical journals or data bases, in complete or abstracted form. These include the National Library of Medicine and other entrepreneurial on-line services. The Computer AIDS Information Network (CAIN), available through Delphi computer service, has an AIDS sections with an abundance of AIDS information.[27]

Various U.S. newspapers have fair to good reputations in reporting news on AIDS and HIV, particularly on medical journal articles about to be published. Some of these, including the New York Times and the Los Angeles Times, have now begun extensive coverage of AIDS and HIV issues. One must keep in mind that newspaper headlines and articles are printed with the intention to sell newspapers. Two caveats: Be sure to read the last paragraphs of the article (including responses from university-affiliated AIDS investigators), and watch the successive days' newspapers for retractions or modifications of the initial article.

SUMMARY

In summary, health care professional education on AIDS and HIV involves problems that are specific to this new disease and epidemic. These include phobias surrounding AIDS (including death and dying), the traditional role of practitioners in providing health information, new concepts in pathobiology relevant to HIV infection, and occupationally related stress and anxiety. Addressing these problems provides the cornerstone for education about AIDS. This education can be accomplished readily through new and traditional means of continuing education, both in hospital and out. When information about AIDS and HIV had been transmitted, and when lay and professional AIDS phobias have been allayed, control of the epidemic will be ascertained more readily. In turn, this will enable improved care for the individual with AIDS and will mitigate negative reactions from the health care professional, family, lover, and community. It should be emphasized that in this author's opinion, traditional means of continuing education for health care providers will fail unless the phobias are resolved.

REFERENCES

1. Moore, M.: Syphilis and public opinion. Archives of Dermatology and Syphilology 1939;39:836–845.

2. Centers for Disease Control (CDC): Update: Acquired immunodeficiency syndrome—United States. Morbidity and Mortality Weekly Report 1986;35:17–21.

3. CDC: Update: Acquired immunodeficiency syndrome—Europe. Morbidity and Mortality Weekly Report 1986;35:35–38, 43–46.

4. Kalman, T. P., et al.: Homophobia among physicians and nurses: An empirical study. Poster 225 presented at the Paris International Conference on AIDS, June 1986.

5. Gallo, R. C., et al.: Frequent detection and isolation of cytopathic retroviruses (HTLV-III) from patients with AIDS and at risk for AIDS. Science 1984;224:500–503.

6. Blattner, W. A., et al.: Epidemiology of human T-lymphotropic virus type III and the risk of the acquired immunodeficiency syndrome. Annals of Internal Medicine 1985;103:665–670.

7. Francis, D.P., et al.: The natural history of infection with the lymphadenopathy-associated virus human T-lymphotropic virus type III. Annals of Internal Medicine 1985;103:719–722.

8. Henderson, D. K., et al.: Risk of nosocomial infection with human T-cell lymphotropic virus type III/lymphadenopathy-associated virus in a large cohort of intensively exposed health care workers. Annals of Internal Medicine 1986;104:644–647.

9. Seeff, L. B., et al.: Type B hepatitis after needlestick exposure: Prevention with hepatitis B immune globulin. Annals of Internal Medicine 1978;88:289–293.

10. Geiseler, P. J., et al.: Tuberculosis in physicians: A continuing problem. American Review of Respiratory Diseases 1986;133:773–776.

11. Lifson, A. R., et al.: National surveillance of AIDS in health care workers. Journal of American Medical Association 1986;256:3231–3236.

12. Gordon, F., et al.: Hospital worker's knowledge, behavior and attitudes towards AIDS. Communication 213:S24e presented at the Paris International Conference on AIDS, June 1986.

13. McKusick, L., et al.: The impact of AIDS on primary practice physicians. Poster 222 presented at the Paris International Conference on AIDS, June 1986.

14. Christ, G.H., et al.: Psychosocial issues in AIDS, in AIDS, V.T. DeVita, et al., eds. Philadelphia: J.B. Lippincott 1985;293–294.

15. Gayling Gee, R. N.: Personal communication.

16. Schaffner, B.: Psychological impact of AIDS upon the social environment (health care

providers, families and friends) and methods of modification. Communication 67:S12k presented at Paris International Conference on AIDS, June 1986.

17. Bartnof, H. S.: Standardized scales and documentation of AIDS-HIV knowledge and prevention for health care professionals and the public. Abstract 194 presented at the 3d International Conference on AIDS, Washington, D.C., June 1987.

18. Braunstein, L., et al.: Bellevue Hospital's administrative response to the AIDS epidemic. Poster 462 presented at the Paris International Conference on AIDS, June 1986.

19. Moynihan, R. T., et al.: Confronting institutional barriers to the treatment of AIDS: A psychosocial support program. Poster 470 presented at the Paris International Conference on AIDS, June 1986.

20. Bartnof, H. S., et al.: AIDS-HIV education for medical, nursing, and pharmacy students at the UCSF School of Medicine. Abstract 224 presented at the 3d International Conference on AIDS, Washington, D.C., June 1987.

21. Bartnof, H. S., et al.: AIDS education for medical and nursing students: Knowledge and attitude correlates. Abstract 203 presented at the 3d International Conference on AIDS, Washington, D.C., June 1987.

22. Bosy, L.: AIDS education is goal of AMA program. American Medical News 1986; Aug. 1: 11.

23. Rucker, R. D., et al.: The role of the United States Public Health Service in educating health professionals about acquired immunodeficiency syndrome. Poster 468 presented at the Paris International Conference on AIDS, June 1986.

24. Broder, S., ed.: "AIDS: Modern Concepts and Therapeutic Challenges." New York: Marcel Dekker, 1987.

25. Ebbesen, P., Biggar, R. J., and Melby, M., eds.: "AIDS: A Basic Clinical Guide for Clinicians." Philadelphia: W.B. Saunders, 1984.

26. DeVita, V. T., Hellman, S., and Rosenberg, S. A., eds.: "AIDS Etiology, Diagnosis, and Prevention." Philadelphia: J. B. Lippincott, 1985.

27. Howard, J. J., et al.: Transmission of AIDS information and education through electronic communication. Poster 706 presented at the Paris International Conference on AIDS, June 1986.

40

Human Immunodeficiency Virus:

Issues in Infection Control

J. Louise Gerberding and M. A. Sande

INTRODUCTION

Transmission of human immunodeficiency virus (HIV) has been extensively evaluated since the epidemic of AIDS first became apparent. Numerous epidemiologic studies of persons at potential risk for exposure have provided important data to establish the modes of HIV transmission, the risk of transmission conferred by various types of exposure, and potential infection control measures to reduce risks. Physicians, nurses, and other health care providers have a responsibility to understand the modes of transmission and rational methods to reduce risk if we are to successfully accomplish our task of curtailing this devastating epidemic.

As early as 1983 it was clear that AIDS was transmitted by sexual contact with infected partners, parenteral exposure to infected blood products, and perinatally to children born of infected mothers. When HIV was proved to be the etiologic agent in 1984, methods became available to identify asymptomatic carriers of the virus so that the extent of transmission within various populations at risk could be further delineated. Current estimates based on these methods indicate that more than 1.5 million Americans are infected with HIV.

HIV had been cultured from nearly all body fluids. It is found in relatively large amounts in the blood and semen of patients with AIDS and ARC.[1,2] It is also frequently detected in the cerebrospinal fluid of patients with neuropsychiatric manifestations of AIDS.[3] It is rarely recovered from vaginal and cervical secretions, tears, saliva, and urine; when present in these fluids, the actual amount of detectable virus is small.[4-7] Only blood, semen, and breast milk have been directly implicated in transmission, although cases of female-to-male transmission suggest that sexual exposure to vaginal or cervical secretions transmits the virus as well.[8]

Despite some similarities between the transmission of HIV and hepatitis B virus, there is currently no evidence that HIV is transmitted to household contacts of infected persons or by casual contact in any environment.[9] The risk to health workers providing care to patients infected with HIV is minimal (see below) even when extensive exposure over long periods of time has occurred.[10-15] Occupational exposure in the non-health care environment has never been implicated in transmission.

RISK OF ACQUIRING HIV FROM SEXUAL ACTIVITY

As with other sexually transmitted diseases, the probability of acquiring HIV from sexual activity is directly proportional to the probability that a given partner is infected; the frequency, duration, and type of contact with an infected partner; and the total number of sexual contacts. Sexual practices associated with the highest rate of transmission in homosexual men include anal-receptive intercourse, fisting, and rimming. Male-to-female transmission accounts for most of the cases of AIDS in heterosexuals reported to the Centers for Disease Control (CDC).[8] Vaginal intercourse is the most likely mode of infection in the majority of patients, although anal intercourse may contribute to risk in a small number of cases. Female-to-male transmission has also been documented but may be a less efficient mechanism for acquiring the virus than is male-to-female transmission.[16] There is no evidence to suggest that exposure to saliva during kissing or during other oral activity is a mode of transmitting HIV.[8]

It is becoming increasingly difficult to determine a priori the probability of HIV infection in sexually active individuals. At the present time, over 50% of homosexual and bisexual men in many urban areas are infected. The prevalence of infection in intravenous drug users is increasing at an alarming rate, and heterosexual transmission in this population is increasing. In the United States, heterosexuals without other risk factors for acquiring the disease currently have an extremely low prevalence of infection. However, in central Africa and in Haiti, heterosexual transmission appears to account for the majority of cases of AIDS.[17-19] Preliminary evidence suggests that the frequency of heterosexual transmission may be increasing in certain locales in this country as well. If this phenomenon extends to other areas, the risk to heterosexuals, particularly those with more than one sexual partner, could increase substantially.

Guidelines for safer practices are based on two premises: (1) the likelihood of acquiring HIV will be reduced if the number of partners is reduced, particularly partners at higher risk of infection, and (2) avoidance of direct mucosal exposure to semen, blood, and vaginal secretions may decrease the risk of acquiring HIV from an infected partner. Most authorities therefore recommend minimizing the number of sexual contacts, avoiding sexual contact with persons at risk for HIV infection, knowing sexual partners sufficiently well to ascertain the likelihood of prior exposure to HIV, and using condoms, other barrier devices, and spermicides containing nonoxynol-9 to prevent direct mucosal inoculation with infected sexual fluids or secretions.[20]

RISKS OF INTRAVENOUS DRUG USERS

Intravenous drug users are known to be at risk for a variety of infectious diseases as a result of direct injection of infected blood. Since HIV is present in the blood, it is not suprising that these individuals are also at risk for AIDS. Obviously, the practice of sharing needles and other drug apparatus promotes the exchange of infected blood. The risk of acquiring the infection is directly related to the probability of infection in a given "donor," the amount of blood injected, and the frequency of shared needle use.

Although intensive campaigns to eliminate intravenous drug use are under way in many urban centers, significant numbers of individuals continue to use a variety of parenteral drugs. Most authorities advocate educational programs for drug users to reduce the prevalence of practices likely to promote the transmission of blood-borne pathogens. In some areas, sterile needles are provided to discourage needle sharing. Drug users who continue to share apparatus should be taught to disinfect needles and other equipment with a 1:100 solution of household bleach or even household detergents. In addition, information about the risk of sexual transmission and maternal-fetal transmission of HIV should be made available.[21]

RISKS TO HEALTH CARE WORKERS

Several large studies of health care workers with occupational exposure to HIV have been performed or are under way.[10-15] These studies have evaluated subjects whose exposures occurred during routine patient care activities, while performing invasive procedures, by handling infected laboratory specimens, and by accidental inoculations with contaminated blood or other body fluids. To determine whether infection has occurred, serum is analyzed for the presence of antibody to HIV, a reliable marker for infection. Detectable levels of antibody may not appear for several weeks following infection. For this reason, most studies of health care workers have included follow-up testing several months after exposure to ensure that adequate time for antibody production has elasped.

Over 4000 health care workers in the United States, including more than 1000 with needle sticks or equivalent exposures, have been enrolled in studies and tested for antibody to HIV.[10-15] Four study subjects have been proved to have acquired HIV as a result of occupational exposure. All four acquired infection through needle-stick injury. The risk to health care workers from a single discrete parenteral exposure to blood infected with HIV is estimated to be 0.13% (4 infections/3000 accidental exposures documented in study subjects). Although this risk has had substantial impact, it confirms earlier impressions that HIV is actually one of the least transmissible occupational pathogens. In contrast, the risk of hepatitis B infection from parenteral exposure is greater than 10%; more than 200 health care providers die each year from the effects of hepatitis infection.[22]

Needle-stick transmission of HIV has also been reported in three other health care workers who were not enrolled in studies.[23-25] Cases of HIV transmission to three female health care workers with non-needle-stick exposure to infected blood have been reported.[26] The exact route of transmission was not ascertained but may have been related to breaks in the exposed skin in two cases or mucosal inoculation in one case. Although these cases affirm the importance of infection control precautions, they do not imply a high degree of risk and must therefore be interpreted in the context of estimated risk found in the cohort studies cited above.

Traditionally, "general" infection control precautions such as hand washing have been advocated for all patients regardless of the probability of infection. Additional "disease-specific" infection control procedures have been developed for patients diagnosed with a particular contagious organism such as hepatitis B virus. The fear of acquiring HIV from exposure to infected patients has stimulated a reevaluation of this approach by many medical centers. Recognition of the asymptomatic carrier state of HIV infection has heightened concerns regarding unprotected exposures to contaminated body fluids from patients with unrecognized infection. Not surprisingly, this concern has prompted a renewed awareness of the potential for exposure to hepatitis B virus and other blood-borne pathogens in patients with asymptomatic infections. As a result, a trend toward basing infection control practices on the type of exposure encountered rather than on the specific diagnosed infection in the involved patient is increasingly evident.

Contemporary standards of infection control are based on the premise that all patients are potentially infected with a transmissible blood-borne pathogen. Infection control guidelines to prevent exposure to blood and other body fluids are therefore *routinely* recommended for *all* patients regardless of the probability of infection with a particular organism such as HIV.[27-29] Screening for evidence of infection is not required for the purpose of implementing infection control measures. The infection control guidelines discussed in the following sections reflect this approach. Implementation and enforcement of these guidelines will afford maximal protection to health care workers by minimizing exposure to contaminated body fluids from patients with clinically evident infections as well as from patients with unsuspected infections. In addition, these practices could have a beneficial impact on reducing the transmission of common nosocomial bacterial pathogens from one patient to another.

Guidelines for Minimizing Exposure to Body Fluids

Hand washing should be performed before and after contact with each patient and after exposure to body fluids or laboratory specimens. Disposable gloves should be worn whenever direct contact with potentially infected substances, body tissues, or environmental surfaces is anticipated. Employees with weeping or exudative skin lesions on the hands or other exposed areas should be excused from direct patient care activities until the condition resolves.

Gowns or other protective garments should be worn if clothing is likely to be soiled with blood, secretions, or excretions. Gowns should not be worn outside of patient care or laboratory areas.

Needles, scalpels, and other sharp disposable objects should be disposed of in conveniently located puncture-resistant containers. Needles should not be resheathed, bent, broken, or manipulated in any manner before disposal.

Masks and protective eye wear are not routinely required. Masks should be worn by coughing patients suspected of having infection with *M. tuberculosis* (or other contagious respiratory disease) until this diagnosis has been excluded or until the patient is no longer contagious. Health care workers and visitors in contact with such patients should also wear masks. Masks and protective eye wear should be worn whenever splatter of saliva, respiratory secretions, amniotic fluid, blood, or other body fluids is anticipated to prevent mucosal inoculation of infected materials.

Contaminated environmental surfaces should be cleaned and then disinfected with a mycobactericidal disinfectant approved by the Environmental Protection Agency or with a 1:100 dilution of 5.25% sodium hypochlorite solution (a 1:10 dilution should be used for heavily contaminated surfaces).

Contaminated wastes should be processed in compliance with existing standards for infectious wastes. Linens and other laundry should be placed in bags for transport and laundered using standard hospital laundry procedures.

Additional infection control guidelines for dentists, laboratory personnel, emergency care providers, and other specialized care providers have been established.[30-32] Although specific recommendations have been detailed, infection control for all health care workers emphasizes prevention of exposure to potentially infected body fluids and tissues.

Management of Accidental Parenteral Exposures

Health care workers who sustain accidental needle-stick exposures, mucosal inoculations, or contact with large amounts of blood for a short time or small amounts for prolonged periods of time should be evaluated by an experienced clinician as soon as possible after the exposure. Hepatitis prophylaxis should be administered when indicated. If the history suggests that the source of the exposure was infected with HIV, the CDC recommends that serum be checked at regular intervals for the presence of antibody to HIV[28] and that the source patient be asked to consent for HIV testing. Hopefully, safe and efficacious postexposure prophylactic therapies will become available in the future to prevent the small number of infections in health care workers that would otherwise occur.

REFERENCES

1. Zagury D, Bernard J, Leibowitch J, et al: HTLV-III in cells cultured from semen of two patients with AIDS. Science 1984;226:449–51.

2. Ho DD, Schooley RT, Rota T, et al: HTLV-III in semen and blood of a healthy homosexual man. Science 1984;226:451–3.

3. Levy JA, Hollander H, Shimabukuro J, et al: Isolation of AIDS-associated retroviruses from cerebrospinal fluid and brain of patients with neurologic symptoms. Lancet 1985;2:586–8.

4. Levy JA, Kaminsky LS, Morrow WJW, et al: Infection by the retrovirus associated with the acquired immunodeficiency syndrome: Clinical, biological and molecular features. Ann Intern Med 1983;103:694–9.

5. Groopman JE, Salahuddin SZ, Sarngadharan MG, et al: HTLV-III in saliva of people with AIDS-related complex and healthy homosexual men at risk for AIDS. Science 1984;226:447–9.

6. Vogt MW, Witt DJ, Craven DE, et al: Isolation of HTLV-III/LAV from cervical secretions of women at risk for AIDS. Lancet 1986;ii:525–7.

7. Wofsy CB, Cohen JB, Hauer LB, et al: Isolation of AIDS-associated retrovirus from genital secretions of women with antibody to the virus. Lancet 1986;ii:527–29.

8. CDC: Heterosexual transmission of human T-lymphotropic virus type III/lymphadenopathy-associated virus. MMWR 1985;34:561–3.

9. Friedland GH, Saltzman BR, Rogers MF, et al: Lack of transmission of HTLV-III/LAV infection to household contacts of patients with AIDS and AIDS related complex with oral candidiasis. N Engl J Med 1986;314:380–2.

10. Hirsch MS, Wormser GP, Schooley RT, et al: Risk of nosocomial infection with human T-cell lymphotropic virus III (HTLV-III). N Engl J Med 1985;312:1–4.

11. Henderson DK, Saah AJ, Zak BJ, et al: Risk of nosocomial infection with human T-cell lymphotropic virus type III/lymphadenopathy-associated virus in a large cohort of intensively exposed health care workers. Ann Intern Med 1986;104:644–7.

12. Gerberding JL, Bryant-LeBlanc CE, Nelson C, et al: Risk of transmitting the human immunodeficiency virus, cytomegalovirus, and hepatitis B virus to health care workers exposed to patients with AIDS and AIDS-related conditions. J Infect Dis 1987;156:1–8.

13. Weiss SH, Saxinger, WC, Rechtman D, et al: HTLV-III infection among health care workers: Association with needlestick injuries. JAMA 1985;254:2089–93.

14. Kuhls TL, Viker S, Paris NB, et al: A prospective cohort study of the occupational risk of AIDS and AIDS-related infections in health care personnel. Clin Res 1986;34:124A (abstract).

15. McCray E, Cooperative Needlestick Group: Occupational risk of the acquired immunodeficiency syndrome among health care workers. N Engl J Med 1986;314:1127–32.

16. Redfield RR, Markham PD, Salahuddin SZ, et al: Heterosexually acquired HTLV-III/LAV disease (AIDS-related complex and AIDS): Epidemiologic evidence for female-to-male transmission. JAMA 1985;254:2094–6.

17. Piot P, Quinn TC, Taelman H, et al: Acquired immunodeficiency syndrome in a heterosexual population in Zaire. Lancet 1984;ii:65–9.

18. Van-de-Perre P, Rouvroy D, Lepage P, et al: Acquired immunodeficiency syndrome in Rwanda. Lancet 1984;ii:62–5.

19. Clumeck N, Guroff R, Van-de-Perre P, et al: Seroepidemiologic studies of HTLV-III antibody prevalence among selected groups of heterosexual Africans. JAMA 1985;254:2599–602.

20. Conant M, Hardy D, Sernatinger J, et al: Condoms prevent transmission of the AIDS-associated retrovirus. JAMA (in press).

21. CDC: Recommendations for assisting in the prevention of perinatal transmission of human T-cell lymphotropic virus type III/lymphadenopathy-associated virus and acquired immunodeficiency syndrome. MMWR 1985;34:721.

22. Werner BJ, Grady GF. Accidental hepatitis-B-surface-antigen-positive inoculations. Use of e antigen to estimate infectivity. Ann Intern Med 1982;97:367–9.

23. Needlestick transmission of HTLV-III from a patient infected in Africa. Lancet 1984;ii:1376–7.

24. Oksenhendler E, Harzig M, Le Roux J, et al: HIV infection with seroconversion following a superficial needlestick injury to the finger. (Letter.) N Engl J Med 1986;315:582.

25. Neisson-Verant C, Arfi S, Mathez D, et al: Needlestick HIV seroconversion in a nurse. Lancet 1986;ii:814.

26. CDC: Update: Human immunodeficiency virus infections in health-care workers exposed to blood of infected patients. MMWR 1987;36:285–9.

27. Gerberding JL, Henderson DK: Design of rational infection control guidelines for human immunodeficiency virus infection. J Infect Dis 1987;156:861–4.

28. CDC: Recommendations for prevention of HIV transmission in health care settings. MMWR 1987;36(Suppl 2S):3S–18S.

29. Gerberding JL, University of California, San Francisco, Task Force on AIDS: Recommended infection-control policies for patients with human immunodeficiency virus infection: An update. N Engl J Med 1986;315:1562–4.

30. CDC: Recommendations for preventing transmission of infection with human T-cell lymphotropic virus type III/lymphadenopathy-associated virus during invasive procedures. MMWR 1986;35:221–3.

31. CDC: Acquired immunodeficiency syndrome (AIDS): Precautions for clinical and laboratory staffs. MMWR 1982;31:577–80.

32. CDC: Recommended infection-control practices for dentistry. MMWR 1986;35:237–42.

IX

POLITICAL ASPECTS

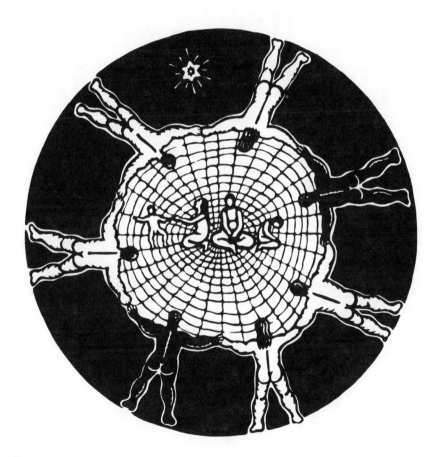

Political Aspects

A group of adults and children with AIDS wait at the center of a web. But the web becomes a net of light, illuminated by the star of hope, when held up by a community which joins hands to meet the needs of persons with AIDS. Once a cure is found, the net will be lowered to the ground and the afflicted will walk out, healed.

41

Public Policy, Federalism, and AIDS

A. E. Benjamin and Philip R. Lee

INTRODUCTION

The epidemic of acquired immune deficiency syndrome (AIDS) has posed a unique challenge to policy makers because of the nature of the disease and the fear it engenders. The responses to this challenge by policy makers at the national, state, and local levels have varied. The initial problem facing policy makers was to determine the nature and magnitude of the AIDS epidemic. AIDS was first recognized in Los Angeles and New York City in 1981 when a small number of homosexual men were diagnosed with a rare form of cancer (Kaposi's sarcoma) and with rare forms of pneumonia (e.g., *Pneumocystis carinii* pneumonia). It has since appeared in individuals who are not homosexual (e.g., IV drug users, transfusion recipients) and in communities in all 50 states and the District of Columbia. Over 28,000 cases of AIDS had been reported in the United States as of January 5, 1987, and it is expected that the cumulative total of AIDS cases will exceed 270,000, with 170,000 deaths, before the end of 1991. The U.S. Public Health Service estimates that 74,000 AIDS patients will be diagnosed in 1991 and an additional 71,000 previously diagnosed patients will be alive at the beginning of that year.[1] It has also been estimated that between 1 million and 1.5 million people in the United States are infected with human immunodeficiency virus (HIV), the causative agent of AIDS, and that from 25% to 50% of those with HIV infection will eventually develop AIDS.[2]

Although the epidemic of AIDS has spread to all 50 states, some cities (e.g., New York, San Francisco, Los Angeles, Houston, Miami) and rural areas (e.g., Belle Glade, FL) have been more heavily affected than others. In addition, neighborhoods within cities such as the Castro neighborhood in San Francisco, the Lower West Side of Manhattan, and areas of West Los Angeles have suffered devastating personal, social, and economic consequences of the AIDS epidemic.

The direct cost of health care for persons with AIDS currently exceeds $1.5 billion annually. The direct costs of health care for persons with AIDS are predicted to range from $8 billion to $16 billion in 1991.[3,4] Although these costs will represent only about 1.2–2.4% of health care expenditures in 1991, the epidemic will pose considerable strain not only on the financing of care but also on the organization and delivery of health care in communities with large numbers of persons with AIDS. The indirect costs are very high, owing to the premature death of so many persons with AIDS. Currently these costs are approximately $7.0 billion, and by 1991 they are estimated to be $55.6 billion.[3]

THE POLICY PROCESS

To address the policy issues posed by the HIV/AIDS epidemic, it is necessary to examine the policy process itself. A distinguishing feature of the political system in the United States is its structure as a three-level federal system with strong constitutional provision for separation of powers among federal, state, and local governments and among executive, legislative, and judicial branches at each level. The result of the distinctive pluralism that characterizes the policy process in the United States is fragmentation, or a wide dispersion of power and ambiguity with respect to authority and responsibility for various functions and programs.

Five dimensions of the policy process are particularly important in understanding the formation and development of public policy in the United States: (1) the relationship of government to the private sector; (2) the relationship of the different levels (federal, state, local); (3) the pluralistic nature of politics; (4) the incremental nature of change in policies; and (5) the making of policy in the process of program implementation.[5]

We will first consider issues related to relationships between the public and private sectors, because the private sector plays the dominant role in health care, and its role must be considered vital in dealing with the AIDS epidemic. The focus of this chapter, however, will be on the relationship of the federal government to state and local governments, because these relationships have had a powerful impact in shaping the nation's response to the epidemic, and the public sector has the primary responsibility to provide leadership in an epidemic. In this review we will not consider in any detail the other three characteristics of the policy process, since they have been less critical in shaping the nation's response to the AIDS epidemic.

Public-Private Relationships

The role of government in the United States, particularly in relation to domestic social programs, has often been to stimulate or support the private sector. This is nowhere more evident than in the area of health, where the bulk of federal and state resources have been used to support activities in the private sector (proprietary and nonprofit). These activities include biomedical research by individuals in private universities, profit-making companies, and nonprofit institutions; construction and modernization of nonprofit hospitals; training of physicians, dentists, nurses, pharmacists, and other health professionals who provide service largely in the private sector; and financing of health care provided by private physicians and hospitals (profit and nonprofit) to Medicare (federal) or Medicaid (state) beneficiaries.

Even more important than the financing of health care for the elderly and the poor through public programs has been the decision to provide health insurance for the general public through the private sector rather than through publicly funded national health insurance. During the past 50 years, private health insurance has grown from a small experiment to the means of financing health care for over 80% of those under the age of 65 years. Private health insurance has been provided through employment, with major tax incentives to both employers and employees to utilize this means of providing protection against the costs of health care. Although private health insurance has provided coverage for the great majority of employed Americans, the number without private health insurance has increased to at least 35 million.[6] This problem will become increasingly serious as the AIDS epidemic spreads and as many more individuals face potentially catastrophic health care costs.

Not only is there a long history of government support for the private sector in the United States, but there has been a long tradition of volunteerism and antipathy to government intervention in domestic affairs. In spite of the antipathy to government, typified by such statements as "He who governs least governs best," Americans have long sought to use the process of government for their own interests. This is evidenced by the growing influence of special interests (e.g., defense contractors, academic medical centers, hospitals) in the United States and the emergence of what has been called single-issue politics (e.g., antiabortion activities, war on cancer). The government response to the AIDS epidemic is, in part, a reflection of the political power of gay males as a special-interest group in some communities. Paradoxically, public policy related to AIDS also reflects equally powerful attitudes (e.g., homophobia) that have limited the capacity of policy makers to deal with a sexually transmitted disease that initially affected stigmatized groups, primarily gay males and IV drug users.

Even more complex than the relationship of the government to private enterprise has been the relationship of the government to individual citizens. The complex nature of this relationship is illustrated by the policy response to the AIDS epidemic. In the United States, policy must respond to the HIV epidemic within the context of the Constitution, the Bill of Rights, and the laws enacted during the past 200 years. How the epidemic will affect the rights of individuals is of increasing importance. Recently, Mills et al.[7] stated the question quite clearly: "AIDS poses the most profound issue of constitutional law and public health since the Supreme Court approved compulsory immunization in 1905." At issue is the individual's interest in liberty and privacy against the public's interest in health and safety. Issues related to quarantine, mandatory HIV antibody testing of high-risk groups (e.g., prostitutes), and confidentiality have arisen, particularly at the state and local levels. Recently, legislators in several states proposed mandatory HIV antibody testing prior to the issuance of a marriage license. This idea and other recommendations for mass testing have been rejected by public health authorities.

In the main, state and local governments have sided with the individual and have limited their regulatory activities to mandatory reporting of AIDS infection, protecting the confidentiality of individuals with AIDS, mandatory HIV antibody testing of all blood donors, general public education, and risk group education. In addition, some state and local governments have taken additional steps to slow the spread of HIV infection. In 1985, an attempt was made by the Director of Public Health in San Francisco to close bathhouses frequented by gay males and considered a threat to public health because of the sexual practices that were permitted and, in some cases, encouraged. The decision by the Director of Public Health was based on his assessment that the risk of spreading HIV infection was sufficiently great to outweigh the rights of the bathhouse owners or their patrons. Although the courts prevented the Director of Public Health from closing the bathhouses, they did require enforcement of strict rules prohibiting high-risk sexual behavior. The result was that many of the bathhouses closed because of the loss of customers, and in those that remained open, the risk of spreading infection was substantially reduced. In New York State a similar effort was made to curb sexual practices that were considered dangerous to public health in bars, bathhouses, and hotels.

In most cases when public health officials have attempted measures to restrict individual liberty to protect the public's health, the individual's rights to liberty and privacy have prevailed, in part because beyond education, behavior change, and protection of the blood supply, effective measures to control the spread of the HIV infection are not available. Although most state public health directors have the power to order quarantine, in the few instances where quarantine was considered for persons with AIDS, the ideal has been rejected, usually by public health officials.

Intergovernmental Relations (Federalism)

"Federalism" is the term commonly used to describe the relationship between the U.S. Government and the 50 state governments. As originally used in the United States, federalism was purely a legal concept to define the constitutional division of authority and responsibility between the national government and the states.[8]

Federalism initially stressed the independence of each level of government from the others and limited the function assigned to the federal government largely to foreign affairs, national defense, the collection of taxes, and efforts to stimulate commerce; other functions, such as public health, police protection, and education, were the responsibility of state and local governments. In the early years of the Republic, public health was the responsibility of local governments, and medical care the responsibility of the private sector, with the payment for medical care resting largely with the individual.[9]

This concept of dual federalism prevailed until the Great Depression of the 1930s. However, even under this concept of strict separation of functions, changes in the federal role began to take place in the 1860s, and federal policies gradually developed in areas that had been the domain of the states. During the period between the Civil War and the Great Depression, the federal government began a process that has continued to this day—the allocation of federal resources to states for national purposes. During the Civil War period, it was the Morrill Act of 1862 that provided grants of federal land to the states to support higher education. Later, cash grants for the establishment of agricultural experiment stations were provided. The federal grants to states made initially during the Civil War began a revolution in federal-state relations.[8] During the next 70 years the role of the federal government increased, and federal policies developed in such areas as regulation of interstate commerce, federal support for state programs in education and agricultural extension, and cash benefits for Civil War veterans and their survivors.[5]

During the Great Depression of the 1930s, major changes in federal-state relations occurred. In response to the Great Depression, the federal government initiated a series of actions designed to save the banks, regulate financial institutions, restore consumer confidence, aid the poor and unemployed, provide social security in old age, and provide federal aid to states for public assistance and public health, including maternal and child health. The most significant domestic social program ever enacted by Congress was the Social Security Act of 1935, which established a new role for the federal government in domestic affairs. After the broadening of the federal role in the 1930s, there was a gradual expansion of the federal role in the 1940s and 1950s.

In the 1960s there was a further transformation in the federal role in domestic social policy. Civil rights, medical care, elementary and secondary education, early childhood development, consumer protection, auto safety regulation, housing and community development, air and water pollution control, and antipoverty programs were among the areas in which the federal role was expanded.

The traditional federal-state relationship was extended to include direct federal support for local governments (cities and counties), nonprofit organizations, and private businesses and corporations in order to carry out a variety of health, education, social service, and community development programs.[10] Over 200 separate grant programs were enacted during the Kennedy and Johnson Administrations (1961–69). In health, programs ranged from Medicaid to rat control, from student loans to air pollution control, from services for the mentally retarded to expanded food and drug regulations. Among the many new health programs initiated during the 1960s, only Medicare (enacted in 1965 as an amendment to the Social Security Act) was directly administered by the federal government.

Although President Nixon placed greater stress on the role of the private sector in meeting domestic needs, there was continued expansion of the federal role, particularly in relation to income support for the elderly and the poor, including food stamps, social services, and health care. Presidents Nixon, Ford, and Carter all placed greater emphasis on the role of state and local governments than had President Johnson. The shift from federal categorical grants to support for state and local government was done through revenue sharing and block grants. During the 1960s and 1970s, voluntary organizations became a major means of providing services at the local level, with funds provided by the federal government, either directly or through block grants to states and revenue sharing with state and local governments.

The AIDS epidemic emerged just as the Reagan Administration was moving to adopt public policies designed to reduce the role of government, particularly the federal government, in domestic social programs. Congress supported the Reagan administration in efforts to decentralize program authority and responsibility ("new federalism") and reduce taxes. The Omnibus Budget Reconciliation Act of 1981, the Tax Equity and Fiscal Responsibility Act of 1982, and the recession of 1981–82 resulted in new relationships and conditions that were to shift the focus of concern and debate. Perhaps the most important was the dramatic reduction in federal taxes in 1982, which cut federal revenues by $750 billion over the next 5 years. These cuts, combined with the massive increase in military spending by the Reagan Administration, produced the largest peacetime federal budget deficit in history. The federal deficit has been the focus of the national policy debate since then, and it has cast a long shadow over efforts to deal with a range of domestic problems—from the care of the homeless and the hungry to the AIDS epidemic.

In the United States the initial federal policy response to the AIDS epidemic in 1981 was shaped by a new set of policy goals advocated by the Reagan Administration: reduced federal spending for domestic social programs or, when this could not be accomplished, a reduced rate of increase in federal spending;

decentralization of program responsibility and authority to state and local governments through block grants (new federalism); deregulation; increased competition; and an expanded role for the private sector.

THE POLICY ISSUES

In considering the policy response of the federal, state, and local governments in the United States to the AIDS epidemic, several questions must be raised. What can be done to prevent the spread of HIV infection and limit the number of future cases of AIDS? What must be done to care for persons with AIDS? How can needed preventive and treatment services be organized and financed? What are the responsibilities of the federal government, state governments, and local governments in dealing with the AIDS epidemic? What is the responsibility of the private sector? Is AIDS a national problem or just a series of local problems? Is the federal role limited primarily to biomedical research, disease surveillance, and technical assistance to state and local governments? What is the federal role in financing health care for AIDS patients? What is the role of the private sector in financing health care for AIDS patients? What is the role of state and local governments?

How governments and the private sector have responded to the AIDS epidemic is related to the magnitude of the epidemic; the groups affected and at risk; the modes of transmission of HIV; the availability, or lack of availability, of effective preventive measures and treatment modalities; sociopolitical factors such as the relationship of the public to the private sector, particularly the nonprofit or voluntary sector; costs; and attitudes, beliefs, and biases. In examining the response of government at the federal, state, and local levels to the AIDS epidemic, it is necessary to examine the full spectrum of activities that must be supported, from basic research to the care of the terminally ill (Table 1).

THE POLICY RESPONSE

Response of the Federal Government

The Initial Response

At the onset of the epidemic in 1981, the U.S. Public Health Service (USPHS)/ Department of Health and Human Services (DHHS) began to record the growing number of cases at the Centers for Disease Control (CDC); it initiated intramural research on AIDS in the National Institutes of Health (NIH) and CDC, and it provided technical assistance to states and local governments. At that point little action was taken by the U.S. Congress, because the potential magnitude of the problem was not recognized.

Soon after the onset of the AIDS epidemic, the USPHS began working with state and local governments, professional associations, and private organizations to develop guidelines related to protection of the nation's blood supply; school attendance, day care, and foster care of children with AIDS; and prevention of AIDS in the workplace. To date, the USPHS has issued 22 separate guidelines on AIDS, largely focused on prevention. The USPHS Plan for the Prevention

Table 1   Health-related AIDS activities requiring support

---

1. Research
2. Epidemiologic surveillance and monitoring
3. Medical care (inpatient, outpatient, physician services, drugs) and long-term care for persons with AIDS and ARC (including skilled nursing care, home care, hospice care)
4. Psychosocial support
5. Mental health services
6. Substance abuse services
7. Health education information for the general public; high school-, junior high school-, and college-aged youth; and persons at increased risk of HIV infection or already infected (e.g., gay males and IV drug users); and risk reduction programs for high-risk groups
8. Health professions education and training
9. Blood screening and testing (blood banks, alternative test sites)
10. Drug and medical device regulation

---

and Control of AIDS (1985), the USPHS Plan for the Prevention and Control of AIDS and the AIDS Virus (1986), the Surgeon General's Report on Acquired Immune Deficiency Syndrome,[11] and the USPHS's Information/Education Plan[12] have provided a broad set of guides for action, particularly for information, education, and risk reduction programs.

In 1983 the Secretary of DHHS declared that AIDS was the Department's No. 1 priority. Three goals received special emphasis by the DHHS: (1) the identification of the causal agent, (2) the development of an antibody test for the virus, and (3) identification of high-risk groups and the routes of transmission. Additional goals included protecting the nation's blood supply, developing a vaccine, and developing and testing drugs. Considerable success has been achieved in reaching the first three goals and in protecting the nation's blood supply. Limited initial success in drug treatment has been achieved with the development and marketing of azidothymidine (AZT), but progress with respect to vaccine development has been slow.

To achieve better planning and coordination of AIDS-related programs, the USPHS established the Executive Task Force on AIDS, chaired by the Assistant Secretary for Health. The Task Force serves as the mechanism by which AIDS-related issues are identified and addressed in a coordinated fashion by the USPHS constituent agencies: the Alcohol, Drug Abuse, and Mental Health Administration (ADAMHA); the CDC; the Food and Drug Administration (FDA); the Health Resources and Services Administration (HRSA); and the National Institutes of Health (NIH). Within the Task Force the CDC has been designated the lead agency in the area of prevention; HRSA in the area of health professions education and training and health care; NIH for biomedical research; FDA for drug and device regulation, including protection of the blood supply; and ADAMHA for issues related to IV drug use and AIDS. The Health Care Financing Administration, responsible for administrating Medicare and Medicaid, is not part of the USPHS Task Force, because it is a separate agency, comparable in organizational status to the USPHS.

Appropriations

Budgets, or appropriations, often reflect priorities. In the early years of the epidemic, the Reagan Administration requested no new funds for AIDS research, training, or services; instead, it transferred monies from other programs to fund these activities. Every year since the epidemic began, Congress has substantially increased the funds requested by the Reagan Administration, particularly the funds for biomedical research (Table 2).

The allocation of resources to AIDS-related programs within the USPHS has been heavily weighted toward basic biomedical research, vaccine development, clinical trials, and epidemiological surveillance. The limited federal funds devoted to public health education, especially for high-risk groups, and to prevention programs are of particular concern. A study conducted by the U.S. Conference of Mayors[13] found that one of the greatest needs at the local level was funding for training and technical assistance in community education, particularly on safe-sex guidelines. The Reagan Administration believes that these services are primarily a local responsibility.

Although much of the factual information available on high-risk groups, modes of transmission, and strategies to prevent the transmission of the AIDS virus has been developed in cooperation with CDC and NIH, the federal government has played a very limited role in the dissemination of information to individuals or groups at risk. During recent years, less than 4% of all USPHS resources for AIDS were appropriated for information dissemination/public affairs. From 1983 to 1986 the USPHS spent $40 million in direct expenditures to inform and educate the public and individuals at high risk of acquiring HIV infection. After the Surgeon General began his vigorous campaign to educate the public on the issue, USPHS funding increased significantly. In 1987 the USPHS will spend $79.5 million for AIDS education, and the President's budget request for fiscal year 1988 included $103.9 million for AIDS education.[12]

Currently no data are available that identify levels and sources of federal expenditures for hospital care, physicians' services, home care, or nursing home care for persons with AIDS. The two largest federal expenditures for these purposes are the federal tax subsidy for the purchase of private health insurance and the share of Medicaid funds used to pay for the care of persons with AIDS.

Because there has been no specific federal policy developed to deal with the catastrophic costs often entailed in the care of AIDS patients, most of the burden has been borne by private health insurance, by state Medicaid programs, by local governments in cities or counties with large numbers of AIDS patients (e.g., New York, San Francisco, and Los Angeles), and by the AIDS patients directly out of pocket.

Table 2   Federal government spending on AIDS 1982–87[a]

Budget (fiscal year)	Amount President requested	Amount appropriated by Congress
1982	NA	$ 5,553,000
1983	$ 8,153,000	$ 28,736,000
1984	$ 39,800,000	$ 61,460,000
1985	$ 54,092,000	$108,000,000
1986	$193,000,000	$244,000,000
1987	$213,000,000	$410,600,000

[a]The figures for federal expenditures related to AIDS do not include federal expenditures for the health care (e.g., Medicaid) provided AIDS patients.

The lack of federal policy with respect to long-term care generally, and particularly for the spectrum of community-based health services (e.g., home health and social services), required by AIDS patients has resulted in only limited funding of demonstration projects in the area. The cost of community-based health and social services falls mainly on afflicted individuals, their families and friends, volunteers, local charitable contributors, and, increasingly, local government.

Planning for the Future

In the summer of 1986 the Assistant Secretary for Health, U.S. DHHS, convened a group of USPHS personnel and advisors in Coolfont, West Virginia, to revise the USPHS plan for the prevention and control of AIDS. The plan now includes three goals:

1. By 1987, reduce transmission of HIV infection.
2. By 1990, reduce increase of incidence of AIDS.
3. By 2000, eliminate transmission of HIV infection.

Five target areas have been identified by the USPHS for action: (1) pathogenesis and clinical manifestations, (2) therapeutics, (3) vaccines, (4) public health control measures, and (5) patient care and health care needs.[1]

Although the plan developed by the USPHS envisioned a substantial expansion of the federal role, it was still a very limited one in terms of financing of health care for persons with AIDS, particularly long-term care. The AIDS budget proposed by the Reagan Administration for fiscal year 1988 did not reflect the expanded role envisioned in the USPHS plan. Although the President's budget proposal of $533 million for all AIDS-related programs in fiscal year 1988 represents an increase above the fiscal year 1987 appropriations, it seems seriously inadequate to groups directly involved in prevention and care. For example, the AIDS Action Council proposed an increase to at least $450 million in fiscal year 1988 for AIDS education, risk reduction, and prevention programs. This would represent a 50% increase in federal funding for these programs and would put the USPHS much closer to the goals recommended by the National Academy of Sciences.[2] The Council recommended a similar level of expenditure—$450 million—for basic biomedical, epidemiological, psychosocial, and other AIDS-related research programs.[14]

Although the USPHS has been constrained in its AIDS prevention, research, training, and service programs, it has moved aggressively, within the limits imposed by the Office of Management and Budget, to assist state and local governments and the private sector in responding to the AIDS epidemic. In its *Information/Education Plan to Prevent and Control AIDS in the United States*[12] the USPHS details the contents of the programs that are needed and roles for federal agencies, state and local governments, and the private sector. The plan addresses four groups: (1) the public; (2) young people, particularly through hotlines, coalitions, advertising campaigns, and a national clearinghouse; (3) persons at increased risk of AIDS, through hotlines, testing and counseling, drug treatment programs and health education, working with state and local governments, university medical centers and national and regional organizations;

and (4) health workers, using symposia, workshops, clearinghouses, training centers, and in-service training.

Response of State Governments

At the state level, markedly different policy, services, and financing responses have emerged in the states with the largest numbers of cases—New York, California, Florida, New Jersey, and Texas. The AIDS epidemic hit these states as the burden of financing health care for the poor was being shifted from the federal government to state and local governments and to the private sector and as the federal government was attempting to shift other health policy responsibilities to state and local governments.

By early 1987, nine states had enacted legislation related to the AIDS epidemic. Among the five states with the greatest number of AIDS cases, only Texas had not enacted any legislation to deal with the epidemic. The AIDS-related legislation enacted at the state level addressed areas ranging from basic biomedical research to income maintenance and housing.

New York, New Jersey, and California have responded more substantially than other states. These three states have funded research, laboratory support, epidemiologic surveillance, information and education programs, and Medicaid services for persons with AIDS. Both New York and New Jersey have begun to develop a comprehensive approach to the HIV/AIDS epidemic.

New York has recently moved to develop a comprehensive approach to the AIDS epidemic, coordinating state policies and programs with those at the local level (Table 3). New York State's comprehensive approach includes the approval of 15 hospitals as AIDS centers that will receive higher levels of payment for services. The 15 AIDS centers link dedicated inpatient and outpatient hospital units with a continuum of community-based services through a case management system. This model was pioneered by the San Francisco Department of Public Health, including its San Francisco General Hospital.

The allocation of funds in California reflects a high priority on research. In fiscal year 1983–84 the California Legislature appropriated $3.4 million for

Table 3 New York State's response to the AIDS epidemic

Department of Health
  1. AIDS Institute
     a. Research
     b. Education/prevention
     c. Testing and counseling for IV drug users
     d. Development/coordination of community-based services
     e. AIDS intervention management system (quality assurance and utilization review)
  2. Comprehensive AIDS care centers
  3. Medicaid
  4. Epidemiologic surveillance and studies
  5. Antibody testing

Division of Substance Abuse Services
  1. Methadone maintenance treatment program
  2. Detoxification
  3. Prevention/education/counseling

AIDS, including more than $1.2 million to the University of California to support research. This increased to $3.9 million in 1984–85 and to $7.59 million in 1985–86, while total AIDS funding increased to $14.76 million. Total AIDS appropriations in California rose to $30.621 million in 1986–87, and the Governor proposed an appropriation of $31.005 million for 1987–88. In fiscal years 1986–87 and 1987–88, funds for research ($15.07 million and $15.646 million, respectively) represented one-half of the budget. In addition, $1.5 million was appropriated in 1986–87 to the San Francisco Department of Public Health to begin plans for a research facility at San Francisco General Hospital. In addition to research, the budget for fiscal year 1987–88 proposed by the Governor will provide epidemiologic surveillance ($2.6 million), HIV antibody testing ($2.0 million), information and education ($4.8 million), and patient care ($1.5 million), but no funding for AIDS-related IV drug abuse programs.[15]

New Jersey, with only 359 cases of AIDS diagnosed between 1981 and 1986 (in contrast to 9272 cases in New York, 6545 in California, 1914 in Florida, and 1791 in Texas), has moved aggressively in the past 2 years to develop prevention and treatment programs. Exclusive of Medicaid expenditures (federal and state), the New Jersey Department of Health's expenditures for AIDS-related programs rose from $144,000 in fiscal year 1985 to $1,969,000 in fiscal year 1986 to $4,954,000 in fiscal year 1987, and the department anticipates expenditures of $7,906,000 in fiscal year 1988. In addition to the state funds, New Jersey has received $809,000 from the Robert Wood Johnson Foundation and $1,196,000 from the federal government. The New Jersey program includes treatment and community support, surveillance, testing and counseling, education and prevention, research (including a study on costs), and laboratory services.[16]

In 1984 California and Florida were among the first states to enact legislation designed to protect the public blood supply, requiring antibody testing by all blood banks and plasma centers. Both states authorized alternative test sites in addition to those at blood banks, and the laws provided means to protect the individuals tested from unauthorized disclosure. Similar legislation has been enacted by all other states.

In 1985 California expanded the scope of its AIDS legislation to include pilot detoxification and treatment programs for IV drug abusers, funds to evaluate the effectiveness of AIDS education and information programs, and funds for a prospective 2-year study concerning medical costs of AIDS. The Governor has not included funds in his fiscal year 1988 budget for a continuation of either of these activities.

According to a recent report of the Intergovernmental Health Policy Project at George Washington University, $117 million in state funds has been spent or obligated specifically for the support of AIDS-related programs since the beginning of 1983.[17] Thirty-three states and the District of Columbia reported spending between $21 million and $22 million of state dollars on surveillance, laboratory services, education and information, outreach, antibody testing, and administration. Another $21.8 million was allocated to research, with the remainder for psychosocial support services and treatment. Recently California, New York, and the District of Columbia have agreed to pay for the cost of AZT prescribed to Medicaid beneficiaries. The bulk of AIDS-related expenditures have been in California, New York, New Jersey, and Massachusetts.

Data have not been gathered nationally on AIDS and the state role in corrections or criminal justice systems, but for New York and New Jersey, this is a major problem, and all states are likely to have to address the issue.

Local Government Response

Like the states, markedly different policy, financing, and administrative responses to the AIDS epidemic have emerged in cities and counties affected by the AIDS epidemic. Many of the political, economic, and public health factors affecting the policy responses at the federal and state levels have also affected the response of local governments.

Problems of organizing, financing, and providing the spectrum of medical, social, and public health services to deal with the AIDS epidemic are complex and therefore costly and difficult to resolve in any community. The services required to care for AIDS patients range from HIV antibody testing to hospice care. In addition, services are required for the education of high-risk groups, for dissemination of information to the general public, for the protection of the blood supply (e.g., HTLV-III antibody testing), for laboratory support, and for epidemiologic surveillance (see Table 1). These services may be provided by public agencies, nonprofit community agencies, volunteers, private practitioners, community hospitals, proprietary home health agencies, and nonprofit or proprietary nursing homes.

New York City and San Francisco (a combined city-county government), which together accounted for more than 40% of all reported AIDS cases in the United States in early 1987, have appropriated significant local tax funds for AIDS services. Los Angeles County, which equals San Francisco in terms of reported cases of AIDS, has appropriated virtually nothing to combat the epidemic. In fiscal year 1986–87, San Francisco will spend more than $10 million in local taxes for such services. New York City's contribution, because it shares part of Medicaid costs, will spend far more. In California, the Medicaid program is funded by federal and state funds. In both New York and San Francisco the local government provides medical care for the indigent who have no source of third-party payment. Each city receives federal and state funds for public health and medical care programs related to AIDS.

A major difference between the cities is how local tax monies have been allocated. It is estimated that more than 90% of local New York City AIDS funds are spent on inpatient hospital care as compared to 25% in San Francisco.[18,19] This difference is due largely to New York City's 25% share of Medicaid expenditures and a direct subsidy to the municipal hospitals (Health and Hospital Corporation) providing care to AIDS patients. But it is also a result of a greater level of hospitalization in New York—the average length of a hospital stay for an AIDS patient in New York was 25 days in 1985 compared to 12 days in San Francisco.[20,21]

Government support of community-based services for persons with AIDS illustrates another key difference in the local policy response between New York City and San Francisco. The response may be related in part to governmental structure. It is certainly related to the political influence of gays in San Francisco. San Francisco is a unique local government in California, because it is a county and a city combined. In contrast, Los Angeles County contains many different cities, including the City of Los Angeles. Because public health and public welfare authority is vested in the state government and county governments in California, the unique government organization of San Francisco as both a city and a county has made the policy response to the AIDS epidemic less complicated than in other California counties and cities.

Community-based services include crisis intervention and counseling, basic home care, hospice care, legal services, entitlements advocacy, group therapy, and education. Although these services have been a major component of the local response in both New York and San Francisco, the sources of funding have been quite different in the two cities. In 1984 the Gay Men's Health Crisis (GMHC) provided the bulk of these services in New York using primarily private (64%) and state funds (33%). Only 3% of the funds were provided by New York City. In sharp contrast, the three largest organizations providing these services in San Francisco—the Shanti Project, the San Francisco AIDS Foundation, and the Hospice of San Francisco—received 62% of their financial resources from the City and County of San Francisco, 30% from private sources, 4% from the state, and 4% from the federal government.[22] San Francisco has allocated more funds directly for AIDS services than any other local government, with spending rising from $180,000 in 1982–83 to $10 million in 1986–87 (Table 4).

Voluntary workers make a highly significant contribution to organizations providing health and social services to individuals with AIDS. Approximately 130,000 volunteer hours were contributed to GMHC in New York City during 1984. This is comparable to the total hours donated to community agencies and groups in San Francisco. The relative dependence of service providers on volunteers vividly illustrates the strength of local commitment to addressing the AIDS epidemic as well as the process by which the burden of dealing with a national public health crisis is continually shifted from the federal to the state level, then to local government, and finally to individuals—either AIDS patients or volunteers.[22]

Local government funding in San Francisco from the Department of Public Health and private donations has been critical for the development of educational, social, psychological, home care, and hospice services in San Francisco. Virtually none of these services are funded by private health insurance, even though they are essential for the adequate care of AIDS patients. As the numbers increase, the city and county will not be able to bear the additional costs.

What of the rest of the country? A survey by the U.S. Conference of Mayors in 1984 assembled information from 55 local governments on their AIDS efforts.[13] Of these, 40% of cities with populations greater than 200,000 and almost

Table 4   City of San Francisco spending on AIDS 1982–87

Fiscal year	Budget
1982–83	$ 180,447
1983–84	$ 4,300,000
1984–85	$ 7,400,000
1985–86	$ 8,800,000
1986–87	$10,000,000

25% of those with less than 200,000 reported some AIDS-related local public spending. Two-thirds of the larger cities had established task forces on AIDS by late 1984. However, the majority of cities and states in both high- and low-incidence areas have not been able to generate the level of support necessary to create service agencies, education programs, and comprehensive approaches to the health needs of people with AIDS. Widespread hostility toward homosexuality and an inhospitable sociopolitical climate have hindered efforts to respond to this public health crisis.

SUMMARY AND CONCLUSION

The AIDS epidemic poses an unprecedented challenge to policy makers at the federal, state, and local levels. To date, the response at the federal level has stressed biomedical research, epidemiological surveillance, protection of the blood supply, and, increasingly, education and information. The tax subsidy for private health insurance and Medicaid funding for the care of persons with AIDS have received very little attention.

Three goals established by the Secretary of DHHS in 1983 have been achieved: the causative agent was identified (in France and the U.S.), the mode of transmission of HIV infection was clarified, and an antibody test was developed and applied to protect the nation's blood supply. In addition, a great deal has been learned about HIV infection and AIDS, and several promising drugs have been developed. Until very recently the most serious deficiency of federal policy has been the lack of an overall plan to combat the epidemic, prevent the spread of HIV infection, and care for those afflicted. Strong federal leadership, beyond the Surgeon General's call for education and prevention, is clearly needed and appears to be gradually developing. The second, equally serious, problem has been the lack of adequate federal funding for research; for education, information, and prevention; for training; and for the financing of acute medical care and long-term care, particularly subacute hospital care, skilled nursing care, and home care.

State policies, with few exceptions, have been very limited in view of the potential magnitude of the epidemic and heavy costs already borne by communities such as New York City, Los Angeles, West Hollywood, San Francisco, Miami, Houston, Baltimore, and more than a dozen other cities or counties. Less than a half a dozen states have responded in any substantial way to the epidemic. Two states, New York and New Jersey, are now providing strong leadership to combat the epidemic. California, which was once in the lead, has devoted almost half of its funds to research, a traditional responsibility of the federal government.

Local government responses, with the exception of San Francisco and New York, have been very limited. Recently, with funding provided by the Robert Wood Johnson Foundation, programs are being strengthened and expanded in 11 cities and counties. In the communities hardest hit, the private sector has responded, particularly through community-based volunteer groups often organized under strong gay male leadership. Much more must be done if the burden borne by persons with AIDS is not to become even greater.

The essential elements of a national AIDS program have been outlined in the Institute of Medicine/National Academy of Sciences' report,[2] the USPHS's

Coolfont report,[3] the Surgeon General's Report,[11] and the USPHS's Information/Education Plan.[12] It is essential that the federal, state, and local governments collectively and cooperatively with the major groups and institutions in the private sector (the insurance industry, hospitals, nursing homes, physicians, nurses, community-based home care agencies, foundations, the pharmaceutical industry, and academic medical centers) move forward to propose national policies, a comprehensive plan, and specific programs to deal effectively with the AIDS epidemic.

REFERENCES

1. Coolfont Planning Conference: Public Health Service plan for prevention and control of AIDS and the AIDS virus. *Public Health Reports* 1986;101:341–348.

2. National Academy of Sciences, Institute of Medicine: *Confronting AIDS: Directions for Public Health, Health Care, and Research*. Washington, DC: National Academy Press, 1986.

3. Scitovsky AA, Rice DP: Estimates of the direct and indirect costs of acquired immunodeficiency syndrome in the United States, 1985, 1986, and 1991. *Public Health Reports* 1987;102(1):5–17.

4. Hardy AM, Rauch K, Echenberg DF, et al: The economic impact of the first 10,000 cases of AIDS in the United States. *JAMA* 1986;255:209–211.

5. Lee PR, Benjamin AE: Health policy and the politics of health care. In Williams SJ, Torrens PR (eds): *Introduction to Health Services*. New York: John Wiley, 1984.

6. Blendon RJ, Aiken LH, Freeman HE, et al: Uncompensated care by hospitals or public insurance for the poor. *N Engl J Med* 1986;314:1160–1163.

7. Mills M, Wofsy CB, Mills J: The acquired immunodeficiency syndrome: Infection control and public health law. *N Engl J Med* 1986;314(14):931–936.

8. Hale GE, Palley ML: *The Politics of Federal Grants*. Washington, DC: Congressional Quarterly Press, 1981.

9. Lee PR, Silver GA: Health planning—a view from the top with specific reference to the USA. In Fry J, Farndale WAJ (eds): *International Medical Care*. Oxford, U.K.: Medical and Technical Publishing, 1972.

10. Reagan MD, Sanzone JG: *The New Federalism*, 2d Ed. New York: Oxford University Press, 1981.

11. U.S. Department of Health and Human Services, U.S. Public Health Service: *Surgeon General's Report on Acquired Immune Deficiency Syndrome*. Washington, DC: U.S. Government Printing Office, 1986.

12. U.S. Department of Health and Human Services, U.S. Public Health Service: *Information/Education Plan to Prevent and Control AIDS in the United States*. Washington, DC: U.S. Government Printing Office, 1987.

13. U.S. Conference of Mayors: *Local Responses to Acquired Immune Deficiency Syndrome (AIDS): A Report of 55 Cities*. Washington, DC: U.S. Government Printing Office, 1984.

14. AIDS Action Council: *AIDS Action Update*, March 1987.

15. California Legislature: *Analyses of the 1987–88 Budget Bill*, Report of the Legislative Analyst to the Joint Legislative Budget Committee, 1987.

16. New Jersey Department of Health: *AIDS in New Jersey*, Report from the Department of Health, March 1987.

17. Intergovernmental Health Policy Project: *An Overview of Specific State Funding for AIDS Programs and Activities*. Washington, DC: George Washington University, July 1986.

18. New York State Comptroller's Office: *Review of New York City's Proposed Financial Plan for Fiscal Years 1986 through 1989* (Report No. 30-86), December 11, 1985.

19. San Francisco Department of Public Health: *San Francisco's Response to AIDS: Status Up-Date*, October 8, 1985.

20. Sencer DJ, Botnick VE: *Report to the Mayor: New York City's Response to the AIDS Crisis*. City of New York, Office of the Mayor, December 1985.

21. West Bay Hospital Conference: *Monthly AIDS Hospital Utilization Report*. San Mateo, CA, October 25, 1985.

22. Arno PS: The nonprofit sector's response to the AIDS epidemic: Community-based services in San Francisco. *Am J Pub Health* 1986;76(11):1325–1330.

42

Estimates of the Direct and Indirect Costs of Acquired Immune Deficiency Syndrome in the United States, 1985, 1986, and 1991

Anne A. Scitovsky and Dorothy P. Rice

INTRODUCTION

Despite the general concern over the financial burden of the AIDS epidemic in the United States, data on use of and expenditures for medical services of persons with AIDS are surprisingly scarce and very limited. Similarly, data on nonpersonal medical costs, such as expenses for research, blood screening and testing, replacement of blood, health education, and support services, are equally difficult to obtain. Finally, only one estimate has been made of the indirect costs of AIDS—the losses incurred by AIDS patients due to time lost from work because of illness, disability, and premature death.

The most frequently cited AIDS cost figure in the United States is an estimate of the lifetime hospital costs and economic losses from disability and premature death (indirect costs) of the first 10,000 patients with AIDS reported in the United States. These estimates were made by Ann Hardy of the national Centers for Disease Control (CDC) and her colleagues and were first presented at a conference on AIDS in Atlanta, GA, in April 1985.[1] They estimated lifetime hospital costs of these patients at $1.473 billion, or $147,000 per AIDS patient. This estimate was based on the assumption of a lifetime use of 168 hospital days, an average survival time of 392 days (or about 13 months), and an average charge (including inpatient professional charges) per hospital day of $878. In the same article, the lifetime indirect costs of these 10,000 cases were estimated at $4.8 billion, almost 3½ times direct hospital costs.

Even today, more than a year after these early estimates, data for estimating the economic costs of the AIDS epidemic in the United States are scarce. Apart from a study of the lifetime medical care costs of AIDS patients in California, based on MediCal (Medicaid) claims data,[2] there have been no systematic stud-

This study was supported by Task Order 282-85-0061 #2 from the Centers for Disease Control (CDC). Norman Axnick, Director, Office of Program Planning and Evaluation, as project officer served as the CDC liaison throughout the study. W. Meade Morgan, PhD, Chief of Statistics and Data Processing Branch, AIDS Program, CDC, supplied the detailed prevalence estimates of AIDS in the 3 years. Mary Cline, BA, Palo Alto Medical Foundation/Research Institute, and Bruce Kieler, MA, MBA, School of Nursing, University of California, San Francisco, served as research assistants and performed much of the detailed data collection. This chapter is a somewhat abbreviated version of an article that appeared in *Public Health Reports*, January/February 1987.

ies. However, additional data on the use and costs of medical services of AIDS patients can be found in unpublished reports by state and city health departments and a few hospital associations. In addition, some hospitals have compiled data on average length of hospital stay and costs or charges per hospital day of AIDS admissions.

In late 1985 the CDC asked us to make new estimates of the direct and indirect economic costs of AIDS in the United States. Our report to the CDC was completed in March 1986,[3] but we have since revised our estimates upward to take account of more recent higher CDC estimates of the incidence and prevalence of AIDS.[4,5] The prevalence estimates we used were prepared by W. Meade Morgan, PhD, Chief of Statistics and Data Processing Branch, AIDS Program, CDC. At our request (because for our estimates we needed the data in this form), he classified all reported AIDS patients alive at any time in 1984, and the estimated number of such persons in the later years, into the following three prevalence categories: (1) those diagnosed in a prior year and alive all 12 months; (2) those who died in the year; and (3) those newly diagnosed and alive at the end of the year.

For 1984, Dr. Morgan also distributed the patients in each of these three categories into three broad diagnostic groups and classified them by age and sex within each diagnostic group. The three diagnostic groups are *Pneumocystis carinii* pneumonia and other infectious diseases, Kaposi's sarcoma, and all other conditions. The year 1984 was selected because it was the first year that health departments in the United States confirmed all cases using the strict definition of AIDS specified by the CDC. In addition, 1984 data are complete, and there are no reporting lags as there would have been had we used 1985 data. For the later years, Dr. Morgan suggested we assume that the distribution of patients within each of the three prevalence categories by diagnosis, age, and sex was the same as in 1984, since there was no adequate basis for forecasting these distributions more accurately. Finally, he advised us to increase all his estimates by 20% to correct for underreporting of AIDS cases.

SUMMARY OF FINDINGS

Table 1 shows the prevalence estimates prepared by Dr. Morgan, increased by 20% for our estimates to take account of underreporting. The total number of persons with AIDS alive at any time during the year is estimated to rise from 9368 in 1984, to 18,720 in 1985, to 31,440 in 1986, and to 172,800 in 1991. This represents an increase in the prevalence rate from 3.96 cases per 100,000 population in 1984 to 68.63 cases per 100,000 population in 1991. The death rate from AIDS is estimated to rise from 1.49 deaths per 100,000 population in 1984 to 25.74 deaths per 100,000 in 1991.

The following costs were estimated:

Direct costs:

• Personal medical care costs; these include expenditures for hospital services, physician inpatient and outpatient services, outpatient ancillary services, and nursing home, home care, and hospice services.

• Nonpersonal costs; these include expenditures for research, blood screening and testing, replacement of blood, health education, and support services.

Table 1 Estimate of prevalence of AIDS, United States. Reported cases for 1984 and estimates for 1985, 1986, and 1991

	Reported cases 1984	Estimates		
Prevalence categories		1985	1986	1991
AIDS patients alive all 12 months but diagnosed prior to year	1,424	3,360	6,240	42,000
AIDS patients who died during year	3,534	6,240	10,800	64,800
AIDS patients diagnosed during year and alive at end of year	4,410	9,120	14,400	66,000
Prevalence (cases)	9,368	18,720	31,440	172,800
Prevalence rate (cases per 100,000 population)	3.96	7.84	13.05	68.63
Death rate (cases per 100,000 population)	1.49	2.61	4.48	25.74

Source: Personal communication, W. Meade Morgan, Ph.D., Chief of Statistics and Data Processing Branch, AIDS Program, CDC. At Dr. Morgan's suggestion, the estimates provided by him have been increased by 20% to take account of underreporting.

Indirect costs:
• Morbidity costs; these are the value of productivity losses due to illness and disability.
• Mortality costs; these are the present value of future earnings lost for those who died prematurely as a result of AIDS.

No attempt was made to estimate the dollar value of social support services and public health information provided by volunteers, although there is evidence that community-based organizations providing such services rely heavily on volunteer labor.[6] Nor did we attempt to estimate the psychological costs due to AIDS, even though it is recognized that these are real and great for the AIDS victims, their friends, and their families.

Because of the many uncertainties about the future course of the AIDS epidemic and the scarcity of data about the medical care costs, nonpersonal costs, and indirect costs of the epidemic, we made three estimates ranging from low to high, which are shown in Table 2. However, we regard our medium estimates as our best estimates. For 1985, our medium estimate of the total direct and indirect costs of AIDS comes to about $4.8 billion in current dollars, of which $630 million is for personal medical care costs, $319 million for nonpersonal direct costs, and $3.9 billion for indirect costs. The corresponding figures for 1986 are a total of $8.7 billion, of which $1.1 billion are for personal medical care costs, $542 million for nonpersonal direct costs, and $7.0 billion for indirect costs. In 1991, they are estimated to rise to a total of $66.5 billion, of which $8.5 billion is for personal medical care expenses, $2.3 billion for nonpersonal direct costs, and almost $56 billion for indirect costs. Thus in all 3 years, indirect costs due to morbidity, and especially premature mortality, account for about 80–84% of the total economic cost of the AIDS epidemic. The reason for the high indirect costs, and especially the high mortality costs, is that most of the victims of AIDS are young, in the 20- to 40-year age bracket, and thus in their most productive years. Thus, although the direct medical care costs of AIDS are not negligible, they are far surpassed by the indirect costs due to premature mortality.

Table 2 Estimated economic costs of AIDS, amounts and percent distributions by type of costs, 1985, 1986, and 1991 (millions of current dollars)

Year	Total direct and indirect	Direct costs			Indirect costs		
		Total	Personal medical	Nonpersonal	Total	Morbidity	Mortality
1985							
Low	$3,766	$647	$402	$245	$3,119	$261	$2,858
Medium	4,836	949	630	319	3,887	261	3,626
High	5,278	1,391	1,072	319	3,887	261	3,626
1986							
Low	6,788	1,166	714	452	5,622	456	5,166
Medium	8,673	1,661	1,119	542	7,012	456	6,556
High	9,457	2,445	1,903	542	7,012	456	6,556
1991							
Low	51,359	6,847	5,452	1,395	44,512	3,315	41,197
Medium	66,464	10,869	8,544	2,325	55,595	3,315	52,280
High	74,000	18,405	14,530	3,875	55,595	3,315	52,280
Percent of total direct and indirect costs							
1985							
Low	100.0	17.2	10.7	6.5	82.8	6.9	75.9
Medium	100.0	19.6	13.0	6.6	80.4	5.4	75.0
High	100.0	26.4	20.3	6.0	73.6	4.9	68.7
1986							
Low	100.0	17.2	10.5	6.7	82.8	6.7	76.1
Medium	100.0	19.2	12.9	6.3	80.8	5.3	75.6
High	100.0	25.9	20.1	5.7	74.1	4.8	69.3
1991							
Low	100.0	13.3	10.6	2.7	86.7	6.5	80.2
Medium	100.0	16.4	12.9	3.5	83.6	5.0	78.7
High	100.0	24.9	19.6	5.2	75.1	4.5	70.6

Estimates of Personal Medical Care Costs

We based our model for estimating the direct personal medical care costs of AIDS patients in the United States on information we gained from a retrospective study of medical care costs of AIDS patients treated at San Francisco General Hospital (SFGH) in 1984.[7] As will be described below, however, the figures used in the model were based on SFGH data only for the low estimates but on data from other areas for the medium and high estimates, because there is considerable evidence that costs of treating AIDS patients are lower in San Francisco than in other areas. In 1984, San Francisco ranked second after New York in the number of AIDS cases in the United States, and about one-half of all San Francisco persons with AIDS were treated at SFGH. Among the data yielded by this study were data on total medical care expenditures of AIDS patients who received all their inpatient and outpatient care at SFGH in 1984. We used the data from this group of patients for our model.

Our data for these patients showed that they fell into the three distinctive prevalence categories described previously, based on their monthly medical expenses. These expenses were lowest ($586) for patients who lived all 12 months; highest ($3660) for those who died and who, on the average, had expenses for 6.4 months of the year; and in between the two ($2617) for those who were newly diagnosed and alive at the end of the year who, on the average, had expenses for 4.6 months. In addition, we found that patients with different initial diagnoses incurred different costs and that, as a result, we had to distinguish between at least the three diagnostic groups (also described previously) within each of the three prevalence categories. Our data showed that patients with *Pneumocystis carinii* pneumonia and other infectious diseases were considerably more expensive to treat than those with Kaposi's sarcoma, who can be treated to quite an extent on an outpatient basis. Data on hospital charges for patients with conditions other than *Pneumocystis carinii* pneumonia, other infectious diseases, and Kaposi's sarcoma suggested that these patients were somewhat less costly to treat than those with Kaposi's sarcoma, although the difference was not substantial.

On the basis of this information, we constructed a simple model to estimate the personal medical care costs of AIDS patients in a given year where the variables determining expenses per case of AIDS were the average number of hospital admissions per case, the average number of hospital days per admission, the average charge per hospital day, and average outpatient charges per case. Total expenses for a given year (for example, 1985) then are:

$$\text{Cost}_{1985} = N_{1985} \times [(a \times b \times c) + d]$$

where N = total number of AIDS cases alive at any time during the year, a = average number of admissions per case, b = average number of hospital days per admission, c = average charge per hospital day, and d = average outpatient charges per case. The average number of admissions per case is the total number of admissions in the year divided by the total number of AIDS cases alive at any time during the year. Similarly, average outpatient charges are total outpatient charges during the year divided by the total number of AIDS patients alive at any time during the year.

As a first step, we used our 1984 SFGH data on these four variables for each of the nine prevalence and diagnosis-specific groups and CDC's distribution of the 1984 cases in the United States among the nine groups to calculate averages for the four variables for the United States as a whole. Because we had only one case with a condition other than *Pneumocystis carinii* pneumonia, other infectious diseases, or Kaposi's sarcoma in the group of patients who received all their inpatient and outpatient care at SFGH in 1984, we assumed costs of these other cases to be similar to those of patients with Kaposi's sarcoma, although data on 177 hospital admissions of such cases suggest that they may be slightly less expensive to treat. Because the estimated distribution of AIDS patients among the three prevalence categories in 1985 and 1986 differs slightly, and in 1991 differs considerably from that in 1984, we repeated these calculations for the later years as well. However, the averages resulting from these calculations were so similar that we used those based on the 1984 distribution of cases. These figures are shown in column 1 of Table 3. The calculations of averages for the four cost variables in our model were necessary, because most of the data on these variables from other sources refer to all AIDS patients and are not prevalence-category and diagnosis-specific.

Using this formula, we made three estimates of the personal medical care costs of AIDS for each of the 3 years, ranging from low to high, varying the cost variables on the basis of data from various sources. The assumptions for the three estimates are shown in columns 2 through 4 of Table 3. All estimates were made in 1984 dollars and then converted to current dollars. As Table 2 shows, the estimates range from $402 million to about $1 billion in 1985, from $714 million to $1.9 billion in 1986, and from $5.5 billion to $14.5 billion in 1991.

The low estimates are based on the data derived from our SFGH study, shown in column 1 of Table 3, except that we have increased average outpatient charges to $4000. We made this adjustment to take account of nonhospital outpatient charges (mainly home health and hospice care), which we estimated on the basis of expenditures of one of the San Francisco voluntary agencies providing home health and hospice care to AIDS patients.

We regard these as the very lowest possible estimates, because they are derived from data from SFGH. Data from other areas suggest that costs of treating AIDS patients in San Francisco are considerably lower than elsewhere, primarily because of a very much shorter hospital stay. Thus these low estimates

Table 3 Model for estimating the personal medical care costs of AIDS in the United States

Cost variables	Averages for 1984 based on SFGH data and U.S. distribution of cases (1)	Low estimate (2)	Medium estimate (3)	High estimate (4)
Average number of hospital admissions per patient	1.7	1.7	1.7	2.2
Average number of hospital days per admission	13	13	20	25
Average charge per hospital day	$740	$740	$850	$950
Average outpatient charges per patient	$2000	$4000	$3000	$2000

can be regarded as estimates of personal medical care costs of AIDS patients if the special conditions existing in San Francisco prevailed elsewhere.

For the other estimates, we made use of data from our review of all other sources that we were able to obtain:

Data on Average Number of Admissions per Case

Data on this variable are extremely scarce. Three unpublished studies showed 1.6 and 1.7 admissions per case, while the California AIDS study[2] implies approximately 2.3 admissions per case. In the absence of any other data, we have used 1.7 admissions per case for our medium estimates and 2.2 for our high estimates, a 30% increase, which brings it close to the rate shown by the State of California data.

Average Length of Hospital Stay

Data on average length of hospital stay range all the way from 12.0 to 72.2 days. However, the stays appear to be clustered in the 15- to 25-day range, and we have therefore chosen 20 and 25 days for our medium and high estimates.

Average Charge per Hospital Day

Average charges per hospital day ranged from $471 to $1038, with a clustering in the $800–1000 range. Accordingly, we chose $850 and $950 as reasonable figures for our medium and high estimates.

Average Outpatient Charges

Data on outpatient charges are practically nonexistent. In addition to our data from SFGH, one unpublished study put outpatient costs at $2668. The California AIDS study estimated outpatient costs at 10% of total costs. In the absence of more data, we used $4000 for our low estimate and decreased the amount in the higher estimates on the assumption that patients with longer hospital stays receive less outpatient care.

Estimates of the Nonpersonal Costs

The spread of the AIDS epidemic has led to the development by the public and private sectors of a variety of nonpersonal services that must be included as part of the direct costs of AIDS. These services include research, conducted mainly by the federal and state governments; blood screening services including screening of blood donors, commercial plasma donors, high-risk groups, sexual contacts of high-risk groups, aliens seeking admission to the United States, and members of and recruit applicants to the U.S. military service; and finally a variety of support services provided by local governments and community-based organizations. Included in these support services are counseling; emotional and spiritual care for patients, their families, and friends; housing; and help with shopping and transportation.

Like the data on personal health care use and expenditures of persons with AIDS, data on nonpersonal costs are difficult to obtain and even more difficult to project. For example, whereas expenditures for research by the federal government are available from the federal budget, state expenditures for research are more problematical, because they are frequently included with other budget items. In the case of many services, much depends on the assumptions one make regarding the number of specific services rendered in a year (e.g., the number of blood samples tested) and of the cost per service. For example, the cost of the ELISA blood screening test is estimated in the range of $5–10; that of the Western blot test, in the range of $40–50. Finally, for education, information, and miscellaneous support services, data on expenditures are frequently combined with expenditures for blood screening and medical care.

In view of these many uncertainties, low and medium-high estimates were made for each of the groups of nonpersonal costs of AIDS for 1985 and 1986. Estimates for the more distant future are practically impossible, because so many factors affect expenditures for these services and because these factors are likely to change over time. For 1991, we therefore assumed that expenditures for nonpersonal services would equal about 27% of personal medical care expenditures, approximately the same as their percentage in our high estimate for 1986, and we made three estimates ranging from low to high. Table 2 shows that estimated costs for nonpersonal medical services range from $245 million to $319 million in 1985 and from $452 million to $542 million in 1986. In 1991, the estimates range from a low of $1.4 billion to a high of $3.9 billion.

Estimates of the Indirect Costs

Indirect costs are the value of lost output because of cessation or reduction of productivity caused by morbidity and mortality. Morbidity costs are wages lost by people who are unable to work because of illness and disability; for persons too sick to perform their usual housekeeping services, an imputed value of these services is included. Mortality costs are the present value of future earnings lost by people who die prematurely.

To estimate the indirect costs of AIDS, the human capital method as developed by Rice was used.[8–10] It is called the human capital method, because an employed person is seen as producing a stream of output over the years that is valued at the individual's earnings.

Morbidity Costs

Calculating morbidity costs involves applying average earnings by age and sex to work-loss years for those currently employed, attaching a dollar value to housekeeping services for those unable to perform these services because of illness, and applying labor force participation rates and earnings to persons who are too sick to be employed. For morbidity costs, a 60% disability rate was assumed for the groups of AIDS patients who lived all 12 months and those who were newly diagnosed and alive at the end of the year. The number of deaths was divided in half on the assumption that they occurred evenly during the year, and it was assumed that these patients were too ill to work at all prior to their death.

There are no hard data on the earnings of persons with AIDS. There is some evidence that male homosexuals have above-average earnings. However, the majority of AIDS victims who are IV drug abusers probably have little or no income or income from illegal sources (drug dealing, theft, and prostitution). In the absence of good data, it was assumed that persons with AIDS had the same average earnings as all others in their age and sex group. Because 1984 data on earnings by age and sex were not available, the 1983 figures were adjusted by a factor of 1.048, the ratio of gross average weekly earnings in 1984 to those in 1983. It was also assumed that labor force participation rates of persons with AIDS were the same as those of all others in their age and sex group. On the basis of these assumptions, morbidity costs were estimated at $261 million in 1985, $456 million in 1986, and $3.3 billion in 1991, as is shown in Table 2.

Mortality Costs

The estimated cost or value to society of premature deaths is the product of the number of deaths and the expected value of a person's future earnings with sex and age taken into account. This method of derivation takes into consideration life expectancy for different age and sex groups, varying labor force participation rates, changing patterns of earnings at successive ages, imputed value for housekeeping services, and the appropriate discount rate to convert a stream of costs or benefits into its present worth. As in the estimates of morbidity costs, it was assumed that persons with AIDS had the same earnings and labor force participation rates as the population as a whole according to their age and sex group. Because the selection of the discount rate makes a considerable difference in discounting future earnings, two estimates were made, a higher one using a 4% discount rate and a lower one using a 6% discount rate.

As Table 2 shows, mortality costs are estimated at $2.9 billion (6% discount rate) and $3.6 billion (4% discount rate) in 1985, and for 1986, $5.2 billion and $6.6 billion (at 6% and 4% discount rates, respectively). For 1991, estimated mortality costs are $41.2 billion and $52.3 billion with the 6% and 4% discount rates, respectively.

COMPARISON WITH OTHER HEALTH CARE COSTS

In conclusion, to give our estimates some perspective, they must be set within the framework of other health care cost data. To begin with the personal medical care costs of AIDS patients, our best estimate of $630 million in 1985 represents 0.2% of 1985 personal health care expenditures in the United States as estimated by the Health Care Financing Administration. Our best estimate of these expenditures in 1991, $8.5 billion, represents 1.4% of estimated 1991 personal health care expenditures.

We can also compare our estimates of medical care expenditures of AIDS patients in 1985 with expenditures of patients suffering from other diseases. In 1980, the Medicare program paid $1.3 billion in reimbursements for patients with end-stage renal disease;[11] in terms of 1985 expenditures, this sum would amount to about $2.2 billion. According to an unpublished study by the U.S. Department of Transportation, persons injured in automobile accidents are estimated to have incurred medical costs of $3.3 billion in 1980. In terms of 1985 expenditures, this would amount to about $5.6 billion. Finally, it has been estimated by the National Center for Health Statistics that in 1980 the medical care costs of persons with cancer of the digestive system amounted to $2.0 billion; those of persons with cancer of the lung, trachea, and bronchus, $1.6 billion; and those with cancer of the breast, $1.3 billion. In terms of 1985 expenses, these figures translate into $3.4 billion, $2.7 billion, and $2.2 billion, respectively.

It must be borne in mind, however, that although data on the number of persons suffering from these other conditions in a given year are not available, it is very likely that the medical care cost *per person* with any of these other conditions is considerably lower than that of a person with AIDS.

Extrapolating 1980 medical expenditures for specific diseases to 1991 is very problematic. But if we assume that the prevalence of and relative medical expenditures for these conditions remain unchanged over time, only medical expenses of victims of automobile accidents will exceed the medical care costs of AIDS patients in 1991, and expenditures of patients with the other conditions will range from about 45% to 70% of those of AIDS patients.

Our best estimates of the indirect costs of AIDS in the United States in current dollars—$3.9 billion in 1985 and $7.0 billion in 1986—represent 1.2% and 2.1% of the estimated total indirect costs of all illness in these 2 years; by 1991, however, they are estimated to represent close to 12% of the estimated total indirect costs of all illness.

To sum up, the annual costs—both direct and indirect—of the AIDS epidemic to date have been relatively low when compared with the economic costs of all illness as well as the costs of some other diseases. These comparisons are in no way intended to belittle the burden that the epidemic imposes on its victims and society in general. Moreover, what has aggravated the situation is that AIDS cases have been concentrated in a few metropolitan centers, which has put and continues to put a serious strain on the resources of these centers, especially on their public hospitals. If the epidemic spreads as forecast by the CDC, however, its burden will be very heavy and will be felt throughout the nation. Thus it is clear that combating the AIDS epidemic requires efforts and financial resources at all levels of the private and public sectors: efforts to reduce the medical care costs by providing alternatives to hospital care; education and information to prevent the spread of the disease, especially for IV drug abusers, since there is considerable evidence that educational efforts aimed at homosexual males have been highly effective; and finally funds for further research to develop a vaccine or a cure for the disease.

LIMITATIONS OF THE ESTIMATES

It must be stressed that our estimates have a number of limitations:

1. *The CDC prevalence estimates.* Uncertainty about the future course of the AIDS epidemic makes forecasts extremely difficult, especially for later years such as 1991. Since the CDC constantly updates its estimates by using the latest information on the progress of the disease, the figures used in our estimates may be superseded in a relatively short time.

2. *Our assumption (suggested by Dr. Morgan of the CDC) that the distribution of AIDS cases between diagnostic groups stays the same as in 1984.* This premise is probably unrealistic. According to Dr. Morgan, it is possible that in 1991, only 10% of all cases, as against almost 20% in 1984, may suffer from Kaposi's sarcoma. Because patients with Kaposi's sarcoma are less expensive to treat than those with *Pneumocystis carinii* pneumonia and other infectious diseases, we have estimated that this would raise direct personal medical care costs by between 4% and 5%.

3. *Our assumption that the average number of months of life in 1984 of AIDS patients who died and of those newly diagnosed and alive at the end of the year was the same for all U.S. patients as for the SFGH patients and that these averages stay the same over time.* Given mortality rates of AIDS cases and the increase in the incidence of AIDS in recent years, our figures seem reasonable for 1985 and 1986 (i.e., about 6 months of expenses for those who died and not quite 5 months for those newly diagnosed who were alive at the end of the year), but they can change, and are likely to change, over time.

4. *Our assumption that medical treatment of AIDS patients remains unchanged.* This assumption is clearly unrealistic. We know that, in the course of the epidemic to date, changes in treatment have already occurred. There is considerable evidence that the average length of hospital stay has declined. For example, in San Francisco Bay Area hospitals, it has declined from 18.2 days in 1982 to 12.3 days in 1984. At M. D. Anderson Medical Center in Houston, the average hospital stay is reported to have gone from 30 days in the early days of the epidemic to 15 days in early 1986. There is also anecdotal evidence that the use of intensive care units for AIDS patients has declined, mainly because it was found that in many cases treatment in an ICU prolonged dying rather than living. Another example is the current practice at SFGH to administer most blood transfusions to severely anemic AIDS patients on an outpatient rather than an inpatient basis, as had been the custom in the earlier years of the epidemic. The effect on medical care costs of a new drug such as the recently introduced AZT is still unclear and may raise or lower costs of treatment. There is little question that further changes will occur in the next few years. Numerous drugs are currently being tested in the laboratory, and others will most likely be developed. Last but not least, if an effective cure or a vaccine is found, the entire cost situation—direct and indirect costs—will change completely.

5. *Our assumptions underlying the estimates of direct nonpersonal costs.* Expenditures for research in 1991 are uncertain; they will depend on progress in research to treat AIDS patients and to develop a vaccine. Other nonpersonal direct costs of AIDS, especially health education, information, and support services, depend on the future community response to the AIDS epidemic.

6. *Our assumption that wage patterns by age and sex remain the same over time.* This too is an unrealistic assumption, considering the changes the American economy has been undergoing, from a manufacturing to a service economy, and the growing number of women in the labor force.

These limitations of our estimates make clear the need for continued and more comprehensive collections of data, especially data on the use and costs of medical services by persons with AIDS. As the epidemic spreads, data will be needed for areas outside the metropolitan centers where it has been concentrated so far. Similarly, as the percentage of persons with AIDS who are IV drug users or sexual partners of IV drug users increases, more use and cost data will be needed for this particular risk group. Changes in treatment methods must also be watched closely, especially as new drugs are being introduced whose effects on the use and costs of medical services are not at all clear at this time. Yet such data are essential if adequate plans are to be made for meeting the medical needs of persons with AIDS and for exploring possible more cost-effective ways of providing care.

REFERENCES

1. Hardy, A.M., et al.: The economic impact of the first 10,000 cases of acquired immuno-deficiency syndrome in the United States. *JAMA* 255:209–215, 1986.

2. Kizer, K., Rodrigues, J., McHolland, G.F., and Weller, W.: *A Quantitative Analysis of AIDS in California.* California Department of Health Services, Sacramento, March 1986.

3. Scitovsky, A.A., Rice, D.P., Showstack, J., and Lee, P.R.: Estimating the direct and indirect economic costs of acquired immune deficiency syndrome, 1985, 1986 and 1990. Final report prepared for the Centers for Disease Control, Task Order 282-85-0061 #2, March 31, 1986. (Unpublished report available on request.)

4. Coolfont Report: A PHS plan for prevention and control of AIDS and the AIDS virus. *Public Health Rep* 101:341–348, 1986.

5. Morgan, W.M., and Curran, J.W.: Acquired immunodeficiency syndrome: Current and future trends. *Public Health Rep* 101:459–465, 1986.

6. Arno, P.S.: The nonprofit sector's response to the AIDS epidemic: Community-based services in San Francisco. *Am J Public Health* 76:1325–1330, 1986.

7. Scitovsky, A.A., Cline, M., and Lee, P.R.: Medical care costs of AIDS patients in San Francisco, *JAMA* 256:3103–3106, 1986.

8. Rice, D.P.: Estimating the cost of illness. DHEW Publication No. (PHS) 947-6. U.S. Government Printing Office, Washington, DC, 1966.

9. Cooper, B., and Rice, D.P.: The economic cost of illness revisited. *Social Security Bull* 39:21–36, 1976.

10. Rice, D.P., Hodgson, T.A., and Hopstein, A.: The economic cost of illness. A replication and update. *Health Care Finc Rev* 7:61–80, 1985.

11. Eggers, P.W.: Trends in Medicare reimbursements for end-stage renal disease: 1974–1979. *Health Care Finc Rev* 6:31–38, 1984.

43

AIDS in the Black Community: The Plague, the Politics, the People

Calu Lester and Larry Saxxon

THE PLAGUE

Black and brown people are quickly being acknowledged for their position in the ranks of those people affected by the acquired immune deficiency syndrome (AIDS) epidemic. Although white gay men have been the focus of the AIDS epidemic, the number of nonwhite people affected is growing at a dangerously high rate.

In *Existentialism, A Theory of Man* by Ralph Harper, the author notes, "The temptation to exhaust reality by universalizing it has been passed through successive inversions of intellectualism down to present popular varieties of cynicism and disrepute, basic insights belong to the individual only and not to the culture, and thinking men find it necessary to clothe even their own ideas in the style of the acceptable past."[1] Here lies the most recent approach to the AIDS epidemic currently raging around the world and striking hardest in the communities of color.

Poverty, ignorance, indifference, and a buy-in to the myth that AIDS is a disease of white gay men have contributed to this situation. According to the Centers for Disease Control (CDC) in Atlanta, between June 1, 1981, and September 8, 1986, a total of 24,576 cases of AIDS were documented.[2] Of this number, 8412 (40%) are black and Hispanic people (25% and 14%), respectively. Also, 80% of women with AIDS are black or brown.[3] Of all children with HIV infection, 80% are black or Hispanic. (*Note*: This figure includes 21,010 persons 13 years and above and 292 children aged 0–12 years.) It has been estimated that 73.1% of the babies diagnosed with AIDS, most of whom are black, have at least one intravenous drug-using parent. Indications are that the IV drug epidemic in the black community has not been lessened but has increased dramatically, and the implications are startling.

Most nonwhite people admit that there is a drug abuse problem in their communities. That AIDS is a blood-borne disease and that substance abuse and needle usage are significant for the transmission of AIDS provides opportunity for the virus to expand rapidly within these particular communities.

The myth that AIDS is a "white gay male disease" has made its way into the black communities and has contributed to a lack of understanding about the disease. This misinformation has delayed the asking of important questions that would provide answers to how the virus affects their lives. This tragedy affects not only those at risk but nonwhite communities in general.

A paucity of effective prevention and education programs within the communities of black and brown people has allowed a virtual time bomb to slowly but steadily tick away. Despite this astounding data, there are, to date, no massive government-sponsored AIDS education and prevention programs in nonwhite communities.

Safe sex practices and information have not been addressed sufficiently as part of prevention in the spread of the AIDS virus in black and brown communities. This leaves an avenue open for the spread of disease.

That nonwhite communities appear to be 2 or 3 years behind in basic AIDS prevention and education is an obstacle to reducing HIV infection in general. As long as this remains the case, the virus will continue to spread.

Going beyond the seropositive stages to what actually happens in many cases with the full-blown AIDS diagnosis, the disease takes a different route within the minority communities. One major difference is survival rates among blacks with AIDS. The average life span following diagnosis is approximately 6 months compared with 18–24 months for Caucasians with AIDS. According to Walter R. Dowdle, AIDS Coordinator for the U.S. Public Health Service, "This phenomenon may be due to the tendency of blacks to postpone medical services until very late in the course of the illness due to economic difficulties."[4] Quality medical attention is an expensive commodity in the United States today, and blacks who exist on the lower rungs of the economic ladder are unable to obtain access to such care. The health care that is available may not be culturally responsive to the needs of blacks.

An important reason why the distribution of infection is vastly out of proportion to the black and Hispanic numbers in the general population is because education and referral agencies have directed their efforts almost exclusively toward the white male gay and bisexual population. This situation is especially problematic for poor women and children.

POLITICS

The proportion of AIDS cases in the black and Hispanic communities is significantly higher than might be expected given their distribution in the U.S. population. Black and Hispanic persons appear in all high-risk behavior categories, which places them at increased risk for developing AIDS. Risk groups include homosexual/bisexual males with and without histories of intravenous drug abuse, heterosexual intravenous drug abusers, heterosexual contacts of persons with AIDS or at increased risk for AIDS, persons with hemophilia and other blood coagulation disorders, recipients of blood or blood products transfusions, and persons with "no known risk."

It is time to discuss the AIDS crisis in ways that will provide and encourage a wider understanding of its impact on *all* Third World communities as well as its devastating repercussions for these communities. The curtain has fallen, setting the backdrop for the second wave of the AIDS epidemic, and its primary target will be people of color. Until recently, nonwhite community leaders have taken a hands-off position, believing that this was solely an issue for white gay men. Yet there are 150 black and brown babies in New York hospitals dying of AIDS; most of these have parents who were simply not aware of the impending danger to their children while using intravenous drugs. Youths in the communities of color are at increased risk for exposure to the virus because many are still using IV drugs and participating in high-risk sexual behavior. Existing AIDS service-providing agencies are not adequately reaching or serving them. Additionally, many youths cannot read or understand the material regarding AIDS prevention.

Gay men of color constitute a significant portion of the total gay population and fall into multiple risk factor categories. As nonwhite gay men, they did not share in the wealth of information that has influenced change in the white gay community. Many gay men of color are isolated in the impoverished inner city and have not been exposed to the basics about how to keep from being exposed to and/or spread the virus. Also, many in this group are the victims of ignorance, denial, and/or drug abuse and rejection by black and brown leaders. This homophobic reaction by black and brown leaders further alienates and isolates those persons of color at risk as well as those already infected with the virus.

This of all times tends to be the moment when racism rears its ugly head, preventing normally eligible citizens from reaping the benefits of much-needed access to support systems that are already established for and often by the gay white male. Scores of clients of color arrive at community-based organizations providing AIDS-related services with virtually no knowledge of the mysterious disease that is literally draining the life from them. They know almost nothing about what is happening within their bodies, because the attending professionals in medical institutions don't bother to assess whether the patient understands standard English. During times of great stress, many patients tend to revert to their native tongues whether that be black vernacular or Spanish or patois.

"Inclusion" and "advocacy" are two key words regarding people of color and AIDS. People of color were not included at the outset of the assessment of groups at risk for AIDS, so they have not been among the initial recipients of the vast amount of information and education available.

Among those who have received excellent hospital, hospice, and grief and bereavement services, the numbers of persons of color with AIDS have been small and for the most part, invisible. The vast majority have died alone without benefit of family (who were usually the last to know and who could only plan and participate in the postmortem activities). This lack of inclusion and dissemination of relevant information has had an impact on mothers and infants as well. There are hospital wards where black and brown babies are dying alone, without stimulation, benefit of loving parents, or discharge plans that would assure that their short lives would at least have some degree of happiness and enjoyment.

Advocate support services have played an exceptional role with gay men confronted with this disease. Volunteers, both men and women, have made a difference in the lives of gay and bisexual men with AIDS through their tireless services and commitment through agencies such as the Shanti Project in San Francisco, the San Francisco AIDS Foundation, New York's Gay Men's Health Crisis, and AIDS Project Los Angeles. Unfortunately, traditional service and advocate groups such as the NAACP, the National Black Social Workers Association, and the Urban League have been reluctant at best to comment and take action on the issue of AIDS. The role of these groups is vital to the education and prevention effort within the nonwhite communities, because they have the established network to educate about the critical issues threatening the existence of black and Hispanic culture. If this text does not provide the motivation to get the leadership of the black and brown communities to respond to this call for action, we challenge them to take one hour of their busy day to visit a pediatric AIDS ward in New York City, Newark, NJ, Miami, or Washington and look into the faces of those helpless brown and black babies who had no choice about being caught in such a horrible situation and say to *them* that they have "no comment."

> The disproportionate number of minorities who are diagnosed with AIDS is inversely proportional to the number of people of color who are involved in the AIDS education and service effort. The AIDS service and education industry's efforts to reach out to minority members of the gay community and to minorities in general have been hampered by a failure to appreciate the unique problems associated with communicating with these individuals.
> Who is at fault here? AIDS service providers for not adequately responding to the peculiar needs of persons of color, or minority communities and their leaders for not spearheading more effective education efforts? Undoubtedly, it's a little of both.
> Whoever is to blame, the fact remains that hundreds of thousands of minority citizens are in grave danger of ignoring or misunderstanding the realities of the AIDS epidemic. As our teachers once told us, the numbers don't lie.[5]

One of the authors became aware of this serious health issue as director of a homeless shelter where he observed attitudes toward health delivery systems among poor and homeless people. As a psychiatric social worker in an AIDS clinic observed, specific problems, such as those described below, become more clear, and the urgent need to address these problems becomes more obvious.

The case of Clotelle, a black woman with AIDS and the mother of 16-month-old Rayvette, who also has the disease, illustrates one of the problems facing mothers and children with AIDS. Clotelle died a year ago in a shelter for homeless people, lying on a cot next to her two older children, ages 7 and 8. Her main worry beyond the pain of fevers and diarrhea was what would happen to her children. Clotelle died without knowing who would care for them. She and her children might have been spared much anguish had the social services system made provision for children whose parents are dying of AIDS.

Rayvette remains alone on a pediatric ward for children with AIDS. Although she receives medical attention for her chronic fevers and bouts with pneumonia and unusual rashes, she has no family member to hold and cuddle her or to provide love, emotional stimulation, or support. The hospital staff does what it can, but it is overworked and does not have the time to give that needed support. Some volunteer programs are trying to recruit older persons to meet this need.

Once a black or Hispanic person has AIDS, he or she can search in vain for culturally sensitive medical treatment or a support network. Hospitals routinely use English for informing Spanish-speaking patients that they have AIDS. Without a thorough understanding and/or awareness of their own affliction, these patients cannot pursue proper medical treatment, let alone process the anger and depression associated with discovery of a terminal illness. Many die in confusion without any understanding of the AIDS virus that has ravaged their immune systems or infected their partners.

The small number of people of color who are social workers, nurses, counselors, and doctors on AIDS wards make it difficult for patients to find a care giver with whom to identify, and medical personnel may have difficulty establishing the rapport necessary to learn a patient's medical, drug, and social history in order to provide proper treatment.

Bud, a 27-year-old black man with a 5-year drug habit, was losing weight for months and suffering unexplained fevers and rashes. His poverty, coupled with a feeling that white doctors treated him with condescension, made him postpone seeking help. He finally went to the emergency room of the county hospital when an AIDS-related lesion that had closed his rectum made it impossible for him to defecate. Although the doctor attending Bud immediately diagnosed him as having AIDS, he gave Bud no explanation. Bud sought help from an AIDS support agency and was accepted in one of the organization's shelter programs. However, the stress of being the only nongay man in the organization's care helped make Bud hostile. To protect the other people in the shelter home, the organization forced Bud to leave. Bud moved into a run-down hotel in the Tenderloin District of San Francisco. He died in his room alone 3 weeks later.

BLACK AND BROWN AIDS IN THE GLOBAL CONTEXT: THE SECOND WAVE

In June of 1986, the International AIDS Conference was held in Paris and attempted to provide a sense of the scope of the AIDS problem in Africa. The data implied that there may be large numbers of people who are seropositive and who have AIDS living in east, central, and west Africa. It is estimated that from 5% to more than 15% of the population in central and equatorial Africa are infected with the virus.[6] However, there were not enough consistent data to describe the epidemiological aspects of its spread because of a lack of diagnostic laboratories for testing and the reluctance of some governments in Africa to collect and report data on AIDS. For example, pediatric AIDS in Africa is confounded by other risk factors: namely, 75–80% of children in central and east Africa have malaria and other immunosuppressive infections. The acute poverty in Africa exacerbates the threat of the AIDS epidemic there. Poor nutrition may also contribute to lower immune system responses to the virus, making it more likely that exposure to the AIDS virus will result in the development of AIDS itself. In Africa, people's immune systems are also compromised by the large number of sexually transmitted diseases. Several studies have documented a high correlation between seropositivity for HTLV-III/LAV antibody and heterosexual promiscuity.[7]

Poverty also impedes the development of adequate health care delivery systems in many African countries. There are inadequate facilities for the sterilization of equipment and for the storage of blood for transfusions and an acute shortage of needles for inoculations. This latter problem has the alarming result of putting many people who depend on rural clinics for their vaccinations in the same risk category as IV drug users. Illiteracy and limited facilities for dissemination of information further complicate the tasks of AIDS education and prevention.

Poverty, malnutrition, and inadequate health and education services that form the backdrop to the AIDS epidemic in Africa are reproduced in the ghettos and pockets of poverty in U.S. urban centers, where an impoverished community of blacks and Hispanics are being infected by the AIDS virus in increasing numbers.

If the second wave of the AIDS epidemic is to be prevented from inundating black and Hispanic communities in the United States, a major national prevention program must be launched. Such a program would have to organize a pool of trainers—preferably people of color—who have a broad-based understanding of how AIDS affects black and Hispanic communities. Culturally and racially sensitive educational materials must be developed for people at risk as well as for service providers. New agencies must be established and old ones expanded so that people of color at risk for AIDS have access to the full range of services and information concerning prevention, treatment, and support. Such a program is dangerously overdue.

REFERENCES

1. Harper, R. *Existentialism, A Theory of Man.* Cambridge, MA: Harvard University Press, 1948, p. 6.
2. CDC. Update: Acquired immunodeficiency syndrome (AIDS)—United States. MMWR 1984;32:688–91.
3. CDC. Update: Acquired immunodeficiency syndrome (AIDS) among blacks and Hispanics— United States. MMWR 1986;35(42):655–6.
4. Dowdle, W.R., AIDS Coordinator for U.S. Public Health Service (personal communication).
5. Kawata, P. *NAN Monitor* 1986;1:9.
6. Chase, M. AIDS has spread 'almost everywhere' in Africa, Zaire doctor tells parley. *Wall Street Journal*, June 24, 1986.
7. Clumeck, N., Robert-Guroff, M., Van de Perre, P., Jennings, A., Sibomana, J., Demol, P., Cran, S., Gallo, R. C. Seroepidemiological studies of HTLV-III antibody prevalence among selected groups of heterosexual Africans. *JAMA* 1985;254:2599–602.

44

Impact of the AIDS Epidemic on the Gay Political Agenda

Jim Foster

Within the gay community the AIDS epidemic is pervasive. It is impossible to avoid it. You cannot go to any gay community meeting without hearing of yet another death or another friend's recent diagnosis.

Five years or ten years ago, no one would have believed that we would attend so many funerals. No one believed that we would worry over every skin blemish, every cough, every headache. No one believed that the simple phrase, "How ya doing" would take on a new and much deeper meaning or that so many of us would be devoting our spare hours to caring for those unfortunate enough to be stricken with the disease.

Five years ago life was wonderful. Life was full of gay bars and bathhouses. Life was a disco party full of beautiful men, all of whom seemed available, if not tonight then tomorrow. Life was psychedelics and other recreational drugs and everyone believed in Peter Pan: I'll never get old. I'll never get sick. I'll never die. The party will last forever.

No matter where you went—San Francisco, New York, Los Angeles, Houston—the party was in full swing and not just in the cities that were known as "gay meccas," but in Atlanta, Philadelphia, Boston, Chicago, Phoenix, Denver, Charleston, Seattle. You could even find a party in Reno, Lubbock, Sioux Falls, or Dubuque, if you knew where to go or whom to ask.

After all, why shouldn't there be a party? Hadn't the sexual revolution of the sixties and seventies freed everyone from the old constraints? In fact, it was healthy to throw your inhibitions away and experiment with new expressions and new people—lots of new expressions and lots of new people. There were, of course, a few bothersome matters that needed to be dealt with, such as Anita Bryant's campaign in Florida to overturn the gay rights ordinance and the Briggs Initiative in California, which would have prohibited gay people from teaching in the schools. The fundamentalists were organizing and using the burgeoning gay rights movement as a focal point; Ronald Reagan's election to the presidency indicated an end to political gains being made at the federal level. Some of us had heard about a strange form of cancer and an unusual pneumonia that seemed to affect only gay men, but no one we knew had it. These were no more than sprinkles on the parade.

Larry Bush, a gay journalist and legislative aide suggests that the role model for gay people prior to the epidemic was the medieval troubadour. An itinerant artist in "glad rags" of lace and codpiece, spontaneous, full of life, and unfettered by convention. The troubadour represented a spirit of individuality and lived in a free zone outside everyday life. His was an individual, not a collective mind-set. There was nothing of yesterday about him. He was not a part of the continuum of history. Indeed, history began the day he was born and each day he was born anew. His was not a case of "Today is the first day of the rest of your life." Today was the only day of his life. Although the troubadour might recognize fellow gay travelers on the road, he recognized them with a wink and a nod as kindred spirits. He was out there doing his own thing and expected everyone else to be doing theirs.

The dynamic of the gay rights political movement reflected the troubadour as a role model, both in its activity and philosophy. The dynamic, simply stated, was: get government off our backs and let us be ourselves.

The decade of the seventies created dramatic improvements in the lives of gay people whether they were self-acknowledged or not. The Stonewall Riot of 1969 changed our lives forever. Gay people had challenged the ability of the police (as guardians of the public morality) to regulate our existence, and what's more, gay people had won. From that moment on, arrests for being gay or being seen in a gay establishment would be fought in court. There was renewed interest in challenging state laws that regulated consensual sexual behavior and in California and several other states those laws were overturned. Cities across the country passed nondiscrimination ordinances. Gay business people successfully challenged city codes and ordinances that had been used in the past to deny them opportunity. Gay people ran for public office and sometimes won. Other gay people were appointed to positions on city commissions and boards. New organizations of gay people sprang up like mushrooms after a rain and although some of them were formed for specific political purposes, such as the Alice B. Toklas Memorial Democratic Club, many more were formed around specific, mutual interests. Groups of lawyers, doctors, insurance agents, social workers, baseball players, bowlers, stamp collectors, Mormons, and Roman Catholics were organized.

In San Francisco, Jon Sims noticed that a Gay Freedom Day Parade had no music. He put up hand-lettered posters on telephone poles in the Castro, Polk, and Folsom Street areas of San Francisco asking people who had experience in marching bands to call him. Within a week he had over 800 phone calls and out of these responses he formed the San Francisco Gay Freedom Day Marching Band, Tap Troupe, and Twirling Corps. Soon there were marching bands in a dozen other cities. The bands were quickly followed by choruses of lesbians and gay men. In short, gay people were discovering themselves and each other and the more discovery that took place, the larger and more diverse the organizations became. Self-help groups were formed to assist gay alcoholics and drug abusers. The Metropolitan Community Church, a Christian body with a special outreach to gay people, became international. The general media began treating gay issues seriously and gay media developed in nearly every major city in America. In San Francisco a group of lesbians in business formed a professional organization that now numbers over 1000 members. Medical clinics were created and staffed by gay medical professionals for gay men and women. Parades to celebrate the victory at Stonewall were held annually in major cities across America. The San Francisco parade attracts a quarter of a million people.

All of this activity had the effect of creating the beginnings of a sense of social community; in addition it brought gay people together as gay people within the larger community. It wasn't possible for a gay politician, for instance, to function alone. He or she had to interact with politicians as a group. A gay lawyer had to interact with the rest of the legal profession and a gay doctor had to deal with the California Medical Association or the American Medical Association. In those places where gay people had organized there was an increasing amount of interaction with other communities. This, in turn, led to putting a human face on homosexuality. Friendships and respect developed, myths and stereotypes were destroyed.

If I were asked the day the party stopped for me, I would have to respond that it was the day that Larry Kramer's open letter to the gay community appeared in *The New York Native* and was later reprinted in many gay newspapers across the country. I suspect it was the day the party stopped for a lot of others as well.

Kramer, who later wrote *The Normal Heart*, one of the first plays to deal with AIDS and the political and social implications of the epidemic, wrote a scathing denunciation of the gay community's denial of a growing epidemic and the indifference of not only the media and the political establishment, but of gay leaders themselves to what was clearly the most dangerous situation we had ever faced. The letter, entitled "1,112 and Counting,"[1] referred to the number of AIDS cases and deaths at that time. Kramer's letter was a clarion call to action and a prophesy of the future. His letter and the production of *The Normal Heart* became the manifesto of a new, gay political dynamic. In the process, a new role model was created—the historical Jew of the holocaust. I do not use the term "holocaust" to mean the specific, historic event that took place in Western Europe in the 1930s and 1940s. I mean it to encompass the Jewish experience.

The new role model is diametrically opposed to the old. If the troubadour sees himself as fundamentally individualistic, the Jew sees himself as part of the collective. He is a link in a chain from the past, which runs through him to the future. He only survives if the community survives. If any part of the organism survives, they all survive. The historical Jew of the holocaust believes that Christian tolerance has before and will again turn against him. The only way to survive in a seemingly hostile world is by adopting the ultimate defensive posture—investing in each other.

In 1982 the Gay Men's Health Crisis published a declaration for survival in *The New York Native*.[2] The advertisement bluntly stated that a crisis existed in the health of gay men and no one would help us except ourselves. We could expect nothing but indifference from the media, the political establishment, and the medical profession. Even the institutions developed in our own community were not prepared or equipped to deal with AIDS. We could expect nothing for education, or research, or the care and treatment of those already afflicted. Therefore, we needed to create a new structure and a new ethic. This was to be our one and only task. The declaration was in effect both an appeal for survival and the method by which it was to be achieved. Apolitical gay people must come together to defend themselves. We must invest in each other because there was no one but ourselves who would do this for us.

In a scene from *The Normal Heart*, Dr. Emma Brookner says to Ned Weeks, a thinly disguised Larry Kramer,

Health is a political issue. Everyone's entitled to good medical care. If you're not getting it, you've got to fight for it. Do you know that this is the only country in the industrialized world besides South Africa that doesn't guarantee health care for everyone? One of my staff told me that you were well known in the gay world and not afraid to say what you think. Is that true? I can't find any gay leaders. I tried calling several gay organizations. No one ever calls me back. Is anyone out there?"

To which Ned Weeks responds,

There aren't any organizations strong enough to be useful, no. Dr. Brookner, no one with a brain gets involved in gay politics. It's filled with the great unwashed radicals of any counterculture. That's why there aren't any leaders the majority will follow.[3]

The pre-epidemic troubadour was able to avoid involvement in the political agenda of the gay rights movement if he so chose—and many did choose non-involvement. In fact, it is safe to say that the vast majority of gay people had either a peripheral interest in or completely ignored the political agenda. For instance, during the Dade County, Florida, campaign to overturn the local gay rights ordinance, many gay people voted against the ordinance, which would have granted them some measure of protection. They felt that the people pressing the issue were "rocking the boat." They agreed with the worst arguments of Anita Bryant that somehow or other the ordinance would allow men in dresses to teach in the public schools. They were resentful that the little secret of their homosexuality might be exposed if there was too much political freedom before there was sufficient social acceptance. Differences of opinion existed about exactly how much freedom was desirable. Many felt that extending rights to those who wore drag or leather was going too far and were uncomfortable being grouped with what the media, in its search for the most extreme and bizarre examples of behavior, characterized as "gay."

Most homosexuals in America today are hidden or "closeted" and until the epidemic, most were able to succeed in their double life. Many are married with families and live in the suburbs of America. Their only communication with the organized gay community is an occasional night out at a bathhouse or a drink at a gay bar after work. According to a recent and unpublished study, 80% of wives of bisexual men in their sample were ignorant of their husband's gay activity.

Much of this bears some resemblance to the experience of the immigrant Jew in this country. There was, for instance, much discrimination among the various groups of Jews themselves. French and German Jews were embarrassed by what they viewed as the excesses of Hasidic Jews from Poland and Russia. Wealthy and middle-class Jews looked askance at the poverty of the Lower East Side in New York and did not wish to be identified with it. Many submerged themselves in the new culture, denied their heritage, and changed their names and religion. Like the early gay rights organizations, Jewish institutions fought to convince Jews to take pride in being Jewish. They ought not hide, change their names, or their religion.

That their efforts were successful is proven by the phenomenal strength of Jewish benevolent institutions and their political ability to protect the state of

Israel as the symbol of their community. The Holocaust in Western Europe during the 1930s and 1940s brought the Jewish people back to the perspective of the historical holocaust and the investment in each other as the ultimate defensive posture. Just as Hitler's S.S. and Gestapo did not differentiate among Jews, the HIV virus does not differentiate among gay men. The S.S. did not care whether you were a French Jew or a Polish Jew. They did not care whether you were a rich merchant or a poor peasant nor did they care if you were an Orthodox, Conservative, or Reform Jew. Indeed, they did not care whether you were a practicing Jew or a Lutheran or Roman Catholic convert.

The HIV virus doesn't discriminate either. It doesn't care whether you wear drag or leather or a three-piece suit. It doesn't care whether you are a famous actor or entertainer or a bartender or department store clerk. It doesn't care whether you live in a gay ghetto or with your wife and family in the suburbs. In short, gay men cannot hide anymore than could the Jews of Europe. They are no longer protected by their wealth, position, or their anonymity. This is having a profound effect on the evolving gay political agenda.

In addition to the growing awareness that the existing gay institutions are not equipped to seek the resources necessary to fund the needs of AIDS patients, a debate has developed over what many gay political activists see as the very basis of the gay political movement—a permissive view of sexual behavior, both in and out of relationships.

Dennis Altman, in his book *AIDS in the Mind of America*, wrote,[4] "The growth of gay assertion and a commercial gay world meant an affirmation of sex outside of relationships as a positive good, a means of expressing both sensuality and community." Altman goes on to say, "I do not think it is too fanciful to see in our preoccupation with public sex both an affirmation of sexuality and a yearning for community, which may be one of the ways we can devise for coming to terms with a violent and severely disturbed society."

By 1982 the need for gay men to significantly change their sexual behavior was being forcefully debated in the gay press. Altman admitted that his former views had caused him some embarrassment as it became clear that the virus was sexually transmitted and that certain sexual acts commonly practiced by gay men carried the greatest risk of transmission.

In an article in *The New York Native* entitled, "Sexual Manners," Neil A. Marks wrote, "The one connection that has made us the unique community that we are leads to the one attack that we all respond to: the attack against life itself."[5]

Later in 1982, Michael Callen and Richard Berkowitz wrote an article for *The New York Native* entitled, "We Know Who We Are." They said, "Disease has changed the definition of promiscuity. What ten years ago was viewed as a healthy reaction to a sex negative culture now threatens to destroy the very fabric of urban gay male life. What we have in the 1980s is a positive political force tied to a dangerous lifestyle. We must recognize the self-hating shortsightedness involved in knowingly or half knowingly infecting our sexual partners with disease, only to have that disease returned to us in exponential form."[6]

Clearly, a major shift was occurring. The debate in the gay press was followed by debates in several cities over the closing of bathhouses and other commercial establishments where sex occurred. These debates pitted gay political activists who for a variety of reasons sincerely believed it was necessary to close down establishments that encouraged multiple, anonymous, high-risk sexual encounters, against other gay political activists who just as sincerely believed that closing the bathhouses constituted a grave violation of civil liberties that could ultimately lead to complete reversals of all the small gains we had won.

Another change was taking place among many leaders of the gay political movement. They were leaving their positions in the old institutions and moving into positions in government and the larger community where they felt they could make a greater contribution to the growing demands of the epidemic. Virginia Apuzzo left as Executive Director of the National Lesbian and Gay Task Force and joined the staff of Governor Mario Cuomo of New York. Larry Bush, a noted gay journalist, joined the staff of Assemblyman Art Agnos of California where he is able to influence state legislation on AIDS. Bill Bogan, a former president of the Gertrude Stein Democratic Club of Washington, D.C., is now a Commissioner of D.C. General Hospital and Vice President of COSMO, a Hispanic health organization. Many others have taken positions with local AIDS organizations where their contacts and political skills have been useful to the fledgling institutions.

Much has been written about the model program for AIDS management in San Francisco and how that came about because of the political clout of the gay community. There is no question that many politicians feel that the gay vote in San Francisco is an important vote and they are careful not to offend a large block of voters, but that isn't the entire story.

The Mayor of San Francisco and most of the Board of Supervisors have very close friends and advisers who are gay. For them, the AIDS epidemic is not something that only affects a minority of people in their city. AIDS is killing their friends. Assemblyman Art Agnos, who represents that portion of San Francisco that includes the Castro district and has the highest number of gay residents in the city, has been the leading legislator in the state capitol for gay rights and AIDS. Agnos is married and the father of two children. He has lost several of his closest friends to the epidemic. His commitment to these issues makes good political sense, but the loss of good friends gives him personal reasons as well for involvement. The mayor and members of the Board of Supervisors also are frequently seen at funerals of people who have died of AIDS or visiting those who are still alive at home or in the hospital. What is remarkable is that 15 or 20 years ago that would not have happened, even in San Francisco. Politicians would not have admitted that they knew any openly gay people and there would not have been any open gay people advising politicians. Indeed, in many parts of the country this is still the case.

In those cities across America where one can find a flourishing gay social life, there has been a discernible decrease in social activity. It would be a mistake, however, to assume that the decrease in social activity indicates a setback in the gay political agenda.

Rick Pacurar, president of the Harvey Milk Democratic Club in San Francisco, sees fewer people attending general meetings, but more people volunteering for specific tasks. Pacurar says there are more and more people saying, "give me something to do." He observes, "We appear to be more united politically than ever before and the AIDS epidemic has strengthened our resolve."

Gay people may have decreased their attendance at bars and bathhouses, but they certainly have not stopped volunteering for work at the various AIDS organizations across the country. They constitute the vast majority of the people who are performing patient services and educating the public about the disease. This is as true in Boston and Atlanta as it is in New York and San Francisco. AIDS organizations such as the Shanti Project and Coming Home Hospice in San Francisco, the Health Crisis Network in Miami, AID/Atlanta to name a very few, were created, staffed, and funded by gay people. Five years later, most of them are still staffed and funded by gay people.

The Gay Men's Health Crisis (GMHC) in New York City has become the largest and wealthiest organization in the country with the word "gay" in its name. GMHC provides education and other services for persons with AIDS in New York. Ironically, although it was founded by Larry Kramer and others to lobby for a political agenda among other things, Kramer has written a scathing denunciation of current GMHC priorities and lack of political action. Kramer accuses the GMHC board of hiding behind their 501(c)(3) tax exemption status as a reason for not engaging both the local and federal governments. In another call to action he writes, "Get off your self-satisfied asses and fight! That's what you were put there for. You continue to deny the political realities of this epidemic. There is nothing in this whole AIDS mess that is not political."

Later in the same letter he returns to the theme of the new role model. "There is no one to do anything, but ourselves. If the Board of GMHC have been cowardly, we have allowed it to become so. If GMHC is on the wrong course, we have allowed it to drift. If Reagan has not uttered the word "AIDS," we have abetted this." He then goes on to link the new role model to a political agenda. "GMHC cannot hope to provide patient services for the dying at the rate they are dying, or preventive education for the potentially infected at the rate they are becoming infected. The only way to force the system to provide these services across the board is by political pressure.

"Our only salvation lies in aggressive scientific research. This will come only from political pressure. Every dime for research that we've had has come from hard political fighting.

"Thus all our solutions can only be achieved through political action. All the kindness in the world will not stem this epidemic. Only political action can change the course of events."[7]

Kramer's second "Call to Arms" will not fall on deaf ears. Across the country, most AIDS organizations are dominated by gay people and their leadership in the epidemic will continue for at least another five or ten years. There is a growing recognition that the epidemic is political. Indeed, there has never been a more political epidemic in the history of this country. The organizations realize that they must develop a more aggressive and sophisticated political structure in order to achieve a partnership with government.

The change taking place between pre- and post-epidemic gay role models is not one that can occur overnight. Indeed, what we are seeing now is the gradual evolution of change. The sort of political activity necessary for success in the face of the epidemic represents a complete reversal from previous political activity. In those pre-epidemic days the major theme of political action was to get government off our backs. Today, the theme is to make government a partner in solving the research, education, and care and treatment issues raised by the epidemic. Yesterday, the movement needed people who could organize marches, rallies, and voter registration drives. Today, in addition to those people, we need grant writers, cost study analysts, and skilled lobbyists who can convince legislators and administrators that it is in the best interests of the country, state, or federal governments to form partnerships with us to find the resources necessary to save lives.

Although there are some areas of the country where this change in theme has occurred—San Francisco comes immediately to mind—most areas have yet to develop the necessary skills to address a new political agenda and strategy. It should be noted also that most other parts of the country have not made as many resources available to their AIDS organizations as is the case in San Francisco.

It is impossible, however, to observe the work done by these AIDS organizations without developing a profound respect for their commitment, dedication, and sacrifice. Often they achieve minor and major miracles in home support services, housing programs, and community education with little or no support from local governmental bodies. Small volunteer groups are coping far beyond their means with death and dying and are hanging by their financial fingernails while doing so. Housing programs for people with AIDS who have lost all their financial resources are minimal, if they exist at all. Local health departments, themselves struggling with reduced funding, throw a little money at some volunteer agency and expect them to educate the entire city or county.

Drastically needed cost analysis studies and strategic planning that could help in the development of government priorities are not being developed in most sections of the country. Small, poorly funded volunteer organizations, composed primarily of gay people, are valiantly attempting to deal with the most severe health crisis this nation has ever seen. Is it any wonder, then, that until they can get some help from their state and local governments there will be no resources available to put into the kind of massive political efforts called for by the new agenda? These groups feel caught in a classic "catch 22" situation. The demands on their time and abilities continue to grow as the epidemic grows, and the daily demands of the epidemic leave no time or resources to deal effectively with the newly emerging political realities. The resources that are needed to hire effective lobbyists, or conduct cost studies, or do strategic planning are more desperately needed to provide the day-to-day needs of AIDS patients.

This situation cannot, of course, go on. Even as this chapter is being written there is considerable movement at the federal level that indicates preparations are being made to assume responsibility for many aspects of the epidemic, which small, local, volunteer agencies have been handling. Since becoming chairman of the Labor and Human Resources Committee of the U.S. Senate, Senator Edward Kennedy has strongly indicated that he intends to make AIDS a major priority. Congresspersons Henry Waxman, Ted Weiss, Barbara Boxer, Ed Roybal, and William S. Natcher (to name just a few) have consistently moved an AIDS agenda in the U.S. House of Representatives. The introduction of the Bowen Bill and the amendments made to it will greatly increase our ability to deal with the care and treatment issues of people with AIDS. It seems likely that there will be tremendous pressure in the 100th Congress to overcome the inertia of the Reagan administration and add much greater funding than the administration has been willing to spend thus far. Significantly, more funds will be made available for education and for care and treatment, the two areas most seriously underfinanced in the past and in which volunteer groups have attempted to fill the gaps. As the epidemic grows, state and local governments will also need to spend more money on education and care and treatment.

During the last California election, I asked a friend of mine, a prominent gay Republican, if he intended to vote for George Deukmajian's reelection. He told me that although he did not want to be quoted by name, he felt very certain that no gay Republican would vote for Deukmajian because of the governor's atrocious record on AIDS funding. He went on to say that although Deukmajian, who is widely believed to have national aspirations, would easily win reelection in California, his sorry record on AIDS funding would hurt him badly among gay Republicans in a national contest.

Certainly the growing numbers of people with AIDS have had an enormous impact on government, but so too have the efforts made by those who have attempted to implement the new gay political agenda. It is no accident that those in public office on the federal level mentioned previously have been the leaders in the effort to secure AIDS funding. They are also representatives that gay people know well and with whom gays have long, established relationships. There is another group that has been quietly working behind the scenes to ensure a new governmental partnership: gay people who work as congressional aides. To date, they are the ones who have done the most effective lobbying, who have prepared the cost studies, who have worked up the budget figures, and who have fought hard and tenaciously for adequate funding.

The epidemic has created strong allies for gay people in the parents, friends, and loved ones of those who have died and are dying of this disease. While this alliance is being forged at a terrible cost, it nevertheless is taking place. Just as it is impossible to observe our institutional response to the epidemic without developing a tremendous respect, so too it is not possible to observe the courage of people with AIDS and their friends and lovers who are caring for them without developing a great respect. This is having a profound impact on parents and relatives who frequently had no previous knowledge of or relationship with gay people. The respect has frequently grown into love and support. I strongly suspect that for every horror story one hears about parents disowning their gay children, there are ten stories of healing and reconciliation.

It would appear that the epidemic has changed the gay political agenda but has not weakened nor destroyed the determination of gay people to seek a guarantee for their place in American life. We have been forced to examine fundamental issues about the nature of being gay and have realized that being gay is as much a sense of identity and connection to other people as it is an expression of our sexuality. Out of this realization is growing a powerful sense of community and a powerful new direction for the gay political agenda.

NOTES

1. Kramer, Larry. "1,112 and Counting." *The New York Native*, March 14, 1983.
2. *The New York Native*, 1982.
3. Kramer, Larry. *The Normal Heart*. New York: New American Library, 1985.
4. Altman, Dennis. *AIDS in the Mind of America*. New York: Anchor Press/Doubleday, 1986.
5. Ibid.
6. Ibid.
7. Kramer, Larry. "Dear Richard." *The New York Native*, January 26, 1987.

X

THE MEDIA AND AIDS

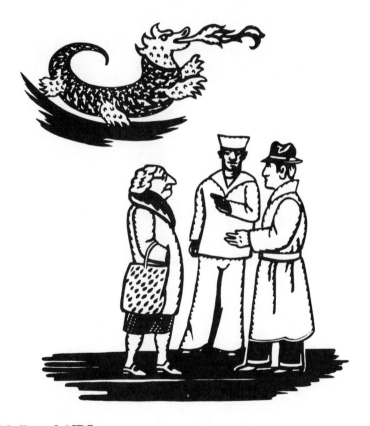

The Media and AIDS
The AIDS dragon snorts fire in the background while a housewife, sailor, and businessman discuss their fears.

45

Public Health, the Press, and AIDS:

An Analysis of Newspaper Articles in London and San Francisco

Lydia Temoshok, Margaret Grade, and Jane Zich

Acquired immune deficiency syndrome (AIDS) is an infectious disease of epidemic proportions. Although numerous treatments are being researched, as yet there is neither a cure nor a vaccine against this frequently fatal disease. Consequently, prevention efforts are of paramount importance. Perhaps the major prevention vehicle is health education aimed at informing the public not only about population risk factors but also about specific behaviors that do or do not modify an individual's risk for contracting AIDS. Studies that document the specific health education needs of various risk groups are essential to develop maximally effective public health education campaigns.

A number of recent publications have examined the current state of behavior change, prevention efforts, and the role of health educators in confronting the AIDS epidemic. These reports have dealt primarily with groups at risk for AIDS—i.e., gay men,[1-3] intravenous drug abusers,[4,5] seropositive blood donors[6]—or minority high-risk individuals. There are only a few studies of knowledge or attitudes about AIDS in groups potentially at risk for AIDS in the near future.[8,9] To our knowledge, there are only two journal articles that have dealt with the general public's knowledge and attitudes about AIDS.[10,11] Public polls reported by the new media appear to be a more fertile source than academic publications for information about the general public's knowledge, concerns, and opinions.[12-14]

The role of the media in public health education—or miseducation—has been discussed by several recent popular books on AIDS.[15-18] These authors have pointed out examples of media coverage that promoted fear and hysteria through misinformation or exaggeration. James Wilkinson, Science Correspondent for BBC Television News,[19] argued in May of 1985 that while Britain's Department of Health has been "tardy" in responding to what is a serious threat

Partial support for this study was provided by the University Research Expeditions Program (UREP), University of California, Berkeley. Dr. Zich's involvement in the research and manuscript preparation was also supported by National Research Service Award 1F32 MH09046, and by Clinical Investigator Award 1 K08 MH00608, both from the National Institute of Mental Health. We thank all the UREP participants who worked on the media aspect of this project, especially Dr. Carl Hopkins, Joy Key, Julia Gregg, Francisca Vanderstaay/Arndt, and Jane Breazzano. Appreciation is due Tony Whitehead, the Terrence Higgins Trust, and Julian Muldren, who provided access to their excellent news files in London. We also thank Anthony Veitch, Harry Coen, and James Wilkinson, who generously spent time in interviews with us. Word processing facilities were generously provided by Dr. Jimmy P. Scott.

to the homosexual community, it is important for both public officials and the press not to overreact or panic.

It is possible, however, that press coverage of *any* kind about AIDS may increase awareness and promote positive health behavior changes. For example, using gonorrhea as a reasonable surrogate index of sexual behavior, a British study[20] reported that decreased incidence of the disease was correlated with increased media coverage of AIDS during a recent 1-year period.

To the extent that information and awareness about health are widely recognized as prerequisites of successful health education, newspapers—which both disseminate information and increase awareness—must be considered part of any public health education process. The aim of the current paper is to explore through both quantitative and qualitative analyses of newspaper accounts in London and San Francisco, which appeared at the time we conducted our knowledge and attitude survey,[11] how the media may have affected public opinion about AIDS. We will first summarize the survey results and then examine the newspaper coverage of AIDS in San Francisco and London during the time the survey was conducted.

THE THREE–CITY SURVEY OF KNOWLEDGE
AND ATTITUDES ABOUT AIDS

In a study by two of the authors (Temoshok and Zich), a survey of knowledge, beliefs, and attitudes about AIDS was administered simultaneously in San Francisco, New York, and London to a total of 399 persons in May and June of 1985.[11] The aim was to investigate how knowledge and attitudes may be influenced by social and cultural contexts as well as by disease epidemiology. Across all samples of the general public (excluding risk group members) in the three cities, general fear of AIDS and antigay attitudes were significantly negatively correlated with knowledge about AIDS.

In the London sample, general fear of AIDS and antigay attitudes were significantly and positively associated with both sexual and general health behavior change. The survey asked respondents whether they had changed their behaviors in response to the threat of AIDS. Because information was not collected on *specific* changes made, it is not possible to determine whether the changes increased, decreased, or had no impact on the person's relative risk for contracting AIDS. Such items should consequently be viewed as indices of motivation to reduce risk rather than as evidence of successful public health education. Sexual behavior change, however, was significantly and positively associated with general fear of AIDS and antigay variables only for the New York sample. Neither of these variables was significantly associated with behavior change of any kind in the San Francisco sample.

We accounted for these intercity differences by proposing a four-stage model of public response to an epidemic over time, which corresponds to how long the general public in a city has been seriously concerned about AIDS and the density of AIDS cases in a city. One implication of our findings is that programs targeted specifically at the general public should be sufficiently tailored to take into account different educational needs and attitudes of particular segments of the general public as well as epidemiologic differences in disease prevalence and risk groups across cities. Such programs for the general public should aim to provide information that will counteract the spread of ignorance, panic, and prejudice as well as spread of the disease.

PUBLIC HEALTH EDUCATION AND THE HEALTH RELIEF MODEL

As a theoretical vantage point from which to view our project, we are adopting the Health Belief Model (HBM), which is derived from several social psychological theories of value expectancy and Lewin's theories about decision making under conditions of uncertainty.[21-23] According to this model, the likelihood of a person taking recommended preventive health action depends on several variables: (1) perceived susceptibility to the health threat (here, contracting AIDS); (2) perceived severity of the consequences of the threat; (3) perceived benefits of taking certain actions; (4) perceived costs of or barriers to possible actions; (5) the presence of cues to take action, such as symptoms or mass media communications; and (6) demographic and sociopsychological factors that may mediate or facilitate action.

While the news media are directly implicated in (5) above, they can also affect the other variables assumed by the model to predict health behavior by providing, for instance, information about the high mortality of AIDS which would presumably affect perceived severity. To take another example, by portraying AIDS as mainly a homosexual, African, or American big-cities phenomenon, the press could influence readers' perceived susceptibility depending on their sexual orientation and demographic characteristics.

METHOD

We considered all AIDS-related articles from Allen's Clipping Service (657 Mission St., San Francisco) and its subcontractor, the International Press Cutting Bureau (70 Newington Causeway, London SE1), published in San Francisco Bay Area and London newspapers from May 1 through June 15, 1985. The clipping service includes comprehensive coverage of the newspapers readily available to the general public. Gay newspapers were not part of the service, but tabloids such as London's *Daily Mirror* were included.

There were 32 Bay Area newspapers sampled from San Francisco, Alameda, San Jose, Marin, Sonoma, and Napa counties. The large majority of articles were from the San Francisco *Chronicle* and *Examiner*. Interestingly, the number of AIDS-related articles was positively correlated with the newspaper's circulation. This was not, however, the case for London, where the corresponding newspapers, the *Times* and the *Guardian*, have a high circulation but not any more AIDS-related articles than any other London area newspaper. All papers sampled from the International Press Cutting Bureau were available in London. Most of the articles were from papers in London proper, although there was an occasional article from as far north as Sheffield and as far west as Gloucester.

Although our public survey of knowledge and attitudes also included New York City, we did not analyze New York newspapers in the present study. The reason for this was that we had limited resources, and responses from New Yorkers generally fell between those from London and San Francisco. Therefore, examining differences between the two most extreme groups in terms of knowledge and attitudes on our AIDS survey seemed the most cost-effective strategy.

Eight content categories (described below) were derived after one of the authors read all the articles and sorted them into various groups on the basis of the kind of information presented. The nonoverlapping categories were confirmed by the first author. Although some articles contained information that could refer to several categories, the dominant theme of an article determined its category assignment. Articles in San Francisco were more likely than those in London to have more than one theme. Although different categories of articles may be particularly likely to influence certain aspects of the HBM, such effects are assumed to be complex and variable across individuals. The categories included:

1. *Statistics.* Articles providing primarily statistical accounts usually conveyed factual information, such as the number of new cases of AIDS or the number of persons who died of AIDS in a given city that month, with little subjective interpretation. This category is assumed to address the variables of perceived severity and perceived risk based on demographic factors in the HBM.

2. *Research.* Into this category fell descriptions of current research on AIDS. These were more than statistical reports; they included summaries of research and usually discussed the wider implications of the findings. It was thought that such articles would not merely provide information but would imply hope—that efforts are under way to treat or prevent AIDS. As such, this might cue people to think in terms of taking action rather than ignoring the threat or resigning oneself to it.

3. *Treatment.* Reports of experimental drugs and therapies, hospital policies on treatment of persons with AIDS, and the attitudes and actions of health care personnel working with AIDS patients were included in this category. As in the research category, articles on experimental treatments are thought to imply that something is being done, that the disease is treatable, and that science has things under control. Alternatively, articles about the limited success of treatment and the discouragement or "burnout" of hospital staff could lead to disillusionment about hopes of a miracle cure. In either case, articles in this category could influence the HBM variable of perceived severity.

4. *Prevention.* This topic is particularly germane to the HBM variable of perceived benefits of taking action as well as to the variable of perceived susceptibility. Most of the articles here concerned "safe sex" criteria, or how to avoid AIDS. Also included in this category were articles about blood testing, which relates indirectly to prevention in that, presumably, persons who test positive for the AIDS virus will curtail certain sexual practices, not donate blood, or have their blood eliminated by blood banks, all of which would contribute to the prevention of AIDS.

5. *Transmission.* Articles that discussed AIDS transmission were often amplifications of more research-based findings. Many were intended as, or included reference to, public health-type "warnings" about various actions that could lead to AIDS transmission. In this latter regard, this category could influence the HBM variables of evaluation of the efficacy of possible behavior, the perceived costs of possible actions, and cues to take action.

6. *Public education.* Many articles in this category announced the availability

and/or plans for formal public education, such as lectures or conferences on AIDS, television documentaries, and other educational campaigns. By implying that knowledge is valuable in the prevention of AIDS, such communications contribute to the HBM variable of cues to action as well as, indirectly, to the variable of the individual's evaluation of the efficacy of possible action.

7. *Funding.* This category included primarily objective rather than subjective reports of support for AIDS research, treatment, or preventive measures as well as announcements of fund-rasing events, the need for funding, and petitions for monies. This category may be related, indirectly, to the variable of perceived susceptibility in the HBM model. For example, if people were to read that the government has appropriated a large amount of money to fight AIDS, they might assume that the problem is, indeed, a serious one. On the other hand, if they read that gay leaders are complaining that not enough money is being devoted to AIDS research, some people who are not part of the gay community might feel it was less of a general problem and believe that the AIDS threat is limited to a minority group to which they do not belong, whereas others might feel concern.

8. *Individual victims.* Articles in this category concerned particular individuals who were symptomatic or had died from AIDS. Tversky and Kahneman[24] have described how any experience that makes a hazard more memorable or imaginable will increase its perceived risk. Thus, articles describing individual AIDS victims in evocative detail could influence the variable of perceived susceptibility in the HBM model.

RESULTS

Quantitative Analysis

Quantitative analyses addressed three variables that were compared between London and San Francisco: (1) number of AIDS-related articles during the study period, (2) average column length for articles, and (3) distribution of articles among the content categories (Table 1). Although interpretations of the impact of the press based on these variables will necessarily be limited and tentative, the quantitative analyses provide another perspective which complements the qualitative analyses to follow.

Statistics are not necessary to underline the fact that there are *four times* the number of AIDS-related newspaper articles in the San Francisco Bay Area than in London during the 6-week period surveyed, despite the fact that articles were drawn from more than twice the number of papers in the London area than in the Bay Area. Equally striking is the average number of column inches devoted to such articles in the San Francisco Bay Area, which was 3.4 times longer than the average number of column inches for London AIDS reports.

The difference between London and San Francisco newspapers in the distribution of articles among the eight categories were tested by the chi-square test for association.[25] Overall, there was a significant difference in the distribution of articles among categories between AIDS-related newspaper articles in the two areas ($\chi^2 = 63.8$, $df = 7$, $p < .001$). Thus, San Francisco and London newspapers were not treating the topic of AIDS in the same manner in terms of attention devoted to the different content areas.

Table 1 Number of newspaper articles and average number of column inches by category for London and San Francisco

	London				San Francisco Bay Area			
Category	Average inches	Number of articles	%	Rank	Average inches	Number of articles	%	Rank
1. Statistics	2.5	22	18.3	3.5	10.0	25	5.1	8
2. Research	6.4	2	1.7	7.5	12.0	39	8.0	6
3. Treatment	4.5	22	18.3	3.5	11.4	84	17.2	2
4. Prevention	2.4	28	23.3	1	17.6	152	31.1	1
5. Transmission	2.3	15	12.5	5	19.3	58	11.9	4
6. Public education	1.5	2	1.7	7.5	12.4	41	8.4	5
7. Funding	10.7	6	5.0	6	21.6	63	12.9	3
8. Individual victims	4.1	23	19.2	2	12.2	26	5.3	7
Overall	4.3	136			14.6	488		

Note: Average inches is the average number of column inches for articles within each category; % refers to percent for each category of the total number of articles; rank refers to ranking of the number of articles in each category.

Qualitative Analysis

Let us turn now, however, to the newspaper reports themselves of May and June of 1985 and look more closely at the categories depicted in Table 1.

Statistics

This was one of two categories in which the number of articles in London (22) approximated the number in the Bay area (25). Nonetheless, the number of column inches devoted to such reports was four times higher in Bay Area than in London papers.

While we might assume that reports in this category are the least vulnerable to subjective or biased interpretation, there were some subtle but important exceptions in our sample. Sixteen of the 22 London articles were based on a study published June 1, 1985, in the respected British medical journal *Lancet*.[26] Based on the prevalence of antibody to HTLV-III (the virus responsible for causing AIDS, now called human immunodeficiency virus, HIV) among British homosexual men attending a London sexually trasmitted disease clinic during 1 week in 1982 as compared to a week in 1984, the authors concluded that the "increasing prevalence of antibody and disease in the U.K. has followed, after a lag period of 3–4 years, that in the USA" and that "at least 2600 homosexual men in London have already been exposed to the virus and most would be symptomless." The findings and conclusions of the *Lancet* study were headlined in the London popular press as "AIDS Virus Hits 3000," "AIDS Increasing Rapidly in London," "AIDS Shock" (followed by "Thousands of men in London have been infected by AIDS"), "Gays at Risk," "More Gays Have AIDS," and "Fresh AIDS Warning" (heading an article which emphasized, "all [homosexuals] are potentially infectious").

No reference was made in the London newspaper accounts to the prevalence or course of AIDS as compared to that in the United States, although another article entitled "AIDS Shock" reported that "Britain now holds second place among European countries with AIDS . . . France being the worst." A different article noted that London itself now accounted for 75% of British AIDS cases. Three other articles in this series were essentially disclaimers, bearing the headlines, "No AIDS Cases in Trent Region," "No AIDS Worry" ("Stroud is AIDS clear . . ."), and "150 Cases in U.K. So Far—Only 1 in Gloucester."

Whereas statistical accounts of AIDS in British papers made no mention of countries other than France, San Francisco Bay Area newspapers discussed the incidence of AIDS in a number of European countries including Britain and in Africa, Japan, Australia, and Brazil. There were no reports of the absence of AIDS in certain cities or countries in Bay Area newspapers. Instead, single articles were devoted to the incidence of AIDS in particular cities and counties including South San Francisco, Marin County, San Mateo County, Fremont, and of course, San Francisco itself. In contrast to the London papers, the course of AIDS, as well as its prevalence, was often discussed.

Nine of the 25 primarily statistical accounts in the San Francisco Bay Area newspapers were based on a press release from the Centers for Disease Control in Atlanta; in each instance, the source was cited. Five of the articles carried the same headline: "The AIDS Case Count Tops 10,000—Nearly Half Dead." The articles themselves featured myriad statistics, including mortality rate (consistently reported as either "nearly one-half" or 49%), expected rate of increased incidence (100% per year), percentages of AIDS victims according to "high-risk" group, percentage according to nationality, and so forth. A wide array of statistics specific to San Francisco were reported, including the number of hospital beds that would be required by 1987. Some reporters evidently could not resist embellishing the statistics with some notable editorializing such as, "With Biblical ferocity the epidemic spread."

Research

A computerized library search revealed a total of 18 articles published on AIDS-related topics in British medical, nursing, epidemiology, public health, or dentistry journals during the month of May 1985 (which would give sufficient time for the material to be picked up by the press by the end of our data collection period, May 1 to June 15, 1985). Of these, 13 articles were published in the better-known and more accessible British Medical Journals, including *Lancet, British Medical Journal, Nature, Community Medicine,* and *Nursing Times.* However, only one article—the one in *Lancet* described above, was picked up by the general press. Two articles (concerning the research of a Scottish veterinary professor whose work with a feline leukemia similar to AIDS was being funded by the American Institute of Health) were devoted to coverage of current research.

By comparison, 63 AIDS-related research reports were published in U.S. medical, nursing, epidemiology, public health, or dentistry journals. Of these, there were 29 research reports in well-known journals more likely to be scanned by the press; i.e., *Journal of the American Medical Association, New England Journal of Medicine, Annals of Internal Medicine, Science, Cancer, American Journal of Public Health, American Journal of Psychiatry, American Journal of Epidemiology, American Journal of Medicine,* and *Mortality and Morbidity Weekly Reports.* Of course, it should be mentioned that some of the well-known British and American journals are subscribed to or read by the science editors of the larger newspapers in both London and San Francisco.

In the San Francisco Bay Area, a large number of articles made secondary reference to research (but were placed in other categories) in addition to the 39 classified as dealing directly and primarily with research. Six of the articles described the importance of a particular, ongoing research project and emphasized the need for increased subject participation. The greatest number of articles (14) concerning a single study during the 6-week sample were devoted to a behavioral study published in The *American Journal of Public Health.*[27] The findings of this study—that there had been substantial reductions in the average number of sexual partners and specific sexual acts believed to be involved in the transmission of AIDS in gay men at risk for AIDS—have direct bearing on several variables in the HBM: perceived susceptibility to a health threat, perceived severity of the consequences of the threat, and evaluation of the efficacy of possible behavior. One of the study's authors, Thomas Coates, was quoted by the newspaper articles as saying, "The decline in sexual activity is probably due to a combination of factors: increased awareness of health guidelines, witnessing of AIDS deaths, the rising number of cases, and an increase in dissemination of scientific information about AIDS."

Treatment

Of the 22 London articles dealing primarily with this topic, seven brief reports concerned an unnamed individual who was discharged from a hospital when it was found that he suffered from AIDS. In all but two articles on interleukin 2 (an experimental immunologic AIDS treatment), the focus of articles in this category was less on treating the AIDS patient than on nursing and hospital care—e.g., how to deal with soiled bedding and patient specimens. By lack of corrective comment, these articles did not dispel the implication that AIDS patients, all their bodily excretions, and items used by them are contagious.

In San Francisco–based reports, the role of the government, the press, and health care professionals in discriminating against AIDS patients was openly addressed. Considerable emphasis was placed on various experimental drugs, including those unavailable in the United States, and the fact that persons with AIDS were "rushing in droves" to Mexico to procure potentially helpful medications. Other articles dealt with alternative health care measures, e.g., vitamins, visualization, and exercise. While barriers to action were identified (i.e., Food and Drug Administration restrictions on legally available drugs, lack of scientific evidence of possible benefits of alternative therapies), the perceived benefits of taking action, in terms of experimental or alternative treatments, were emphasized in these articles.

Prevention

This category accounted for the largest percentage of articles in both London and San Francisco. A significant difference between the two cities, however, was that although criteria for "safe sex" were directly and repeatedly reported in Bay Area papers, no mention was made within London papers of sexual practices, safe or not (with the exception of one article which said that "a change of sexual behavior [among homosexuals] could still have a major impact" in preventing AIDS). Londoners were simply not informed by the press as to what actions they could take to prevent AIDS. Instead, they were told in 16 of the 28 reports that a "Guide to Avoiding AIDS" had been distributed to family practitioners. Three additional articles mentioned the availability of a "hotline" for the "gay disease." There were six articles on blood testing in London papers, compared to 41 in the Bay Area.

Transmission

Newspapers in both London and San Francisco were prone to fear-promoting and negatively biased treatment of the topic. While San Francisco reports were generally more responsible in their content, hysterical coloring was often added to the facts. For example, the facts regarding transmission of AIDS were referred to as "chilling," and "only the tip of the iceberg" in one article. The implication here is that the routes and means of transmission would extend far beyond those already identified, exposing many more persons to AIDS. Without discussion or disclaimer, one San Quentin prison officer was quoted as saying (with reference to concern about AIDS within the criminal justice system), "One chance in a million is more than enough for me and my members—just think of the danger to a prison officer if an AIDS sufferer slashes his wrists."

This quote was reported in San Francisco newspapers seven times, and in all instances, the quote stood alone without corrective comment (citing, for example, the observation known at that time that for all the health care personnel who were exposed to blood and other bodily products of AIDS patients, no health care provider had developed AIDS as a result of this exposure). There were other unfortunate instances in which an article implied that AIDS could be easily contracted. It was reported that a plastic bag with needles was found by a street cleaner and that "a prick could have led to hepatitis or possibly AIDS." Other articles warned about "travel AIDS" (presumably travel to Africa, involving exchange of bodily fluids with an infected person) and the risk of being exposed to AIDS during open heart surgery or blood transfusion.

Ten of the 15 London-based articles concerned the assumed fact that the African ape was responsible for AIDS (a conjecture that has since been put to rest). One particularly problematic article was introduced by the boldest-print headline of any London AIDS article, with letters 1.7 inches high. The headline read, "Swinging Capital Out of Bounds for Lovers." The body of the article began with, "Don't have sex with anyone from London was the warning yesterday from a charity set up to stop the spread of AIDS." According to the article, the warning was issued by the Terrence Higgins Trust, a voluntary, primarily gay service and education charity in London. A member of that organization was quoted as saying, "We want a ban on anyone from outside London having sex with people from London. The spread of AIDS has become such a serious worry that we do not think this is too extreme." The implication of the article was that no one (i.e., including heterosexuals) should have sex with anyone in London, but a closer examination for the article indicated that the Terrence Higgins Trust was probably referring to homosexuals only.

Public Education

In the San Francisco Bay Area, newspapers announced lectures, ongoing education forums, upcoming television documentaries, and the formation of "awareness groups." These educational efforts were sponsored not only by educational institutions and AIDS groups but also by groups of firemen, dentists, and bartenders. Strong pleas were made for wide-reaching prevention education efforts, with explicit note of the need to educate the general public, not just groups at high risk for the disease.

In London, a conference on AIDS sponsored by the Royal Society of Health was announced. Another article reported that a Town Hall was preparing "a campaign to tell its workers about the killer disease, AIDS."

Funding

There were over 10 times the number of articles concerning funding of AIDS research and services in San Francisco Bay Area newspapers than in London. During the identified period of time, 22 fund-raising events, ranging from a "Closet Ball" to a Bike-a-Thon to a formal ball at which San Francisco's Mayor Diane Feinstein was hostess, were announced in Bay Area newspapers. Only two comparable events were announced in London: "a terribly witty and outrageous ball" put on by a 15-year-old girl whose parents were less concerned "she'd bring the disease home, but for the possible debt she might run up," and gay athletic games which were actually only in the planning stages when announced. Nineteen articles published in the Bay Area were devoted to either the need for monies, petitions for monies, or monies granted; five comparable articles appeared in London papers.

We might surmise that of all the categories, this one was the most dependent on what was happening in the two cities and thus the least influenced by selection and editorializing by the press. There was at least one exception in London, however: of all the funding articles published in London during this period, the one with the boldest headline print (1-inch-high letters) was entitled, "High Expense of the Fight Against AIDS." The article then read, "Keeping AIDS out of Mersey Region could cost the taxpayer more than £328,000 this year."

Individual Victims

This was the category in which the press could exercise most poetic license, because the articles were less often immediate news reports than feature stories. Although the absolute numbers of stories were similar in the two cities, the average numbers of column inches per story were significantly discrepant: an average of 12.2 in the Bay Area versus 4.1 in London. In the San Francisco articles, the large majority of individuals were named; sympathetic descriptions of their life histories and of them as individuals were frequently included. In 13 of the articles there were pictures of the individuals. In contrast, no corresponding pictures appeared in London newspapers, and individuals were rarely named. Most significantly, the vast majority of the articles dealt with foreigners: an unnamed Italian man living in London ("Drug Man Has AIDS," "Addict Gives Himself AIDS"), and a 9-year-old Swedish hemophiliac who had received American-made plasma. The deaths of two British hemophiliacs were reported.

DISCUSSION

Limitations of the Study

There are some limitations to our methods that restrict the interpretations and generalizations that can be made from our findings. First, we do not know how many people were reached in each city by the newspapers in our survey. Circulation figures probably underestimate the number of people picking up tabloids, in particular, from newspaper stands and checkout counters. In addition, an unknown number of persons read headlines and parts of articles as they stand in checkout lines in grocery stores, glimpse them through clear plastic newspaper boxes (more in San Francisco), or read headlines of papers that serve as advertisements on newspaper stands (in London). Compounding the problem, we don't know how many people who pick up the newspapers in question actually read the article. For example, even in 1985, we overheard people saying, more in San Francisco than in London, that they were "tired" of AIDS stories, that the articles were "too depressing," and that they weren't going to read AIDS-related material anymore.

Other caveats should be noted in terms of interpreting our quantitative and qualitative findings. For example, while the difference is striking between the average number of column inches devoted to AIDS-related articles in San Francisco Bay Area and that London area newspapers, we have not analyzed the average number of column inches for other non-AIDS-related articles, medical or general, in the two geographic areas. Such an analysis would be beyond the scope of the current paper, which is focused on comparing AIDS-related articles in London and San Francisco Bay Area newspapers. What we are able to say on the basis of the threefold difference in average column inches in San Francisco versus London newspapers is that there is the opportunity in that increased length to discuss at greater length reports of AIDS research, treatment, prevention, and transmission. The qualitative analyses revealed that articles in San Francisco often provided more detail and interpretation of research reports, which would, we believe, aid the reader in drawing accurate conclusions from the information presented.

We have also not analyzed qualitatively how other medical issues have been discussed in London or San Francisco papers. For example, we were told by Anthony Veitch, Science Editor of the respected London *Guardian*, that British newspapers have always been conservative and even prudish about printing any direct sexual terminology and are often reluctant to go into details about other medical problems such as cancer.

Finally, it is not clear to what extent readers are influenced by the articles they read. For example, we were informed by a number of people in London that everyone takes the tabloids "with a large grain of salt." It was also mentioned that the hysterical and fear-promoting stories in the London tabloids in February 1985 produced an opposite reaction in other journalistic quarters. More responsible newspapers, such as the *Guardian*, began a campaign to provide corrective and objective information about AIDS. Television journalists were particularly aware of the problem of the February fiasco and produced a number of informative and responsible documentaries and news briefs around the time of our study. This observation raises another question, which is how much the general public is exposed to and influenced by newspaper articles compared with television news stories.

Thus, for all these reasons, it is difficult to assess to what extent the numbers of articles, the number of column inches, and/or the content of the newspaper articles in London and San Francisco actually influenced the inhabitants of the respective areas, particularly in terms of impact on attitudes, knowledge, and actual behavior change relevant to preventing AIDS. Nevertheless, we can hypothesize that there is some correspondence between the numbers of articles in newspapers and the numbers of articles read, and that the content of the articles will have some impact on knowledge and attitudes about AIDS.

Numbers and Lengths of Articles in the Two Cities

The large differences between the numbers and average lengths of articles in London and the San Francisco Bay Area may be attributable to the numbers or densities of AIDS cases in the two areas. At the time of the study in May and June of 1985, there were only 150 cases reported in England, nearly all in London (a density of 2.2 per 100,000 people in London), compared to 1235 cases in the San Francisco Bay Area (a density of 105.6 per 100,000 people). The relatively high number and particularly the density of AIDS cases in the San Francisco Bay Area may help explain the greater "newsworthiness" of AIDS there and thus the greater number and length of articles.

The lower number and density of AIDS cases in London contributed, we feel, to the epidemic of fear-generating, attention-grabbing headlines and stories, primarily in the tabloids, that plagued London about 6 months before our study was undertaken. When something is unknown and unfamiliar, it tends to be more frightening.[28] In this sense, we might consider the London newspaper stories in February 1985 as *reflecting* fears and attitudes of the general public as well as *amplifying* them. Some examples of such headlines include:

"AIDS Death Shock at BBC: 'Take action now' " (*Sunday Mirror* Feb. 17, 1985)
"Ban on 'Deadly' Kiss of Life; We believe we are all at risk, say firemen" (*Sunday Mirror*, Feb. 17, 1985)
"Gay Plague Kills Man at Beeb" (*News of the World*, Feb. 17, 1985)
"Boys Jail Chaplain Dies of AIDS" (*Daily Mirror*, Feb. 1, 1985)

Discussion of Results in Terms of the Health Belief Model

In all the categories except public education and funding, newspaper articles in San Francisco, compared with those in London, were judged more potentially facilitative of the HBM variables of perceived susceptibility to a health threat, perceived severity of the consequences, perceived benefits of taking certain actions, and the presence of cues to action.

Prevention

Of our eight content categories, prevention seems to be the most pertinent to public health education and the HBM. It is also the category to which the press has potentially the most to contribute in terms of public health education. After all, the overwhelming majority of a paper's readers will be those who need to know how to avoid AIDS, not how to treat it. While our quantitative analysis revealed this to be the most popular area for newspaper stories in both cities, qualitative analyses showed that London newspapers, in sharp contrast to those in San Francisco, were not informative about specific sexual practices that were either "safe" or "unsafe" in terms of contracting AIDS.

According to Anthony Veitch and Harry Coen of the *Guardian* in London, there had been quite a battle between science writers and the editorial staff over whether to mention anal (or rectal) intercourse in direct and precise terms when describing sexual practices particularly conducive to transmission of the virus.[29] The science writers had only recently convinced the editors of the importance of citing specific dangerous sex practices, but these terms were still often deleted by night editors. Mention of specific behaviors to be adopted or changed to prevent AIDS is relevant to the HBM variable of presence of cues to action. We feel this is an important area for the press to emphasize in direct, accurate, and objective reports.

Evidently, public health officials in Great Britain thought so as well. In March 1986, an information campaign was presented in certain newspapers. For example, a full-page, large-print message in the *Sunday Observer*[30] presented in outline form answers to the following questions: What is AIDS? Is AIDS spread through normal contact with other people? Does AIDS only attack homosexuals? Is AIDS spread by objects touched by infected persons? Are blood transfusions safe? How is AIDS spread? How do you know if you are at risk? What is safe sex? What is risky sex?

Portrayals of Individual Victims

We believe that the news media can do a great deal more in the area of increasing perceived susceptiblity and enhancing public openness to public health education/prevention through empathetically engaging articles about individual "victims." Nisbett and Ross[31] have summarized research and written extensively about the impact of vivid writing on people's perceptions of themselves and their fellow humans and society at large. According to these authors, information is likely to attract and hold our attention to the extent that it is (1) emotionally interesting, (2) concrete and imagery-provoking, and (3) proximate in a sensory, temporal, or spatial way. The more vivid the information is, the greater its impact can be on recognition and recall.

Research demonstrating the superiority of pictures to words or sentences is germane to our observation that there were no photographs of individual persons with AIDS in London, in contrast to San Francisco–based newspapers during this same period.[32] Of course, the nature of the photograph is important. What the San Francisco photographs showed were usually attractive, intelligent-looking human beings. The vivid and sympathetic portrayals of the "nice boy next door" in the San Francisco papers would be more likely to evoke empathetic engagement in the reader than the stark, abstract, unsympathetic British reports about drug-addicted foreigners. Thus, we would hypothesize that the San Francisco articles would do much more to enhance perceived susceptibility in the reader (e.g., "That poor guy could be my brother/son/co-worker/friend! I guess AIDS can hit anyone . . . maybe even me!") and facilitate openness to behavioral changes that could prevent AIDS.

Other studies have demonstrated that even a single vivid description can influence social attitudes in ways unadorned statistics do not, even though statistics provide a sounder base of evidence from which to make accurate judgements.[33,34] Reading about the personal and financial hardships, prejudice, and pain encountered by one person diagnosed with AIDS makes the disease an emotional reality that goes beyond the factual reality of how many cases were diagnosed in a certain area this month. It is often such emotional insight that precipitates behavior change.

Emotional reactions to AIDS may, however, be a barrier as well as a facilitator, in terms of the HBM model. Reviews of the fear-arousal literature indicate that no blanket statement can be made concerning the value of fear as a motivator of health behavior.[35] However, some reports have demonstrated that moderate levels of anxiety may be optimal for health prevention or early detection campaigns.[36,37] When the emotional response to risk information is minimal, motivation to change may be lacking. On the other hand, if emotion, particularly fear, is too high, persons are apt to try to reduce their fear by avoiding the distressing topic. This may include avoiding important information as well as avoiding behavior change. In such cases fear becomes an obstacle to health promotion.

A major goal of public health education should be to prevent an epidemic of fear and to promote responsible depictions of the real problem of AIDS. By portraying persons with AIDS as human beings, often admirable and courageous ones, with families, jobs, hopes, fears, and dreams, the news media can help to change some of the unfortunate attitudes borne of prejudice and fear.

Relationship of the Press Articles to the Knowledge and Attitude Survey

We conducted the present analysis of newspaper articles appearing in London and the San Francisco Bay Area from May 1 to June 15, 1985, partly in order to explore any relationship with the surveys of knowledge and attitudes about AIDS, which were administered to the general public in London and San Francisco (as well as New York City) during the same time period. We recognized that it would be impossible to establish any causal relationship—that, for example, coverage by the press influenced public knowledge or attitudes about AIDS. It is far more likely that, as with most psychosocial phenomena, there are ever shifting, complex interactions among demographic, sociocultural, and epidemiologic (in terms of incidence and prevalence of the disease) factors, public opinion, and the media. It is probably impossible to determine for any particular instance whether public opinion is a reflection of, a consequence of, or a contributor to demographic, sociocultural, epidemiologic, or media factors. Thus, our analysis must be more historical than scientific in its method.

With these cautionary notes in mind, we can speculate that there is a relationship between London–San Francisco differences in the general public's knowledge and attitudes about AIDS and London–San Francisco differences in newspaper coverage of AIDS. For example, we found that the San Francisco public was significantly more knowledgeable about AIDS and less generally fearful about AIDS than was the London public sampled.[11] Certainly, the fact that there were over four times as many articles about AIDS in San Francisco than in London papers might have some bearing on the public's knowledge about how AIDS is caused, transmitted, and prevented.

Similarly, the hysteria-promoting headlines that occurred in London 3 months before the survey, and the tendency even during the time of the survey for London headlines and articles to be more alarmist, particularly around the issue of transmission, could be associated with the higher level of fear of AIDS in London than in San Francisco. Elsewhere,[11] we suggested that some of the cross-cultural differences found in our study comparing public response to AIDS in London, San Francisco, and New York could be attributed to differences in information and attitudes communicated through the news media in these three cities. It was our impresssion, confirmed by interviews with medical personnel, persons with AIDS, and media representatives, that the newspapers in London were markedly more fear-promoting and sensationalizing about AIDS than were the newspapers in San Francisco.

In our survey, we also found that the heterosexual public's fear of AIDS and antigay attitudes were significantly correlated with sexual behavior change in London but not in San Francisco.[11] As previously noted, we do not have information on the specific changes made. Therefore, we do not know whether the changes would reduce, increase, or have no effect on a person's risk for contracting AIDS. However, because both more fear of AIDS and more antigay attitudes were significantly correlated with less knowledge about AIDS, we might hypothesize that the sexual changes made were not based on accurate knowledge about what is effective to prevent contracting AIDS.

We suspect there is a relationship between the London–San Francisco survey differences in the public's knowledge and attitudes about AIDS, and the differences in quantity and content of AIDS-related press in London versus San Francisco. Because our study was not prospective, we are unable to demonstrate a causal relationship. One explanation for our results is that the news media is a mere reflection of public opinion. However, it is equally plausible that the press can be a powerful tool—for good or for ill—to influence public health education regarding AIDS.

CONCLUSION AND FURTHER COMMENT

Since our 1985 study, the British government appears to have recognized and harnessed some of the potential power of the press in the fight to prevent AIDS. In March 1986 the British government, as part of a national campaign strategy, placed a full-page advertisement about AIDS, introduced by a preamble by medical officials, in every national newspaper. An evaluation of this effort[38] concluded, however, that the health education campaign had little or no impact on attitudes, desire for information, intended behavior, or anxiety. The government then initiated a week-long campaign of newspaper advertisements and television announcements in November 1986.[39] In January, 1987, the government, as part of its new $30 million education campaign against AIDS, began broadcasts on BBC radio, along with other education campaign strategies.[39] According to a recent newspaper poll, such campaigns may be finally paying off, as young single persons report more use of condoms, and married people report fewer extramarital affairs.[39]

A well-respected science writer has said that neither the scientists nor the journalists should be in the business of deciding paternalistically what is in the best interest of the public to be published.[40] However, it would seem that in the interests of social responsibility, both scientists and journalists must be concerned not only that their data are accurate and objectively presented but that their articles have some social value that is clearly communicated. Public health educators, who are in the business of prevention, should be more aware of the powers of the press to inform or misinform readers, to motivate health-promoting action, to lull one into complacency, or to incite hysterical reaction. It is beyond the scope of this paper for us to make specific suggestions about utilizing the press in public health education. We hope, however, that our study may suggest areas in which the press can be allied with public health educators to communicate information that will be helpful in AIDS prevention.

REFERENCES

1. Martin, J.L. (1986). AIDS risk reduction recommendations and sexual behavior patterns among gay men: A multifactoral categorical approach to assessing change. *Health Education Quarterly, 13*, 347–358.

2. Stall, R., McKusick, L., Wiley, J., Coates, T.J., & Ostrow, D.G. (1986). Alcohol and drug use during sexual activity and compliance with safe sex guidelines for AIDS: The AIDS Behavioral Research Project. *Health Education Quarterly, 13*, 359–372.

3. Emmons, C.A., Joseph, J.G., Kessler, R.C., Wortman, C.B., Montgomery, S.B., & Ostrow, D.G. (1986). Psychosocial predictors of reported behavior change in homosexual men at risk for AIDS. *Health Education Quarterly, 13,* 331–346.

4. Friedman, S.R., Des Jarlais, D.C., & Sotheran, J.L. (1986). AIDS health education for intravenous drug users. *Health Education Quarterly, 13,* 383–394.

5. Ginzburg, H.M., French, J., Jackson, J., Hartsock, P.I., MacDonald, M.G., & Weiss, S.H. (1986). Health education and knowledge assessment of HTLV-III diseases among intravenous drug users. *Health Education Quarterly, 13,* 373–382.

6. Cleary, P.D., Rogers, T.F., Singer, E., Avorn, J., Van Devanter, N., Perry, S., & Pindyck, J. (1986). Health education about AIDS among seropositive blood donors. *Health Education Quarterly, 13,* 317–330.

7. Williams, L.S. (1986). AIDS risk reduction: A community health education intervention for minority high risk group members. *Health Education Quarterly, 13,* 407–422.

8. Price, A.H., Desmond, S., & Kukulka, G. (1985). High school students' perceptions and misperceptions of AIDS. *Journal of School Health, 55,* 107–109.

9. DiClemente, R.J., Zorn, J., & Temoshok, L. (1986). *American Journal of Public Health, 76,* 1443–1445.

10. Bausell, R.B., Damrosch, S., Parks, P., & Soeken, K. (1986). Public perceptions regarding the AIDS epidemic: Selected results from a national poll. *AIDS Research, 2,* 253–258.

11. Temoshok, L., Sweet, D.M., & Zich, J. (1987). A three-city comparison of the public's knowledge and attitudes about AIDS. *Psychology & Health: An International Journal, 1,* 43–60.

12. Steinbrook, R. (1985, Dec. 18). Majority see their risk of contracting AIDS as low. *Los Angeles Times.*

13. Harris, M. (1986, Jan. 7). AIDS called top health issue. *San Francisco Chronicle.*

14. CBS News and *New York Times* (1985, Sept.). Poll on AIDS.

15. Altman, D. (1986). *AIDS in the Mind of America: The Social, Political, and Psychological Impact of a New Epidemic.* New York: Doubleday.

16. Brandt, A.M. (1985). *No Magic Bullet: A Social History of Venereal Disease in the United States since 1880,* New York: Oxford University Press.

17. Fettner, A.G., & Check, W.A. (1985). *The Truth about AIDS: Evolution of an Epidemic.* New York: Holt, Rinehart & Winston.

18. Patton, C. (1985). *Sex and Germs: The Politics of AIDS.* Boston: South End Press.

19. Wilkinson, J. (1985, March). A narrow line between complacence and alarmism. *Listener,* 30–31.

20. Weller, I.V., Hindley, D.J., & Adler, M.W. (1984). Gonorrhoea in homosexual men and media coverage of AIDs in London 1982–3. *British Medical Journal 289,* 1041.

21. Becker, M.H. (ed.). (1974). *The Health Belief Model and Personal Health Behavior.* Thorofare, NJ: Slack.

22. Maiman, L.A., & Becker, M.H. (1974). The health belief model: Origins and correlates in psychological theory. *Health Education Monographs 2,* 236–253.

23. Becker, M.H., & Maiman, L.A. (1983). Models of health-related behavior. In D. Mechanic (ed.), *Handbook of Health, Health Care, and the Health Professions,* New York: Free Press.

24. Tversky, A., & Kahneman, D. (1974). Judgement under uncertainty: Heuristics and biases. *Science 185,* 1124–1131.

25. Siegel, S. (1956). *Nonparametric Statistics for the Behavioral Sciences.* New York: McGraw-Hill.

26. Carne, C.A., Weller, I.V.D., Sutherland, S., Cheinsong-Popov, R., Ferms, R.B., Williams, P., Mindel, A., Tedder, R., & Adler, M.W. (1985). Rising prevalence of human T-lymphotropic virus type III (HTLV-III) infection in homosexual men in London. *Lancet i,* 1261–1262.

27. McKusick, L., Horstman, W., & Coates, T.J. (1985). AIDS and sexual behavior reported by gay men in San Francisco. *American Journal of Public Health 75,* 493–496.

28. Douglas, M. (1966). *Purity and Danger: An Analysis of Concepts of Pollution and Taboo.* London: Routedge & Kegan Paul.

29. Veitch, A., & Coen, H. (1985, May 3). Personal communication.

30. Acheson, D., Crompton, G., MacDonald, I.S., & Weir, R.J. (1986, March 16). Are you at risk for AIDS? *Sunday Observer,* p. 4.

31. Nisbett, R., & Ross, L. (1980). *Human Inference: Strategies and Shortcomings of Social Judgement.* Englewood Cliffs, NJ: Prentice-Hall.

32. Gehring, R.E., Toglia, M.P., & Kimble, G.A. (1976). Recognition memory for words and pictures at short and long retention intervals. *Memory and Cognition, 4,* 256–260.

33. Hamill, R., Wilson, T.D., & Nisbett, R.E. (1979). *Ignoring Sample Bias: Inferences about Collectivities from Atypical Cases.* Unpublished manuscript, University of Michigan.

34. Borgida, E., & Nisbett, R.W. (1977). The differential impact of abstract vs. concrete information on decisions. *Journal of Applied Social Psychology, 7,* 258–271.

35. Sutton, S.R. (1982). Fear-arousing communications: A critical examination of theory and research. In J.F. Eiser (ed.), *Social Psychology and Behavioral Medicine.* Chichester, U.K.: John Wiley.

36. Leventhal, H., Singer, R., & Jones, S. (1965). The effects of fear and specificity of recommendations. *Journal of Personality and Social Psychology 2,* 20–25.

37. Temoshok, L., DiClemente, R.J., Sweet, D.M., Blois, M.S., & Sagebiel, R.W. (1984). Factors related to patient delay in seeking medical attention for cutaneous malignant melanoma. *Cancer 54,* 3048–3053.

38. Sher, L. (1987). An evaluation of the UK government health education campaign on AIDS. *Psychology & Health: An International Journal, 1,* 61–72.

39. Moseley, R. (1987, Jan. 11). British now fight AIDS with ads. *San Francisco Sunday Examiner and Chronicle* (originally *Chicago Tribune*), pp. A13, 18.

40. Russell, C. (1985, Feb. 13). Science in the eye of the storm: Conflicts in communicating research to the public. The Fifth Chancellor's Distinguished Lectureship for the Public Understanding of Science, University of California, San Francisco.

46

Questions from the Public

David Watts

House Calls is a 60-min radio call-in program broadcast on KQED in San Francisco and hosted by Dr. David Watts, Associate Clinical Professor of Medicine at the University of California, San Francisco. Programs on *House Calls* have included such topics as problems of aging, cancer prevention, osteoporosis, stroke, and depression. On February 25, 1985, Dr. Watts introduced the topic of AIDS to his radio listeners. On September 18, 1985, Dr. Watts invited two experts in the field of AIDS to join him on *House Calls*. A transcript of this program follows to indicate the types of questions of concern to the San Francisco Bay Area listeners at that time.

Watts: Hello and welcome to this special edition of *House Calls*. This is Dr. David Watts, the host of this program. We are giving you a follow-up to the national call-in program that you may have just heard coming out of Washington NPR. Our guests are Paul Volberding, Chief of Oncology and Director of AIDS Activities at San Francisco General Hospital. Also with us is Holly Smith, who is Media Relations Coordinator of the San Francisco AIDS Foundation. Paul, let's begin with the CDC policy on attendance in schools. Is it safe to have someone who has AIDS go to school and have casual contact, as it is called, with individuals who are participating in the same classes?

Volberding: Well, in response I think we have to admit that we all share some concerns, some fears about this disease. On the other hand, at this point in time, we have a great deal of information, and all of the information says that casual contact as would occur in the workplace and in the schools does not transmit this disease, so I think essentially all AIDS experts would agree with these CDC guidelines.

Smith: I think it's important to reiterate that, as part of the CDC guidelines, they are clear to communicate that it's on a case-by-case basis that a student, a young child who has AIDS, is admitted to school because sometimes it's inappropriate, they may be too ill to attend school. And so, it's very important to understand that the CDC is not saying that every child should go to school who is antibody-positive or has AIDS, but that those, there's no fear for people to worry about.

Caller No. 1: Hello, I would like a comment on the fact that AIDS is also related to the effects of dioxins, which also suppress the immune system.

Watts: O.K. We'll turn that one over to Paul.

Volberding: It's an interesting question. I haven't been asked it in a long time. At first it was one of the things that people were concerned about. Actually, we did a study. One of the international dioxin experts from Sweden, Leonard Hardell, was a visitor in our clinic for about 6 months and did a study of our patients and could find no evidence that our patients had any more substantial history of exposure than anyone else in the population. We don't think, at least it's not an important factor.

Watts: So your feeling is that dioxin has nothing or perhaps very little to do with the AIDS epidemic.

Volberding: Yes, very little, if any.

Caller No. 1: Is it possible for a fragment of the dioxin molecule to be impregnated in the virus at all?

Volberding: No, I don't think so.

Watts: O.K. Thank you very much for your question. Now, we're going to be talking to caller No. 2. Hello, do you have a question for us?

Caller No. 2: Yes, I do. It's somewhat involved. I live in kind of a communal household with two gay individuals along with my son and his mother. An associate of theirs died of AIDS last year, and since it is kind of a communal situation, I am wondering if we are in any possible danger of my son or myself contracting that. Should we have a test? I'm concerned about things like sharing a joint, you know dishes, bathroom, taking baths, and things of that sort since they are commonly used. Is there any danger there?

Smith: The types of activities you are describing are what we term casual contact, the types of activities that do not seem to be effective transmitters of the virus. We show no evidence in the pattern of close to 13,000 cases now diagnosed in the United States to show that casual contact is an issue in transmission, and you should put your mind to rest about those common everyday issues that you were discussing just now."

Caller No. 2: May I interject one thing. I've heard at one time, I don't know if this is still true about saliva possibly carrying it. Now, if we're smoking a joint, sharing that, is there a possibility there, or if one puts a spoon in food, for example, in their mouth, and then puts it in again. That's somewhat more than casual; it becomes more intimate in a sense.

Watts: That's a good question because it's been brought up many times with regard to specific cases that are being looked at very carefully now.

Volberding: Well, the virus is in the saliva. The virus is probably in every part of the body, in cells in every part of the body. So it's not surprising that it's in the saliva, that it's been reported in the tears and the rest. But the real question is what is the evidence that it is transmitted by that fluid, and the evidence, in fact, is nonexistent. There are no confirmed cases of transmission by saliva, and in San Francisco, I think it's remarkable and reassuring that the disease has remained so concentrated in the same risk groups that it has been for 4 years. If that sort of spread was possible, or at all probable, we would have seen many cases of people who had shared joints or shared coffee cups or shared bathroom facilities with someone who either has the virus or has the disease. So, I think we can be very reassured that that is not a reality.

Caller No. 2: Maybe I should bring out the point that associating with homosexuals, since they are in a high-risk group, whether they have it or not, doesn't present any particular danger to anyone?

Smith: Absolutely!

Volberding: Oh, I think it presents no danger at all.

Watts: It also brings out an important principle of medicine, which I think can be pieced out, that just because a virus is present in a certain particular tissue or exposure doesn't mean that it's going to transmit the disease. I think there are other factors involved. There may be a certain load of viruses one needs to be in contact with just before the disease actually takes place. Does this figure in at all to what you just said?

Volberding: Greatly, I think the feeling now is the virus is necessary to cause AIDS and that you can't get AIDS without the virus. There's growing evidence that there are many other factors involved as well. I think a healthy person who is exposed to this virus, especially by means of saliva, which we think is very low risk, is much more able to fight off the virus and less likely to get infected.

Caller No. 2: May I ask one final question?

Watts: O.K. What's your question?

Caller No. 2: It's about the new test. Is it an AIDS test to find out if you have been exposed to it? Would that test be advisable for me, my son, or his mother to have? I would think for homosexuals to have, too? I don't know if they had that or not, but is that helpful? What does that mean if it is a positive result or a negative? Can you discuss that?

Smith: The test you are referring to is the HTLV-III antibody test. It is commonly referred to in the media as the "AIDS Test," and that is merely a media shorthand. It is not a diagnostic or a predictor test of the AIDS issue. It merely detects whether or not you came in contact with the virus and your system developed an antibody. An antibody is somewhat like a chemical marker, that you came in contact with a foreign invader.

Caller No. 2: Does that mean you can be immune to it?

Watts: Not necessarily.

Smith: Not necessarily, unfortunately not. You develop all sorts of antibodies whenever you have a foreign contact with viruses. Some antibodies are ones that fight off the diseases; some are just those chemical markers. This is a test that measures that chemical marker, that you've had contact with the virus.

Watts: Don't forget that this is not predictive of getting AIDS, as she has said.

Caller No 2: What does it serve us exactly? It doesn't exactly put your mind at rest either way.

Watts: No, the test was designed to provide an extra safety measure for the nation's blood supply. It is very effective for what it was designed to do, ensure safety of that blood donation bank. When you talk about using it outside of that system, there is controversy about its values and its nonvalues. There are some values, whatever we're talking about, in a clinical setting for trying to rule out some kinds of problems that people are facing. It is valuable whenever you are talking about high-risk persons who are considering entering into pregnancy, because we know the virus can be transmitted via mother to child, and it may have other kinds of values, but the decision to take the test is really one that each individual must make for himself. So you need to become very educated as to what it does and does not mean, what are the possible harassment and discrimination factors you might face, given a possible positive result.

Caller No. 2: It should be confidential results, I think though?

Smith: In San Francisco we have a testing process at the alternative testing sites, where you can go and get this test, become educated, and your test result will be completely anonymous. They do not take your name, there is no identifying information that is taken, and your confidentiality is totally guaranteed.

Watts: Paul, did you have something you wanted to add?

Volberding: Just the comment that I think I understand Holly's point about the test not being predictive, but at the same time, I don't think we should let the impression come across that the test means nothing. A positive test means that you have been exposed. It means that your possibility of transmitting the virus to a sexual partner is very reasonable and clearly increases your risk of developing AIDS. We think the risk is somewhere between 5% and 20%. We don't have enough data to say that. But it clearly does indicate one is at risk.

Caller No. 2: But if you were to come down with a positive test, would it take 5 or 10 years to come down with the disease? You wouldn't even know when you contracted the disease?

Volberding: Exactly. If you know when you become positive, then we think the incubation period after that is 1–5 years, in most cases. But there is absolutely no way to predict.

Watts: We have some other callers waiting, so we'll have to go. Now we're talking with caller No. 3.

Caller No. 3: I'd like to ask about the safety of the blood supply. I understand that the test they are giving for the screening has a significant false-negative result, that, for example, people are exposed but take some time to develop the antibodies. I wondered if there is any quantitative information on exactly what that false-negative rate is and how really safe the blood supply is.

Watts: O.K. For that answer, we'll turn to Paul Volberding.

Volberding: The data have actually been presented at several national meetings including one in March at the FDA that I was at. I went very skeptical, having heard the same concerns about false positives and false negatives. In fact, I was amazed at how accurate the test is. The test is extremely accurate, and for the purposes it was designed for, extremely useful, and I think it clearly is helping ensure the safety of the blood supply. I point out that even before the test was introduced, the blood supply was safe, that all evidence was that gay men had already stopped donating blood at the blood banks. In fact, the number of positive donors that they are finding now that they are doing the test is much less than one of 1% of all people coming to the blood banks, so the blood was already safe. The test will make it even safer, because the test is in fact very accurate.

Caller No. 3: Is there any quantitative number on that one in thousand for the false-negative rate?

Volberding: The sensitivity of the test, the ability to pick up somebody who is truly positive is greater than 99%. The ability to prove that someone is actually negative is very close to that, in the 98% range."

Caller No. 3: I heard on another AIDS hotline program or call-in program, somebody was saying, and I didn't understand this, that for some reason the test is much less accurate when it is given to people who are not in the high-risk group. What's that mean?

Volberding: It's exactly right in a sense. It's right in the sense, and it's not right. The accuracy of the test is the same no matter where it's used, but the problem is if you use a test like this, and it's a convoluted statistical argument that I barely understand anymore. But basically, if you are using a screening test like this, even a very good one like this, in a situation where very few people actually have the antibody, then occasionally and actually very frequently, when the test is positive, it is going to be falsely positive. So the real problem in this test in the blood banks isn't that we're missing people who are truly positive, but that in the situation we are possibly telling someone they are positive when in fact they are not.

Caller No. 3: So there are no false negatives?

Volberding: It's not so much the false-negative problem.

Caller No. 3: O.K. Fine!

Watts: Thank you very much for your question. I have with us today Paul Volberding, who is Chief of Oncology and Director of AIDS Activities at San Francisco General Hospital. Also with us is Holly Smith, Media Relations Coordinator of the San Francisco AIDS Foundation. We were talking about casual contact. Let's take that one step further. What about needle stick? Are we safe from needle stick from AIDS patients?"

Volberding: One of the ways viruses are spread in the medical environment, it is especially true of hepatitis B virus, is by contaminated needle stick. When you've drawn blood from someone, and in the process of disposing the needle, you accidentally puncture your own skin. That clearly transmits hepatitis; it's a real risk for medical staff. With the AIDS virus, the evidence is really very strong. It's hard to convince the public of this at times, but the evidence is really strong that the virus isn't transmitted even by that very direct exposure. We think that the virus is present in almost none of the blood cells, that only about one in 10,000 to one in 1 million cells are infected with the virus. Transmitting the virus would require a lot more blood than you get with a needle stick.

Watts: O.K. Let's go to caller No. 4. Do you have a question for us?

Caller No. 4: Yes. It's my understanding that the AIDS patient that is dying is dying of diseases acquired because of his reduced immunity. My question is, aside from the question of contracting the AIDS virus, does the victim of AIDS pose a risk to the community because of these other diseases that might be contracted?

Watts: You're talking about the diseases of infection of the lungs, Kaposi's sarcoma?

Caller No. 4: What are those dangers?

Watts: Do they spread those illnesses to other, immune-competent, individuals?

Volberding: It's an excellent question, and it's one that bothered us at first, but as we have learned more and more about the infections that people with AIDS get, we have learned that they are actually infections that reactivated from within their own bodies. These are infections that all of us are carrying around, but our immune system is able to keep them under control. With AIDS, the immune system breaks down and allows those infections to appear, but they don't transmit to another person whose immune system is intact. And we don't even see evidence of substantial risk of transmission of one of those infections from one AIDS patient to another, because these patients are often waiting in the clinic waiting rooms and in support groups, and we don't see epidemics of these infections even in that compromised situation, so I think the answer is that there is really no risk at all.

Watts: It's important to remember that we carry around organisms with us all the time and potentially lethal ones, in our gut, in our throat, on our skin.

It's our immune system that protects us against these organisms at all times, except when, under the circumstances of AIDS or other things, our immune system is somewhat compromised, those can take over and cause problems.

Caller No. 4: Thank you very much.

Watts: Let's now move back to San Francisco. Caller No. 5, you are on *House Calls.*

Caller No. 5: I have heard that in Africa, East Africa, where they have a great incidence of AIDS, up to 50% in all age groups, male and female, homosexual and heterosexual. I'm wondering, is there any idea how it has become so widespread? Because children are born with it, or what? What is the idea?

Smith: The belief is that AIDS has existed for some period of time in Africa, that it may in fact have been an animal-borne disease previously, perhaps in the monkey community, and it was transmitted from that community to humans. Currently it is transmitted like it is here in the United States, through direct sexual contact with partners and through the exchange of blood products between two individuals. Here, we talk about IV drug use and the sharing of needles. In Africa, we're talking about very different medical practices where needles are used more than once, so you can come in contact with blood easily from another person, or from ritual tribal customs where blood is exchanged because of sanctification processes, but it is the same basic two issues. Sexual contact and direct exchange of blood or blood products.

Watts: To follow up on that for a moment, if I may, caller No. 5 asked a question that's kind of interesting. In Africa, more women seem to have AIDS than in America. Is that not the case, and is it a different disease, expressed differently in Africa, or are we really dealing with essentially the same problem?

Volberding: No, it's essentially the same problem. The spectrum of infections to some degree differs in different parts of the world depending on which organisms are common in those areas. When you get AIDS, you get what's common in that environment. In Africa, it's a little bit different than in the United States. It appears that malaria may be much more common in patients in Africa, but the disease is the same. And I agree with Holly completely, I think the evidence of transmission is the same in Africa as it is here, at the same time admitting that there are a number of social and cultural factors in Africa that haven't been very well clarified yet.

Watts: O.K. Thank you very much for your call. Yes, you want to say something more?

Caller No. 5: Yes, the malaria just brought to mind something else. I believe in Florida there's a city where everything is very run down, a lot of swamps, and mosquito infestation, and doctors there believe that people who had no history of homosexuality or IV drug use, etc., etc. were coming down with AIDS, and they thought it was due to this mosquito problem.

Watts: Can mosquitoes transmit AIDS? That's the question. What do you think, Holly?

Smith: There is no current evidence to indicate that mosquitoes transmit AIDS. One of the researchers in Belgrade is looking at the relationship between tropical-borne diseases that are transmitted via insects, and as a cofactor, where these people have been bombarded with infections over time, have extreme poverty, very low economic conditions, that their immune systems are already depressed to such a point that they are susceptible to exposure and infection when they come in contact with the AIDS virus. But she's talking about, and everybody is still talking about, that it's still sexual transmission and blood contact, and again it's not just homosexual sexual activity. Any sexual activity, that is, if of an unsafe nature.

Watts: All right. Thank you very much for your questions, and let's now talk with caller No. 6.

Caller No. 6: I know that this is a bit of a political hotcake, but it seems to me that the public at large, in order to protect themselves from exposure to AIDS, have only one choice of being absolutely sure, which is to become sexually abstinent or celibate. And, I'm wondering whether, I hesitate to say this, because it's a politically very charged question, but will there ever be a time when a test will be available, over the counter, like a pregnancy test, that if somebody wanted to engage in sexual activity with somebody else, would they be able to ask them to take the test to know whether they were going to be exposed or not?

Volberding: Well, it's an interesting point. I've actually heard people discussing the possibility of AIDS-free clubs, where you would gain entry if you could prove that you were negative. I think the problems are many, and it brings up all of the issues of the antibody testing and possible negative social consequences of having your test done, especially if it's not done in a totally confidential way. I believe there should be a lot of opposition to that. At least with what we know now, and at least with the current political situation, I would agree that the only absolutely safe way to conduct your life is to be abstinent, but that is not something we can easily recommend to people. It is not realistic.

Watts: Nor is it likely to happen.

Volberding: Exactly.

Smith: That's also why there are organizations throughout the Bay Area that are committed to teaching people how to change their behavior from high-risk activity to the safer sexual activity and expression so that they are not either risking exposure or transmission to the people that they care for.

Volberding: I'd also, as long as we're beating this one to death, say at this point, heterosexual activity, although while we do think there needs to be concern in education devoted to it, it is extremely low risk. All of the evidence now is that heterosexuals have remained, at least right now, almost exclusively free of this virus, so it is time to learn about it, but I think you can relax to some degree about your risk, that every contact isn't going to give you AIDS.*

Smith: But, adding a little to that, it's important to understand that with multiple exposures, with lots of different partners, you risk the chance of coming in contact with either the virus for the first time or reaching that viral load that we talked about a little earlier. So we do recognize that as much as we are not seeing it in the greater Bay Area, a tremendous rise in the heterosexual-transmitted cases, we do recognize, for the future, because we're talking about a disease that incubates for up to 5 years, perhaps, don't go out and just decide that you can just do anything you want to.

Volberding: I agree with that.

Smith: Learn what safe precautions you can take, incorporate communication in your contacts with partners, take a look at how you can be healthy overall— that's very important.

Note: This was the belief about heterosexual transmission in 1985.

Watts: It pays to use good common sense. Thank you for your comments, and thank you, caller No. 6.

Caller No. 6: I just wanted to say that what concerns me is when my children get to be college age, which is 8 or 10 years down the line, in which case, I think if no cure is found, the disease might be found to be much more prevalent in the heterosexual community than it is now. I wonder if parents of teenage and college-age children are not more concerned?

Volberding: I think you have touched on a critical thing. And there should be growing appreciation of the points you've made, that education, especially as the virus spreads to broader and broader populations, is the only way to prevent the epidemic at this point, in that that education should start early, before somebody is extremely sexually active. We favor and I'm sure the AIDS Foundation is working with school districts to incorporate AIDS prevention education as part of their curriculum.

Smith: Absolutely. It's very important, and it has a lot of rather hot issues associated with it, because we're talking about sexuality and drug use and sexual preference, and those are already controversial issues that parents have some degree, sometimes, of difficulty whenever we're talking about incorporating that into the educational system. We believe that it is necessary, because, in fact, teenage years are the times when we see many individuals experimenting widely, both sexually and with drug use, and we want to get to people before they learn bad habits and behaviors. We don't want that to happen and have to go back to try to change behaviors. That's very hard to do.

Watts: You've been listening to *House Calls,* a special edition. I'd like to thank our guests for being with us. We've been talking with Dr. Paul Volberding, who is Chief of Oncology and Director of AIDS Activities at San Francisco General Hospital, and we've also been talking with Holly Smith, Media Relations Coordinator of the San Francisco AIDS Foundation. Thank you for listening, and take care of yourself.

XI

THE FUTURE

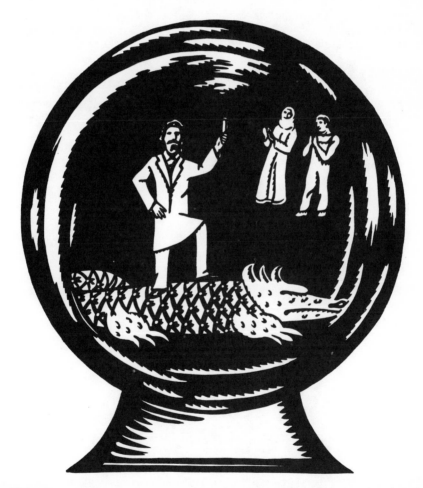

The Future
The AIDS dragon is slain. The men and women of science have found a cure and the world applauds in gratitude.

47

Prospects for the Future

Donald P. Francis

Human immunodeficiency virus type I (HIV) has infected people in most, if not all, countries of the world. Yet because of its restricted transmission patterns, it has affected people in some areas more than others. As a result, some geographic areas have very high prevalences of infection, and others have very low prevalences. Furthermore, within any infected country, there are population subgroups that, because of their behaviors or their medical therapeutic requirements, have much higher rates of infection than others. For example, in San Francisco and Melbourne, it is homosexual men that predominate; in Newark and Milan, it is intravenous drug users; in New York City, it is both of the above; and in Kinshasa and Nairobi, it is female prostitutes who have the highest infection prevalences.

Like glowing coals, HIV seems to be searching the globe for dry grass to ignite and, once ignited, the wind of multiple sexual or needle-sharing partners rapidly spreads the infection. Indeed, the rates of new infections in homosexual men in San Francisco in the early 1980s (20% per year) or Nairobi prostitutes in 1985 (over 50% per year) or intravenous drug users in the United States or Europe (10% per year) attest to the remarkable ability of this virus to spread. Once the virus has been introduced into one of these amplification groups, it extends more slowly to other sexual contacts and to babies of infected women.

Estimates of 1–2 million people in the United States and 5–10 million people worldwide infected with HIV have been made. If, as currently thought, over 50% of these will develop AIDS, at least 5 million deaths can be expected over the next decade. In addition, an equal number of other HIV-related diseases, such as HIV-induced tuberculosis, will also occur.

Fortunately, not all the news is bad. Through research our knowledge of HIV and its transmission offers means to limit its devastation. Important is the limited transmission of the virus, which spreads only by sexual intercourse, by sharing blood, and from infected mothers to their babies. Since most of this transmission is through consensual relationships, the possibility of limiting transmission by behavior change is real. Also, our knowledge of the entire gene sequence of the virus, the proteins that make up its structure, and some information of its pathogenesis offer potentials for prevention by vaccine and treatment of clinical conditions.

TREATMENT

Let us first examine the possibility of therapeutic intervention. Research on possible therapeutic agents for AIDS began early and has made substantial progress. Despite early failures of a variety of modern biologic agents such as interferons, which act nonspecifically, more recent work on therapeutic agents that act specifically on the causative virus look far more promising. Specifically, several chemical compounds have been shown to inhibit the replication of HIV in the laboratory, and two have been shown to have some positive effect when given to clinically ill humans. The most widely publicized compound, azidothymidine (AZT), has been given a license for marketing and is being used in thousands of patients now. The problem with this drug and many other antiviral compounds is that to inhibit the growth of viruses (which use the cell's machinery to grow), compounds often adversely affect normal cell functions. For example, AZT has a marked effect on bone marrow production of erythrocytes, and treated patients often become anemic and require transfusions. Such an adverse effect is perhaps tolerable for treatment of severely afflicted patients, like those with AIDS, but it may not be acceptable for asymptomatic or mildly ill individuals.

Will these compounds, or other therapeutics, have a major effect in the next 5 or so years? No one can really say, but considering the progress to date, there is real hope that some therapeutic compound will be produced that will have beneficial effects without producing unacceptable side reactions. However, it seems unlikely, even with more novel approaches, including direct effects on the genome of the virus, that any real cure for this infection will be available in the next 5 years. This is not to say that various agents will not have some impact, however. It is clear that some drugs will have an effect on prolonging the lives of some patients. It is also clear that these drugs will be used, even if they have substantial side reactions. Considering the grim outlook for those who develop AIDS, most patients are willing to risk considerable side reactions for some prolongation of life. If nothing else, such agents will give some ray of hope to those who are suffering from this disease.

But another effect will be economic. With the urgency of the AIDS issue, developmental drugs have been brought to the market with unusual expediency. However, as with any new product, the costs are high. In addition, with the desperation of AIDS patients, the use of such drugs is going to be considerably broader than those recommended by disease experts and the package inserts. As a result, the cost of these new drugs together with the cost of treating the expected complications of therapy will be considerable.

PREVENTION

Another possible hope to alleviate the scourge of HIV is a vaccine. The existence of a vaccine for AIDS would considerably ease the apprehension of the world's population and quell some of the resulting chaos. But, although the possibility remains open, there is no candidate vaccine in mid-1988 that seems definitely effective. As a matter of fact, all early attempts at producing an effective vaccine by various techniques have so far failed to protect chimpanzees. Even if we did have a prototype vaccine in hand now, it would take at least 2 years to test its efficacy and begin large-scale production.

Without a vaccine or highly effective vaccine, what can we predict for the near future? We can reasonably predict that during the next 5 years the cases of AIDS will continue to grow at an alarming rate as people, already infected today, develop symptoms. In addition, other people will be infected by the ever-increasing pool of carriers. These will be the cases of the future.

Who will comprise the future cases? Like the geographic blurring of incidence boundaries that has occurred over the past few years, the definitions of "risk groups" will also begin to blur. No doubt the preponderance of cases over the next 5 years will continue to be in "first-wave" groups (homosexual men, IV drug users, and their sexual contacts) as clinical disease continues to develop in those infected in years past. But as the virus extends into more sexually active heterosexual men and women, the actual chains of transmission traceable to members of established risk groups will become more diffuse. If individuals do not take action to protect themselves from being infected, more cases will begin to surface in the "general population" whose source of infection cannot be traced exactly. Eventually, heterosexually active men and women will make up the majority of cases. As more women of childbearing age become infected, more perinatal transmission will become evident. Exactly when this future scenario will occur is only a guess—possibly in a decade or two.

Using the example of another blood-borne and sexually transmitted virus, hepatitis B virus (HBV), we can make additional predictions as to the ultimate spread of HIV in the U.S. population. These two viruses have remarkably similar epidemiology, although HBV produces a chronic (infectious) carrier state in only 10% of those infected compared to nearly 100% for HIV. This discrepancy could well mean that HIV will surpass HBV in terms of the proportion of the population who will become infected. Realizing this potential difference we can, nevertheless, make minimum estimates for HIV in the United States. Left without control, it would not be surprising if eventually 10% of Americans were infected with HIV.

As it is now, the infection would not be evenly distributed around the country. Existing risk groups would continue to have high rates. The major emerging group would be the lower socioeconomic, inner-city populations where needle use and casual sexual encounters are more prevalent. This distribution is already being seen in the New York–New Jersey area of the United States. In Africa and other areas where traditional village cultures have been urbanized, increased transmission can also be expected.

How widespread HIV infection will become in the world's population depends significantly on what individuals do to prevent becoming infected. This depends to a large extent on how successful prevention programs are in instilling protective behavior changes in the society. The determinants of the success or failure of prevention programs will depend on both their quality and their quantity together with the support of society for their goals. Indeed, it is the support of society for AIDS prevention that is the key for the ultimate success of AIDS prevention. Society must be convinced that because of the severity of the AIDS problem it is willing to pay the price of AIDS prevention—both in terms of resources to hire staff to undertake such an extensive program and in terms of dealing with the difficult issues raised by the AIDS epidemic. Clearly, neither resources (funding) nor maturity in dealing with difficult matters such as sex, including homosexual sex, and drug use has highlighted AIDS prevention to date.

Most of the AIDS deaths in the next 5 years are destined, because these people have already been infected. Additional deaths from ongoing transmission will be in excess of these. A feeling for the future climate surrounding AIDS can be gained by hypothetically changing the incubation period for AIDS from years (as we know it to be) to weeks (as is common for other infectious diseases). Just suppose that *today* 5 million people have developed AIDS since 1978, half have died, and many of those alive are clogging the halls of existing hospitals and nursing facilities. Although horrible, this is a very real way to prepare one for the future impact of AIDS. Indeed, considering the slow process of planning, funding, and fielding prevention and treatment programs, we probably would be far better off if we were to plan using the type of scenario that incorporates infection information together with natural history data instead of pure case counting.

Given this scenario, what can we see ahead in terms of the world's reaction to AIDS? To answer this we need to examine not only the "problem," as shown above, but any possible solutions that would have great impact on the disease.

THE FUTURE

The National Academy of Sciences' Institute of Medicine Report[1] and the Surgeon General's Report on AIDS[2] issued in early 1987 form the basis of AIDS prevention, treatment, and research plans. These reports clearly recognize the risk of HIV to the American public, and the NAS report calls for substantial increases in funding for all aspects, including $1 billion for prevention per year.

What should we do? On the clinical side, the burden will certainly grow. Again, how well that burden is handled depends on our ability to plan and convince those in positions responsible for funding that proactive action can be both economically and humanly beneficial. Seldom have we been in a position to be able to plan so well for an epidemic. Although the long incubation period of AIDS adversely affects the prevention program, because the seriousness of the problem is not recognized until years have passed, it is beneficial in terms of hospital and home care planning. By knowing the prevalence of infection in the community and the proportion of infected people who will require medical care by year postinfection, advanced planning can be made for inpatient, outpatient, and extended-care facilities as well as for the financing of these facilities.

The plans for medical care of HIV-infected individuals must take into account all stages of infection. Asymptomatic carriers require clinical follow-up for immune status. They need information on preventing transmission to others, information on what the early signs are that require immediate treatment, and support for the considerable anxiety associated with infections. Patients with AIDS-related conditions require a variety of medical and dental services that range from minimal to extensive. Finally, AIDS patients require extensive inpatient and outpatient services that require a high level of expertise from all members of the health care team. Perhaps the greatest challenge in the United States currently regarding AIDS is the home care, nursing care issue. These traditionally weak links in health care in the United States are being highlighted by AIDS. Hopefully, the AIDS crisis will give us the opportunity to strengthen these weak areas.

Unfortunately, the unending chaos of AIDS in and around hospitals, like that in the prevention field, has consumed much of the time of those who could influence the planning process. Indeed, the burden of patient care and the frustrations of support services have taken a toll in the medical community itself. The emotional and physical burdens of AIDS patient care are considerable and preclude or limit those knowledgeable providers from being able to commit the time and energy necessary to educate others and to develop long-term strategic plans. This limitation on the resources that can be mobilized to plan, educate, and develop policy based on actual experience with AIDS patient care must be addressed immediately through increased resources and support for health care providers.

On the prevention side, there is little doubt that populations around the world will insist on effective and aggressive programs. The question is how long will it take for such programs to be fielded by responsible authorities. The answer to this depends on the leadership of individual countries. Those leaders who decide early to deal with AIDS through scientifically well-founded prevention programs will, no doubt, save countless numbers of their countrymen. Those who choose the more convenient approach and postpone aggressive programs will face an even greater crisis in the future. Because of the high proportion of HIV-infected people who become carriers of the virus and thus reservoirs of infection for others, the later a country's leaders institute prevention programs, the more difficult it is to stop transmission.

Universally, it has been difficult for politicians to move ahead with AIDS prevention programs. In many countries the political climate has directed governments, whose responsibility includes public health, away from any new activities that require additional resources. The difficulties in dealing with issues of sex, sex education, intravenous drug use, and homosexuality linked with a resistance to committing already scarce resources have driven most governments toward choosing the convenient rather than the wise approach. The result has been that most have chosen to do as little as possible and still maintain a veneer of public responsibility. It is clear that such approaches are shortsighted and will ultimately be more costly. It is also clear that shortsighted officials will be judged very severely by the history of this important and devastating outbreak.

Overall, countries and locales that deal with AIDS prevention as early as possible via aggressive and scientifically well-founded programs will fare better than those that do not. Similarly, individuals within these countries and locales who heed the message of AIDS prevention and modify their behavior are not likely to become infected with HIV. In this way AIDS is one of many tests of basic Darwinian principles. As Dr. Jonas Salk says, "Survival of the wisest."

It is clear from those areas where community concern and prevention programs have worked together to spread the relatively simple words of AIDS prevention that dramatic effects have been realized. Thus, AIDS prevention can work. The data are most striking for the male homosexual community, where at-risk sexual practices have decreased markedly. Yet the motivation for behavior change has been greatest in this community because of the early introduction of virus into this group before the infectious nature of this disease was even known. As a result, the number of AIDS cases has been substantial, and the personal impact of knowing someone with AIDS and seeing the inexorable progression of this disease to death has in itself been an important factor in motivating behavior change.

Such a motivational factor will not be so available (hopefully) as prevention programs are spread wider. Yet with appropriate messages and delivery modalities, it should be possible to instill the wisdom necessary to foster behavior changes. No doubt such changes will be most readily realized in the educated, media-contacting segments of society and will be progressively more difficult to achieve as one moves down the socioeconomic and age ladders. Certainly the most difficult populations in which to effect change will be those inner-city groups (especially the youth) who probably are at the greatest risk for long-term endemicity of HIV infection.

Several additional issues regarding AIDS in the United States are worth dealing with here. One is male homosexuality. There exists in the American society a confrontation of two extreme views that could profoundly affect the future of AIDS prevention. The two polarized extremes are represented by extreme antihomosexual factions and extremists from the male homosexual community. The former, for whatever reasons, cannot deal with male homosexuality in any way other than to "eliminate it." They refuse to accept the current scientific belief that homosexuality is to a large extent inherent in the human species and is not an acquired behavior. They have hoped to use AIDS as a means by which all homosexuals could be isolated from the rest of society. In their own right and in response to the antihomosexual extreme, members of the homosexual community have resisted many AIDS prevention efforts, claiming that such efforts might violate their civil rights. The extremists of the homosexual community have claimed that several standard disease prevention methods like case reporting, serologic testing, and contact tracing/notification are all potential violations of the civil rights of the individual and should be resisted.

The resolution of the homosexual-antihomosexual conflict in the future could have a major effect on the ability of our societies to mount an effective AIDS prevention program. I predict that as the years progress reason will win out but that the road to reason will not be smooth, nor will it be realized without strong and sensitive national and local leadership. We will, no doubt, see a continuation of the attempts by extremist fringe groups (best represented by the Proposition 64 and 69 campaigns in California by the La Rouche group) to implement highly repressive and even hostile forms of transmission control. However, several things will balance these attempts. First, the tragedy afflicting the gay community will increasingly become personally obvious to everyone as national leaders, friends, and acquaintances develop AIDS. As a result, the society that by and large tolerates homosexuality, as long as it is not discussed, will develop an increasing familiarity with the homosexual community as a whole.

As generalized knowledge increases, more individuals will recognize personal acquaintances, neighbors, friends, teachers, etc., who are homosexual. Surrounding the pressing issues of the moment, more open discussion of homosexuality will occur. This should help dissolve much of the mystique (and fear) of homosexuality and increase both the tolerance of homosexual men and increase sympathy for their AIDS plight. Second, as more nonhomosexual members of the society become infected and that infection is recognized either through serologic testing or disease occurrence, wider resistance to scientifically unfounded repressive community actions will surface. This resistance from a wider political constituency will be an extremely strong force against extremist actions. Finally, our understanding of HIV transmission and the absence of risk for those not exposed to blood or having sexual relations will become more widely accepted. This will further erode the substrate of ignorance on which fear campaigns of the past have been based.

Another issue is serologic testing. Tests of serum for antibodies to HIV were initially developed to screen donated blood and plasma to prevent transfusion and blood product–associated AIDS. These assay systems have been so refined over the years that they are accepted to be nearly perfect in their accuracy. Yet controversy abounds regarding their use. They have been castigated for having no public health or medical value. Many gay organizations have actively discouraged men from taking the tests, fearing everything from emotional collapse to mass quarantine of seropositive individuals.

On the other hand, many of us in the public health and medical sector have encouraged serologic testing for those who choose, claiming that a state of knowledge is better than a state of ignorance and that knowledge of one's infection status could have a positive effect on both the treatment and prevention of AIDS. A major misinterpretation of this recommendation has been that serologic testing is in itself a panacea for AIDS prevention. This misinterpretation has led many to see testing as an end in itself and that by recommending widespread testing they feel they can control HIV transmission. Such quick-fix approaches could actually be counterproductive, especially if they are explicitly or implicitly linked to inappropriate discrimination practices or use up the limited AIDS prevention resources. Clearly no quick-fix approach is going to stop HIV transmission. Only a long-term, intensive, and high-quality program based on scientific principles will succeed, and medical and public health leaders will have to continue to guide the less informed in that direction.

In practical terms, thousands of people at risk including gay men and heterosexual men and women are coming forth to be tested—at both public and private testing facilities. A consensus is developing, which will solidify over the next year or two, that the test is useful for many people who think they might have been exposed. For these people, centers should exist where efficient and highly trained staff can provide services to those who desire them. These services must protect the privacy of the client and must include information, counseling, medical, social, and support group services or referrals.

In summary, the future of the AIDS epidemic will depend on two major areas of human endeavor. First will be our ability as world societies and individuals in those societies to take responsibility for ourselves and our fellow citizens to keep ourselves from getting infected with this virus. Second will be our abilities in the technological arena to discover and apply therapeutic and preventive agents to reduce the AIDS epidemic. Success can be expected in both of these areas. However, the extent of that success will depend greatly on the maturity of local, national, and international leaders and their abilities to mount the necessary effort to stem the tide of this epidemic.

REFERENCES

1. Institute of Medicine, National Academy of Sciences. *Confronting AIDS: Directions for public health, health care, and research.* Washington, DC: National Academy Press, 1986.

2. U.S. Department of Health and Human Services. *Surgeon General's report on acquired immune deficiency syndrome.* Washington, DC: author, 1986.

Epilogue

After his death, this letter written by Ori Sherman to a friend was shared with us. It captures his appreciation of life and living and reminds each of us that any consideration of the AIDS pandemic needs to return to a focus on the individual, the person with HIV disease. Ori's letter provides his vision of how each of us can transform our worlds by getting in touch with the nobility within us, as he did.

May 30, 1987

Dear

After our talk yesterday I realized how much you mean to me as a friend, and out of the strictest self-interest I decided to try and pump a little joie-de-vivre into your bleak soul this morning. Not an easy task, I realized, for everything you are going through is legitimate cause for anguish, but, I want to make it clear, not for despair.

What is the difference between anguish and despair, you might ask. Don't they go hand in hand? Well, not necessarily. In my view, anguish is a natural response to pain. But after the wringing of the hands and the shedding of the tears, it *is* possible to take a big deep breath, look around, realize, "Hey! I'm still alive. What do I do now?", and get on with the business of living. Despair means that you refuse to take the big deep breath and get on with it. Even with pain and suffering, there are substantial rewards to be had just by being in the world: the enjoyment of friendship, of nature, a good meal, a hot shower, a good book. You name it. The list is limitless. But often it is desperately hard to see the light through the trees, to mix a metaphor, and God knows I've been there myself, seeing no light at all.

If I've learned anything from this illness, it's a degree of patience. Pain and suffering are not permanent conditions. They come in waves. The darkest night gives way to morning light and that is always worth remembering. Nobody says you have to enjoy the pain you are going through, but in order to get through it with a minimum of stress, it is useful to remember that even with the most intractable pain, there are moments of remission. To be patient means to realize that, and not panic each time a fresh symptom or a new ache appears. They will come but they will also go. Some symptoms will get worse, others will get better, some will reappear after an absence, others will disappear completely. The important thing is not to get too hooked into this transitory parade of symptoms. Observe them, do what you can to alleviate them, but realize that they are only one small part of your life and not the whole of it.

You are infinitely more than your symptoms. Though you may not think so right now, your inner resources are enormous, more than adequate to the task

571

ahead of you. You have intelligence, passion, compassion, and a sense of humor. With a head, a heart, and a soul, and a body which is not entirely useless, there is no reason on earth why the same passions that have engaged your interest in the past shouldn't continue to do so.

One other thing you are is a mentor, a teacher, not alone to your students but also to your friends and to your lover. The way you handle yourself at this time in your life will not go unnoticed by any of them. You have a tremendous opportunity to be a powerful exemplar in people's lives right now. You can choose to see your cup of life as half full or half empty. It is a crucial distinction which only you can make. But remember, whichever way you choose to view your life from now on, half full or half empty, lots of eyes will be on you. As a teacher, this is the greatest class you will ever teach, how you live your life, affirming life or denying it. It seems to me, having known you for years, that all your political passions, whether they be getting Jews and Arabs to be nice to one another or giving El Salvadoreans a respite from grief and war, have had to do with affirming life and justice and decency. You haven't changed fundamentally just because you are not feeling well right now. All of those issues are still crucially important and need your energy and passion. You have that passion, and even though you are full of fear right now, I have every confidence that your life-affirming instincts will win the day.

Remember, finally, dear friend, you are not alone. You are surrounded by the love of friends and family. We look to you to love yourself as much as we love you.

Index